# 2007
# YEAR BOOK OF
# CARDIOLOGY®

# The 2007 Year Book Series

Year Book of Anesthesiology and Pain Management™: Drs Chestnut, Abram, Black, Gravlee, Lee, Mathru, and Roizen

Year Book of Cardiology®: Drs Gersh, Cheitlin, Elliott, Graham, Sundt, and Waldo

Year Book of Critical Care Medicine®: Drs Dellinger, Parrillo, Balk, Bekes, Dorman, and Dries

Year Book of Dentistry®: Drs McIntyre, Belvedere, Buhite, Davis, Henderson, Johnson, Ohrbach, Olin, Scott, Spencer, and Zakariasen

Year Book of Dermatology and Dermatologic Surgery™: Drs Thiers and Lang

Year Book of Diagnostic Radiology®: Drs Osborn, Abbara, Birdwell, Dalinka, Elster, Gardiner, Levy, Oestreich, and Rosado de Christenson

Year Book of Emergency Medicine®: Drs Hamilton, Bruno, Handly, Quintana, and Werner

Year Book of Endocrinology®: Drs Mazzaferri, Bessesen, Clarke, Howard, Kennedy, Leahy, Meikle, Molitch, Rogol, and Schteingart

Year Book of Family Practice®: Drs Bowman, Apgar, Bouchard, Dexter, Neill, Scherger, and Zink

Year Book of Gastroenterology™: Drs Lichtenstein, Chang, Dempsey, Drebin, Jaffe, Katzka, Kochman, Makar, Morris, Osterman, Rombeau, Shah, and Stein

Year Book of Hand and Upper Limb Surgery®: Drs Chang and Steinmann

Year Book of Medicine®: Drs Barkin, Berney, Frishman, Garrick, Loehrer, Mazzaferri, Phillips, and Snydman

Year Book of Neonatal and Perinatal Medicine®: Drs Fanaroff, Ehrenkranz, and Stevenson

Year Book of Neurology and Neurosurgery®: Drs Kim and Verma

Year Book of Nuclear Medicine®: Drs Coleman, Blaufox, Royal, Strauss, and Zubal

Year Book of Obstetrics, Gynecology, and Women's Health®: Dr Shulman

Year Book of Oncology®: Drs Loehrer, Arceci, Glatstein, Gordon, Hanna, Morrow, and Thigpen

Year Book of Ophthalmology®: Drs Rapuano, Cohen, Eagle, Flanders, Hammersmith, Myers, Nelson, Penne, Sergott, Shields, Tipperman, and Vander

Year Book of Orthopedics®: Drs Morrey, Beauchamp, Peterson, Swiontkowski, Trigg, and Yaszemski

Year Book of Otolaryngology-Head and Neck Surgery®: Drs Paparella, Gapany, and Keefe

Year Book of Pathology and Laboratory Medicine®: Drs Raab, Parwani, Bejarano, and Bissell

Year Book of Pediatrics®: Dr Stockman

Year Book of Plastic and Aesthetic Surgery™: Drs Miller, Bartlett, Garner, McKinney, Ruberg, Salisbury, and Smith

Year Book of Psychiatry and Applied Mental Health®: Drs Talbott, Ballenger, Buckley, Frances, Jensen, and Markowitz

Year Book of Pulmonary Disease®: Drs Phillips, Barker, Lewis, Maurer, Tanoue, and Willsie

Year Book of Rheumatology, Arthritis, and Musculoskeletal Disease™: Drs Panush, Furst, Hadler, Hochberg, Lahita, and Paget

Year Book of Sports Medicine®: Drs Shephard, Cantu, Feldman, Jankowski, McCrory, Nieman, Pierrynowski, Rowland, and Shrier

Year Book of Surgery®: Drs Copeland, Bland, Daly, Eberlein, Fahey, Jones, Mozingo, Pruett, and Seeger

Year Book of Urology®: Drs Andriole and Coplen

Year Book of Vascular Surgery®: Dr Moneta

2007

# The Year Book of
# CARDIOLOGY®

Editor in Chief

**Bernard J. Gersh, MB, ChB, DPhil, FRCP**

*Professor of Medicine, Mayo Clinic College of Medicine; Consultant on Cardiovascular Diseases, Mayo Clinic, Rochester, Minnesota*

Editors

**Melvin D. Cheitlin, MD, MACC**

*Emeritus Professor of Medicine, University of California, San Francisco; Former Chief of Cardiology, San Francisco General Hospital, San Francisco, California*

**Thomas P. Graham, MD**

*Professor of Pediatrics, Vanderbilt University School of Medicine; Division of Cardiology/Vanderbilt Children's Hospital, Nashville, Tennessee*

**William J. Elliott, MD, PhD**

*Professor of Preventive Medicine, Internal Medicine, and Pharmacology, RUSH Medical College; Attending Physician, RUSH University Medical Center, Chicago, Illinois*

**Thoralf M. Sundt III, MD**

*Professor of Surgery, Mayo College of Medicine; Consultant, Division of Cardiovascular Surgery, Mayo Clinic, Rochester, Minnesota*

**Albert L. Waldo, MD**

*The Walter H. Pritchard Professor of Cardiology, Professor of Medicine and Professor of Biomedical Engineering, Case Western Reserve University School of Medicine; Associate Chief of Cardiology for Academic Affairs, University Hospitals Case Medical Center, Cleveland, Ohio*

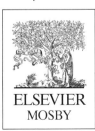

ELSEVIER
MOSBY

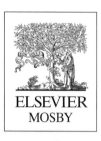

## ELSEVIER
## MOSBY

*Vice President, Continuity:* John A. Schrefer
*Developmental Editor:* Yonah Korngold
*Supervisor, Electronic Year Books:* Donna M. Adamson
*Illustrations and Permissions Coordinator:* Linda Jones

Printed in the United States of America
Composition by Thomas Technology Solutions, Inc.
Printing/binding by Sheridan Books, Inc.

Editorial Office:
Elsevier
1600 John F. Kennedy Blvd.
Suite 1800
Philadelphia, PA 19103-2899

International Standard Serial Number: 0145-4145
International Standard Book Number: 978-0-323-04667-1

# Table of Contents

# Journals Represented

Journals represented in this YEAR BOOK are listed below.

American Heart Journal
American Journal of Cardiology
American Journal of Epidemiology
American Journal of Hypertension
American Journal of Kidney Diseases
American Journal of Medicine
American Journal of Physiology–Renal Physiology
Annals of Internal Medicine
Annals of Thoracic Surgery
Archives of Disease in Childhood. Fetal and Neonatal Edition
Archives of Internal Medicine
Archives of Surgery
British Medical Journal
Cardiology in the Young
Cardiovascular Pathology
Circulation
Diabetes Care
Europace
European Heart Journal
Heart
Hypertension
International Journal of Cardiology
Journal of Cardiac Failure
Journal of Cardiovascular Electrophysiology
Journal of Clinical Hypertension
Journal of Electrocardiology
Journal of Heart and Lung Transplantation
Journal of Hypertension
Journal of Pediatrics
Journal of Stroke and Cerebrovascular Diseases
Journal of Thoracic and Cardiovascular Surgery
Journal of Urology
Journal of the American College of Cardiology
Journal of the American Geriatrics Society
Journal of the American Medical Association
Kidney International
Lancet
Mayo Clinic Proceedings
Medicine and Science in Sports and Exercise
National Institute for Health and Clinical Excellence
New England Journal of Medicine
Pharmacotherapy
Proceedings of the National Academy of Sciences
Stroke
Transplantation
Ultrasound in Obstetrics and Gynecology

STANDARD ABBREVIATIONS

The following terms are abbreviated in this edition: acquired immunodeficiency syndrome (AIDS), cardiopulmonary resuscitation (CPR), central nervous system (CNS), cerebrospinal fluid (CSF), computed tomography (CT), deoxyribonucleic acid (DNA), electrocardiography (ECG), health maintenance organization (HMO), human immunodeficiency virus (HIV), intensive care unit (ICU), intramuscular (IM), intravenous (IV), magnetic resonance (MR) imaging (MRI), ribonucleic acid (RNA), and ultrasound (US).

NOTE

The YEAR BOOK OF CARDIOLOGY is a literature survey service providing abstracts of articles published in the professional literature. Every effort is made to assure the accuracy of the information presented in these pages. Neither the editors nor the publisher of the YEAR BOOK OF CARDIOLOGY can be responsible for errors in the original materials. The editors' comments are their own opinions. Mention of specific products within this publication does not constitute endorsement.

To facilitate the use of the YEAR BOOK OF CARDIOLOGY as a reference tool, all illustrations and tables included in this publication are now identified as they appear in the original article. This change is meant to help the reader recognize that any illustration or table appearing in the YEAR BOOK OF CARDIOLOGY may be only one of many in the original article. For this reason, figure and table numbers will often appear to be out of sequence within the YEAR BOOK OF CARDIOLOGY.

# 1 Hypertension

## Introduction

The field of hypertension had few surprises during 2006. Although the American Heart Association updated its recommendations for dietary measures to lower blood pressure, the most important new set of guidelines came from the British National Institute for Health and Clinical Excellence, which recommended initial therapy with either an ACE-inhibitor (for young white patients) or a calcium antagonist (for older or black patients), and relegated beta-blockers to fourth-line therapy for patients with uncomplicated hypertension. Excellent reviews of resistant (or "refractory") hypertension, ambulatory blood pressure monitoring, Cushing's syndrome, and recent controversies in hypertension were published in important journals.

More studies showed that the prevalence, awareness, and control of hypertension continue to increase, both in the United States and all countries. Some of the shortfall in blood pressure control in the United States has been blamed on physicians who fail to intensify treatment, and avoid chlorthalidone, the best-studied, inexpensive thiazide-like diuretic, which was superior to hydrochlorothiazide in a small head-to-head trial. Discontinuation rates for initial antihypertensive drugs differed across drug classes in British general practitioners, as they have in several other countries. Home blood pressure monitoring was associated with improved adherence to prescribed medications in one study, and lower adherence rates were linked to increased healthcare resource utilization in Indianapolis. A large epidemiological study from Tennessee showed a higher risk of major congenital malformations in babies born to women who were prescribed ACE-inhibitors, validating information required in the product information for these drugs since 1986. Two studies suggested that elevated systolic blood pressure in people age 85 years and older does not impact their mortality. Conclusions from clinical trials in secondary stroke prevention were questioned by a review of characteristics of patients with strokes in Birmingham, UK. In the largest epidemiological study of its type, diuretics and beta-blockers were synergistically associated with a higher risk of new-onset diabetes.

Two studies showed an elevated risk for cardiovascular events, including death, in prehypertension (blood pressure between 120/80 and 139/89 mm Hg), compared to normal blood pressure (<120/70 mm Hg). Several new studies confirmed and extended the prognostic value of ambulatory blood pressure monitoring for heart failure, stroke, and all cardiovascular events. A formal cost-effectiveness analysis of "The Polypill®" suggested that an in-

1

expensive, low-dose, multi-drug combination could halve the burden of cardiovascular disease worldwide, and would fulfill the requirements of the World Health Organization for use in countries with low economic resources.

Although traditional "secondary hypertension" had less emphasis in 2006 compared to prior years, attention was focused on hypertension related to shock-wave lithotripsy, lower nephron number and birth weight in African Americans, rofecoxib (compared to other selective inhibitors of cyclooxygenase-2), short sleep duration, and obesity and diabetes in Native Americans. Conversely, the benefits of bariatric surgery on blood pressure were reported in 347 patients with an initial body-mass index of about 50 kg/m².

Three major clinical trials were reported in 2006: The TRial Of Preventing HYpertension (TROPHY) compared candesartan 16 mg/d with placebo in 809 patients with prehypertension, and showed that active treatment delayed the onset of hypertension, even for 2 years after the drug had been stopped; thus drug treatment of prehypertension is feasible. Support for both a target blood pressure of <140/90 mm Hg and the use of calcium antagonists as second-line drugs came from the Felodipine EVEnts Reduction (FEVER) trial, which randomized 9711 Chinese patients with baseline blood pressures >140/90 mm Hg on 12.5 mg/d of hydrochlorothiazide to either placebo or felodipine, and showed major significant reductions in nearly all cardiovascular events among those given the latter. The Conduit Artery Function Evaluation (CAFÉ) substudy of the Anglo-Scandinavian Cardiac Outcomes Trial (ASCOT) not only provided further evidence favoring amlodipine±perindopril over atenolol±bendroflumethiazide, but also suggested that part of the reason an initial beta-blocker may be less effective in preventing cardiovascular events in high-risk hypertensive patients is that it does not reduce central aortic pressure as much as brachial artery pressure. Useful meta-analyses included the beneficial effects of calcium antagonists (compared to other drugs) in reducing carotid intima-medial thickness (a potential explanation of how they might be better in preventing stroke), and lifestyle modifications to lower blood pressure. The Antihypertensive and Lipid Lowering to prevent Heart Attack Trial (ALLHAT) Research Group published several detailed analyses of their study's results, including subgroups by baseline estimated glomerular filtration rate, a post-hoc analysis of lisinopril versus amlodipine, and hyperglycemia, which was more common among those receiving chlorthalidone, but did not translate into a higher risk of cardiovascular events in their 4.9 years of average follow-up. Two other reports of incident diabetes showed a lower risk with an initial ACE-inhibitor, but in the study designed primarily for this purpose, ramipril did not achieve statistical significance over placebo. The INternational VErapamil/Trandolapril (INVET) trial results were reanalyzed twice: one study reported an increased risk of the primary event with most established cardiovascular risk factors, but a decreased risk with lower blood pressure and combination antihypertensive drugs; the other suggested that achieving diastolic blood pressure lower than 84 mm Hg was associated with increased risk of myocardial infarction, but not stroke. A well-done, nearly double-blind, clinical trial of acupuncture showed little improvement in blood pressure, but an equally well-done "cluster" randomized trial showed better improvement in blood pressure control with patient education than with either provider education or when it was combined with an "alert" at the point of care. An unusual meta-analysis claimed no specific benefit of agents that block the renin-angiotensin system on renal endpoints independent of blood pressure reduction, but a Chinese trial of benazepril and the first trial of high- versus low-dose angiotensin receptor blockers on proteinuria and loss of renal function (as well as those of the African American Study of Kidney Disease and hypertension [AASK] and the Irbesartan Diabetes Nephropathy Trial [IDNT]) made these conclusions very controversial.

In sum, the field of hypertension advanced in 2006, with a new set of British guidelines that are quite different from the American Seventh Report of the Joint National Committee on Prevention, Detection, Evaluation, and Treatment of High Blood Pressure (issued in 2003), the demonstration that drug therapy can prevent the progression from prehypertension to hypertension, and much more information about how blood pressure control can be achieved in large numbers of patients. Whether this information will be incorporated into new treatment guidelines in the United States seems unlikely soon.

**William J. Elliott, MD, PhD**

## Guidelines and Overviews

**Dietary Approaches to Prevent and Treat Hypertension: A Scientific Statement From the American Heart Association**
Appel LJ, Brands MW, Daniels SR, et al (Johns Hopkins Univ; Med College of Georgia; Cincinnati Children's Hosp, Ohio; et al)
*Hypertension* 47:296-308, 2006                                          1–1

A substantial body of evidence strongly supports the concept that multiple dietary factors affect blood pressure (BP). Well-established dietary modifications that lower BP are reduced salt intake, weight loss, and moderation of alcohol consumption (among those who drink). Over the past decade, increased potassium intake and consumption of dietary patterns based on the "DASH diet" have emerged as effective strategies that also lower BP. Of substantial public health relevance are findings related to blacks and older individuals. Specifically, blacks are especially sensitive to the BP-lowering effects of reduced salt intake, increased potassium intake, and the DASH diet. Furthermore, it is well documented that older individuals, a group at high risk for BP-related cardiovascular and renal diseases, can make and sustain dietary changes. The risk of cardiovascular disease increases progressively throughout the range of BP, beginning at 115/75 mm Hg. In view of the continuing epidemic of BP-related diseases and the increasing prevalence of hypertension, efforts to reduce BP in both nonhypertensive and hypertensive individuals are warranted. In nonhypertensive individuals, dietary changes can lower BP and prevent hypertension. In uncomplicated stage I hypertension (systolic BP of 140 to 159 mm Hg or diastolic BP of 90 to 99 mm Hg), dietary changes serve as initial treatment before drug therapy. In those hypertensive patients already on drug therapy, lifestyle modifications, particularly a reduced salt intake, can further lower BP. The current challenge to healthcare providers, researchers, government officials, and the general public is developing and implementing effective clinical and public health strategies that lead to sustained dietary changes among individuals and more broadly among whole populations.

▶ This Scientific Statement from the American Heart Association is an update of previous reviews by these and other authors[1-3] that has now been subjected to the scrutiny of, and approved by, the Science and Advisory Committees of the American Heart Association.

As with most Scientific Statements from the American Heart Association, this review breaks no new ground but does reinforce what is already known. The Clinical and Public Health Advisory Statement from the National High Blood Pressure Education Program from 2002 is now a bit out of date, and so this more-recent summary can and does provide many of the references and much of the more-current research than was available in 2002. The summary about weight loss and sodium restriction is particularly good, but this review takes the position that restriction of alcohol intake in those who consume more than 2 drinks per day has a beneficial effect on blood pressure. Sadly, no mention is made of the largest randomized clinical trial that directly evaluated this strategy. The Prevention and Treatment of Hypertension study did not show a significant reduction in blood pressure with an intense cognitive-behavioral approach to reducing alcohol consumption, probably because (before the intervention was started) the control group reduced their self-reported consumption nearly as much as the intervention group did.[4] More discussion is provided in this summary about potassium supplementation, "whole dietary patterns" (including vegetarian diets as well as the DASH diet), and "special populations" than in other recent summaries. As the authors indicate, it is a large challenge to health care providers, researchers, governmental officials, and the general public to change longstanding dietary habits and then maintain healthy lifestyles (including diets) in both individuals and in broad populations.

**W. J. Elliott, MD, PhD**

*References*

1. Erlinger TP, Vollmer WM, Svetkey LP, et al: The potential impact of nonpharmacologic population-wide blood pressure reduction on coronary heart disease events: Pronounced benefits in African Americans and hypertensives. *Prev Med* 37:327-333, 2003.
2. Miller ER Jr, Erlinger TP, Young DR, et al: Lifestyle changes that reduce blood pressure: Implementation in clinical practice. *J Clin Hypertens (Greenwich)* 1:191-198, 1999.
3. Whelton PK, He J, Appel LJ, et al: Primary prevention of hypertension: Clinical and public health advisory from the National High Blood Pressure Education Program. *JAMA* 288:1882-1888, 2002.

4. Cushman WC, et al for the PATHS Group: The Prevention and Treatment of Hypertension Study (PATHS): Effects of an alcohol treatment program on blood pressure. *Arch Intern Med* 152:1197-1207, 1998.

**Hypertension: Management of hypertension in adults in primary care: partial update**
National Institute for Health and Clinical Excellence ([British] National Collaborating Centre for Chronic Conditions, England; British Hypertension Society, England; Newcastle Guideline Development and Research Unit, England)
*NICE* :i-94, 2006                                                                                              1–2

*Introduction.*—This National Institute for Health and Clinical Excellence (NICE) guideline provides recommendations for the primary care management of raised blood pressure (BP). It includes recommendations on approaches to identifying patients with persistently raised BP and managing hypertension (including lifestyle advice and use of BP-lowering drugs).

*Methods.*—This NICE guideline on the management of hypertension is based on the best available evidence. A multidisciplinary Guideline Development Group carefully considered evidence of both the clinical effectiveness and cost effectiveness of treatment and care in developing these recommendations. The draft guideline was then modified in the light of 2 rounds of extensive consultation with the relevant stakeholder groups, including National Health Service organizations, health care professionals, patient/caregiver groups, and manufacturers.

*Results.*—The previous NICE recommendations for measuring BP, instituting and maintaining lifestyle modifications, and estimating cardiovascular risk have not changed; only those pertaining to drug treatment have been updated. Drug therapy should be offered to patients with persistent high BP of 160/100 mm Hg or more and patients at raised cardiovascular risk (10-year risk of cardiovascular disease of 20% or more or existing cardiovascular or target-organ damage) with persistent BP of more than 140/90 mm Hg. In hypertensive patients aged 55 years or older or black patients of any age, the first choice for initial therapy should be either a calcium-channel blocker or a thiazide-type diuretic. For this recommendation, black patients are considered to be those of African or Caribbean descent, not mixed-race, Asian, or Chinese. In hypertensive patients younger than 55 years, the first choice for initial therapy should be an angiotensin-converting enzyme inhibitor (or an angiotensin-II receptor antagonist if an angiotensin-converting enzyme inhibitor is not tolerated). An annual review of care should be provided to monitor blood pressure, provide patients with support, and discuss their lifestyle, symptoms, and medication.

*Conclusions.*—The British National Health Service will use these guidelines and their associated audit parameters to assess and improve the quality of care provided by general practitioners.

▶ These new British guidelines for general practitioners may well have been influenced by the Anglo-Scandinavian Cardiac Outcomes Trial (ASCOT).[1] Although there was no significant difference in the primary end point in ASCOT (fatal or nonfatal coronary heart disease, as in the American Antihypertensive and Lipid-Lowering treatment to prevent Heart Attack Trial [ALLHAT][2]), the group randomized to amlodipine (followed by perindopril, as required) experienced fewer of several secondary outcomes than the group randomized to atenolol (followed by bendroflumethiazide, as required). These recommendations, however, were ostensibly derived from a series of economic analyses based on the entire British population and acquisition costs of antihypertensive drugs that are much different than those for the same or similar drugs in the United States. Because the health care expenditures for diabetics are 2- to 3-fold higher than nondiabetics, the economic analyses may have been swayed somewhat by the higher incidence of type 2 diabetes mellitus associated with diuretics and/or β-blockers,[3] which may be one reason why these guidelines recommend drugs that seem not to be associated with an increased risk of new-onset diabetes. Data from ALLHAT and several other studies have not shown a higher cardiovascular risk among those who became diabetic while taking antihypertensive therapy,[4-6] but limited statistical power makes this controversial in both Britain and in the United States.

TABLE.—Acquisition Costs of Commonly Used Antihypertensive Agents in the United Kingdom or the United States

| Drug used in NICE Economic Analyses | UK Cost ($/year*) | US Cost ($/year) |
| --- | --- | --- |
| Ramipril 10 mg | 57 | 840 |
| Losartan 100 mg | 410 | 910 |
| Atenolol 100 mg | 25 | 60 |
| Amlodipine 10 mg | 132 | 828 |
| Bendroflumethiazide 2.5 mg | 32 | 60 |

*Based on exchange rate of 1£ = $US 1.89 (on Sept. 15, 2006).

Unlike American guidelines that seem to have little impact on long-term prescribing practices of antihypertensive drugs,[7] these guidelines are expected to shape hypertension and its treatment in the United Kingdom. The British National Health Service has initiated a program that rewards general practitioners who adopt and implement the NICE guidelines in their practices with as much as a 40% increment over their usual salaries. The idea of "pay for performance" has only recently been proposed in the United States, and despite the controversy associated with it, has not been adopted by the largest governmental payer (The Centers for Medicare and Medicaid Services). It will be interesting to see how practice patterns change in the United Kingdom during the next several years, perhaps due to these new guidelines.

**W. J. Elliott, MD, PhD**

*References*

1. Dahlöf B, Sever PS, Poulter NR, et al: Prevention of cardiovascular events with an antihypertensive regimen of amlodipine adding perindopril as required versus atenolol adding bendroflumethiazide as required, in the Anglo-Scandinavian Cardiac Outcomes Trial-Blood Pressure Lowering Arm (ASCOT-BPLA): A multicentre randomised controlled trial. *Lancet* 366:895-906, 2005.
2. Major outcomes in high-risk hypertensive patients randomized to angiotensin-converting enzyme inhibitor or calcium channel blocker vs. diuretic: The Antihypertensive and Lipid Lowering Treatment to Prevent Heart Attack Trial (ALLHAT). The ALLHAT Officers and Coordinators for the ALLHAT Collaborative Research Group. *JAMA* 288:2981-2997, 2002.
3. Elliott WJ: Differential effects of antihypertensive drugs on new onset diabetes? *Curr Hypertens Rep* 7:249-256, 2005.
4. Kostis JB, Wilson AC, Freudenberger RS, et al: Long-term effect of diuretic-based therapy on fatal outcomes in subjects with isolated systolic hypertension with and without diabetes. *Am J Cardiol* 95:29-35, 2005.
5. Qiao Q, Jousilahti P, Eriksson J, et al: Predictive properties of impaired glucose tolerance for cardiovascular risk are not explained by the development of overt diabetes during follow-up. *Diabetes Care* 26:2910-2914, 2003.
6. Eberly LE, Cohen JD, Prineas R, et al: Impact of incident diabetes and incident nonfatal cardiovascular disease on 18-year mortality: The Multiple Risk Factor Intervention Trial experience. *Diabetes Care* 26:848-854, 2003.
7. Stafford RS, Monti V, Furberg CD, et al: Long-term and short-term changes in antihypertensive prescribing by office-based physicians in the United States. *Hypertension* 48:213-218, 2006.

**Ambulatory Blood-Pressure Monitoring**

Pickering TG, Shimbo D, Haas D (Columbia Presbyterian Med Ctr, New York; Mount Sinai School of Medicine, New York)
*N Engl J Med* 354:2368-2374, 2006                    1–3

*Background.*—Ambulatory blood pressure monitoring (ABPM) was developed more than 4 decades ago as a research tool. Its use has expanded over the years, and it is now used in many patients, particularly for an initial evaluation. Medicare reimbursement is available in some cases, and norms have been developed to determine whether drug therapy should be instituted to reduce a person's cardiovascular risk. The differences between the various ambulatory blood pressure monitoring techniques available were reviewed; results were described of clinical studies showing that ABPM is better than office measurements for predicting clinical outcomes; and reimbursement issues and potential future applications were analyzed.

*Overview.*—ABPM has been used most widely to determine average blood pressure, and it is the only method available for determining the circadian rhythm of blood pressure. Patients whose blood pressure does not fall by 10% to 20% during sleep have a worse prognosis, as do patients who have a brisk rise in blood pressure on awakening. APBM is also useful for the evaluation of so-called white-coat hypertension, which may be present in some persons with resistant hypertension. In addition, APBM is the only method available for diagnosing masked hypertension, a condition in which the blood pressure is normal when measured in the office, but target-organ damage is present and attributable to hypertension outside the medical office. ABPM may also be useful in some patients with postural hypertension because this technique may help decide how best to manage blood pressure. ABPM has also been used in clinical trials of antihypertensive drugs and is being introduced to some clinical practices. Medicare will pay between $56 and $122 per 24-hour recording session, depending on where the monitoring is performed, but only in cases of suspected white-coat hypertension. Patients with this diagnosis do not receive antihypertensive drug treatment, but they may undergo ABPM annually. It has been estimated that if all patients with newly diagnosed hypertension were to undergo ABPM, fewer drug treatments—at an annual cost of at least $300—would be necessary, providing a net reduction in the cost of managing hypertension.

*Conclusions.*—ABPM has been used in a minority of patients with hypertension, but its use is increasing, particularly in newly diagnosed hypertensive patients. The monitors are reliable, convenient to wear, and generally accurate. ABPM has been shown to be a better predictor of clinical outcome than conventional blood pressure measurements.

▶ This is the best short review of ABPM in the recent medical literature. Rather than presenting all the research data on a particular question related to the procedure and its interpretation, this article summarizes the conclusion in a brief fashion and provides at least one leading reference to one of the most salient studies on the topic. Particularly important in today's health care setting is the issue of reimbursement for the procedure, which is well explained, and currently ranges from $56 to $122 depending on the geographic region in the United States. Payment is not authorized if the patient has target-organ damage or if the specific requirements summarized above are not documented in the medical record.[1] Several cost-effectiveness analyses have shown that an overall cost savings would result if every newly diagnosed patient with hypertension were to have ABPM.[2,3]

The take-home message from this review is that the results of ABPM correlate better with both target-organ damage and prediction of cardiovascular events than do office blood pressure measurements. More research is needed to see how the results of blood pressures measured by ABPM versus home readings (which do not require the expensive equipment needed for ABPM) compare for these purposes.[4,5]

**W. J. Elliott, MD, PhD**

*References*

1. Tunis S, Kendall P, Londner M, et al: *Ambulatory blood pressure monitoring (#CAG-00067N): Decision memo,* 2001, www.cms.hhs.gov/mcd/viewdecision memo.asp?id=5, accessed June 3, 2006.

2. Yarows SA, Khoury S, Sowers JR: Cost effectiveness of 24-hour ambulatory blood pressure monitoring in evaluation and treatment of essential hypertension. *Am J Hypertens* 7:464-468, 1994.

3. Krakoff LR, Schechter C, Fahs M, et al: Ambulatory blood pressure monitoring: Is it cost-effective? *J Hypertens* 9(suppl):S28-S30, 1991.

4. O'Brien E, Asmar R, Beilin L, et al: European Society of Hypertension recommendations for conventional, ambulatory and home blood pressure measurement. *J Hypertens* 21:821-848, 2003.

5. Cappuccio FP, Kerry SM, Forbes L, et al: Blood pressure control by home monitoring: Meta-analysis of randomised trials. *BMJ* 329:145, 2004.

---

**Controversies in hypertension**
Kaplan NM, Opie LH (Univ of Texas Southwestern Med Ctr, Dallas; Univ of Cape Town Med School, South Africa)
*Lancet* 367:168-176, 2006                                                    1–4

---

Hypertension remains the most common risk factor for cardiovascular morbidity and mortality. Its incidence is rising in both ageing and obese populations, but its control remains inadequate worldwide. We address several persisting controversies that may interfere with appropriate management of hypertension. They include: the reasons behind the increasing incidence of hypertension and the possible ways to slow the process, especially by lifestyle changes; the need for overall cardiovascular risk assessment; the major issues in the decision to institute drug therapy and the choice of drugs; and the importance of screening for various identifiable causes. We provide the background for these controversies, followed by some opinions on how to guide practitioners to offer more effective management of hypertension.

▶ This brief discussion of many of the current controversies in hypertension is reassuring in that the reader learns that the authoritative figures on hypertension in 2 different continents frequently disagree. It is likely that neither author would agree with many opinions recently expressed by authorities in Europe, either!

These authors end each of their 5 major topic areas with a section entitled "Opinion," which is meant to summarize their recommendations for practicing physicians. These briefly include the following: (1) Lifestyle modifications should be promoted for all societies,[1] but blood pressure–lowering drugs given to those individuals who are above a threshold blood pressure (eg, 160/100 mm Hg)[2]; (2) With the exception of an initial β-blocker,[3] achieving the blood pressure target is likely to be more important than which antihypertensive drug is used to begin the process[4]; (3) Whether certain drugs ought to be preferred to prevent specific types of events (eg, diabetes, stroke, heart failure) is too controversial for the 2 authors to agree about; and (4) Most hypertensive patients should not be routinely screened for secondary hypertension unless they have sufficient "clinical clues" for a specific condition to warrant such testing.[2]

**W. J. Elliott, MD, PhD**

*References*

1. Appel LJ, Brands MW, Daniels SR, et al: Dietary approaches to prevent and treat hypertension: A scientific statement from the American Heart Association. *Hypertension* 47:296-308, 2006.
2. Chobanian AV, Bakris GL, Black HR, et al: The seventh report of the Joint National Committee on Prevention, Detection, Evaluation, and Treatment of High Blood Pressure: The JNC 7 Report. *JAMA* 289:2560-2572, 2003.
3. Lindholm LH, Carlberg B, Samuelsson O: Should β-blockers remain first choice in the treatment of primary hypertension? A meta-analysis. *Lancet* 366:1545-1553, 2005.
4. Blood Pressure Lowering Treatment Trialists' Collaboration: Effects of different blood-pressure-lowering regimens on major cardiovascular events: Results of prospectively-designed overviews of randomised trials. *Lancet* 362:1527-1535, 2003.

## Resistant or Difficult-to-Control Hypertension

Moser M, Setaro JF (Yale Univ School of Medicine, New Haven, Conn)
*N Engl J Med* 355:385-392, 2006                                    1–5

*Introduction.*—Resistant (or refractory) hypertension can be defined as a blood pressure of 140/90 mm Hg or greater (or 130/80 mm Hg or greater in a diabetic or person with chronic kidney disease) despite adherence to treatment with full doses of at least 3 antihypertensive medications, including a diuretic. However, the information available about this condition is sparse.

*Methods.*—Although few data are available about the prevalence of resistant hypertension, and few clinical trials are available that enrolled only patients with this condition, new data have been published from several large series derived from specialty clinics where this diagnosis is more common. These have led to a differential diagnosis, suggested evaluation, and recommended drug treatment algorithm.

*Results.*—A cause can be identified in the vast majority of patients with resistant hypertension: unusual aspects of blood pressure measurement (eg, "white-coat hypertension"), nonadherence to prescribed medications, interfering substances (eg, nonsteroidal antiinflammatory drugs), obesity/metabolic syndrome, and secondary causes of hypertension (especially primary aldosteronism and sleep apnea). Many multidrug strategies have demonstrated an improvement in blood pressure in about 50% to 70% of initially resistant patients.

*Conclusions.*—Resistant hypertension is an important clinical problem that has only recently been systematically studied. The algorithm suggested here or consultation with a hypertension specialist is likely to improve blood pressure control in affected patients.

▶ This is the best recent review of resistant (or refractory) hypertension in the peer-reviewed medical literature. The authors are well-known experts on hypertension. The former has written a great deal on resistant hypertension,[1,2] and latter was chair of the First Report of the Joint National Committee on Detection, Evaluation, and Treatment of High Blood Pressure in 1977.[3] While the differential diagnosis of resistant hypertension described in this report is not novel,[4-6] the useful list of possibilities has been validated (and relative prevalence assessed) in several large series.[4-7]

Many different approaches to intensification of antihypertensive drug therapy have been recommended in resistant hypertension. Unfortunately, only 2 drugs have been specifically tested in this patient population. After an unacceptably high rate of angioedema was found with omapatrilat (compared with enalapril),[8] consideration was briefly given to testing it in patients with refractory hypertension, in whom the risks may have been outweighed by the benefits. Such a study has recently been completed with darusentan, a specific endothelin-1A inhibitor.[9] Although no longer recommended as an initial drug, doxazosin has shown antihypertensive efficacy (as a third-, fourth-, or fifth-line agent) in a short-term clinical trial[10] and in the Anglo-Scandinavian Cardiac Outcomes Trial (ASCOT).[11]

The take-home message from this and other studies on this important topic is that, after suitable evaluation and appropriate changes to the medication regimen, at least 50% to 70% of people with resistant hypertension can have their blood pressures controlled.[5,6]

**W. J. Elliott, MD, PhD**

*References*

1. Setaro JF, Black HR: Refractory hypertension. *N Engl J Med* 327:543-547, 1992.
2. Setaro JF: Resistant hypertension. In Black HR, Elliott WJ, eds: *Hypertension: A companion text to Braunwald's heart disease,* Philadelphia, 2007, Elsevier, pp 498-511.
3. The Joint National Committee on Detection Evaluation and Treatment of High Blood Pressure: Report of the Joint National Committee on Detection, Evaluation, and Treatment of High Blood Pressure: A Cooperative Study. *JAMA* 237:255-261, 1977.
4. Yakovlevitch M, Black HR: Resistant hypertension in a tertiary care clinic. *Arch Intern Med* 151:1786-1792, 1991.
5. Vidt DG: Contributing factors in resistant hypertension. Truly refractory disease is rarely found in a properly-conducted workup. *Postgrad Med* 107:57-60, 2000.
6. Garg JP, Elliott WJ, Folker A, et al: Resistant hypertension revisited: A comparison of two university-based cohorts. *Am J Hypertens* 18:619-626, 2005.
7. Elliott WJ: Resistant hypertension. In: Lip GHY, Hall J, eds: *Comprehensive hypertension.* New York, 2006, Elsevier.
8. Kostis JB, Packer M, Black HR, et al: Omapatrilat and enalapril in patients with hypertension: The Omapatrilat Cardiovascular Treatment vs. Enalapril (OCTAVE) trial. *Am J Hypertens* 17:103-111, 2004.
9. Black HR, El Shahawy M, Weiss RJ, et al: Darusentan: Antihypertensive effect in patients with resistant systolic hypertension [abstract]. *J Am Coll Cardiol* 47:299A, 2006.
10. Black HR, Sollins JS, Garofalo JL: The addition of doxazosin to the therapeutic regimen of hypertensive patients inadequately controlled with other antihypertensive medications: A randomized, placebo-controlled study, *Am J Hypertens* 13:468-474, 2000.

11. Dahlöf B, Sever PS, Poulter NR, et al: Prevention of cardiovascular events with an antihypertensive regimen of amlodipine adding perindopril as required versus atenolol adding bendroflumethiazide as required, in the Anglo-Scandinavian Cardiac Outcomes Trial-Blood Pressure Lowering Arm (ASCOT-BPLA): A multicentre randomised controlled trial. *Lancet* 366:895-906, 2005.

## Epidemiological Studies

### Blood pressure and the global burden of disease 2000. Part II: Estimates of attributable burden

Lawes CMM, Vander Hoorn S, Law MR, et al (Univ of Auckland, New Zealand; Queen Mary's School of Medicine and Dentistry, London; Imperial College of Science Technology and Medicine, London; et al)
*J Hypertens* 24:423-430, 2006                                                    1–6

*Objectives.*—To provide estimates of the global burden of disease attributable to non-optimal blood pressure by age and sex for adults aged $\geq$ 30 years, by WHO subregion.

*Methods.*—Estimates of attributable burden were made using population impact fractions, which used data on mean systolic blood pressure levels, disease burden [in deaths and/or disability-adjusted life years (DALYs)] and relative risk corrected for regression dilution bias. Estimates were made of burden attributable to a population distribution of blood pressure with a mean systolic blood pressure of greater than 115 mmHg.

*Results.*—Globally, approximately two-thirds of stroke and one-half of ischaemic heart disease were attributable to non-optimal blood pressure. These proportions were highest in the more developed parts of the world. Worldwide, 7.1 million deaths (approximately 12.8% of the global total) and 64.3 million DALYs (4.4% of the global total) were estimated to be due to non-optimal blood pressure. Overall approximately, two-thirds of the attributable burden of disease occurred in the developing world, approximately two-thirds in the middle age groups (45–69 years) and approximately one-half occurred in those with systolic blood pressure levels between 130 and 150 mmHg.

*Conclusions.*—The burden of non-optimal blood pressure is almost double that of the only previous global estimates, which is largely explained by the correction for regression dilution adopted in these analyses. High blood pressure is a leading cause of global burden of disease, and most of it occurs in the developing world.

▶ This report confirms, extends, and reemphasizes the conclusions of previous work done by the Global Burden of Disease group, which estimated that as the health gap between developed and developing nations is reduced by good sanitation and other worthwhile measures, hypertension and its related cardiovascular diseases will soon take over the first position in causes of death and disability worldwide.[1,2] Earlier estimates had suggested that the burden of hypertension will largely come from developing nations, but these data suggest that the incidence of cardiovascular events that is attributable to "suboptimal blood pressures" will increase, even in developed nations.[3] The 29,972-patient INTERHEART study suggested that a history of hypertension had a population-attributable risk of only 17.9% for myocardial infarction, but these data were derived from a case-control registry.[4] These data continue to support WHO's sustained call for improvements in detection, awareness, and control of blood pressure as well as the development and distribution of inexpensive but effective antihypertensive medications. These goals will not easily be met, as the pace of development and regulatory approval of new antihypertensive medications has slowed greatly, in the United States and globally, since the turn of the millennium.

**W. J. Elliott, MD, PhD**

*References*

1. Lopez AD, Mathers CD, Ezzati M, et al: Global and regional burden of disease and risk factors, 2001: Systematic analysis of population health data. *Lancet* 367:1747-1757, 2006.
2. Ezzati M, et al and the Comparative Risk Assessment Collaborating Group: Selected major risk factors and global and regional burden of disease. *Lancet* 360:1347-1360, 2002.
3. Kearney PM, Whelton M, Reynolds K, et al: Global burden of hypertension: Analysis of worldwide data. *Lancet* 365:217-223, 2005.
4. Yusuf S, Hawken S, Ounpuu S, et al: Effect of potentially modifiable risk factors associated with myocardial infarction in 52 countries (the INTERHEART study): Case-control study. *Lancet* 364:937-952, 2004.

---

**Prevalence, Awareness, Treatment, and Control of Hypertension: United States National Health and Nutrition Examination Survey 2001-2002**

Cheung BMY, Ong KL, Man YB, et al (Univ of Hong Kong, China)
*J Clin Hypertens* 8:93-98, 2006                    1–7

---

The prevalence, awareness, treatment, and control of hypertension in the United States are analyzed using the National Health and Nutrition Examination Survey (NHANES) database covering the period 1988-2002. Mean body mass index was $26.1\pm0.1$ kg/m$^2$ in 1988–1991 and $27.9\pm0.2$ kg/m$^2$ in 2001–2002 ($p<0.001$). In the same period, the prevalence of diabetes mellitus increased from 5.0% to 6.5% ($p=0.03$). Diastolic blood pressure was $73.3\pm0.2$ mm Hg in 1988–1991 and $71.6\pm0.4$ mm Hg in 2001–2002 ($p<0.001$). Among the 18–39 years and 60 years and older age groups, the prevalence of hypertension increased significantly since 1988–1991. Multiple regression shows age, body mass index, and being non-Hispanic black were significantly associated with hypertension. In the period 1988–2002, the percentage receiving treatment and the percentage with blood pressure controlled increased significantly. In 2001–2002, significantly more people with hypertension and diabetes reached a blood pressure target of <130/85 mm Hg. Overall, the control rates were low, especially among middle-aged Mexican-American men (8%).

▶ Although these data have been analyzed previously,[1,2] the focus of this study (with regression analyses that attempt to attribute the increase in hypertension prevalence and control of blood pressure in diabetics to less than 130/85 mm Hg) is different than other recent studies derived from the same population-based US national survey. These authors' calculations are even a little different than those from a very important study that analyzed data from NHANES 1988 to 2000.[3] All of these authors and national public health officials have been heartened by the big improvement in hypertension control rates seen in the United States since 1988. Data from several managed care organizations submitted to the National Center for Quality Assurance suggest that control rates in excess of 50% were achieved during 2001 to 2002. Similar control rates (49.4%) have been reported from the largest managed care organization in the world, the US Department of Veterans Affairs.[4]

These authors are also encouraged by the improvement in blood pressure control among diabetics, which soared from a nadir of 41.6% and 17.2% in 1991 to 1994 to the 56.5% and 35.9% in 2001 to 2002 (for control at less than 140/90 mm Hg or less than 130/85 mm Hg, respectively). Unfortunately, the less than 130/85 mm Hg target was recommended by JNC VI in 1997[5] and has since been superceded by less than 130/80 mm Hg in JNC 7.[6] The guidelines of all national authoritative groups now agree with the less than 130/80 mm Hg target.[7,8] One presumes that the reason the authors don't report control rates at the now-recommended target of less than 130/80 mm Hg is that JNC 7 was presented and published in 2003, after the data were collected. It is likely that the proportion of diabetics achieving the current goal blood pressure is in the low to mid-teens. Recent data from the US Department of Veterans Affairs also show hypertension control rates of greater than 40% among diabetics.[9]

The racial/ethnic disparities discussed by the authors of this report corroborate the improvement (compared with historical data, also seen in other studies[1,2]) in the awareness, treatment, and control of hypertension among African Americans, but a somewhat worse performance in Mexican Americans. These are important issues that continue to be closely scrutinized by national public health authorities. The age-related disparities in blood pressure control may be ameliorated by the new Medicare Part D drug benefit, which may assist some Medicare beneficiaries in purchasing expensive antihypertensive drugs.

These data about inadequate hypertension control rates (especially compared with Healthy People 2010, which has a target of 50% controlled hypertension) should cause American public health officials to reinvigorate their efforts.

**W. J. Elliott, MD, PhD**

*References*

1. Glover MJ, Greenlund KJ, Ayala C, et al: Racial/ethnic disparities in prevalence, treatment and control of hypertension-United States, 1999-2002. *MMWR* 54:7-9, 2005.
2. Hertz RP, Unger AN, Corneel JA, et al: Racial disparities in hypertension prevalence, awareness and management. *Arch Intern Med* 165:2098-2104, 2005.
3. Hajjar I, Kotchen TA: Trends in prevalence, awareness, treatment, and control of hypertension in the United States, 1988-2000. *JAMA* 290:199-203, 2003.
4. Rehman SU, Hutchison FN, Hendrix K, et al: Ethnic differences in blood pressure control among men at Veterans Affairs clinics and other health care sites. *Arch Intern Med* 165:1041-1047, 2005.
5. The sixth report of the Joint National Committee on Prevention, Detection, Evaluation, and Treatment of High Blood Pressure (JNC VI). *Arch Intern Med* 157:2413-2446, 1997.
6. Chobanian AV, Bakris GL, Black HR, et al: The seventh report of the Joint National Committee on Prevention, Detection, Evaluation, and Treatment of High Blood Pressure: The JNC 7 Report. *JAMA* 289:2560-2572, 2003.
7. K/DOQI clinical practice guidelines on hypertension and antihypertensive agents in chronic kidney disease. *Am J Kidney Dis* 43(5 suppl 2):1-290, 2004.
8. American Diabetes Association: Hypertension management in adults with diabetes. *Diabetes Care* 27(suppl 1):S65-S67, 2004.
9. Greenberg JD, Tiwari A, Rajan M, et al: Determinants of sustained uncontrolled blood pressure in a national cohort of persons with diabetes. *Am J Hypertens* 19:161-169, 2006.

**Large Increases in Hypertension Diagnosis and Treatment in Canada After a Healthcare Professional Education Program**

Onysko J, for the Canadian Hypertension Education Program (Public Health Agency of Canada, Ottawa, Ont, Canada; et al)
*Hypertension* 48:853-860, 2006                                                  1–8

This study was conducted to compare the self-reported prevalence and treatment of hypertension in adult Canadians before and subsequent to the implementation of the Canadian Hypertension Education Program in 1999. Data were obtained from 5 cycles of the Canadian Health Surveys between 1994 and 2003 on respondents aged ≥20 years. Piecewise linear regression was used to calculate the average annual increase in rates, before and after 1999. Between 1994 and 2003, the percentage of adult Canadians aware of being diagnosed with hypertension increased by 51% (from 12.37% to 18.74%; $P<0.001$), and the percentage prescribed antihypertensive drugs increased by 66% (from 9.57% to 15.86%; $P<0.001$). After 1999, there was approximately a doubling of the annual rate of increase in the diagnosis of hypertension (from 0.52% of the population per year before 1999 to 1.03% per year after 1999; $P<0.001$) and the percentage prescribed antihypertensive drugs (from 0.54% of the population per year before 1999 versus 0.98% per year after 1999; $P<0.001$). The proportion of those aware of the diagnosis of hypertension but not being treated with drugs was reduced by half between 1994 and 2003 (from 31.47% untreated to 15.34% untreated; $P<0.001$). There was a greater increase in awareness of hypertension and use of antihypertensive drugs among men compared with women after 1999. The large increase in the diagnosis and treatment of hypertension in Canada between 1994 and 2003 is consistent with an overall beneficial effect of the Canadian Hypertension Education Program, including a reduced gender gap in hypertension care.

▶ In several population-based surveys over the years, Canada has had lower rates of awareness, treatment, and control of hypertension than its southern neighbor.[1] The National High Blood Pressure Education Program started in the United States in 1972, but the Canadian Hypertension Education Program began only in 1999, in part in response to the lower rates seen there for several years. Part of the improvement in blood pressure awareness, treatment, and control in the United States since 1972 has been attributed to the National High Blood Pressure Education Program.[2,3] This study provides circumstantial evidence for the temporal association of the beginning of the Canadian Hypertension Education Program and the subsequent near doubling of the rates of antihypertensive drug utilization. The Canadian surveys are based on self-reports, unlike the National Health And Nutrition Examination Surveys in the United States, so there is some concern that awareness, treatment, and control may be underreported in Canada (compared with the United States). Nonetheless, the national campaign to educate health care providers and the public seems to have been successful, but getting 50% of hypertensives under control (as in the US Healthy People 2010) may prove to be more difficult.

**W. J. Elliott, MD, PhD**

*References*

1. Wolf-Maier K, Cooper RS, Banegas JR, et al: Hypertension prevalence and blood pressure levels in 6 European countries, Canada, and the United States. *JAMA* 289:2363-2369, 2003.
2. Roccella EJ, Lenfant C: Considerations regarding the cost and effectiveness of public and patient education programmes. *J Hum Hypertens* 6:463-467, 1992.
3. Lenfant C: Reflections on hypertension control rates: A message from the Director of the National Heart Lung and Blood Institute. *Arch Intern Med* 162:131-132, 2002.

---

**Therapeutic Inertia Is an Impediment to Achieving the Healthy People 2010 Blood Pressure Control Goals**

Okonofua EC, Simpson KN, Jesri A, et al (Med Univ of South Carolina, Charleston; Ralph H Johnson Veterans Affairs Med Ctr, Charleston, SC)
*Hypertension* 47:345-351, 2006                                                    1–9

---

Therapeutic inertia (TI), defined as the providers' failure to increase therapy when treatment goals are unmet, contributes to the high prevalence of uncontrolled hypertension ($\geq$140/90 mm Hg), but the quantitative impact is unknown. To address this gap, a retrospective cohort study was conducted on 7253 hypertensives that had $\geq$4 visits and $\geq$1 elevated blood pressure (BP) in 2003. A 1-year TI score was calculated for each patient as the difference between expected and observed medication change rates with higher scores reflecting greater TI. Antihypertensive therapy was increased on 13.1% of visits with uncontrolled BP. Systolic BP decreased in patients in the lowest quintile of the TI score but increased in those in the highest quintile ($-6.8\pm0.5$ versus $+1.8\pm0.6$ mm Hg; $P<0.001$). Individuals in the lowest TI quintile were $\approx33$ times more likely to have their BP controlled at the last visit than those in highest quintile (odds ratio, 32.7; 95% CI, 25.1 to 42.6; $P<0.0001$). By multivariable analysis, TI accounted for $\approx19\%$ of the variance in BP control. If TI scores were decreased $\approx50\%$, that is, increasing medication dosages on $\approx30\%$ of visits, BP control would increase from the observed 45.1% to a projected 65.9% in 1 year. This study confirms the high rate of TI in uncontrolled hypertensive subjects. TI has a major impact on BP control in hypertensive subjects receiving regular care. Reducing TI is critical in attaining the Healthy People 2010 goal of controlling hypertension in 50% of all patients.

▶ Although these data are derived from a sample of physician practices in the Southeast United States (in "The Stroke Belt") that are unlikely to be representative of the country as a whole, there are several important observations in this study. The first is that medications were intensified in about 13% of visits during which uncontrolled blood pressures were measured. This compares favorably with about 6% of visits in a much earlier series from New England Department of Veterans' Affairs Medical Centers.[1] It is no surprise that individuals in the lowest quintile of TI (who were given significantly more antihypertensive medications over the year) had about a 33-fold increased risk of having controlled hypertension than did those in the highest quintile (who actually received less medication after a year's observation).

Perhaps the most important (yet disappointing) aspect of this report is the roster of risk factors for TI. Hypertensive patients with older age, previously diagnosed cardiovascular disease (including heart failure), diabetes, or dyslipidemia were significantly less likely to have their medication regimens intensified. These are attributes of those at higher absolute risk of hypertension-related complications, including stroke, myocardial infarction, and cardiovascular death.

The authors predict that only mild increases in the fraction of physician-patient encounters that result in intensification of antihypertensive drug therapy would have a big positive effect on both the proportion of patients with controlled hypertension in the country (currently only 34%)[2] and the public health. The accompanying editorial suggests that there is not yet enough scientific information to support large interventions to remind physicians to consider intensification of antihypertensive drug therapy when faced with a patient with blood pressure of 140/90 mm Hg or greater,[3] but several completed and ongoing studies will likely support both physician education about the importance of intensifying therapy, and (perhaps more effective) direct computer-based reminders delivered at the point of care.[4,5] When integrated into the electronic medical record, these sorts of programs appear to be quite effective and may become the wave of the future.

**W. J. Elliott, MD, PhD**

*References*

1. Berlowitz DR, Ash AS, Hickey C, et al: Inadequate management of blood pressure in a hypertensive population. *N Engl J Med* 339:1967-1963, 1998.
2. Cheung BMY, Ong KL, Man YB, et al: Prevalence, awareness, treatment and control of hypertension: United States National Health and Nutrition Examination Survey, 2001-2002. *J Clin Hypertens* 8:93-98, 2006.
3. Fine LJ, Cutler JA: Hypertension and the treating physician: Understanding and reducing therapeutic inertia [editorial]. *Hypertension* 47:319-320, 2006.
4. Roumie CL, Elasy TA, Greevy R, et al: Improving blood pressure control through provider education, provider alerts, and patient education: A cluster randomized trial. *Ann Intern Med* 145:165-175, 2006.
5. Bosworth HB, Olsen MK, Goldstein MK, et al: The Veterans' study to improve the control of hypertension (V-STITCH). *Contemp Clin Trials* 26:155-168, 2005.

---

## Long-Term and Short-Term Changes in Antihypertensive Prescribing by Office-Based Physicians in the United States

Stafford RS, Monti V, Furberg CD, et al (Stanford Univ, Palo Alto, Calif; Wake Forest Univ School of Medicine, Winston-Salem, NC)

*Hypertension* 48:213-218, 2006                                                    1–10

---

Medication choices for the treatment of elevated blood pressure have a large potential impact on both patient outcomes and health care costs. Historic trends of prescribing for hypertension will advance the understanding of physician practice of evidence-based medicine. This study describes both long- and short-term trends in US antihypertensive prescribing from 1990 through 2004. Data were extracted from the National Disease and Therapeutic Index, a continuing survey of a national sample of US office-based physicians. Cox and Stuart and z tests were performed. Diuretics ranked among the top 3 antihypertensive drug classes throughout the entire study time span. Angiotensin-converting enzyme (ACE) inhibitors and calcium channel blockers (CCBs) were preferred over diuretics beginning in 1993, with diuretics surpassing CCBs in 2000. β-blockers were consistently the fourth most common class until 2002, when exceeded by angiotensin II receptor antagonists (ARBs). Most recent trends indicated an immediate but short-lived increase in the prescription of thiazide diuretics after the new clinical evidence released in December 2002 demonstrating clinical equivalence of thiazides to ACE inhibitors and CCBs. In contrast, prescription of ACE inhibitors declined, accompanied by continuation of a pre-existing increase in the prescription of ARBs, whereas prescription of CCBs remained essentially stable after the new evidence was released. The recorded long- and short-term trends indicate that evidence-based clinical recommendations had an impact on antihypertensive prescribing practices, but the magnitude of impact may be smaller and of more limited duration than desired.

▶ These data must be disappointing to the authors, one of whom served as chair of the steering committee of the Antihypertensive and Lipid Lowering to prevent Heart Attack Trial (ALLHAT),[1] which is not referred to by name in the abstract (and the acronym of which is misspelled in the body of this article). Prior work by many of these authors had demonstrated a major decrease in the prescribing and dispensing of α-blockers[2] that was temporally related to, and occurred shortly after, the early termination of the doxazosin arm of ALLHAT.[3] Those analyses were unfortunately confounded by the near-simultaneous loss of patent protection, drug marketing, free sampling, and "generic erosion" of doxazosin, but were corroborated (at least in part) by data for other α-blockers. The authors may be justifiably proud of the fact that the final ALLHAT results did increase the popularity of thiazide diuretics,[4,5] which their data suggest was a temporary phenomenon.

One of the other reasons for the apparently persistent effects of ALLHAT on α-blocker prescribing, but not thiazide diuretic prescribing, was the recurring publication of several iterations of the data from the doxazosin arm of ALLHAT. The initial publication was followed by at least 3 further reports providing validation and further analyses of the data, all of which reinforced the initial conclusion and received widespread media attention.[6-8] These results were never contradicted by any other clinical trial results. On the other hand, the final results of ALLHAT regarding the superiority of chlorthalidone (over both an angiotensin-converting enzyme inhibitor and a calcium antagonist) were not corroborated by the 2 subsequent clinical trials of initial antihypertensive therapy, one of which alleged superiority of the angiotensin-converting enzyme inhibitor over a different thiazide diuretic,[9] and the other of which was stopped early because of early mortality in the β-blocker arm (± thiazide diuretic) compared with the calcium antagonist (± angiotensin-converting enzyme inhibitor) arm.[10]

It is difficult to argue with the authors that there are at least 4 reasons why thiazide diuretics are not prescribed as often as clinical trial evidence and guidelines would suggest. (1) Not all guidelines and not all studies support the universal recommendation to use a thiazide-type or thiazide-like diuretic as first-line therapy. (2) Some continue to be concerned about potential adverse metabolic effects of thiazides. (3) Other drugs are certainly effective in lowering blood pressure and may be suitable alternatives to thiazides in those in whom the latter are contraindicated, or in whom the former have "compelling indications." (4) Other drug classes are more heavily marketed, advertised, and distributed as free samples and may be attractive to those physicians and patients who prefer "newer" therapies. Which of these, if any, may account for the fact that the increase in prescribing of thiazides for hypertension that occurred immediately after the ALLHAT results, and was not sustained, is still uncertain.

**W. J. Elliott, MD, PhD**

*References*

1. Major outcomes in high-risk hypertensive patients randomized to angiotensin-converting enzyme inhibitor or calcium channel blocker vs. diuretic: The Antihypertensive and Lipid Lowering Treatment to Prevent Heart Attack Trial (ALLHAT). The ALLHAT Officers and Coordinators for the ALLHAT Collaborative Research Group. *JAMA* 288:2981-2997, 2002.

2. Stafford RS, Furberg CD, Finkelstein SN, et al: Impact of clinical trial results on national trends in alpha-blocker prescribing, 1996-2002. *JAMA* 291:54-62, 2004.
3. The ALLHAT Collaborative Research Group: Major cardiovascular events in hypertensive patients randomized to doxazosin vs. chlorthalidone: The Antihypertensive and Lipid-Lowering Treatment to Prevent Heart Attack Trial (ALLHAT). *JAMA* 283:1967-1975, 2000.
4. Xie F, Pettiti DB, Chen W: Prescribing patterns for antihypertensive drugs after the Antihypertensive and Lipid-Lowering to prevent Heart Attack Trial: Report of experience in a health-maintenance organization. *Am J Hypertens* 18:464-469, 2005.
5. Austin P, Mamdani MM, Tu K, et al: Changes in prescribing patterns following publication of the ALLHAT trial [letter]. *JAMA* 291:45-47, 2004.
6. Validation of heart failure events in the Antihypertensive and Lipid-Lowering treatment to prevent Heart Attack Trial (ALLHAT) participants assigned to doxazosin and chlorthalidone. *Curr Cont Trials in Cardiovasc Med* 3:10, 2002.
7. Davis BR, Cutler JA, Furberg CD, et al: Relationship of antihypertensive treatment regimens and change in blood pressure to risk for heart failure in hypertensive patients randomly assigned to doxazosin or chlorthalidone: Further analyses from the Antihypertensive and Lipid-Lowering Treatment to Prevent Heart Attack Trial. The ALLHAT Collaborative Research Group. *Ann Intern Med* 137:313-320, 2002.
8. ALLHAT Officers and Coordinators for the ALLHAT Collaborative Research Group. Diuretic versus alpha-blocker as first-step antihypertensive therapy: Final results from the Antihypertensive and Lipid-Lowering Treatment to Prevent Heart Attack Trial (ALLHAT). *Hypertension* 42:239-246, 2003.
9. Wing LMH, Reid CM, Ryan P, et al: A comparison of outcomes with angiotensin-converting-enzyme inhibitors and diuretics for hypertension in the elderly. Second Australian National Blood Pressure Study Group. *N Engl J Med* 348:583-592, 2003.
10. Dahlöf B, Sever PS, Poulter NR, et al: Prevention of cardiovascular events with an antihypertensive regimen of amlodipine adding perindopril as required versus atenolol adding bendroflumethiazide as required, in the Anglo-Scandinavian Cardiac Outcomes Trial-Blood Pressure Lowering Arm (ASCOT-BPLA): A multicentre randomised controlled trial. *Lancet* 366:895-906, 2005.

## Antihypertensive Medication Use Among US Adults With Hypertension

Gu Q, Paulose-Ram R, Dillon C, et al (Harris Corp, Falls Church, Va; Centers for Disease Control and Prevention, Hyattsville, Md)
*Circulation* 113:213-221, 2006                                                    1–11

*Background.*—High blood pressure can be controlled through existing antihypertensive drug therapy. This study examined trends in prescribed antihypertensive medication use among US adults with hypertension and compared drug utilization patterns with recommendations of the Sixth Joint National Committee on Prevention, Detection, Evaluation, and Treatment of High Blood Pressure.

*Method and Results.*—Persons aged ≥18 years from the National Health and Nutrition Examination Surveys were identified as hypertensive on the basis of either a blood pressure ≥140/90 mm Hg or self-reported current treatment for hypertension with a prescription medication. In 1999–2002, 62.9% of US hypertensive adults took a prescription antihypertensive medication compared with 57.3% during 1988–1994 ($P<0.01$). Men had the greatest increase in antihypertensive medication use (47.5%, 1988–1994 versus 57.9%, 1999–2002 [*P*<0.001]). In both surveys, antihypertensive medication use increased with age, was lower among men than among women, and was lower among Mexican Americans than among non-Hispanic whites and blacks. Multiple antihypertensive drug use increased from 29.1% to 35.8% (*P*<0.001). Polytherapy with a calcium channel blocker, β-blocker, or angiotensin-converting enzyme inhibitor significantly increased by 30%, 42%, and 68%, respectively, whereas monotherapy with a diuretic or β-blocker significantly decreased. For hypertensives with diabetes, congestive heart failure, or a prior heart attack, the utilization patterns closely followed the Sixth Joint National Committee guideline recommendations.

*Conclusions.*—Antihypertensive medication use and multiple antihypertensive medication use among US hypertensive adults increased over the past 10 years, but disparities by sociodemographic factors continue to exist.

▶ This report summarizes somewhat reassuring data regarding the antihypertensive drug-taking patterns of Americans (and the prescribing patterns of their physicians) after JNC VI.[1] These data are perhaps more interesting than similar figures drawn from America's pharmacy data, which show essentially the same trends and a very similar rank ordering of drug use by number of prescriptions.[2-4] For the years 2000 to 2002, pharmacies reported that the top 5 antihypertensive drugs (by numbers of prescriptions dispensed) were atenolol (9.4%), lisinopril (8.7%), metoprolol (8.4%), furosemide (7.9%), and amlodipine (7.1%).[2-4] According to the current study, the top 5 antihypertensive drugs taken by people surveyed in NHANES 1999 to 2002 were lisinopril (13.6%), atenolol (11.5%), hydrochlorothiazide (10.4%), metoprolol (10.1%), and amlodipine (9.3%); these are the same "top 5" drugs that were dispensed by US pharmacies in 2002.[4] Both the pharmacy data and the NHANES data are potentially confounded by indication; that is, some people who have heart failure, rather than hypertension, take lisinopril but would be counted as hypertensive in the NHANES dataset because they take a pill that lowers blood pressure.

The fact that fewer Mexican Americans took antihypertensive drugs in NHANES 1999 to 2002 than their non-Hispanic white or African American counterparts is no doubt part of the explanation for recent survey data showing lower rates of blood pressure control in this growing demographic subgroup.[5] The growing use of fixed-dose combination antihypertensive drug products (which are not identified as such in NHANES surveys, as the individual components are counted separately) is likely attributable to at least 2 contemporary trends: the change in marketing focus from older (branded) single antihypertensive agents to branded "line extensions" (eg, lisinopril being replaced by branded lisinopril + hydrochlorothiazide) and the realization that antihypertensive drug monotherapy has a low probability of achieving the blood pressure target.[6] It is still reassuring to know that, in NHANES 1999 to 2002, physicians were prescribing specific antihypertensive drugs that usually matched the "compelling indications" (taken from JNC VI) that they diagnosed in their patients. Whether the national trend of adherence to clinical practice guidelines for hypertension will continue after ALLHAT[7] and the JNC VII[8] will be interesting to see.

**W. J. Elliott, MD, PhD**

*References*

1. The Sixth Report of the Joint National Committee on Prevention, Detection, Evaluation, and Treatment of High Blood Pressure (JNC VI). *Arch Intern Med* 157:2413-2446, 1997.
2. *Drug Topics,* January 1, 2006, www.drugtopics.com/drugtopics/content/printContentPopup.jsp?id=104549, accessed June 5, 2006.
3. *Drug Topics,* March 2, 2002, www.drugtopics.com/drugtopics/content/printContentPopup.jsp?id=116557, accessed June 5, 2006.
4. *Drug Topics,* March 13, 2003, www.drugtopics.com/drugtopics/content/printContentPopup.jsp?id=110839, accessed June 5, 2006.
5. Glover MJ, Greenlund KJ, Ayala C, et al: Racial/ethnic disparities in prevalence, treatment and control of hypertension—United States, 1999-2002. *MMWR* 54:7-9, 2005.
6. Elliott WJ: Should there be any reluctance to initiate combination antihypertensive therapy in patients with blood pressure of 160/100 mm Hg or higher? In Bakris GL, editor: *Therapeutic Strategies in Hypertension,* Oxford, England, 2006, Clinical Publishing, pp 85-102.
7. Major outcomes in high-risk hypertensive patients randomized to angiotensin-converting enzyme inhibitor or calcium channel blocker vs. diuretic: The Antihypertensive and Lipid Lowering Treatment to Prevent Heart Attack Trial (ALLHAT). The ALLHAT Officers and Coordinators for the ALLHAT Collaborative Research Group. *JAMA* 288:2981-2997, 2002.
8. Chobanian AV, Bakris GL, Black HR, et al: Seventh Report of the Joint National Committee on Prevention, Detection, Evaluation and Treatment of High Blood Pressure. National High Blood Pressure Education Program Coordinating Committee. *Hypertension* 42:1206-1252, 2003.

---

**Discontinuation of antihypertensive drugs among newly diagnosed hypertensive patients in UK general practice**

Burke TA, Sturkenboom MC, Lu S, et al (Univ of Medicine and Dentistry of New Jersey, Piscataway; Erasmus Univ Med Ctr, Rotterdam, The Netherlands; Analytic Consulting Solutions, Wakefield, RI)
*J Hypertens* 24:1193-1200, 2006                                    1–12

---

*Objectives.*—To evaluate antihypertensive drug discontinuation among newly diagnosed hypertensive patients.

*Methods.*—This was a population-based cohort study using the UK General Practice Research Database (GPRD). Patients newly diagnosed with hypertension between 1991 and 2001 and subsequently treated with antihypertensive drugs were included. Overall antihypertensive drug discontinuation was evaluated from a patient's first-ever antihypertensive prescription. Class-specific discontinuations were evaluated from a patient's first-ever prescriptions of angiotensin-converting enzyme (ACE) inhibitors (ACE-I), alpha antagonists, angiotensin-2 antagonists (AIIA), β blockers, calcium-channel blockers (CCB), miscellaneous, potassium-sparing diuretics, and thiazides. Discontinuation occurred when no antihypertensive prescription was issued within 90 days following the most recent prescription expiration.

*Results.*—The study population comprised 109 454 patients, with 223 228 antihypertensive drug-class episodes contributing to the class-specific analysis. Overall antihypertensive drug discontinuation was 20.3% [95% confidence interval (CI): 20.0, 20.5%] at 6 months and 28.5% (95% CI: 28.2, 28.7%) at 1 year, with a median time to discontinuation of 3.07 years. The median time to antihypertensive class discontinuation was longest for AIIAs (2.90 years) followed by ACE-I (2.24), CCB (1.86), β blockers (1.50), thiazides (1.50), alpha antagonists (1.35), potassium-sparing diuretics (0.40), and miscellaneous (0.39). One-year discontinuation ranged from 29.4% (95% CI: 28.0, 30.7) for AIIAs to 64.1% (95% CI: 62.1, 66.3) for potassium-sparing diuretics. Forty-four percent who discontinue their first-ever antihypertensive drug class failed to switch to a different drug class within 90 days of discontinuation.

*Conclusion.*—It is important that general practitioners (GPs) monitor patients closely in the first year following antihypertensive drug initiation, due to the high early risk of discontinuation, and the low percentage of patients who switch to a different antihypertensive drug class after a drug-class discontinuation. AIIA, followed by ACE-I and CCB, had the lowest risk of discontinuation among antihypertensive drug classes.

▶ The data regarding differential "persistence" (ie, continuous pharmacy refills) across classes of antihypertensive drugs are similar to those from the largest pharmacy benefits manager in the United States,[1,2] Italy,[3] and Canada.[4] Although some data of this type suggest that there are even differences across individual drugs of the same class,[5] angiotensin receptor blockers appear to have the highest refill rates. Some have suggested that this is because this class of drugs typically has fewer and less severe adverse effects (or side effects) than do other types of antihypertensive drugs.[6] The major positive attributes of this study were that the sample size is very large and probably broadly representative of the entire English population, and the prescribing physicians were all GPs (and did not include specialists, who would be more likely to treat patients with comorbidities).

TABLE 1.—Year Discontinuation Rates for Classes of Antihypertensive Drugs in Large Numbers of Newly Diagnosed Patients

| | England (n = 109,454) | US (n = 21,723)[1] | US (n = 15,175)[2] | Europe (n = 2416)[5] | Canada (n = 20,531)[4] | Italy (n = 16,783)[3] |
|---|---|---|---|---|---|---|
| ARB | 29% | 29% | 33% | 26% | — | 42% |
| ACE inhibitor | 38% | 33% | 39% | 34% | 17% | 60% |
| α-Blocker | 45% | — | — | — | — | — |
| β-Blocker | 44% | 50% | 54% | 29% | 26% | 62% |
| CCB | 41% | 41% | 46% | 31% | 22% | 69% |
| Diuretic (thiazide) | 44% | 56% | 79% | 34% | 30% | 70% |

*ARB*, Angiotensin receptor blocker.

Although there are few head-to-head comparisons, English patients taking their first-ever drug for hypertension appear to "persist" with the therapy longer than patients from other countries. It is difficult to know what factors might contribute to these differences; the generally lower numbers of patients who were prescribed angiotensin receptor blockers (vs other drugs), 30- or 90-day periods without a refill (to define "persistence"), and systems of health care delivery may all be important.

The disturbing thing about these sorts of data is the high proportion of patients who abandon antihypertensive therapy altogether after not receiving a refill for their originally prescribed medication. This may be a major contributor to the relatively high proportion of people with diagnosed, but untreated, hypertension, which was found in 10% of the American hypertensive population in the National Health and Nutrition Examination Survey 2001-2002.[7]

**W. J. Elliott, MD, PhD**

*References*

1. Bloom BS: Continuation of initial antihypertensive medication after 1 year of therapy. *Clin Ther* 20:671-681, 1998.
2. Conlin PR, Gerth WC, Fox J, et al: Four-year persistence patterns among patients initiating therapy with the angiotensin II receptor antagonist losartan versus other antihypertensive drug classes. *Clin Ther* 23:1999-2010, 2001.
3. Degli Esposti E, Sturani A, Di Martino M, et al: Long-term persistence with antihypertensive drugs in new patients. *J Hum Hypertens* 16:439-444, 2002.
4. Marentette MA, Gerth WC, Billings DK, et al: Antihypertensive persistence and drug class. *Can J Cardiol* 18:649-656, 2002.
5. Hasford J, Mimran A, Simons WR: A population-based European cohort study of persistence in newly diagnosed hypertensive patients. *J Hum Hypertens* 16:569-575, 2002.
6. Law MR, Wald NJ, Morris JK, et al: Value of low-dose combination treatment with blood pressure-lowering drugs: Analysis of 354 randomised clinical trials. *BMJ* 326:1427-1431, 2003.
7. Cheung BMY, Ong KL, Man YB, et al: Prevalence, awareness, treatment and control of hypertension: United States National Health and Nutrition Examination Survey, 2001-2002. *J Clin Hypertens* 8:93-98, 2006.

---

**Association of Refill Adherence and Health Care Use Among Adults with Hypertension in an Urban Health Care System**
Stroupe KT, Teal EY, Tu W, et al (Northwestern Univ, Chicago; Indiana Univ, Indianapolis; Univ of North Carolina, Chapel Hill)
*Pharmacotherapy* 26:779-789, 2006                                                1–13

---

*Study Objectives.*—To determine the rates of undersupply, appropriate supply, and oversupply of antihypertensive drugs, as measured by refill adherence, among patients with complicated and uncomplicated hypertension (i.e., patients who have and have not, respectively, experienced hypertension-related target organ damage), and to examine the association of refill adherence with hospitalization and health care costs among these patients.

*Design.*—Retrospective analysis of electronic medical records.

*Setting.*—An urban, public health care system.

*Patients.*—A total of 15,206 patients aged 18 years or older whose electronic medical records indicated a clinical diagnosis of hypertension based on the *International Classification of Diseases, Ninth Revision, Clinical Modification* codes, and who had received at least one prescription of an antihypertensive drug from 1995–2001.

*Measurements and Main Results.*—We used multivariable analyses to investigate the association of refill adherence with hospitalization and costs. On average, 53% of patients had appropriate supplies (80–120% of supplies needed), 7% had undersupplies, and 40% had oversupplies of drug annually. For patients with complicated hypertension, an undersupply of drug was associated with a 15% greater probability (p=0.009) and an oversupply with a 16% greater probability (p<0.0001) of hospitalization. Among those with uncomplicated hypertension, oversupply was associated with an 11% greater probability (p=0.0002) of hospitalization; undersupply was not associated with greater probability of hospitalization. Total health care costs were lower for patients with undersupplies and higher for those with oversupplies of drug.

*Conclusion.*—Among adults in an urban health care system with complicated hypertension, both undersupply and oversupply of drug were associated with increased hospitalization rates. Monitoring refill adherence of patients, particularly those with low income, minority status, and complicated hypertension, may be useful for targeting patients with undersupplies of drug to encourage refill adherence and identifying patients with oversupplies, who are at high risk of hospitalization.

▶ This retrospective analysis of a large, publicly supported hospital system in Indianapolis reaffirms a conclusion drawn by many others: after a year, only about 50% of hypertensive patients take their drug or drugs as prescribed.[1,2] These authors analyzed their data using the medication possession ratio, a standard method of calculating what proportion of days a medication was available to the patient given the date of dispensing, the number of pills dispensed, and the frequency of pill taking. Other investigators have analyzed similar data using drug persistence: the proportion of people who continue to refill the initially prescribed drug over the long term (typically 1 year).[3-5] Amazingly enough, 50% is the average for either parameter in several large populations.

The authors' data about the dispensing of different classes of antihypertensive drugs are interesting. There were significant differences across classes for those with uncomplicated versus complicated hypertension, with β-blockers being more commonly dispensed to the latter. The overall use of the different drug classes (angiotensin-converting enzyme inhibitors, 28%; calcium channel blockers and diuretics, 25%; β-blockers, 15%; α-blockers, 4%; and angiotensin receptor blockers, 4%) was not much different than use in the US population during the same time period.[6]

While it is probably not surprising that subjects in this study who had undersupplies of antihypertensive drugs (ie, those who were not "persistent") had a significantly higher risk of hospitalization than those whose supplies were deemed adequate, the surprising finding was that those with "oversupplies" of antihypertensive drugs had an even slightly higher risk of hospitalization. One possible way for a subject to obtain an oversupply of drug that is not well addressed by these authors is an interim visit to the physician, which might occur before the previously dispensed drug supply was exhausted. Any change to the patient's regimen would then be added (and increase the medication/possession ratio) to the drug that had been previously dispensed. This phenomenon could explain a higher-than-expected drug utilization rate and would presumably be a marker for a subject at higher risk for hospitalization, as the intensity of treatment would have been increased.

Base on these data, the authors call for increased efforts by pharmacists and physicians to encourage hypertensive patients to refill and take their prescribed medications, but also suggest that efforts by payers to restrict extraneous dispensing might also be enhanced since their data show that subjects who were oversupplied with antihypertensive medications also had significantly more hospitalizations and consumed more health care resources.

**W. J. Elliott, MD, PhD**

*References*

1. McDonald HP, Garg AX, Haynes RB: Interventions to enhance patient adherence to medication prescriptions: Scientific review. *JAMA* 288:2868-2879, 2002.
2. Osterberg L, Blaschke T: Drug therapy: Adherence to medication. *N Engl J Med* 353:487-497, 2005.
3. Conlin PR, Gerth WC, Fox J, et al: Four-year persistence patterns among patients initiating therapy with the angiotensin II receptor antagonist losartan versus other antihypertensive drug classes. *Clin Ther* 23:1999-2010, 2001.
4. Caro JJ, Speckman JL, Salas M, et al: Effect of initial drug choice on persistence with antihypertensive therapy: The importance of actual practice data. *CMAJ* 160:41-60, 1999.
5. Jones JK, Gorkin L, Lian JF, et al: Discontinuation of and changes in treatment after start of new courses of antihypertensive drugs: A study of a United Kingdom population. *BMJ* 311:293-296, 1995.
6. Stafford RS, Monti V, Furberg CD, et al: Long- and short-term changes in antihypertensive prescribing by office-based physicians in the United States. *Hypertension* 48:213-218, 2006.

---

**Efficacy of a home blood pressure monitoring programme on therapeutic compliance in hypertension: the EAPACUM–HTA study**

Márquez-Contreras E, for the Compliance Group of the Spanish Society of Hypertension (SEE) (La Order Health Centre, Huelva, Spain; et al)
*J Hypertens* 24:169-175, 2006
1–14

---

*Objective.*—To evaluate the efficacy of a programme of home blood pressure measurement (HBPM) on therapeutic compliance in mild-to-moderate hypertension.

*Design.*—A prospective controlled multicentre clinical trial.

*Setting.*—Forty primary care centres in Spain, with a duration of 6 months.

*Patients.*—A total of 250 patients with newly diagnosed or uncontrolled hypertension were included.

*Interventions.*—The patients were randomly selected and distributed in two groups: (1) the control group (CG) who received standard health intervention; (2) the intervention group (IG): the patients in this group received an OMRON in their homes for a programme of HBPM.

*Main Outcome Measure.*—Four visits were scheduled, for the measurement of blood pressure (BP). They were provided with an electronic monitor for measuring compliance (monitoring events medication system; MEMS). Therapeutic compliance was defined as a drug consumption of 80–110%. A number of variables were calculated using the MEMS. The mean BP were calculated and the percentage of controlled patients.

*Results.*—A total of 200 patients completed the study (100 in each group). Compliance was observed in 74 and 92%, respectively, in the CG and IG [95% confidence interval (CI) 63.9–84.1 and 86.7–97.3; $P = 0.0001$], the mean percentage compliances were 87.6 and 93.5% (95% CI 81.2–94 and 80.7–98.3; $P = 0.0001$), the percentages of correct days were 83.6 and 89.4%, the percentages of subjects who took the medication at the prescribed time were 79.89 and 88.06%, and the levels of therapeutic cover were 86.7 and 93.1%. The number needed to treat to avoid one case of noncompliance was 5.6 patients. The differences in the mean decreases in BP were significant for diastolic BP, with a greater decrease observed in the IG.

*Conclusions.*—An HBPM programme using electronic monitors is effective in improving compliance in arterial hypertension, measured using the MEMS.

▶ A number of previous studies have attempted to link HBPM with improved medication adherence (the currently accepted term for what these authors call "compliance"). A recent nonquantitative systematic review of this topic concluded that the evidence in favor of this relationship was mixed,[1] primarily because most prior studies used multifactorial interventions, and only a few included HBPM. This report is probably the best of its type because it randomized newly diagnosed subjects, followed them for 6 months, and used the MEMS monitor as the gold standard measure of medication adherence.[2] These virtues probably outweigh the limitations: losing 20% of the individuals during the 6-month follow-up period, measuring office blood pressure (using an automated device) only twice before randomization, and some apparent imbalances at randomization that may have favored the intervention group (eg, baseline blood pressures were 155.6 ± 14.6/91.0 ± 9.0 mm Hg in the control group versus 159.1 ± 16.6/92.4 ± 10.8 mm Hg in the intervention group). The use of a MEMS device has been shown to improve blood pressure control, even without medication changes, probably because individuals know that their pill-taking habits are being measured.[3]

One of the more interesting aspects of the study was the finding that the final office blood pressures were not significantly different across randomized groups (136.7 ± 11.2/81.3 ± 7.6 mm Hg in the control group vs 135.6 ± 13.8/

79.5 ± 8.4 mm Hg in the intervention group), despite the significant difference in adherence.[4] The authors explain this by providing data about "white coat adherence" (also known as "the toothbrush effect," as dentists report that their patients brush more commonly in the few days preceding an appointment). In the 3 days before the final visit in this study, adherence rates were 96.2% and 97.0% in the control and intervention groups, respectively.

These data support the view that HBPM should be recommended for every hypertensive person,[5] although some individuals can become so obsessed with the data that the process becomes burdensome to them, their families, and their physicians. Others recommend monitoring of medication adherence (using the MEMS monitor) for every patient with resistant hypertension.[6]

**W. J. Elliott, MD, PhD**

*References*

1. Ogedegbe G, Schoenthaler A: A systematic review of the effects of home blood pressure monitoring on medication adherence. *J Clin Hypertens (Greenwich)* 8:174-180, 2006.
2. Osterberg L, Blaschke T: Drug therapy: Adherence to medication. *N Engl J Med* 353:487-497, 2005.
3. Nuesch R, Schroeder K, Dieterle T, et al: Relation between insufficient response to antihypertensive treatment and poor compliance with treatment: A prospective case-control study. *BMJ* 323:142-146, 2001.
4. Wetzels GWC, Nelemans P, Schouten JS, et al: Facts and fiction of poor compliance as a cause of inadequate blood pressure control: A systematic review. *J Hypertens* 22:1849-1855, 2004.
5. Yarows SA, Julius S, Pickering TG: Home blood pressure monitoring. *Arch Intern Med* 160:1251-1257, 2000.
6. Burnier M, Santschi V, Favrat B, et al: Monitoring compliance in resistant hypertension: An important step in patient management. *J Hypertens* 21(suppl 2):S37-S42, 2003.

---

**Major Congenital Malformations after First-Trimester Exposure to ACE Inhibitors**
Cooper WO, Hernandez-Diaz S, Arbogast PG, et al (Vanderbilt Univ School of Medicine, Nashville; Boston Univ)
*N Engl J Med* 354:2443-2451, 2006                                            1–15

---

*Background.*—Use of angiotensin-converting–enzyme (ACE) inhibitors during the second and third trimesters of pregnancy is contraindicated because of their association with an increased risk of fetopathy. In contrast, first-trimester use of ACE inhibitors has not been linked to adverse fetal outcomes. We conducted a study to assess the association between exposure to ACE inhibitors during the first trimester of pregnancy only and the risk of congenital malformations.

*Methods.*—We studied a cohort of 29,507 infants enrolled in Tennessee Medicaid and born between 1985 and 2000 for whom there was no evidence of maternal diabetes. We identified 209 infants with exposure to ACE inhibitors in the first trimester alone, 202 infants with exposure to other antihypertensive medications in the first trimester alone, and 29,096 infants with no exposure to antihypertensive drugs at any time during gestation. Major congenital malformations were identified from linked vital records and hospitalization claims during the first year of life and confirmed by review of medical records.

*Results.*—Infants with only first-trimester exposure to ACE inhibitors had an increased risk of major congenital malformations (risk ratio, 2.71; 95 percent confidence interval, 1.72 to 4.27) as compared with infants who had no exposure to antihypertensive medications. In contrast, fetal exposure to other antihypertensive medications during only the first trimester did not confer an increased risk (risk ratio, 0.66; 95 percent confidence interval, 0.25 to 1.75). Infants exposed to ACE inhibitors were at increased risk for malformations of the cardiovascular system (risk ratio, 3.72; 95 percent confidence interval, 1.89 to 7.30) and the central nervous system (risk ratio, 4.39; 95 percent confidence interval, 1.37 to 14.02).

*Conclusions.*—Exposure to ACE inhibitors during the first trimester cannot be considered safe and should be avoided.

▶ Precise estimates of the incidence of congenital anomalies in infants born to women who took an ACE inhibitor during the second and/or third trimesters of pregnancy are not available because of the longstanding warning that these exposures result in oligohydramnios, renal dysplasia (and aplasia), anuria, renal failure, pulmonary hypoplasia, joint contractures, intrauterine growth retardation, hypocalvaria (and other associated defects of the skull and brain), and fetal death.[1,2] These authors undertook the daunting challenge of identifying infants whose mothers took ACE inhibitors during the first trimester of pregnancy to see if they had an increased risk of major congenital anomalies. Fortunately, they had already done much of the legwork for a similar study involving maternal exposures to antibiotics,[3] so the marginal effort to study this question was not as great as it could have been if they had begun de novo.

Many had previously assumed that first-trimester exposure to ACE inhibitors was not particularly harmful, primarily because the drug could be stopped shortly after the first missed menstrual period or positive pregnancy test. It is, of course, difficult to put into perspective the 7.3% incidence (18 of 209 babies) found in this study of congenital anomalies for women who were exposed to ACE inhibitors during the first trimester of pregnancy, but 7.3% is certainly higher than 0% (the desired level). There were only 3 affected infants whose mothers were exposed to ACE inhibitors only during the first month after a missed menstrual period; 2 had an atrial-septal defect and a patent ductus arteriosus and the other had hypospadias. Since most authorities believe that a patent ductus arteriosus is a somewhat less serious major congenital malformation than many others, an exposure during the first month after a missed period could be thought of as perhaps not quite as bad.

The authors' work to tease out this relatively infrequent adverse effect (7.3%) of a hopefully rare exposure (0.07%: 209 of 29,507 women) is truly remarkable. The process of obtaining waivers of informed consent to examine birth records, pharmacy databases, and physician and hospital records must have been grueling and is unlikely to be easily repeated since the Health Insurance Portability and Accountability Act. This is probably why the time period they surveyed was 1985 to 2000. Their unusual definition of the first trimester of pregnancy (the 90 days after the last normal menstrual period, which in most cases includes the 14 days before conception) probably did not confound their findings. Their extra care to attempt to exclude diabetic mothers from their analyses is particularly noteworthy. Since both ACE inhibitors and angiotensin receptor blockers are very widely prescribed, these data should remind physicians of the need to be judicious regarding prescribing these potentially troublesome drugs to potentially pregnant women.

**W. J. Elliott, MD, PhD**

*References*

1. Postmarketing surveillance for angiotensin-converting enzyme inhibitor use during the first trimester of pregnancy-United States, Canada and Israel. *JAMA* 277:1193-1194, 1997.
2. Friedman JM: ACE inhibitors and congenital anomalies [editorial]. *N Engl J Med* 354:2498-2500, 2006.
3. Cooper WO, Ray WA, Griffin MR: Prenatal prescription of macrolide antibiotics and infantile hypertrophic pyloric stenosis. *Obstet Gynecol* 100:101-106, 2002.

---

**In a population-based prospective study, no association between high blood pressure and mortality after age 85 years**
van Bemmel T, Gussekloo J, Westendorp RGJ, et al (Leiden Univ Med Centre, The Netherlands)
*J Hypertens* 24:287-292, 2006                                                    1–16

---

*Objective.*—To study the impact of a history of hypertension and current blood pressure on mortality in the oldest old.

*Design.*—An observational population-based cohort study.

*Setting.*—Community city of Leiden, The Netherlands.

*Participants.*—Five hundred and ninety-nine inhabitants of the birthcohort 1912–1914 were enrolled on their 85th birthday. There were no selection criteria related to health or demographic characteristics.

*Interventions.*—The mean follow-up was 4.2 years. Medical histories were obtained from general practitioners. Medication histories were obtained from the participant's pharmacist. Blood pressure was measured twice at baseline.

*Main Outcome Measures.*—All cause and cardiovascular mortality.

*Results.*—Five hundred and seventy-one participants were included, 39.2% had a history of hypertension. During follow-up 290 participants died, 119 due to cardiovascular causes. Compared to participants without a history of hypertension, those with a history of hypertension had increased mortality from cardiovascular causes [relative risk (RR) 1.60, confidence interval (CI) 1.06–2.40] but equal mortality from all causes (RR 1.19, CI 0.91–1.55). High blood pressure at baseline (age 85) was not a risk factor for mortality. Baseline blood pressure values below 140/70 mmHg ($n = 48$)

were associated with excess mortality, predominantly in participants with a history of hypertension.

*Conclusion.*—In the oldest old, high blood pressure is not a risk factor for mortality, irrespective of a history of hypertension. Blood pressure values below 140/70 mmHg are associated with excess mortality.

▶ This report rekindles the controversy regarding blood pressure (and its treatment) in individuals older than 80 or 85 years and suggests that since blood pressure is not correlated directly to mortality in the "oldest old," there would seem little reason to treat it. This conclusion disagrees with that of the INDANA group, which found significant reductions in both stroke (by 36%) and heart failure (by 38%, albeit with a slight and nonsignificant 6% increase in mortality) among 1670 participants older than 79 years in 7 trials of antihypertensive drug therapy versus placebo/no treatment.[1] The authors' data also support the "J-shaped curve" hypothesis, which suggests that lowering blood pressure may be harmful, in that a higher risk of mortality was found in those older than 84 years with blood pressures lower than 140/70 mm Hg. This phenomenon has been long and widely debated[2,3] despite being seen in many (even untreated) population-based cohorts and was not observed in the only clinical trial designed to test the hypothesis (the Hypertension Optimal Treatment study).[4]

Although the results of the Hypertension in the Very Elderly Trial (HYVET) Pilot Study did not convincingly demonstrate a benefit of drug treatment in hypertensive people older than 80 years,[5] it is expected that the main HYVET trial, with about 2100 subjects, should provide an answer to this question in the next few years.[6] It will be interesting to learn if the clinical trial provides evidence that contradicts the conclusions of this study, which are based on only 2 baseline blood pressure readings and only 40 deaths among the group having blood pressures below 140/70 mm Hg. Whether this reflects a longer duration of treated hypertension than those with higher blood pressure at baseline is unclear.

**W. J. Elliott, MD, PhD**

*References*

1. Gueyffier F, et al, for the INDANA Group: Antihypertensive drugs in very old people: A subgroup meta-analysis of randomised controlled trials. *Lancet* 353:793-796, 1999.
2. Farnett L, Mulrow CD, Linn WD, et al: The J-curve phenomenon and the treatment of hypertension. Is there a point beyond which pressure reduction is dangerous? *JAMA* 265:489-495, 1991.
3. Fletcher AE, Bulpitt CJ: How far should blood pressure be lowered? *N Engl J Med* 326:251-254, 1992.
4. Hansson L, Zanchetti A, Carruthers SG, et al: Effects of intensive blood pressure lowering and low-dose aspirin in patients with hypertension: Principal results of the Hypertension Optimal Treatment (HOT) randomised trial: The HOT Study Group. *Lancet* 351:1755-1762, 1998.
5. Bulpitt CJ, Beckett NS, Cooke J, et al: Results of the pilot study for the Hypertension in the Very Elderly Trial (HYVET-pilot). *J Hypertens* 21:2409-2417, 2003.
6. Bulpitt C, Fletcher A, Beckett N, et al: Hypertension in the Very Elderly Trial (HYVET): Protocol for the main trial. *Drugs Aging* 18:151-164, 2001.

### Association Between Blood Pressure and Survival over 9 Years in a General Population Aged 85 and Older

Rastas S, Pirttilä T, Viramo P, et al (Lohja Hosp, Finland; Univ of Kuopio, Finland; Oulu Deaconess Inst, Finland; et al)
*J Am Geriatr Soc* 54:912-918, 2006                                    1–17

*Objectives.*—To investigate the association between blood pressure and mortality in people aged 85 and older.

*Design.*—Population-based prospective study with 9-year follow-up.

*Setting.*—Department of Neuroscience and Neurology and Department of Public Health and General Practice, University of Kuopio, and Department of Clinical Neurosciences, Helsinki University Hospital.

*Participants.*—Of all 601 people living in the city of Vantaa born before April 1, 1906, whether living at home or in institutions and alive on April 1, 1991, 521 were clinically examined and underwent blood pressure measurement.

*Measurements.*—Blood pressure was measured using a standardized method in the right arm of the subject after resting for at least 5 minutes. Information on medical history for each participant was verified from a computerized database containing all primary care health records. Death certificates were obtained from the National Register; the collection of death certificates was complete.

*Results.*—After adjusting for age, sex, functional status, and coexisting diseases (earlier-diagnosed myocardial infarction, congestive heart failure, dementia, cancer, stroke, or hypertension), low systolic blood pressure (BP) was associated with risk of death.

*Conclusion.*—Low systolic BP may be partially related to poor general health and poor vitality, but the very old may represent a select group of individuals, and the use of BP-lowering medications needs to be evaluated in this group.

▶ This study stokes further the controversy regarding blood pressure (and its treatment) in individuals older than 85 years and suggests that lower blood pressure is associated with a higher mortality rate in the oldest old. The silent implication is that treatment of high blood pressure may be unwarranted in this age group. This conclusion agrees with another recent Dutch study[1] but disagrees somewhat with that of the INDANA group, which found significant reductions in both stroke (by 36%) and heart failure (by 38%, albeit with a slight and nonsignificant 6% increase in mortality) among 1670 participants older than 79 years in 7 trials of antihypertensive drug therapy versus placebo/no treatment.[2] The authors' data also support the J-shaped curve hypothesis, which suggests that lowering blood pressure may be harmful, in that a higher risk of mortality was found in those older than 84 years with blood pressures lower than 140/70 mm Hg. This phenomenon has been long and widely debated[2-5] despite being seen in many (even untreated) population-based cohorts and was not observed in the only clinical trial designed to test the hypothesis (the Hypertension Optimal Treatment study).[6]

The major difficulty with the authors' conclusions is that they did not stratify their data according to whether or not the individual was taking antihypertensive medication. This might have allowed them to implicate more closely antihypertensive drug therapy with an increased risk of death, particularly since their population included about 50% of individuals at each level of systolic blood pressure who were drug treated. They performed a very large number of subgroup analyses, but none compared mortality rates in those who were drug treated versus those who took no antihypertensive agents.

These and other epidemiologic data are interesting[1] but will likely pale in comparison to the results of the main Hypertension in the Very Elderly Trial (HYVET), with about 2100 subjects.[7] The randomized clinical trial ranks higher in the hierarchy of medical evidence than cohort studies, and HYVET will likely be the best answer to the question of whether hypertensive individuals older than 85 years should be considered differently than individuals who are otherwise identical, just younger in age. It will be interesting if HYVET contradicts the conclusions of this study, which are based on a single blood pressure reading by an attending neurologist.

**W. J. Elliott, MD, PhD**

*References*

1. van Bemmel T, Gussekloo J, Westendorp RGJ, et al: In a population-based prospective study, no association between high blood pressure and mortality after age 85 years. *J Hypertens* 24:287-292, 2006.
2. Gueyffier F, et al, for the INDANA Group: Antihypertensive drugs in very old people: A subgroup meta-analysis of randomised controlled trials. *Lancet* 353:793-796, 1999.
3. Farnett L, Mulrow CD, Linn WD, et al: The J-curve phenomenon and the treatment of hypertension. Is there a point beyond which pressure reduction is dangerous? *JAMA* 265:489-495, 1991.
4. Fletcher AE, Bulpitt CJ: How far should blood pressure be lowered? *N Engl J Med* 326:251-254, 1992.
5. Messerli FH, et al, for the International Verapamil-Trandolapril Study Investigators. Dogma disputed: can aggressively lowering blood pressure in hypertensive patients with coronary artery disease be dangerous? *Ann Intern Med* 144:884-893, 2006.
6. Hansson L, Zanchetti A, Carruthers SG, et al: Effects of intensive blood pressure lowering and low-dose aspirin in patients with hypertension: Principal results of the Hypertension Optimal Treatment (HOT) randomised trial: The HOT Study Group. *Lancet* 351:1755-1762, 1998.
7. Bulpitt C, Fletcher A, Beckett N, et al: Hypertension in the Very Elderly Trial (HYVET): Protocol for the main trial. *Drugs Aging* 18:151-164, 2001.

---

**Applicability to primary care of national clinical guidelines on blood pressure lowering for people with stroke: cross sectional study**

Mant J, McManus RJ, Hare R (Univ of Birmingham, England)
*BMJ* 332:635-637, 2006
1–18

---

*Objective.*—To compare the characteristics of patients with cerebrovascular disease in primary care with those of the participants in the

PROGRESS trial, on which national guidelines for blood pressure lowering are based.

*Design.*—Population based cross sectional survey of patients with confirmed stroke or transient ischaemic attack.

*Setting.*—Seven general practices in south Birmingham, England.

*Participants.*—All patients with a validated history of stroke (n = 413) or transient ischaemic attack (n = 107).

*Main Outcome Measures.*—Patient characteristics: age, sex, time since last cerebrovascular event, blood pressure, and whether receiving antihypertensive treatment.

*Results.*—Patients were 12 years older than the participants in PROGRESS and twice as likely to be women. The median time that had elapsed since their cerebrovascular event was two and a half years, compared with eight months in PROGRESS. The systolic blood pressure of 315 (61%) patients was over 140 mm Hg, and for 399 (77%) it was over 130 mm Hg. One hundred and forty seven (28%) patients were receiving a thiazide diuretic, and 136 (26%) were receiving an angiotensin converting enzyme inhibitor.

*Conclusions.*—Important differences exist between the PROGRESS trial participants and a typical primary care stroke population, which undermine the applicability of the trial's findings. Research in appropriate populations is urgently needed before the international guidelines are implemented in primary care.

▶ This report claims that because of important demographic and clinical differences between patients with a prior stroke in the South Birmingham Primary Care Trust and those who were enrolled in the PROGRESS (Perindopril Protection Against RECURRENT Stroke Study),[1] the clinical practice guidelines for antihypertensive drug therapy (angiotensin-converting enzyme inhibitor plus thiazide diuretic) derived from PROGRESS may not be relevant and can be ignored. These authors call for more studies, particularly in patients with similar baseline characteristics, to what is seen in South Birmingham before these international guidelines are implemented in primary care.

Another way to view the authors' data is to consider the fact that, on average, the patients in South Birmingham were 2.5 years out from their first stroke. This could be interpreted as a missed opportunity for secondary prevention since PROGRESS enrolled patients who were between 2 weeks and 5 years out from their first stroke (on average, 8 months). The average blood pressure of the patients with a prior stroke in South Birmingham was 148/80 mm Hg, higher than the British Hypertension Society's target,[2] while fully 38% had blood pressure of 160/90 mm Hg or greater and only 68% were receiving antihypertensive drug therapy.

The PROGRESS investigators were sensitive to the regional variation in stroke risk and performed several analyses to assess whether significant differences were present, such as in Australia versus China (where in 2000, 21% of the deaths were attributed to stroke).[3] They found no significant inhomogeneity in their results when the subjects were subgrouped by blood pressure,[1] age, gender, and country of residence.[4] In addition, the South Birmingham Primary Care Trust should be reminded that several other studies in poststroke patients show a significantly reduced risk of cardiovascular events among those randomized to active antihypertensive drug therapy. The Post-stroke Antihypertensive Therapy Study (PATS) showed a 29% reduction in second stroke and a 25% reduction in cardiovascular events in those randomized to indapamide rather than placebo.[5] The Heart Outcomes Prevention Evaluation (HOPE) study included 1013 individuals with a prior stroke; they had about 2.4 times the risk of stroke as those without a prior history of stroke.[6] Those randomized to placebo had about a 15% reduction in the risk of a second stroke, although this did not reach statistical significance (perhaps because of limited statistical power).[6] Using an angiotensin receptor blocker acutely in patients admitted to hospital with stroke improved outcomes compared with placebo in the Acute Candesartan Cilexetil Evaluation in Stroke Survivors (ACCESS) trial.[7] An epidemiological study of 2435 people with cerebrovascular disease showed a direct correlation between usual systolic and diastolic blood pressures and the risk of recurrent stroke.[8] A recent systematic review of antihypertensive drug therapy and secondary stroke prevention also shows a significant correlation between the differences in achieved blood pressures between randomized groups and the absolute reduction in a second stroke, indicating that the lower the blood pressure, the lower the risk of recurrent stroke.[9] While it is difficult to argue against further research to define optimal blood pressure treatment to prevent a second stroke, most authorities recommend effective antihypertensive drug therapy as part of a multifactorial program (including antiplatelet agents and lipid-lowering therapy) in patients with known cerebrovascular disease.[10,11]

**W. J. Elliott, MD, PhD**

*References*

1. PROGRESS Collaborative Group: Randomised trial of a perindopril-based blood-pressure-lowering regimen among 6105 individuals with previous stroke or transient ischaemic attack. *Lancet* 358:1033-1041, 2001.
2. Williams B, Poulter NR, Brown MJ, et al: British Hypertension Society guidelines for hypertension management 2004 (BHS-IV): Summary. *BMJ* 328:634-640, 2004.
3. He J, Gu D, Wu X, et al: Major causes of death among men and women in China. *N Engl J Med* 353:1124-1129, 2005.
4. PROGRESS Collaborative Group: Perindopril-based blood pressure lowering in individuals with cerebrovascular disease: consistency of benefits by age, sex and region. *J Hypertens* 22:653-659, 2004.
5. PATS Collaborating Group: Post-stroke antihypertensive treatment study. A preliminary result. *Chinese Med J* 108:710-717, 1995.
6. Bosch J, Yusuf S, Pogue J, et al: Use of ramipril in preventing stroke: Double blind randomised trial. *BMJ* 324:699-702, 2002.
7. Schrader J, Luders S, Kulschewski A, et al: The ACCESS Study: Evaluation of Acute Candesartan Cilexetil Therapy in Stroke Survivors. *Stroke* 34:1699-1703, 2003.
8. Rodgers A, MacMahon S, Gamble G, et al: Blood pressure and risk of stroke in patients with cerebrovascular disease. The United Kingdom Transient Ischaemic Attack Collaborative Group. *BMJ* 313:147, 1996.
9. Rashid P, Leonardi-Bee J, Bath P: Blood pressure reduction and secondary prevention of stroke and other vascular events: A systematic review. *Stroke* 34:2741-2748, 2003.

10. Sacco RL, Adams R, Albers G, et al: Guidelines for prevention of stroke in patients with ischemic stroke or transient ischemic attack: A statement for healthcare professionals from the American Heart Association/American Stroke Association Council on Stroke: Co-sponsored by the Council on Cardiovascular Radiology and Intervention: The American Academy of Neurology affirms the value of this guideline. *Circulation* 113:e409-e449, 2006.
11. Gorelick PB, Broder MS, Crowell RM, et al: Determining the appropriateness of selected surgical and medical management options in recurrent stroke prevention: A guideline for primary care physicians from the National Stroke Association Work Group on Recurrent Stroke Prevention. *Cerebrovasc Dis* 13:196-207, 2004.

**Antihypertensive Medications and the Risk of Incident Type 2 Diabetes**
Taylor EN, Hu FB, Curhan GC (Harvard Med School; Harvard School of Public Health, Boston)
*Diabetes Care* 29:1065-1070, 2006                                     1–19

*Objective.*—The purpose of this study was to examine the association between the use of different classes of antihypertensive medications and the risk of incident type 2 diabetes.

*Research Design and Methods.*—We conducted a prospective study of three cohorts: the Nurses' Health Study (NHS) I and II and the Health Professionals Follow-up Study (HPFS). Antihypertensive medication use was ascertained by biennial questionnaires. After excluding participants who reported a history of diabetes at baseline, 41,193 older women (NHS I), 14,151 younger women (NHS II), and 19,472 men (HPFS), all with hypertension, were followed for 8, 10, and 16 years, respectively.

*Results.*—We documented 3,589 incident cases of diabetes. After adjustment for age, BMI, physical activity, the use of other antihypertensive medications, and other risk factors, the multivariate relative risk (RR) of incident diabetes in participants taking a thiazide diuretic compared with those not taking a thiazide was 1.20 (95% CI 1.08–1.33) in older women, 1.45 (1.17–1.79) in younger women, and 1.36 (1.17–1.58) in men. The multivariate RR in participants taking a β-blocker compared with those not taking a β-blocker was 1.32 (1.20–1.46) in older women and 1.20 (1.05–1.38) in men. ACE inhibitors and calcium channel blockers were not associated with risk.

*Conclusions.*—Thiazide diuretic and beta-blocker use were independently associated with a higher risk of incident diabetes. Increased surveillance for diabetes in patients treated with these medications may be warranted.

▶ The conclusions of this large observational study agree quite closely with those drawn from randomized clinical trials comparing these drugs with any other antihypertensive drug: thiazide diuretics increase the risk of incident diabetes by about 25% (95% CI, 11%-38%) and β-blockers by about 19% (95% CI, 10%-27%).[1] This is surprising because the meta-analyses compare each drug with any other antihypertensive drug with which it was compared in clinical trials, and the observational studies compare the risk with and without the individual drugs, after statistical adjustment for any other antihypertensive drug that the person reported taking. Even more interesting is the similarity of the estimate of risk from these observational studies when compared with the more complex "network meta-analysis," which suggests that the diuretic increases the risk (compared with placebo) by 30% (95% CI, 7%-58%), whereas a β-blocker increases the risk (compared with placebo) by 17% (95% CI, −2% to 40%).[2] These meta-analyses are not able to provide gender-specific estimates, as the observational study does.

Two major caveats remain regarding these sorts of data. Although some have advocated believing the results of large, long-term observational studies, since they sometimes lead to similar point estimates of risk compared with randomized clinical trials,[3-4] the example of postmenopausal hormone replacement therapy reminds us that observational studies can, in fact, be contradicted by well-done clinical trials,[5,6] which have a higher position in the hierarchy of medical evidence promulgated by the Cochrane Collaboration and other proponents of evidence-based medicine.[7]

The other warning that is most appropriate at this time is that the clinical consequences of type 2 diabetes mellitus that arise after treatment with antihypertensive drugs are uncertain. The ALLHAT investigators (who have the most outcomes data) remind us that individuals who developed hyperglycemia after being randomized to chlorthalidone did not have an increase in cardiovascular risk during an average of 3 years of follow-up.[8] There are now several other studies that corroborate this assertion,[9-11] and only one Italian study that disagrees, which was unable to link the increased risk of cardiovascular events to an initial diuretic.[12]

Despite the uncertain clinical consequences of new-onset diabetes associated with antihypertensive drugs, there is little doubt that health care expenditures are increased in these individuals, given the lower blood pressure and LDL cholesterol targets that come in play with a new diagnosis of type 2 diabetes. This is apparently part of the reason the new British NICE (National Institute for Health and Clinical Excellence) guidelines for hypertension suggest avoiding the combination of a diuretic and a β-blocker because of the economic consequences of the increased risk of new-onset diabetes.[13]

**W. J. Elliott, MD, PhD**

*References*

1. Elliott WJ: Differential effects of antihypertensive drugs on new-onset diabetes? *Curr Hypertens Rep* 7:249-256, 2005.
2. Elliott WJ, Meyer PM: Incident diabetes in clinical trials of antihypertensive drugs: A network meta-analysis [abstract]. *J Clin Hypertens (Greenwich)* 8:A46, 2006.
3. Benson K, Hartz AJ: A comparison of observational studies and randomized, controlled trials. *N Engl J Med* 342:1878-1886, 2000.
4. Concato J, Shah N, Horwitz RI: Randomized, controlled trials, observational studies, and the hierarchy of research designs. *N Engl J Med* 342:1887-1892, 2000.
5. Rossouw JE, Anderson GL, Prentice RL, et al: Writing Group for the Women's Health Initiative Investigators. Risks and benefits of estrogen plus progestin in healthy postmenopausal women: Principal results From the Women's Health Initiative randomized controlled trial. *JAMA* 288:321-333, 2002.

6. Anderson GL, Limacher M, Assaf AR, et al: Women's Health Initiative Steering Committee. Effects of conjugated equine estrogen in postmenopausal women with hysterectomy: The Women's Health Initiative randomized controlled trial. *JAMA* 291:1701-1712, 2004.
7. Sackett DL, Rosenberg WM, Gray JA, et al: Evidence based medicine: What it is and what it isn't. *BMJ* 312:71-72, 1996.
8. Barzilay JI, et al for the ALLHAT Collaborative Research Group. Fasting glucose levels and incident diabetes mellitus in older nondiabetic adults randomized to receive 3 different classes of antihypertensive treatment: A report from the Antihypertensive and Lipid-Lowering Treatment to Prevent Heart Attack Trial (ALLHAT). *Arch Intern Med* 166:2191-2201, 2006.
9. Kostis JB, Wilson AC, Freudenberger RS, et al: Long-term effect of diuretic-based therapy on fatal outcomes in subjects with isolated systolic hypertension with and without diabetes. *Am J Cardiol* 95:29-35, 2005.
10. Qiao Q, Jousilahti P, Eriksson J, et al: Predictive properties of impaired glucose tolerance for cardiovascular risk are not explained by the development of overt diabetes during follow-up. *Diabetes Care* 26:2910-2914, 2003.
11. Eberly LE, Cohen JD, Prineas R, et al: Impact of incident diabetes and incident nonfatal cardiovascular disease on 18-year mortality: The Multiple Risk Factor Intervention Trial experience. *Diabetes Care* 26:848-854, 2003.
12. Verdecchia P, Reboldi G, Angeli F, et al: Adverse prognostic significance of new diabetes in treated hypertensive subjects. *Hypertension* 43:963-969, 2004.
13. National Institute for Health and Clinical Excellence: *Hypertension: Management of hypertension in adults in primary care, a partial update of NICE clinical guideline 18*, www.nice.org.uk/page.aspx?o-cg034NICEguideline, accessed July 4, 2006.

# Hypertension and Cardiovascular Risk

### Blood Pressure Usually Considered Normal Is Associated with an Elevated Risk of Cardiovascular Disease

Kshirsagar AV, Carpenter M, Bang H, et al (Univ of North Carolina at Chapel Hill; Cornell Univ, New York; Univ of Mississippi Med Ctr, Jackson)
*Am J Med* 119:133-141, 2006                                                          1–20

*Purpose.*—Research on the risk of cardiovascular disease among individuals with prehypertension (blood pressure 120/80 to 139/89 mm Hg) is incomplete. Additional information among individuals with a high risk of cardiovascular disease complications may help to focus current and future efforts.

*Subjects and Methods.*—We performed a prospective cohort analysis among 8960 middle-aged adults in the Atherosclerosis Risk in Communities (ARIC) study. The exposure variables were blood pressure levels: high normal blood pressure, systolic blood pressure 130-139 mm Hg or diastolic blood pressure 85-89 mm Hg; and normal blood pressure, systolic blood pressure 120-129 mm Hg or diastolic blood pressure 80-84 mm Hg. The outcome was incident cardiovascular disease defined as fatal/nonfatal coronary heart disease, cardiac procedure, silent myocardial infarction, or ischemic stroke. Subgroup analysis was performed among blacks, diabetics, individuals aged 55-64 years, individuals with renal insufficiency, and among individuals with varying levels of low-density lipoprotein (LDL) cholesterol and body mass index (BMI).

*Results.*—Compared with optimal blood pressure (systolic blood pressure <120 mm Hg and diastolic blood pressure <80 mm Hg), the relative risk (RR) of cardiovascular disease for high normal blood pressure was 2.33 (95% confidence interval [CI], 1.85-2.92), and RR for normal blood pressure was 1.81 (1.47-2.22); among blacks: RR for high normal blood pressure was 3.29 (95% CI, 1.68-6.45); among diabetics: RR for high normal blood pressure 4.10 (95% CI, 2.26-7.46); age 55-64 years: RR for high normal blood pressure 2.41 (95% CI, 1.75-3.30) among individuals with renal insufficiency: RR for high normal blood pressure was 1.90 (95% CI, 1.34-2.70); among individuals with BMI >30 kg/m$^2$: RR for high normal blood pressure was 3.56 (95% CI, 1.99-6.35); and among individuals with LDL >160 mg/dL, RR for high normal blood pressure was 1.85 (95% CI, 1.26-2.72).

*Conclusions.*—Individuals with prehypertensive levels of blood pressure have an increased risk of developing cardiovascular disease relative to those with optimal levels. The association is pronounced among blacks, among individuals with diabetes mellitus, and among those with high BMI.

▶ Although previous prospective observational studies (including both the Framingham Heart Study[1] and a nationally representative sample of adults in 1972-1977[2]) have shown an increased risk of cardiovascular events among those with prehypertension, this study further defines the characteristics of those at greatest risk. As with hypertensives, African American, diabetic, and obese prehypertensives were those with the highest risk for cardiovascular events.

From their biracial cohort of 15,792 middle-aged individuals recruited from 1987 to 1989 from 4 US communities (Forsyth County, NC; Jackson, Miss; and suburbs of Minneapolis, Minn, and Washington County, Md), the authors excluded those with known cardiovascular disease or hypertension, leaving 5622 with "optimal" blood pressure, 2059 with "normal" blood pressure, and 1279 with "high-normal" blood pressure (using now-outdated JNC VI terminology).[3] During an average of 11.6 years, there were 772 incident cardiovascular events (most of which were coronary heart disease events). This provided sufficient statistical power to test the association of both "normal" and "high-normal" blood pressures with incident cardiovascular events in their subgroups.

The finding that diabetics were at higher risk with prehypertensive levels of blood pressure is not really a surprise and validates many sets of current guidelines that recommend a blood pressure of less than 130/80 mm Hg for diabetics.[4-6] The finding of increased risk of cardiovascular events among African Americans with prehypertensive levels of blood pressure corroborates a set of guidelines from the International Society on Hypertension in Blacks[7] that recommended a target of less than 130/85 mm Hg for this population before JNC 7 was released. Whether obesity itself imparts an increased risk of cardiovascular events, or is tied to increased LDL cholesterol levels, glucose intolerance, and other associated traditional cardiovascular risk factors, is somewhat less clear.

Although the conclusions of this study are not surprising, they do reinforce the rationale for lowering blood pressure, not only in those with hypertension, but also in those with prehypertension. Whether this is best done by lifestyle modifications[8,9] or pharmacological therapy[10] is a question that should be answered by future research.

**W. J. Elliott, MD, PhD**

*References*

1. Vasan RS, Larson MG, Leip EP, et al: Impact of high-normal blood pressure on the risk of cardiovascular disease. *N Engl J Med* 345:1291-1297, 2001.
2. Liszka HA, Mainous AG III, King DE, et al: Prehypertension and cardiovascular morbidity. *Ann Fam Med* 3:294-299, 2005.
3. The sixth report of the Joint National Committee on Prevention, Detection, Evaluation, and Treatment of High Blood Pressure (JNC VI). *Arch Intern Med* 157:2413-2446, 1997.
4. Chobanian AV, Bakris GL, Black HR, et al: The seventh report of the Joint National Committee on Prevention, Detection, Evaluation, and Treatment of High Blood Pressure: The JNC 7 Report. *JAMA* 289:2560-2572, 2003.
5. American Diabetes Association: Clinical practice recommendations, 2004. *Diabetes Care* 27(suppl 1):S1-S153, 2004.
6. Whitworth JA, for the World Health Organization, International Society of Hypertension Writing Group: 2003 World Health Organization (WHO)/International Society of Hypertension (ISH) statement on management of hypertension. *J Hypertens* 21:1983-1992, 2003.
7. Douglas JG, Bakris GL, Epstein M, et al: Hypertension in African Americans Working Group of the International Society on Hypertension in Blacks. Management of high blood pressure in African Americans: Consensus statement of the Hypertension in African Americans Working Group of the International Society on Hypertension in Blacks. *Arch Intern Med* 163:525-541, 2003.
8. Appel LJ, Brands MW, Daniels SR, et al: Dietary approaches to prevent and treat hypertension: A scientific statement from the American Heart Association. *Hypertension* 47:296-308, 2006.
9. Appel LJ, Champagne CM, Harsha DW, et al: Writing Group of the PREMIER Collaborative Research Group. Effects of comprehensive lifestyle modification on blood pressure control: Main results of the PREMIER clinical trial. *JAMA* 289:2083-2093, 2003.
10. Julius S, Nesbitt SD, Egan B, et al: Feasibility of treating prehypertension with an angiotensin receptor blocker. *N Engl J Med* 354:1685-1697, 2006.

## Are Blood Pressure Predictors of Cardiovascular Disease Mortality Different for Prehypertensives Than for Hypertensives?

Greenberg (Brooklyn College of the City Univ of New York)
*Am J Hypertens* 19:454-461, 2006                                          1–21

*Background.*—The ability of diastolic, systolic, mean arterial, and pulse pressures to predict cardiovascular disease (CVD) morality has not been assessed for persons with prehypertension (diastolic pressure 80 to 89 mm Hg or systolic pressure 120 to 139 mm Hg).

*Methods.*—Cox's regression analyses were conducted using 4849 subjects aged 33 to 87 years from the First National Health and Nutrition Examination Survey Epidemiologic Follow-up Study. A correction was made for the regression–dilution bias.

*Results.*—There were 327 cardiovascular disease and 258 coronary heart-disease deaths during an average follow-up of 8.6 years. For nonelderly prehypertensives, systolic blood pressure (BP) was a stronger predictor than diastolic BP. The multivariate single predictor hazard ratios (95% confidence interval) for CVD mortality were 1.43 (0.65–3.14) and 2.11 (1.28–3.49), for a 10 mm Hg increment diastolic and systolic BP, respectively. For elderly prehypertensives, it was reversed. The equivalent results were 1.53 (1.10–2.13) and 1.25 (0.89–1.60), respectively. For nonelderly hypertensives, diastolic BP was a stronger predictor than systolic BP, and for elderly hypertensives it was reversed. Diastolic and systolic BP provided as much as or more predictive information than pulse and mean arterial pressure in all analyses.

*Conclusions.*—For nonelderly prehypertensives, systolic BP was the strongest predictor, whereas for hypertensives the strongest predictor was diastolic BP. For elderly subjects this pattern was reversed.

▶ At face value, these data about prehypertension contradict what is now widely understood about hypertension[1]: systolic BP is the more powerful prognostic indicator of cardiovascular events (including death) in older individuals,[2,3] whereas diastolic BP may be somewhat more important in youth.[4] The reason or reasons for the fact that this dataset contradicts prior knowledge about hypertension are not explored in the report, but several possibilities come to mind. The NHANES I Epidemiological Follow-Up Study contains 2 sets of BP measurements, taken about 10 years apart, and the author was therefore able to adjust for a regression-dilution bias in this dataset (which is seldom possible with most cross-sectional epidemiological studies). This adjustment was performed for the data collected by the Prospective Studies Collaborative,[2] however, so it probably doesn't account for the difference in conclusions. The more likely possibility is that, in the prehypertensives, there is a range of possible usual blood pressure values of only 9 mm Hg diastolic but 19 mm Hg systolic. As a result, there is greater statistical power to find a difference for systolic than diastolic, assuming that the usual blood pressure values are rather normally distributed. This would be expected more in the younger group (which had an average usual blood pressure of 124.4/79.0 mm Hg) but is less likely in the older group (with an average usual blood pressure of 130.3/75.3 mm Hg) because the distribution is more likely skewed toward the upper ranges in the older group. The third possible explanation is that there were only 473 prehypertensives in the older age group compared with 1405 in the younger age group, but it is unclear how many of each group experienced the end point, cardiovascular death. A fourth possibility is that the author performed Cox analyses with 327 cardiovascular deaths across 2 age groups and 3 blood pressure groupings, with 11 other covariates in each model. One wonders if this model had sufficient end points to withstand such a great degree of statistical adjustment; typically statisticians like to see 10 events in every cell (group × covariate), and this seems unlikely.

Nonetheless, others have also reported the importance of systolic BP as a significant prognostic factor for cardiovascular death among younger subjects, both in this dataset[5] as well as in others.[6,7] Controlling systolic BP is therefore an important treatment objective for both older and younger individuals.

**W. J. Elliott, MD, PhD**

*References*

1. Chobanian AV, Bakris GL, Black HR, et al: Seventh Report of the Joint National Committee on Prevention, Detection, Evaluation and Treatment of High Blood Pressure. National High Blood Pressure Education Program Coordinating Committee. *Hypertension* 42:1206-1252, 2003.
2. Age-specific relevance of usual blood pressure to vascular mortality: A meta-analysis of individual data for one million adults in 61 prospective studies. Prospective Studies Collaborative. *Lancet* 360:1903-1913, 2002.
3. Izzo JL Jr, Levy D, Black HR: Clinical advisory statement: Importance of systolic blood pressure in older Americans. *Hypertension* 35:1021-1024, 2000.
4. National High Blood Pressure Education Program Working Group on High Blood Pressure in Children and Adolescents: The Fourth Report on the Diagnosis, Evaluation and Treatment of High Blood Pressure in Children and Adolescents. *Pediatrics* 114:555-576, 2004.
5. Fang J, Madhavan S, Alderman MH: Pulse pressure: A predictor of cardiovascular mortality among young normotensive subjects. *Blood Press* 9:260-266, 2000.
6. Rosenman RH, Sholtz RI, Brand RJ: A study of comparative blood pressure measures in predicting risk of coronary heart disease. *Circulation* 54:51-58, 1976.
7. McCarron P, Davey-Smith G, Oksasha M, et al: Blood pressure in young adulthood and mortality from cardiovascular disease. *Lancet* 355:1430-1431, 2000.

---

**Diurnal Blood Pressure Pattern and Risk of Congestive Heart Failure**
Ingelsson E, Björklund-Bodegård K, Lind L, et al (Uppsala Univ, Sweden; AstraZeneca Research and Development, Mölndal, Sweden)
*JAMA* 295:2859-2866, 2006                                    1–22

---

*Context.*—High blood pressure is the most important risk factor for congestive heart failure (CHF) at a population level, but the relationship of an altered diurnal blood pressure pattern to risk of subsequent CHF is unknown.

*Objectives.*—To explore 24-hour ambulatory blood pressure characteristics as predictors of CHF incidence and to investigate whether altered diurnal blood pressure patterns confer any additional risk information beyond that provided by conventional office blood pressure measurements.

*Design, Setting, and Participants.*—Prospective, community-based, observational cohort in Uppsala, Sweden, including 951 elderly men free of CHF, valvular disease, and left ventricular hypertrophy at baseline between 1990 and 1995, followed up until the end of 2002. Twenty-four-hour ambulatory blood pressure monitoring was performed at baseline, and the blood pressure variables were analyzed as predictors of subsequent CHF.

*Main Outcome Measure.*—First hospitalization for CHF.

*Results.*—Seventy men developed heart failure during follow-up, with an incidence rate of 8.6 per 1000 person-years at risk. In multivariable Cox proportional hazards models adjusted for antihypertensive treatment and established risk factors for CHF (myocardial infarction, diabetes, smoking, body mass index, and serum cholesterol level), a 1-SD (9–mm Hg) increase in nighttime ambulatory diastolic blood pressure (hazard ratio [HR], 1.26; 95% confidence interval [CI], 1.02-1.55) and the presence of "nondipping" blood pressure (night-day ambulatory blood pressure ratio ≥1; HR, 2.29; 95% CI, 1.16-4.52) were associated with an increased risk of CHF. After adjusting for office-measured systolic and diastolic blood pressures, nondipping blood pressure remained a significant predictor of CHF (HR, 2.21; 95% CI, 1.12-4.36 vs normal night-day pattern). Nighttime ambulatory diastolic blood pressure and nondipping blood pressure were also significant predictors of CHF after exclusion of all participants who had an acute myocardial infarction before baseline or during follow-up.

*Conclusions.*—Nighttime blood pressure appears to convey additional risk information about CHF beyond office-measured blood pressure and other established risk factors for CHF. The clinical value of this association remains to be established in future studies.

▶ This report adds CHF to the list of adverse cardiovascular[1-5] and renal events[6] about which ambulatory blood pressure monitoring provides prognostic information above and beyond office blood pressure readings. Although only 70 men in this study were hospitalized for CHF, and many statistical adjustments were made, the conclusions were robust and withstood all this extra testing. Diagnosis of CHF in the outpatient department is usually more challenging than the in-hospital diagnosis,[7] which nearly always includes an echocardiogram or another measure of left ventricular ejection fraction.[8] For this reason, their choice of hospitalization for heart failure as the primary end point was probably wise, but one wonders how many men died from CHF (without being hospitalized). Only 64 men (of whom only 11 who developed CHF) had left ventricular hypertrophy at baseline, so the statistical power for evaluating the relationship between ambulatory blood pressures and heart failure in men with left ventricular hypertrophy was very limited. Nonetheless, these data suggest that the nondipping blood pressure pattern is associated with future heart failure in older men.

**W. J. Elliott, MD, PhD**

*References*

1. Staessen JA, Thijs L, Fagard R, et al: Predicting cardiovascular risk using conventional vs. ambulatory blood pressure in older patients with systolic hypertension. *JAMA* 282:589-596, 1999.
2. Verdecchia P, Reboldi G, Porcellati C, et al: Risk of cardiovascular disease in relation to achieved office and ambulatory blood pressure control in treated hypertensive subjects. *J Am Coll Cardiol* 39:878-885, 2002.
3. Ohkubo T, Hozawa A, Yamaguchi J, et al: Prognostic significance of the nocturnal decline in blood pressure in individuals with and without high 24-h blood pressure: The Ohasama study. *J Hypertens* 20:2183-2189, 2002.

4. Clement DL, De Buyzere ML, De Bacquer DA, et al: Prognostic value of ambulatory blood-pressure recordings in patients with treated hypertension. *N Engl J Med* 348:2407-2415, 2003.
5. Björklund K, Lind L, Zethelius B, et al: Prognostic significance of 24-hour ambulatory blood pressure characteristics for cardiovascular morbidity in a population of elderly men. *J Hypertens* 22:1691-1697, 2004.
6. Lurbe E, Redon J, Kesani A, et al: Increase in nocturnal blood pressure and progression to microalbuminuria in type 1 diabetes. *N Engl J Med* 347:797-805, 2002.
7. Messerli FH: ALLHAT, or the soft science of the secondary end point. *Ann Intern Med* 139:777-780, 2003.
8. Hunt SA, Baker DW, Chin MH, et al: ACC/AHA guidelines for the evaluation and management of chronic heart failure in the adult: Executive summary. *Circulation* 104:2996-3007, 2001.

## Ambulatory Blood Pressure Monitoring and Risk of Cardiovascular Disease: A Population Based Study

Hansen TW, Jeppesen J, Rasmussen S, et al (Research Ctr for Prevention and Health, Copenhagen; Glostrup Univ Hosp, Copenhagen; Bispebjerg Univ Hosp, Copenhagen)
*Am J Hypertens* 19:243-250, 2006

1–23

*Background.*—Information on the relationship between ambulatory blood pressure (BP) and cardiovascular disease in the general population is sparse.

*Methods.*—Prospective study of a random sample of 1700 Danish men and women, aged 41 to 72 years, without major cardiovascular diseases. At baseline, ambulatory BP, office BP, and other risk factors were recorded. The end point was a combined end point consisting of cardiovascular mortality, ischemic heart disease, and stroke.

*Results.*—After a mean follow-up of 9.5 years, 156 end points were recorded. In multivariate models, the relative risk (95% confidence interval) associated with increments of 10/5 mmHg of systolic/diastolic ambulatory BP were 1.35 (1.21–1.50) and 1.27 (1.16–1.39). The corresponding figures for office BP were 1.18 (1.09–1.29) and 1.11 (1.03–1.19). Compared with normotension (office BP <140/90 mm Hg; daytime BP <135/85 mm Hg) the relative risks associated with isolated office hypertension (office BP ≥140/90 mm Hg; daytime BP <135/85 mm Hg), isolated ambulatory hypertension (office BP <140/90 mm Hg; daytime BP ≥135/85 mm Hg), and sustained hypertension (office BP ≥140/90 mm Hg; daytime BP ≥135/85 mm Hg) were 0.66 (0.30–1.44), 1.52 (0.91–2.54), and 2.10 (1.45–3.06), respectively. A blunted BP decrease at night was a risk factor ($P = .02$) in subjects with daytime ambulatory hypertension, but not in subjects with daytime ambulatory normotension ($P = .13$).

*Conclusions.*—Ambulatory BP provided prognostic information about cardiovascular disease better than office BP. Isolated office hypertension was not a risk factor and isolated ambulatory hypertension tended to be associated with increased risk. A blunted BP decrease at night was a risk factor in subjects with daytime ambulatory hypertension.

▶ In a previous publication using the same dataset, these authors showed that the results of ambulatory BP monitoring predicted both cardiovascular and all-cause mortality better than did traditional office BP readings.[1] Because cardiovascular morbid events had not been previously linked to ambulatory BP monitoring results, they examined their data using the combined cardiovascular end point of coronary heart disease, stroke, or cardiovascular death. In addition, these analyses examined the association of "isolated office hypertension" (often known as "white coat hypertension") and "dipping" versus "nondipping" diurnal patterns of BP in hypertensive people.

The major virtues of these analyses include the random sample of a population-based cohort, the relative completeness of end point data for both morbid and mortal events (which is much easier for researchers in Denmark than it is in the United States), and the straightforward and traditional methods of analyses of the end points. The limitations include the 32% of the original cohort that were excluded from these analyses (typically due to poor-quality ambulatory BP monitoring data), the fact that only 2 office readings were obtained at a single visit (rather than the more traditional 3 readings at 2 or more visits before hypertension is diagnosed), the known problem with reproducibility of "dipper versus nondipper status" from a single ambulatory BP monitoring session, and the lack of ethnic minorities in this Danish sample.

These data nonetheless extend previous studies showing a better correlation between ambulatory BP monitoring data and outcomes than with other methods of BP measurement,[2-5] and the findings that white-coat hypertension and nondipping hypertension have a better and worse prognosis, respectively, than the more common dipping hypertensive patient.[6,7] These data support the growing push outside the United States for at least 1 ambulatory BP monitoring session for every newly diagnosed hypertensive patient, which is thought to be too expensive for most traditional American health plans, outside the Department of Veterans Affairs Medical Centers and similar settings that have decades-long continuous enrollment of participants.

**W. J. Elliott, MD, PhD**

*References*

1. Hansen TW, Jeppesen J, Rasmussen S, et al: Ambulatory blood pressure and mortality: A population-based study. *Hypertension* 45:499-504, 2005.
2. Verdecchia P, Porcellati C, Schillaci G, et al: Ambulatory blood pressure: An independent predictor of prognosis in essential hypertension. *Hypertension* 24:793-801, 1994.
3. Staessen JA, Thijs L, Fagard R, et al: Predicting cardiovascular risk using conventional vs. ambulatory blood pressure in older patients with systolic hypertension. *JAMA* 282:589-596, 1999.
4. Clement DL, De Buyzere ML, De Bacquer DA, et al: Prognostic value of ambulatory blood-pressure recordings in patients with treated hypertension. *N Engl J Med* 348:2407-2415, 2003.

5. Dolan E, Stanton A, Thijs L, et al: Superiority of ambulatory over clinical blood pressure measurement in predicting mortality: The Dublin outcome study. *Hypertension* 46:156-161, 2005.

6. Verdecchia P, Reboldi GP, Angeli F, et al: Short- and long-term incidence of stroke in white-coat hypertension. *Hypertension* 45:203-208, 2005.

7. Ohkubo T, Kikuya M, Metoki H, et al: Prognosis of "masked" hypertension and "white-coat" hypertension detected by 24-h ambulatory blood pressure monitoring: A 10-year follow-up from the Ohasama study. *J Am Coll Cardiol* 46:508-515, 2005.

## Prognostic Significance for Stroke of a Morning Pressor Surge and a Nocturnal Blood Pressure Decline: The Ohasama Study

Metoki H, Ohkubo T, Kikuya M, et al (Tohoku Univ, Sendai, Japan; Ohasama Hosp, Iwate, Japan)
*Hypertension* 47:149-154, 2006                                     1–24

There is continuing controversy over whether the pattern of circadian blood pressure (BP) variation that includes a nocturnal decline in BP and a morning pressor surge has prognostic significance for stroke risk. In this study, we followed the incidence of stroke in 1430 subjects aged ≥40 years in Ohasama, Japan, for an average of 10.4 years. The association between stroke risk and the pattern of circadian BP variation was analyzed with a Cox proportional hazards model after adjustment for possible confounding factors. There was no significant association between total stroke risk and the nocturnal decline in BP (percentage decline from diurnal level) or between total stroke risk and the morning pressor surge. The cerebral infarction risk was significantly higher in subjects with a <10% nocturnal decline in BP as compared with subjects who had a ≥10% nocturnal decline in BP ($P=0.04$). The morning pressor surge was not associated with a risk of cerebral infarction. On the other hand, an increased risk of cerebral hemorrhage was observed in subjects with a large morning pressor surge (≥25 mm Hg; $P=0.04$). Intracerebral hemorrhage was also observed more frequently in extreme dippers (those with a ≥20% nocturnal decline in BP) than dippers (those with a 10% to 19% decline; $P=0.02$). A disturbed nocturnal decline in BP is associated with cerebral infarction, whereas a large morning pressor surge and a large nocturnal decline in BP, which are analogous to a large diurnal increase in BP, are both associated with cerebral hemorrhage.

▶ These data, drawn from a prospective, population-based epidemiological study, are reminiscent of but go beyond those obtained from a cohort of elderly Japanese patients with established cerebrovascular disease.[1] Both studies showed a significantly higher risk of subsequent stroke with altered patterns of nocturnal "dipping" of blood pressure. However, Kario et al[1] did not find a significant association between stroke and the early morning surge in blood pressure, but instead the increased risk was said to arise from "extreme dipping" or "reverse dipping" patterns. In some ways, these observations were confirmed in this dataset, but, in addition, the effects of the early morning surge in blood pressure were associated with an increased risk of hemorrhagic (but not ischemic) stroke. Studies done outside Japan had previously reported either an increase[2] or decrease[3] in the risk of cardiovascular events associated with the early morning surge in blood pressure.

One of the other reasons for the apparently persistent effects of ALLHAT on α-blocker prescribing, but not thiazide diuretic prescribing, was the recurring publication of several iterations of the data from the doxazosin arm of ALLHAT.[4,5] The initial publication was followed by at least 3 further studies providing validation and further analyses of the data, all of which reinforced the initial conclusion and received widespread media attention.[6-8] These results were never contradicted by any other clinical trial results. On the other hand, the final results of ALLHAT regarding the superiority of chlorthalidone (over both an ACE inhibitor and a calcium antagonist) were not corroborated by the 2 subsequent clinical trials of initial antihypertensive therapy, one of which alleged superiority of the ACE inhibitor over a different thiazide diuretic,[9] and the other of which was stopped early because of early mortality in the β-blocker (± thiazide diuretic) arm compared with the calcium antagonist (± ACE inhibitor) arm.[10]

It is difficult to argue with the authors that there are at least 4 reasons why thiazide diuretics are not prescribed as often as clinical trial evidence and guidelines would suggest: (1) Not all guidelines and not all studies support the universal recommendation to use a thiazide-type or thiazide-like diuretic as first-line therapy; (2) Some continue to be concerned about potential adverse metabolic effects of thiazides; (3) Other drugs are certainly effective in lowering blood pressure and may be suitable alternatives to thiazides in those in whom the latter are contraindicated or in whom the former have compelling indications; and (4) Other drug classes are more heavily marketed, advertised, distributed as free samples, and may be attractive to those who prefer "new" therapies. Which of these, if any, may account for the fact that the increase in prescribing of thiazides for hypertension that occurred immediately after the ALLHAT results, and was not sustained, is still uncertain.

**W. J. Elliott, MD, PhD**

*References*

1. Kario K, Pickering TG, Umeda Y, et al: Morning surge in blood pressure as a predictor of silent and clinical cerebrovascular disease in elderly hypertensives: A prospective study. *Circulation* 107:1401-1406, 2003.
2. Gosse P, Lasserre R, Minifié C, et al: Blood pressure surge on rising. *J Hypertens* 22:1113-1118, 2004.
3. Staessen JA, Thijs L, Fagard R, et al: Predicting cardiovascular risk using conventional vs. ambulatory blood pressure in older patients with systolic hypertension. *JAMA* 282:589-596, 1999.
4. Xie F, Pettiti DB, Chen W: Prescribing patterns for antihypertensive drugs after the Antihypertensive and Lipid-Lowering to prevent Heart Attack Trial: Report of experience in a health-maintenance organization. *Am J Hypertens* 18:464-469, 2005.
5. Austin P, Mamdani MM, Tu K, et al: Changes in prescribing patterns following publication of the ALLHAT trial [letter]. *JAMA* 291:45, 2004.
6. Validation of heart failure events in the Antihypertensive and Lipid-Lowering treatment to prevent Heart Attack Trial (ALLHAT) participants assigned to doxazosin and chlorthalidone. *Curr Cont Trials in Cardiovasc Med* 3:10, 2002.

7.  Davis BR, Cutler JA, Furberg CD, et al: Relationship of antihypertensive treatment regimens and change in blood pressure to risk for heart failure in hypertensive patients randomly assigned to doxazosin or chlorthalidone: Further analyses from the Antihypertensive and Lipid-Lowering Treatment to Prevent Heart Attack Trial. The ALLHAT Collaborative Research Group. *Ann Intern Med* 137:313-320, 2002.
8.  ALLHAT Officers and Coordinators for the ALLHAT Collaborative Research Group. Diuretic versus alpha-blocker as first-step antihypertensive therapy: Final results from the Antihypertensive and Lipid-Lowering Treatment to Prevent Heart Attack Trial (ALLHAT). *Hypertension* 42:239-246, 2003.
9.  Wing LMH, Reid CM, Ryan P, et al: A comparison of outcomes with angiotensin-converting-enzyme inhibitors and diuretics for hypertension in the elderly. Second Australian National Blood Pressure Study Group. *N Engl J Med* 348:583-592, 2003.
10. Dahlöf B, Sever PS, Poulter NR, et al: Prevention of cardiovascular events with an antihypertensive regimen of amlodipine adding perindopril as required versus atenolol adding bendroflumethiazide as required, in the Anglo-Scandinavian Cardiac Outcomes Trial-Blood Pressure Lowering Arm (ASCOT-BPLA): A multicentre randomised controlled trial. *Lancet* 366:895-906, 2005.

## Cardiovascular disease prevention with a multidrug regimen in the developing world: a cost-effectiveness analysis

Gaziano TA, Opie LH, Weinstein MC (Harvard Med School; Univ of Cape Town, South Africa; Harvard School of Public Health, Boston)
*Lancet* 368:679-686, 2006                                                 1–25

*Background.*—Cardiovascular disease is the leading cause of death, with 80% of cases occurring in developing countries. We therefore aimed to establish whether use of evidence-based multidrug regimens for patients at high risk for cardiovascular disease would be cost-effective in low-income and middle-income countries.

*Methods.*—We used a Markov model to do a cost-effectiveness analysis with two combination regimens. For primary prevention, we used aspirin, a calcium-channel blocker, an angiotensin-converting-enzyme inhibitor, and a statin, and assessed them in four groups with different thresholds of absolute risks for cardiovascular disease. For secondary prevention, we assessed the same combination of drugs in one group, but substituted a β blocker for the calcium-channel blocker. To compare strategies, we report incremental cost-effectiveness ratios (ICER), in US$ per quality-adjusted life-year (QALY).

*Findings.*—We recorded that preventive strategies could result in a 2-year gain in life expectancy. Across six developing World Bank regions, primary prevention yielded ICERs of US$746–890/QALY gained for patients with a 10-year absolute risk of cardiovascular disease greater than 25%, and $1039–1221/QALY gained for those with an absolute risk greater than 5%. ICERs for secondary prevention ranged from $306/QALY to $388/QALY gained.

*Interpretation.*—Regimens of aspirin, two blood-pressure drugs, and a statin could halve the risk of death from cardiovascular disease in high-risk patients. This approach is cost-effective according to WHO recommendations, and is robust across several estimates of drug efficacy and of treatment cost. Developing countries should encourage the use of these inexpensive drugs that are currently available for both primary and secondary prevention.

▶ These data put some economic teeth into the theoretical constructs and proposal of Wald and Law (patented by them as The Polypill in the United Kingdom) to make widespread use of a single pill containing 5 drugs: low-dose (75 mg) aspirin, half-usual doses of a diuretic, β-blocker, angiotensin converting-enzyme inhibitor, and an HMG-CoA reductase inhibitor, along with 400 µg of folic acid.[1] Many originally considered this to be only a facetious proposal without any direct experimental data to justify it.[2] Others claimed that aspirin insensitivity (thought to occur in up to 20% of the general population), the high prevalence of asthma (an absolute contraindication to a β-blocker) in some populations, and a small risk (0.7%) of potentially fatal angioedema[3] made the population-wide distribution of this pill a public health threat.

These authors have refined the concept of the "polypill" somewhat (perhaps in an attempt to avoid patent infringement?) and propose 2 such pills, one for primary prevention (with a calcium antagonist replacing the β-blocker) and the other for those with existing cardiovascular disease. Their calculations suggest that this population-wide preventive strategy may well be economically feasible, especially in countries with few economic resources. In wealthier countries, a "polymeal" strategy (combining the benefits of several health-promoting foodstuffs) has been advocated.[4]

The proof that this concept will actually prevent cardiovascular events is currently lacking, but a large multinational study (known best by its acronym, PILL: Program to Improve Life and Longevity) has been organized to test a similar single-pill strategy (to be manufactured by Reddy in India).[5,6] Unfortunately, the United States will not contribute study subjects, as the National Institute of Health has insufficient funds to support the many clinics that would carry out the international protocol.

This report may be of greatest interest to wealthy philanthropic organizations that proclaim an interest in inexpensive methods of improving the public health of developing countries. Perhaps even developed nations can be convinced to use such population-wide measures if the clinical trial has positive results.

**W. J. Elliott, MD, PhD**

*References*

1. Wald NJ, Law MR: A strategy to reduce cardiovascular disease by more than 80%. *BMJ* 326:1419-1425, 2003.
2. Rogers A: A cure for cardiovascular disease [editorial]? *BMJ* 326:1407-1408, 2003.
3. Kostis JB, Packer M, Black HR, et al: Omapatrilat and enalapril in patients with hypertension: The Omapatrilat Cardiovascular Treatment vs. Enalapril (OCTAVE) trial. *Am J Hypertens* 17:103-111, 2004.
4. Franco OH, Bonneaux L, de Laet C, et al: The Polymeal: A more natural, safer, and probably tastier (than the Polypill) strategy to reduce cardiovascular disease by more than 75%. *BMJ* 329:1147-1150, 2004.

5. Krishnan GS: Compound cure. *Businessworld*, www.drreddys.com/newsroom/pdf/bworld_03apr2006.pdf, accessed October 23, 2006.
6. *New projects of the Cardiovascular Research Division of the George Institute for International Health*, www.thegeorgeinstitute.org/research/cardiovascular/cardiovascular_home.cfm#New, accessed October 23, 2006.

# "Causes" of Hypertension

## Cushing's Syndrome

Newell-Price J, Bertagna X, Grossman AB, et al (Univ of Sheffield, England; Université Paris 5; Queen Mary School of Medicine and Dentistry, London)

*Lancet* 367:1605-1617, 2006                                                                            1–26

*Introduction.*—Cushing's syndrome results from lengthy and inappropriate exposure to excessive glucocorticoids. Untreated, it has significant morbidity and mortality. The syndrome remains a challenge to diagnose and manage.

*Methods.*—We searched MEDLINE from January 2000 to October 2005, using "Cushing's" or "Cushing's" and "Syndrome," and then selected publications, including older publications, review articles, and book chapters, to highlight recent developments and areas of controversy regarding the biology of Cushing's syndrome, its diagnosis, differential diagnosis, and management.

*Results.*—Traditionally, Cushing's syndrome has an incidence of about 0.7 to 2.4 per million population per year, but recent screening of obese patients with poorly controlled diabetes put it at 2% to 5% in this population. About 80% to 85% of cases are corticotropin dependent (formerly adrenocorticotrophic hormone), and about 80% of these are caused by the classic basophilic adenoma in the pituitary. About 60% of the corticotropin-independent cases are attributable to autonomously functioning adrenal adenomas. The recommended screening tests for Cushing's syndrome are 3 24-hour urinary collections for free cortisol, low-dose dexamethasone suppression test, and/or assessment of midnight plasma cortisol or late-night salivary cortisol levels. Recently, a serum corticotropin level has been recommended over the high-dose dexamethasone suppression test. Other diagnostic tests include the recombinant human (or the ovine sequence) corticotropin-releasing hormone stimulation test and computed axial tomographic scanning of the pituitary and adrenal glands. Between 60% and 80% of pituitary adenomas have an initial remission after surgery, but many different medical, surgical, and radiotherapy options are effective when an adenoma is not present or recurs.

*Conclusions.*—Diagnosis and management of Cushing's syndrome remain a considerable challenge, even in tertiary referral centers. The outcome of treatment for the most common cause of Cushing's syndrome, Cushing's disease, remains disappointing, and further developments are needed in this area.

▶ This report is the best current summary of recent developments in the presentation, diagnostic evaluation, and pitfalls associated with testing for Cushing's syndrome, first described by Harvey Williams Cushing in 1932.[1] Major recent developments in this area include the much higher prevalence in obese diabetics with persistent hyperglycemia,[2] the use of late-night salivary cortisol levels as a screening test (which appears to be much more popular in Britain than in the USA),[3] and the deemphasis of the high-dose dexamethasone suppression test as the classic confirmatory test for a basophilic adenoma.[4] The relatively widespread availability of serum corticotropin levels are said to be more helpful,[5] particularly since about 80% of patients with a pituitary adenoma who are given 8 × 2 mg of dexamethasone every 6 hours will suppress their postdose cortisol level to less than 50% of the basal level. Except when petrosal sinus sampling is too dangerous or unavailable, these authors no longer recommend the high-dose dexamethasone suppression test because its positive predictive value is about the same as the pretest probability of Cushing's disease in a person with hypercortisolemia.

The authors also review the short- and long-term outcomes in patients with various forms of Cushing's syndrome, which are somewhat less optimistic than in prior years. It is highly likely, however, that the literature contains many more reports of diagnostic and therapeutic failures than the more routine successes; the several large series from referral centers cited among the 199 references tend to bear this out. Since mortality rates are said to be about 8-fold higher in patients with Cushing's syndrome, and the recent relative epidemic in obese diabetics, physicians will likely be seeing more patients with this syndrome in the near future.

**W. J. Elliott, MD, PhD**

*References*

1. Cushing HW: The basophil adenomas of the pituitary body and their clinical manifestations (pituitary basophilism). *Bull Johns Hopkins Hosp* 50:137-195, 1932.
2. Catargi B, Rigalleau V, Poussin A, et al: Occult Cushing's syndrome in type-2 diabetes. *J Clin Endocrinol Metab* 88:5808-5813, 2003.
3. Viardot A, Huber P, Puder J, et al: Reproducibility of nighttime salivary cortisol and its use in the diagnosis of hypercortisolism as compared to urinary free cortisol and overnight dexamethasone suppression test. *J Clin Endocrinol Metab* 90:5730-5736, 2005.
4. Aron DC, Raff H, Findling JW: Effectiveness versus efficacy: The limited value in clinical practice of high dose dexamethasone suppression testing in the differential diagnosis of adrenocorticotropin-dependent Cushing's syndrome. *J Clin Endocrinol Metab* 82:1780-1785, 1997.
5. Reimondo G, Paccotti P, Minetto M, et al: The corticotrophin-releasing hormone test is the most reliable noninvasive method to differentiate pituitary from ectopic ACTH secretion in Cushing's syndrome. *Clin Endocrinol (Oxf)* 58:718-724, 2003.

### Hypertension, glomerular number, and birth weight in African Americans and white subjects in the southeastern United States

Hughson MD, Douglas-Denton R, Bertram JF, et al (Univ of Mississippi Med Ctr, Jackson; Monash Univ, Clayton, Victoria, Australia; Univ of Queensland, Brisbane, Australia)
*Kidney Int* 69:671-678, 2006                                              1–27

---

Low nephron number has been related to low birth weight and hypertension. In the southeastern United States, the estimated prevalence of chronic kidney disease due to hypertension is five times greater for African Americans than white subjects. This study investigates the relationships between total glomerular number ($N_{glom}$), blood pressure, and birth weight in southeastern African Americans and white subjects. Stereological estimates of $N_{glom}$ were obtained using the physical disector/fractionator technique on autopsy kidneys from 62 African American and 60 white subjects 30–65 years of age. By medical history and recorded blood pressures, 41 African Americans, and 24 white subjects were identified as hypertensive and 21 African Americans and 36 white subjects as normotensive. Mean arterial blood pressure (MAP) was obtained on 81 and birth weights on 63 subjects. For African Americans, relationships between MAP, $N_{glom}$, and birth weight were not significant. For white subjects, they were as follows: MAP and $N_{glom}$ ($r=-0.4551$, $P=0.0047$); $N_{glom}$ and birth weight ($r=0.5730$, $P=0.0022$); MAP and birth weight ($r=-0.4228$, $P=0.0377$). For African Americans, average $N_{glom}$ of 961 840±292 750 for normotensive and 867 358±341 958 for hypertensive patients were not significantly different ($P=0.285$). For white subjects, average $N_{glom}$ of 923 377±256 391 for normotensive and 754 319±329 506 for hypertensive patients were significantly different ($P=0.03$). The data indicate that low nephron number and possibly low birth weight may play a role in the development of hypertension in white subjects but not African Americans.

▶ These authors investigated 2 interesting hypotheses regarding the pathogenesis (and perhaps even embryogenesis) of hypertension. In 1988, Brenner et al postulated that a decreased glomerular filtration surface (typically quantitated thereafter as the number of nephrons) was associated with the risk of hypertension.[1] This hypothesis gathered support from a European autopsy study that found a significantly lower glomerular number ($N_{glom}$) and mean glomerular volume ($V_{glom}$) in hypertensive accident victims.[2] A more recent hypothesis linked low birth weight to subsequent hypertension and has also received some support.[3-5] These authors therefore extended their previous study of both of these factors in a series of autopsied adults from the Southeastern United States, where hypertension (and end-stage renal disease) is particularly common, especially among African Americans.[6]

Their first major conclusion was that low nephron number and low birth weight were significantly associated with hypertension in whites but not in African Americans. There are many challenges to interpreting their data, including the wide confidence intervals in $N_{glom}$ (due to the huge numbers of glomeruli in only 140 autopsied adults), the lack of blood pressure (51 subjects) or birth weight data (63 subjects), and African American and white women with hypertension (18 or 11, respectively).

The second somewhat surprising finding was that the hypertensive African Americans didn't have a lower number of nephrons or birth weight than the whites. Because birth weight has been previously associated with both higher blood pressures and an increased risk of end-stage renal disease in both African Americans and Australian aborigines, it was thought likely that the relationship would be stronger in the 62 African Americans studied in this report. The fact that 41 were hypertensive (leaving only 21 with normal blood pressures) and only 37 had birth weights may have limited their statistical power to see the expected relationship.

In sum, these data support the relationship of low birth weight and low nephron number with hypertension in whites from the Southeastern United States ("the Stroke Belt"), where hypertension and end-stage renal disease are very prevalent. But whether these relationships are really not present, or just unable to be teased out from the available autopsy specimens in African Americans, is as yet unclear.

**W. J. Elliott, MD, PhD**

*References*

1. Brenner BM, Garcia DL, Anderson S: Glomeruli and blood pressure: Less of one, more of the other? *Am J Hypertens* 1:335-347, 1988.
2. Keller G, Zimmer G, Mall G, et al: Nephron number in patients with primary hypertension. *N Engl J Med* 348:101-108, 2003.
3. Law CM, Shiell AW: Is blood pressure inversely related to birth weight? The strength of evidence from a systematic review of the literature. *J Hypertens* 14:935-941, 1996.
4. Huxley RR, Shiell AW, Law CM: The role of size at birth and postnatal catch-up growth in determining systolic blood pressure: A systematic review of the literature. *J Hypertens* 18:815-831, 2000.
5. Huxley R, Neil A, Collins R: Unraveling the fetal origins hypothesis: Is there really an inverse association between birthweight and subsequent blood pressure? *Lancet* 31:659-665, 2002.
6. Hoy WE, Douglas-Denton RN, Hughson MD, et al: A stereological study of glomerular number and volume: Preliminary findings in a multiracial study of kidneys at autopsy. *Kidney Int* 63(suppl):S31-S37, 2003.

---

**Diabetes Mellitus and Hypertension Associated With Shock Wave Lithotripsy of Renal and Proximal Ureteral Stones at 19 Years of Followup**

Krambeck AE, Gettman MT, Rohlinger AL, et al (Mayo Clinic College of Medicine, Rochester, Minn)
*J Urol* 175:1742-1747, 2006 1–28

---

*Purpose.*—SWL has revolutionized the management of nephrolithiasis and it is a preferred treatment for uncomplicated renal and proximal ureteral calculi. Since its introduction in 1982, conflicting reports of early adverse effects have been published. However, to our knowledge the long-term medical effects associated with SWL are unknown. We evaluated these adverse medical effects associated with SWL for renal and proximal ureteral stones.

*Materials and Methods.*—Chart review identified 630 patients treated with SWL at our institution in 1985. Questionnaires were sent to 578 patients who were alive in 2004. The response rate was 58.9%. Respondents were matched by age, sex and year of presentation to a cohort of patients with nephrolithiasis who were treated nonsurgically.

*Results.*—At 19 years of followup hypertension was more prevalent in the SWL group (OR 1.47, 95% CI 1.03, 2.10, p = 0.034). The development of hypertension was related to bilateral treatment (p = 0.033). In the SWL group diabetes mellitus developed in 16.8% of patients. Patients treated with SWL were more likely to have diabetes mellitus than controls (OR 3.23, 95% CI 1.73 to 6.02, p <0.001). Multivariate analysis controlling for change in body mass index showed a persistent risk of diabetes mellitus in the SWL group (OR 3.75, 95% CI 1.56 to 9.02, p = 0.003). Diabetes mellitus was related to the number of administered shocks and treatment intensity (p = 0.005 and 0.007).

*Conclusions.*—At 19 years of followup SWL for renal and proximal ureteral stones was associated with the development of hypertension and diabetes mellitus. The incidence of these conditions was significantly higher than in a cohort of conservatively treated patients with nephrolithiasis.

▶ This single-center experience with SWL followed patients seen in 1985, the first year such therapy was available in the United States, and concluded that, after 19 years, those who had SWL had a significantly higher rate of developing both diabetes and hypertension. Earlier reports had shown higher risk of both hypertension and diabetes acutely after SWL,[1,2] but the literature about medium-term risk has been less worrisome.[3,4]

The authors acknowledge several major weaknesses with their study. They obtained follow-up information from those who received SWL by mailed questionnaire (that had only a 49.8% response rate, with another 15% who were deceased at the time of attempted follow-up and were not included in the results); about 82% of those who responded never returned for follow-up. Data about the control subjects were obtained from medical chart reviews (rather than by questionnaire) of individuals who continued follow-up at The Mayo Clinic. Ascertainment bias may therefore be responsible for some of their findings. The authors apparently did not perform time-to-event analyses of their data', perhaps because they did not ascertain when the new diagnoses of hypertension or diabetes were made. The authors did not mention the significant difference in hypertension prevalence in 1985 between the SWL group and the control group (28 of 288 vs 48 of 288, $P < 0.014$ by $\chi^2$); the finding of a higher incidence of hypertension in the former group may therefore be a regression to the mean. A further confounder for both incident hypertension and diabetes (which was not evaluated in this study) might have been the use of thiazide-type diuretics, which would be expected to be common in both groups to prevent hypercalciuria and subsequent stone formation since 78% of those who received SWL had calcium-containing stones. Those who used thiazide diuretics for this indication could have been perceived as hypertensive (as they were treated with a drug commonly used to lower blood pressure) and would have been more likely to develop diabetes in the long term.[5-7]

The authors' view (supported by prior work[4,8]) is that the shock waves used in lithotripsy can damage both the kidneys and the pancreas, which is consistent with a higher risk of hypertension in those who underwent bilateral SWL, and by a graded relationship between the intensity of SWL and the risk of future diabetes. Thus, it appears that SWL deserves a place among the potential causes of hypertension, although it is unlikely that any specific therapy (beyond the usual low-dose thiazide diuretic) would be useful for it.

**W. J. Elliott, MD, PhD**

*References*

1. Montgomery BS, Cole RS, Palfrey EL, et al: Does extracorporeal shock wave lithotripsy cause hypertension? *Br J Urol* 64:567-571, 1989.
2. Smith LW, Drach G, Hall P, et al: National High Blood Pressure Education Program (NHBPEP) review paper on complications of shock wave lithotripsy for urinary calculi. *Am J Med* 91:635-641, 1991.
3. Jewett MAS, Bombardier C, Logan AG, et al: A randomized controlled trial to assess the incidence of new onset hypertension in patients after shock wave lithotripsy for asymptomatic urinary calculi. *J Urol* 160:1241-1243, 1998.
4. Lingeman JE, Woods JR, Toth PD: Blood pressure changes following extracorporeal shock wave lithotripsy and other forms of treatment for nephrolithiasis. *JAMA* 263:1789-1794, 1990.
5. Opie LH, Schall R: Old antihypertensives and new diabetes. *J Hypertension* 22:1453-1458, 2004.
6. Padwal R, Laupacis A: Antihypertensive therapy and incidence of type 2 diabetes. *Diabetes Care* 27:247-255, 2004.
7. Elliott WJ: Differential effects of antihypertensive drugs on new-onset diabetes? *Curr Hypertens Rep* 7:249-256, 2005.
8. Hassan I, Zietlow SP: Acute pancreatitis after extracorporeal shock wave lithotripsy for a renal calculus. *Urology* 60:1111, 2002.

## Adverse Effects of Cyclooxygenase 2 Inhibitors on Renal and Arrhythmia Events: Meta-analysis of Randomized Trials

Zhang J, Ding EL, Song Y (Harvard Med School; Harvard School of Public Health, Boston)

*JAMA* 296:1619-1632, 2006                                        1–29

*Context.*—Adverse effects of selective cyclooxygenase 2 (COX-2) inhibitors on renal events and arrhythmia have been controversial, with suggestions of a class effect.

*Objective.*—To quantitatively evaluate adverse risks of renal events (renal dysfunction, hypertension, and peripheral edema) and arrhythmia events and to explore drug class effects and temporal trends of apparent effects of the COX-2 inhibitors: rofecoxib, celecoxib, valdecoxib, parecoxib, etoricoxib, and lumiracoxib.

*Data Sources.*—A systematic search of EMBASE and MEDLINE (through June 2006), bibliographies, US Food and Drug Administration reports, and pharmaceutical industry clinical trial databases.

*Study Selection.*—From relevant reports, 114 randomized double-blind clinical trials were included.

*Data Extraction.*—Information on publication year, participant characteristics, trial duration, drug, control, dose, and events were extracted using a standardized protocol.

*Data Synthesis.*—Results were pooled via random-effects models and meta-regressions. Of 116 094 participants from 114 trial reports including 127 trial populations (40 rofecoxib, 37 celecoxib, 29 valdecoxib + parecoxib, 15 etoricoxib, and 6 lumiracoxib), there were a total of 6394 composite renal events (2670 peripheral edema, 3489 hypertension, 235 renal dysfunction) and 286 arrhythmia events. Results indicated significant heterogeneity of renal effects across agents (*P* for interaction = .02), indicating no class effect. Compared with controls, rofecoxib was associated with increased risk of arrhythmia (relative risk [RR], 2.90; 95% confidence interval [CI], 1.07-7.88) and composite renal events (RR, 1.53; 95% CI, 1.33-1.76); adverse renal effects increased with greater dose and duration (both *P*≤.05). For all individual renal end points, rofecoxib was associated with increased risk of peripheral edema (RR, 1.43; 95% CI, 1.23-1.66), hypertension (RR, 1.55; 95% CI, 1.29-1.85), and renal dysfunction (RR, 2.31; 95% CI, 1.05-5.07). In contrast, celecoxib was associated with lower risk of both renal dysfunction (RR, 0.61; 95% CI, 0.40-0.94) and hypertension (RR, 0.83; 95% CI, 0.71-0.97) compared with controls. Other agents were not significantly associated with risk. Time-cumulative analyses indicated that for rofecoxib the adverse risks for peripheral edema and hypertension were evident by the end of year 2000 and for risk of arrhythmia by 2004.

*Conclusions.*—In this comprehensive analysis of 114 randomized trials with 116,094 participants, rofecoxib was associated with increased renal and arrhythmia risks. A COX-2 inhibitor class effect was not evident. Future safety monitoring is warranted and may benefit from an active and continuous cumulative surveillance system.

▶ This report summarizes the world's literature about selective COX-2 inhibitors and hypertension, edema, renal dysfunction, and cardiac arrhythmias and concludes that rofecoxib has a significantly higher risk than other agents of this type. These conclusions validate those of a previous meta-analysis[1] and are consistent with the idea that blood pressure elevation may have played a role in the increased cardiovascular risk seen in long-term randomized controlled trials of rofecoxib.[2,3] Two previous meta-analyses of celecoxib trials suggested that there was not a significantly increased risk of cardiovascular events (compared with traditional, nonselective, nonsteroidal anti-inflammatory drugs [NSAIDs]),[4,5] except possibly for the very highest doses (800 mg/d).[6,7] Two earlier identically designed, but independently executed, head-to-head studies of rofecoxib versus celecoxib had shown a significantly higher risk of development of both edema and "clinically important hypertension" (defined for these studies as blood pressure of 140/90 mm Hg or greater and an increase in systolic blood pressure by 20 mm Hg compared with baseline) with rofecoxib.[8,9]

These data indicate that rofecoxib had a higher risk of hypertension than other COX-2 selective agents, but the US Food and Drug Administration and those who market these drugs insist that "Any NSAID can lead to the onset of new hypertension or worsening of preexisting hypertension, either of which may contribute to the increased incidence of cardiovascular events. Fluid retention and edema have been observed in some patients taking NSAIDs, so NSAIDs should be used in caution in patients with fluid retention or heart failure." These seem to be appropriate caveats to the use of these once very popular drugs.

**W. J. Elliott, MD, PhD**

*References*

1. Aw T-J, Haas SJ, Liew D, et al: Meta-analysis of cyclooxygenase-2 inhibitors and their effects on blood pressure. *Arch Intern Med* 165:490-496, 2005.
2. Bombardier C, Laine L, Reicin A, et al: VIGOR Study Group. Comparison of upper gastrointestinal toxicity of rofecoxib and naproxen in patients with rheumatoid arthritis. *N Engl J Med* 343:1520-1528, 2000.
3. Bresalier RS, Sandler RS, Quan H, et al: Cardiovascular events associated with rofecoxib in a colorectal adenoma chemoprevention trial. *N Engl J Med* 352:1092-1102, 2005.
4. White WB, Faich G, Borer JS, et al: Cardiovascular thrombotic events in arthritis trials of the cyclooxygenase-2 inhibitor, celecoxib. *Am J Cardiol* 92:411-418, 2003.
5. Caldwell B, Aldington S, Weatherall M, et al: Risk of cardiovascular events and celecoxib: A systematic review and meta-analysis. *J Royal Soc Med* 99:132-140, 2006.
6. Solomon SD, McMurray JJV, Pfeffer MA, et al: Cardiovascular risk associated with celecoxib in a clinical trial for colorectal adenoma prevention. *N Engl J Med* 352:1071-1080, 2005.
7. Arber N, Eagle CJ, Spicak J, et al: Celecoxib for the prevention of colorectal adenomatous polyps. PreSAP Trial Investigators. *N Engl J Med* 355:885-895, 2006.
8. Whelton A, Fort JG, Puma JA, et al: SUCCESS VI Study Group. Cyclooxygenase-2-specific inhibitors and cardiorenal function: a randomized controlled trial of celecoxib and rofecoxib in older hypertensive osteoarthritis patients. *Am J Ther* 8:85-95, 2001.
9. Whelton A, White WB, Bello AE, et al: SUCCESS-VII Investigators. Effects of celecoxib and rofecoxib on blood pressure and edema in patients greater than or equal to 65 years of age with systemic hypertension and osteoarthritis. *Am J Cardiol* 90:959-963, 2002.

---

**Short Sleep Duration as a Risk Factor for Hypertension: Analyses of the First National Health and Nutrition Examination Survey**
Gangwisch JE, Heymsfield SB, Boden-Albala B, et al (Columbia Univ, New York; Merck Research Labs, Rahway, NJ; Netherlands Inst for Brain Research, Amsterdam; et al)
*Hypertension* 47:1-7, 2006                                                        1–30

---

*Introduction.*—Depriving healthy subjects of sleep has been shown to acutely increase blood pressure and sympathetic nervous system activity. Prolonged short sleep durations could lead to hypertension through extended exposure to raised 24-hour blood pressure and heart rate, elevated sympathetic nervous system activity, and increased salt retention. Such forces could lead to structural adaptations and the entrainment of the cardiovascular system to operate at an elevated pressure equilibrium. Sleep disorders are associated with cardiovascular disease, but we are not aware of any published prospective population studies that have shown a link between short sleep duration and the incidence of hypertension in subjects without apparent sleep disorders.

*Methods.*—We assessed whether short sleep duration would increase the risk for hypertension incidence by conducting longitudinal analyses of the first National Health and Nutrition Examination Survey (n = 4810) using Cox proportional hazards models and controlling for covariates. Hypertension incidence (n = 647) was determined by physician diagnosis, hospital record, or cause of death over the 8- to 10-year follow-up period between 1982 and 1992.

*Results.*—Sleep durations of ≤5 hours per night were associated with a significantly increased risk of hypertension (hazard ratio, 2.10; 95% CI, 1.58 to 2.79) in subjects between the ages of 32 and 59 years, and controlling for the potential confounding variables only partially attenuated this relationship. The increased risk continued to be significant after controlling for obesity and diabetes, which was consistent with the hypothesis that these variables would act as partial mediators.

*Conclusion.*—Short sleep duration could, therefore, be a significant risk factor for hypertension.

▶ Epidemiological information from representative samples of the American population has shown an increase in the prevalence of hypertension and, concomitantly, a decrease in the average sleep duration in adults.[1,2] Sleep deprivation studies in both normotensive and hypertensive subjects (including house physicians after a night on call) have demonstrated an acute rise in blood pressure after as little as 1 night with little sleep.[3,4] The pathophysiology of, and attendant cardiovascular risk associated with, sleep apnea and sleep-disordered breathing also suggest that shortened sleep duration should, and perhaps may well, increase the risk of developing hypertension and its cardiovascular sequelae.[5,6] These authors therefore interrogated a publicly available database that originally contained records from 14,407 subjects, but only 4810 were used in this analysis because of missing data and other problems. Compared with those who reported a "normal" 7 to 8 hours of sleep (on average), individuals who reported sleeping only 5 or fewer hours per night had the highest risk of incident hypertension, which was most marked in those between 32 and 59 years of age. Older individuals did not show this pattern, and the effect diminished as more covariates were added to the regression model.

Only 647 cases of incident hypertension (or 13% of the cohort) were identified by the authors during a mean follow-up of about 9 years. This number is lower than most estimates in previous work and could be confounded by the fact that about a third of hypertensive Americans were unaware of their hypertension in the period of 1982 to 1992 because blood pressure was not as commonly measured as it is today. The small number of incident cases also limits the statistical power of the study to link short sleep durations with cardiovascular events and sequelae of hypertension, which is the focus of ongoing research. Other limitations of the authors' data include the use of reported average sleep duration (rather than an objective measure), variability in sleep duration over a decade of follow-up, the possible influence of insomnia, and known difficulties with overlap between insomnia and other psychosocial stressors that increase cardiovascular risk.[7] The authors do not discuss older information that links mortality to shorter (and longer) durations of sleep.[8,9]

Nonetheless, these data are consistent with a growing body of work suggesting that a good night's sleep is important for health and now includes high blood pressure as one of the consequences for those individuals who do not follow their mother's advice on this topic.

**W. J. Elliott, MD, PhD**

*References*

1. Cheung BMY, Ong KL, Man YB, et al: Prevalence, awareness, treatment and control of hypertension: United States National Health and Nutrition Examination Survey, 2001-2002. *J Clin Hypertens (Greenwich)* 8:93-98, 2006.
2. National Sleep Foundation: *"2002 Sleep in America" poll,* Washington, DC, 2002, National Sleep Foundation.
3. Lusardi P, Mugelini A, Preti P, et al: Effects of a restricted sleep regimen on ambulatory blood pressure monitoring in normotensive subjects. *Am J Hypertens* 9:503-505, 1996.
4. Lusardi P, Zoppi A, Preti P, et al: Effects of insufficient sleep on blood monitoring in hypertensive patients: A 24-hour study. *Am J Hypertens* 12:63-68, 1999.
5. Wolk R, Shamsuzzaman ASM, Somers VK: Obesity, sleep apnea and hypertension. *Hypertension* 42:1067-1074, 2003.
6. Marin JM, Carrizo SJ, Vicente E, et al: Long-term cardiovascular outcomes in men with obstructive sleep apnea-hypopnea with or without treatment with continuous positive airway pressure: An observational study. *Lancet* 365:1046-1053, 2005.
7. Appels A, Schouten E: Waking up exhausted as risk indicator of myocardial infarction. *Am J Cardiol* 68:395-398, 1991.
8. Wingard DL, Berkman LF: Mortality risk associated with sleeping patterns among adults. *Sleep* 6:102-107, 1983.
9. Kojima M, Wakai K, Kawamura T, et al: Sleep patterns and total mortality: A 12-year follow-up study in Japan. *J Epidemiol* 10:87-93, 2000.

---

**Risk Factors for Arterial Hypertension in Adults With Initial Optimal Blood Pressure: The Strong Heart Study**
de Simone G, for the Strong Heart Study Investigators (Cornell Univ, New York; et al)
*Hypertension* 47:162-167, 2006                                           1–31

---

Whether metabolic factors and their change over time influence development of arterial hypertension in adults with initially optimal blood pressure (BP) is unknown. We analyzed associations of BP in the optimal range (<120/80 mm Hg), metabolic risk factors, and their changes over 4-year follow-up, with 8-year incident hypertension, in a cohort of American Indians with a high prevalence of obesity. At baseline, 967 participants with optimal BP and no prevalent cardiovascular disease (69.5% women; mean age, 54±7 years) were evaluated and reexamined after 4 (second examination) and 8 years to evaluate predictors of 8-year incident arterial hypertension. In participants with normal glucose tolerance, baseline BP and decrease in high-density lipoprotein cholesterol from baseline to the second examination were the most potent predictors of 8-year arterial hypertension (both $P<0.0001$), with additional effects of baseline waist circumference and its increase, increase in BP, and presence of diabetes at the second examination (all $P<0.04$). In participants with impaired glucose tolerance or diabetes, the most potent predictor of 8-year incident hypertension was diabetes at the second examination ($P<0.0001$) followed by a increase in BP and LDL cholesterol over the first 4 years (both $P<0.001$). Thus, incident arterial hypertension can be predicted by initial metabolic profile and unfavorable metabolic variations over time, in addition to initial BP. At optimal levels of initial BP, increasing abdominal obesity, and abnormal lipid profile are major predictors of development of arterial hypertension. Possible implications of these findings for primary cardiovascular prevention should be tested in prospective studies.

▶ These data predict an increase in the prevalence of not only hypertension, but also cardiovascular disease events over the coming decades in the United States.[1,2] Although these data were garnered from the largest study ever of Native Americans regarding their risk factors for cardiovascular disease, emerging data suggest that those descended from immigrant American populations (eg, those unrelated to Native Americans, or as they are currently named in Canada, First Nation Peoples) are beginning to emulate those who initially inhabited this geographical area. Americans are gradually becoming more overweight/obese and are more likely to have the metabolic syndrome, over the last few decades.[1,2]

In the nondiabetic Native Americans in this study, the most important predictors of hypertension were waist circumference, systolic blood pressure, the presence of either hypertension or diabetes after the first examination, and the change in systolic blood pressure, HDL cholesterol, and waist circumference after the interim examination (at 4 years). In those who were either frankly diabetic or who had impaired fasting glucose at baseline, the most important predictors of hypertension were not much different: male gender, initial systolic blood pressure, the presence of either hypertension or diabetes at baseline, or the change in either systolic blood pressure or LDL cholesterol from baseline.

The incontrovertible message from this and other studies on this important topic is that efforts (especially those involving lifestyle modifications[3-5]) to mitigate and prevent[3,5] the inexorable effects of the metabolic syndrome should be undertaken not only by Native Americans, but also by all Americans.

**W. J. Elliott, MD, PhD**

*References*

1. Hedley AA, Ogden CL, Johnson CL, et al: Prevalence of overweight and obesity among U.S. children, adolescents, and adults, 1999-2002. *JAMA* 291:2847-2850, 2004.
2. Flegal KM, Graubard BI, Williamson DF, et al: Excess deaths associated with underweight, overweight, and obesity. *JAMA* 293:1861-1867, 2005.
3. Appel LJ, Brands MW, Daniels SR, et al: Dietary approaches to prevent and treat hypertension: A Scientific Statement from the American Heart Association. *Hypertension* 47:296-308, 2006.
4. Chobanian AV, Bakris GL, Black HR, et al: Seventh Report of the Joint National Committee on Prevention, Detection, Evaluation and Treatment of High Blood Pressure. National High Blood Pressure Education Program Coordinating Committee. *Hypertension* 42:1206-1252, 2003.
5. Whelton PK, He J, Appel LJ, et al: Primary prevention of hypertension: Clinical and public health advisory from the National High Blood Pressure Education Program. *JAMA* 288:1882-1888, 2002.

## Long-term Changes in Blood Pressure in Extremely Obese Patients Who Have Undergone Bariatric Surgery

Fernstrom JD, Courcoulas AP, Houck PR, et al (Univ of Pittsburgh School of Medicine, Pa)
*Arch Surg* 141:276-283, 2006                                    1–32

*Hypothesis.*—Systolic and diastolic pressure and the incidence of hypertension in very obese patients decline after bariatric surgery and do not rebound.

*Design.*—Chart review.

*Setting.*—Surgical practice in a university medical center.

*Patients.*—Women and men, 18 years or older, with a body mass index (BMI) (calculated as weight in kilograms divided by the square of height in meters) of 40 or greater, having no previous surgical intervention for extreme obesity.

*Intervention.*—Vertical-banded gastroplasty or Roux-en-Y gastric bypass.

*Main Outcome Measures.*—Systolic and diastolic blood pressure, BMI, and antihypertensive medications.

*Results.*—Patients underwent Roux-en-Y gastric bypass (n = 285; mean initial BMI, 55.7) or vertical banded gastroplasty (n = 62; mean initial BMI, 48.5); half of each group was hypertensive at evaluation. The BMI dropped in both groups after surgery and stabilized at about 35 within 18 months. Systolic pressure changes were generally modest, although diastolic pressure declined significantly after surgery. In patients with untreated stage 1 hypertension, marked reductions in systolic and diastolic pressures occurred after surgery. Many patients taking antihypertensive medications before surgery discontinued them after surgery and remained normotensive.

*Conclusions.*—Blood pressure reductions that occur after bariatric surgery and substantial weight loss depend on the blood pressure status of patients before surgery: normotensive patients and hypertensive patients taking antihypertensive medications show small postsurgical pressure reductions, while patients with elevated blood pressure before surgery show notable postsurgical pressure drops. The overall incidence of hypertension after bariatric surgery declines substantially and remains low.

▶ This single-center, unblinded, uncontrolled retrospective review of medical records from a cohort of individuals who successfully underwent 1 (and only 1) surgical procedure for obesity observed a major average reduction in BMI (about 10 to 15 kg/m² or about 30 to 50 kg overall over 18 months of follow-up) and an apparently significant drop only in diastolic blood pressure (BP). For unclear reasons, the authors' analyses compared outcomes across the 2 surgical procedures and included both duration of time after the procedure and a procedure × time interaction term. The exact overall BP changes are not given in the report but were noted to be only about 5 to 6 mm Hg, on average. After the procedure, 35 (34%) of 103 patients who were initially taking antihypertensive medications stopped doing so (and did not resume them). Those who were initially hypertensive (89 of 244 patients) but who were not taking antihypertensive medications had a larger drop in BP after the procedure (∼16/9 mm Hg, from a baseline of about 145/87 mm Hg) compared with those without hypertension before the operation (drop of ∼0/2 mm Hg from a baseline of 125/79 mm Hg). A further analysis of those who were hypertensive but unmedicated before the operation indicated that 65 of 89 individuals had BPs below 140/90 mm Hg at 2 of 3 of the last clinic visits. In this series, 192 of 347 patients were hypertensive before the procedure (including 103 who were treated with antihypertensive medications) compared with only 92 of 347 who remained hypertensive afterwards (including 68 taking at least 1 antihypertensive medication). No information is given about individuals who may have had a reduction in the number of antihypertensive prescriptions after the procedure.

Other limitations of the authors' conclusions include a high degree of attrition during follow-up (only 124 of the original cohort of 347, or 36%, had BPs measured 18 months after surgery) and a single measurement of BP at each follow-up visit.

This report differs from a prior series that suggested that the decline in BP after bariatric surgery reverses after about 1 or 2 years of follow-up.[1] Another controlled series of 73 obese patients who underwent laparoscopic gastric banding noted a significant drop in the numbers of patients developing either hypertension or diabetes at 4 years, compared with 49 who refused surgery.[2] The authors call for a prospective, randomized, controlled trial to monitor the changes in BP after bariatric surgery, which seems to be wise before advocating surgery to improve BP in obese individuals.

**W. J. Elliott, MD, PhD**

*References*

1. Sjöström CD, Peltonen M, Wedel H, et al: Differentiated long-term effects of intentional weight loss on diabetes and hypertension. *Hypertension* 36:20-25, 2000.

2. Pontiroli AE, Folli F, Paganelli M, et al: Laparoscopic gastric banding prevents type 2 diabetes and arterial hypertension and induces their remission in morbid obesity. *Diabetes Care* 28:270-279, 2005.

## Clinical Trials

### Feasibility of Treating Prehypertension with an Angiotensin-Receptor Blocker

Julius S, for the Trial of Preventing Hypertension (TROPHY) Study Investigators (Univ of Michigan, Ann Arbor; et al)
*N Engl J Med* 354:1685-1697, 2006                               1–33

*Background.*—Prehypertension is considered a precursor of stage 1 hypertension and a predictor of excessive cardiovascular risk. We investigated whether pharmacologic treatment of prehypertension prevents or postpones stage 1 hypertension.

*Methods.*—Participants with repeated measurements of systolic pressure of 130 to 139 mm Hg and diastolic pressure of 89 mm Hg or lower, or systolic pressure of 139 mm Hg or lower and diastolic pressure of 85 to 89 mm Hg, were randomly assigned to receive two years of candesartan (Atacand, AstraZeneca) or placebo, followed by two years of placebo for all. When a participant reached the study end point of stage 1 hypertension, treatment with antihypertensive agents was initiated. Both the candesartan group and the placebo group were instructed to make changes in lifestyle to reduce blood pressure throughout the trial.

*Results.*—A total of 409 participants were randomly assigned to candesartan, and 400 to placebo. Data on 772 participants (391 in the candesartan group and 381 in the placebo group; mean age, 48.5 years; 59.6 percent men) were available for analysis. During the first two years, hypertension developed in 154 participants in the placebo group and 53 of those in the candesartan group (relative risk reduction, 66.3 percent; P<0.001). After four years, hypertension had developed in 240 participants in the placebo group and 208 of those in the candesartan group (relative risk reduction, 15.6 percent; P<0.007). Serious adverse events occurred in 3.5 percent of the participants assigned to candesartan and 5.9 percent of those receiving placebo.

*Conclusions.*—Over a period of four years, stage 1 hypertension developed in nearly two thirds of patients with untreated prehypertension (the placebo group). Treatment of prehypertension with candesartan appeared to be well tolerated and reduced the risk of incident hypertension during the study period. Thus, treatment of prehypertension appears to be feasible.

▶ This landmark clinical trial has several important implications. The most obvious is that it showed that prehypertension can be treated with well-tolerated antihypertensive agents and that doing so delays the onset of hypertension. It therefore opens the door for potential drug treatment of an estimated 25 million Americans who have blood pressures in the 130 to 139 mm Hg diastolic and 85 to 89 mm Hg systolic range (formerly called high-normal blood pressure, but now the top half of what is called prehypertension).[1,2] Because Americans are getting both older and more obese,[3,4] despite strong public health messages extolling the virtues of "lifestyle modifications" to prevent or treat hypertension,[5,6] physicians may now have another modality in the struggle to prevent hypertension that is probably simpler, more convenient, and perhaps even less costly than major modifications of diet or daily exercise. Most impressive, perhaps, is the fact that only 3.7 subjects in TROPHY had to be treated for 2 years to prevent 1 from developing hypertension. Similarly, only 76 subjects needed to be treated for 4 years to prevent 1 cardiovascular hospitalization. The major concern is that there was a much higher than expected transition from prehypertension to hypertension in the placebo-treated group, suggesting that the lifestyle modification advice received by all subjects was suboptimal.

The somewhat unusual study design of TROPHY was chosen to parallel experiments that showed long-term prevention of hypertension in rats that were treated with an angiotensin-converting enzyme inhibitor for a 6-week period during weeks 6 to 12 of life.[7] No such effect was seen when the rats were treated later in life.[8] One possible interpretation of the rather parallel incidence rates for the primary end point among those randomized to placebo for the first 2 years of TROPHY and the subjects given 2 years of placebo after 2 years of candesartan is that the subjects were too mature and their blood pressure too far advanced to see an effect similar to that observed in very young rats.

Another important observation of the TROPHY study is that adverse effects (both hospitalizations and side effects) were more common among those treated with placebo rather than with candesartan. Whether the economic cost of giving drug treatment to many people with prehypertension can be offset by an improvement in their well-being and the observed reduction in hospitalizations is not yet clear. However, if one uses the 2006 retail cost of candesartan, the cost of preventing 1 person from developing hypertension in 2 years was about $4900. The cost of preventing 1 cardiovascular hospitalization over 4 years was a little less than $100,000; the cost of preventing 1 hospitalization was about $54,000 during 4 years. These last 2 amounts are not much different than those pertaining to treatment of hypertension with the same type of drug.

**W. J. Elliott, MD, PhD**

Editor's Note: Dr Elliott was a TROPHY Study investigator and made the first public commentary about the study at the American College of Cardiology Meeting in Atlanta on March 14, 2006, when the data were first presented.

*References*

1. Wang Y, Wang QJ: The prevalence of prehypertension and hypertension among US adults according to the new Joint National Committee guidelines. *Arch Intern Med* 164:2126-2134, 2004.
2. Greenlund KJ, Croft JB, Mensah GA: Prevalence of heart disease and stroke risk factors in persons with prehypertension in the United States, 1999-2000. *Arch Intern Med* 164:2113-2118, 2004.

3. Cheung BMY, Ong KL, Man YB, et al: Prevalence, awareness, treatment and control of hypertension: United States National Health and Nutrition Examination Survey, 2001-2002. *J Clin Hypertens (Greenwich)* 8:93-98, 2006.
4. Hedley AA, Ogden CL, Johnson CL, et al: Prevalence of overweight and obesity among U.S. children, adolescents, and adults, 1999-2002. *JAMA* 291:2847-2850, 2004.
5. Chobanian AV, Bakris GL, Black HR, et al: The seventh report of the Joint National Committee on Prevention, Detection, Evaluation, and Treatment of High Blood Pressure: The JNC 7 Report. *JAMA* 289:2560-2572, 2003.
6. Whelton PK, He J, Appel LJ, et al: Primary prevention of hypertension: Clinical and public health advisory from the National High Blood Pressure Education Program. *JAMA* 288:1882-1888, 2002.
7. Harrap SB, van der Merwe WM, Griffin SA, et al: Brief angiotensin converting enzyme inhibitor treatment in young spontaneously hypertensive rats reduces blood pressure long term. *Hypertension* 16:603-614, 1990.
8. Wu JN, Berecek KH: Prevention of genetic hypertension by early treatment of spontaneously hypertensive rats with the angiotensin converting enzyme inhibitor captopril. *Hypertension* 22:139-146, 1993.

---

**The Felodipine Event Reduction (FEVER) Study: a randomized long-term placebo-controlled trial in Chinese hypertensive patients**
Liu L, for the FEVER Study Group (Chinese Academy of Medical Sciences, Beijing; et al)
*J Hypertens* 23:2157-2172, 2005                                     1–34

---

*Objective.*—To compare the incidence of stroke and other cardiovascular events in hypertensive patients receiving a low-dose diuretic and low-dose calcium antagonist combination with those receiving low-dose diuretic monotherapy, and assess the effects of a small blood pressure difference at achieved levels lower than those achieved in previous placebo-controlled trials.

*Methods.*—The Felodipine Event Reduction (FEVER) trial was an investigator-designed, prospective, multicentre, double-blind, randomized, placebo-controlled, parallel group trial. It enrolled 9800 Chinese patients, of either sex, aged 50–79 years, with one or two additional cardiovascular risk factors or disease, whose blood pressure, 6 weeks after switching from previous antihypertensive therapy to low-dose (12.5 mg a day) hydrochlorothiazide, was in the range 140–180 mmHg (systolic) or 90–100 mmHg (diastolic). These patients were randomly assigned either to low-dose felodipine extended release or placebo, and followed at 3-month intervals for an average of 40 months.

*Results.*—The intention-to-treat analysis included 9711 randomly selected patients with only 30 (0.3%) lost to follow-up. A total of 31 842 patient-years of follow-up were accumulated, with 85.9% of patients remaining on blinded randomized treatment. Add-on therapy was given to 33.9% of the hydrochlorothiazide–felodipine patients and to 42.3% of the hydrochlorothiazide–placebo patients. In the felodipine group, systolic blood pressure (SBP)/diastolic blood pressure (DBP) decreased (from randomization to study end) from 154.2/91.0 to 137.3/82.5 mmHg, and in the placebo group from 154.4/91.3 to 142.5/85.0 mmHg, with an average difference throughout the trial of 4.2/2.1 mmHg. In the felodipine group, the primary endpoint (fatal and non-fatal stroke) was reduced by 27% ($P$ = 0.001). Among secondary endpoints, all cardiovascular events were reduced by 27% ($P$ < 0.001), all cardiac events by 35% ($P$ = 0.012), death by any cause by 31% ($P$ = 0.006), coronary events by 32% ($P$ = 0.024), heart failure by 30% ($P$ = 0.239), cardiovascular death by 33% ($P$ = 0.019), cancer by 36% ($P$ = 0.017) in the felodipine group. No significant differences were found in new-onset diabetes. Both treatments were very well tolerated.

*Conclusions.*—In moderately complicated hypertensive patients from China even a difference in SBP/DBP as small as 4/2 mmHg, such as that induced by adding low-dose felodipine to low-dose hydrochlorothiazide, is associated with very substantial reductions in the incidence of most types of cardiovascular events. As the SBP achieved in the felodipine group was below the recommended goal of less than 140 mmHg, and SBP in the placebo group was slightly above that level, FEVER provides the required evidence in support of the guidelines recommended goal, even for a hypertensive population not entirely consisting of patients with diabetes or previous cardiovascular events.

▶ This study is important for several reasons. Perhaps the most important is that FEVER validates the SBP target of less than 140 mm Hg for uncomplicated hypertensive patients, recommended by JNC 7 and other authoritative groups.[1-3] The evidence for this derives from the post-hoc analysis of achieved blood pressures; those who received only the thiazide diuretic had a mean blood pressure during follow-up of 142.5/85.0 mm Hg, whereas those who received the diuretic and felodipine had it lowered to an average of 137.3/82.5 mm Hg. Although randomization in FEVER was not to a target blood pressure, as was the case in the Hypertension Optimal Treatment (HOT) study,[4] the FEVER data show that those who, on average, achieved the SBP less than 140/90 mm Hg experienced a 28% reduction in stroke (the primary end point) and a significant prevention of many other cardiovascular events as well.

The second important message from FEVER is that the combination of a calcium antagonist and a thiazide diuretic not only lowers blood pressure, but also is associated with significant improvement in cardiovascular events compared with using a diuretic alone. Years ago, some authors believed that the combination of a calcium antagonist and a diuretic was ineffective in lowering blood pressure.[5] This thesis was roundly dispelled by the first "factorial design" study of diltiazem and hydrochlorothiazide, which showed a significant and independent blood pressure–lowering effect of both therapies,[6] but the combination was never marketed. This led many physicians to believe the allegation that the 2 drug classes did not lower blood pressure any better than either alone. The FEVER data, and those of the recent REIN-2 trial,[7] which also added felodipine extended-release tablets to a regimen containing a low-dose angiotensin-converting enzyme inhibitor, show that there is a significant blood pressure lowering when felodipine is added to another antihypertensive agent.

A third, although perhaps less important, point is that the FEVER study is one of the first clinical trials to be done in China that included randomization of subjects to initial therapy. Previous studies in Chinese hypertensives (including the Shanghai Trial Of Nifedipine in the Elderly [STONE][8] and Systolic Hypertension in China [Syst-China][9]) assigned the initial drug treatment by "sequential allocation" because of local customs that made assigning treatment purely by chance unacceptable. Because these earlier studies were not randomized, many subsequent meta-analyses did not accept or include their data,[10-12] although they appear to be as rigorously collected and analyzed as any Western clinical trial.

**W. J. Elliott, MD, PhD**

*References*

1. Chobanian AV, Bakris GL, Black HR, et al: The seventh report of the Joint National Committee on Prevention, Detection, Evaluation, and Treatment of High Blood Pressure: The JNC 7 Report. *JAMA* 289:2560-2572, 2003.
2. Williams B, Poulter NR, Brown MJ, et al: British Hypertension Society guidelines for hypertension management 2004 (BHS-IV): Summary. *BMJ* 328:634-640, 2004.
3. 2003 European Society of Hypertension-European Cardiology guidelines for the management of arterial hypertension. Guidelines Committee. *J Hypertension* 21:1011-1053, 2003.
4. Hansson L, Zanchetti A, Carruthers SG, et al: Effects of intensive blood pressure lowering and low-dose aspirin in patients with hypertension: Principal results of the Hypertension Optimal Treatment (HOT) randomised trial: The HOT Study Group. *Lancet* 351:1755-1762, 1998.
5. Nicholson JP, Resnick LM, Laragh JH: Hydrochlorothiazide is not additive to verapamil in treating essential hypertension. *Arch Intern Med* 149:125-128, 1989.
6. Burris J, Weir M, Oparil S, et al: An assessment of diltiazem and hydrochlorothiazide in hypertension. *JAMA* 263:1507-1512, 1990.
7. Ruggenenti P, Perna A, Loriga G, et al: Blood-pressure control for renoprotection in patients with non-diabetic chronic renal disease (REIN-2): multicentre, randomised controlled trial. *Lancet* 365:939-946, 2005.
8. Gong L, Zhang W, Zhu Y, et al: Shanghai trial of nifedipine in the elderly (STONE). *J Hypertens* 14:1237-1245, 1996.
9. Liu L, et al for the Systolic Hypertension in China (Syst-China) Collaborative Group. Comparison of active treatment and placebo in older Chinese patients with isolated systolic hypertension. *J Hypertens* 16:1823-1829, 1998.
10. Blood Pressure Lowering Treatment Trialists' Collaboration. Effects of different blood-pressure-lowering regimens on major cardiovascular events: Results of prospectively-designed overviews of randomised trials. *Lancet* 362:1527-1535, 2003.
11. Staessen JA, Wang J-G, Thijs L: Cardiovascular prevention and blood pressure reduction: A quantitative overview updated until 01 March 2003. *J Hypertension* 21:1005-1076, 2003.
12. Psaty BM, Lumley T, Furberg CD, et al: Health outcomes associated with various antihypertensive therapies used as first-line agents: A network meta-analysis. *JAMA* 289:2534-2544, 2003.

### Differential Impact of Blood Pressure–Lowering Drugs on Central Aortic Pressure and Clinical Outcomes: Principal Results of the Conduit Artery Function Evaluation (CAFE) Study

Williams B and the CAFE Investigators, for the Anglo-Scandinavian Cardiac Outcomes Trial (ASCOT) Investigators (Univ of Leicester, England; et al)
*Circulation* 113:1213-1225, 2006                                                                 1–35

*Background.*—Different blood pressure (BP)–lowering drugs could have different effects on central aortic pressures and thus cardiovascular outcome despite similar effects on brachial BP. The Conduit Artery Function Evaluation (CAFE) study, a substudy of the Anglo-Scandinavian Cardiac Outcomes Trial (ASCOT), examined the impact of 2 different BP lowering-regimens (atenolol±thiazide-based versus amlodipine±perindopril-based therapy) on derived central aortic pressures and hemodynamics.

*Method and Results.*—The CAFE study recruited 2199 patients in 5 ASCOT centers. Radial artery applanation tonometry and pulse wave analysis were used to derive central aortic pressures and hemodynamic indexes on repeated visits for up to 4 years. Most patients received combination therapy throughout the study. Despite similar brachial systolic BPs between treatment groups ($\Delta 0.7$ mm Hg; 95% CI, $-0.4$ to 1.7; $P=0.2$), there were substantial reductions in central aortic pressures with the amlodipine regimen (central aortic systolic BP, $\Delta 4.3$ mm Hg; 95% CI, 3.3 to 5.4; $P<0.0001$; central aortic pulse pressure, $\Delta 3.0$ mm Hg; 95% CI, 2.1 to 3.9; $P<0.0001$). Cox proportional-hazards modeling showed that central pulse pressure was significantly associated with a post hoc–defined composite outcome of total cardiovascular events/procedures and development of renal impairment in the CAFE cohort (unadjusted, $P<0.0001$; adjusted for baseline variables, $P<0.05$).

*Conclusions.*—BP-lowering drugs can have substantially different effects on central aortic pressures and hemodynamics despite a similar impact on brachial BP. Moreover, central aortic pulse pressure may be a determinant of clinical outcomes, and differences in central aortic pressures may be a potential mechanism to explain the different clinical outcomes between the 2 BP treatment arms in ASCOT.

▶ This study, a 5-center substudy of ASCOT, was designed originally to compare the central aortic systolic and pulse pressures across the 2 randomized treatment arms in about 500 hypertensive patients.[1] The CAFE investigators recognized that this would be a very small subset of the ASCOT trial population and therefore enrolled 2199 patients after they had been randomized in ASCOT. The original CAFE study plan included comparisons of the randomized groups for each of the primary and secondary outcomes of ASCOT, but this was not the original primary objective of CAFE. The authors reported the results of Cox proportional hazards modeling for the post hoc end point chosen by the ASCOT investigators after ASCOT was completed: total cardiovascular events and procedures, presumably because this outcome measure had the highest number of participants who experienced it, thus maximizing statistical power.[2]

Despite these unusual features, the results of this study (taken in conjunction with 2 recent meta-analyses[3,4]) have convinced several editorialists[5,6] and even the National Institute for Clinical Excellence in the United Kingdom to relegate β-blockers to be only "add-on" drugs for hypertension, unless it is complicated by another condition that has a specific indication for a β-blocker. The central tenet of their argument is that β-blockers reduce brachial blood pressure, but not central aortic blood pressure, which correlates more closely with clinical outcomes.

**W. J. Elliott, MD, PhD**

*References*

1. Dahlvf B, Sever PS, Poulter NR, et al: Prevention of cardiovascular events with an antihypertensive regimen of amlodipine adding perindopril as required versus atenolol adding bendroflumethiazide as required, in the Anglo-Scandinavian Cardiac Outcomes Trial-Blood Pressure Lowering Arm (ASCOT-BPLA): A multicentre randomised controlled trial. *Lancet* 366:895-906, 2005.
2. Poulter NR, Wedel H, Dahlvf B, et al: Role of blood pressure and other variables in the differential cardiovascular events rates noted in the Anglo-Scandinavian Cardiac Outcomes Trial-Blood Pressure Lowering Arm (ASCOT-BPLA). *Lancet* 366:907-913, 2005.
3. Lindholm LH, Carlberg B, Samuelsson O: Should β-blockers remain first choice in the treatment of primary hypertension? A meta-analysis. *Lancet* 366:1545-1553, 2005.
4. Carlberg B, Samuelson O, Lindholm LH: Atenolol in hypertension: Is it a wise choice? *Lancet* 364:1684-1689, 2004.
5. Oparil S, Izzo JL Jr: Pulsology rediscovered: Commentary on the Conduit Artery Function Evaluation (CAFE) study [editorial]. *Circulation* 113:1162-1163, 2006.
6. Wilkinson IB, McEniery CM, Cockcroft JR: Atenolol and cardiovascular risk: An issue close to the heart [Commentary]. *Lancet* 367:627-628, 2006.

---

**Carotid Intima-Media Thickness and Antihypertensive Treatment: A Meta-Analysis of Randomized Controlled Trials**

Wang J-G, Staessen JA, Li Y, et al (Univ of Leuven, Belgium; Shanghai Jiaotong Univ, China; Univ of Ghent, Belgium; et al)
*Stroke* 37:1933-1940, 2006                                      1–36

---

*Background and Purpose.*—Hypertension promotes carotid intima-media thickening. We reviewed the randomized controlled trials that evaluated the effects of an antihypertensive drug versus placebo or another antihypertensive agent of a different class on carotid intima-media thickness.

*Methods.*—We searched the PubMed and the Web of Science databases for randomized clinical trials, published in English before 2005, and included 22 trials.

*Results.*—In 8 trials including 3329 patients with diabetes or coronary heart disease, antihypertensive treatment initiated with an angiotensin-converting enzyme (ACE) inhibitor, a β-blocker, or a calcium-channel blocker (CCB), compared with placebo or no-treatment, reduced the rate of intima-media thickening by 7 µm/year ($P=0.01$). In 9 trials including 4564 hypertensive patients, CCBs, ACE inhibitors, an angiotensin II receptor blocker or an α-blocker, compared with diuretics or β-blockers, in the presence of similar blood pressure reductions, decreased intima-media thickening by 3 µm/year ($P=0.03$). The overall beneficial effect of the newer over older drugs was largely attributable to the decrease of intima-media thickening by 5 µm/year ($P=0.007$) in 4 trials of CCBs involving 3619 patients. In 5 trials including 287 patients with hypertension or diabetes, CCBs compared with ACE inhibitors did not differentially affect blood pressure, but attenuated intima-media thickening by 23 µm/year ($P=0.02$). The treatment induced changes in carotid intima-media thickness correlated with the changes in lumen diameter ($P=0.02$), but not with the differences in achieved blood pressure ($P>0.53$).

*Conclusions.*—CCBs reduce carotid intima-media thickening. This mechanism might contribute to their superior protection against stroke.

▶ Many have argued the question of whether specific antihypertensive drugs or drug classes have benefits beyond blood pressure control.[1,2] Some believe that calcium antagonists offer superior protection against stroke compared with ACE inhibitors[3] or an initial diuretic or β-blocker,[2] but others have attributed these differences to better achieved blood pressure control in the group receiving the calcium antagonist.[2,4]

These authors therefore explored clinical trial data that might identify another potential mechanism by which the calcium antagonists may be beneficial in long-term protection against stroke: reducing the progression of carotid intima-media thickness, which has been associated in many studies with an increase in risk for future stroke. Although the authors' analysis of differential effects of antihypertensive drugs on blood pressure was not significant, they saw significant differences across drug classes (calcium antagonists were greater than ACE inhibitors, which were greater than diuretic/β-blockers were approximately the same as placebo/no treatment) in progression of carotid intima-media thickness. Although these differences achieved traditional levels of statistical significance ($0.007 < P < 0.02$, without adjustment for multiple comparisons), there were no significant differences in any major cardiovascular end point across the different antihypertensive drugs when all the clinical trials were meta-analyzed. These data therefore support the hypothesis of Fleckenstein et al[5] and early animal data of Henry and Bentley[6] that calcium antagonists may have beneficial effects on atherosclerosis but hardly prove that their effects are independent of their lowering of blood pressure, which (in other meta-analyses and meta-regressions) is also greatest (compared with placebo) of any class of antihypertensive drug.[4]

**W. J. Elliott, MD, PhD**

*References*

1. Sever PS, Poulter NR: Management of hypertension: Is it the pressure or the drug? *Circulation* 113:2754-2763, 2006.

2. Elliott WJ, Jonsson MC, Black HR: It's NOT Beyond the Blood Pressure, It IS the Blood Pressure. *Circulation* 113:2763-2772, 2006.

3. Verdecchia P, Reboldi G, Angeli F, et al: Angiotensin-converting enzyme inhibitors and calcium channel blockers for coronary heart disease and stroke prevention. *Hypertension* 46:386-392, 2006.

4. Turnbull F, for the Blood Pressure Lowering Treatment Trialists' Collaboration: Effects of different blood-pressure-lowering regimens on major cardiovascular events: Results of prospectively-designed overviews of randomised trials. *Lancet* 362:1527-1535, 2003.

5. Fleckenstein A, Frey M, Thimm M, et al: Excessive mural calcium overload? A predominant causal factor in the development of stenosing coronary plaques in humans. *Cardiovasc Drug Ther* 4:1005-1014, 1990.

6. Henry PD, Bentley KI: Suppression of atherogenesis in cholesterol-fed rabbits treated with nifedipine. *J Clin Invest* 68:1366-1369, 1981.

## Lifestyle interventions to reduce raised blood pressure: a systematic review of randomized controlled trials

Dickinson HO, Mason JM, Nicolson DJ, et al (Univ of Newcastle upon Tyne, England; Univ of Durham, Stockton-on-Tees, England; Univ of Leeds, England; et al)

*J Hypertens* 24:215-233, 2006
1–37

*Purpose.*—To quantify effectiveness of lifestyle interventions for hypertension.

*Data Sources.*—Electronic bibliographic databases from 1998 onwards, existing guidelines, systematic reviews.

*Study Selection and Data Abstraction.*—We included randomized, controlled trials with at least 8 weeks' follow-up, comparing lifestyle with control interventions, enrolling adults with blood pressure at least 140/85 mmHg. Primary outcome measures were systolic and diastolic blood pressure. Two independent reviewers selected trials and abstracted data; differences were resolved by discussion.

*Results.*—We categorized trials by type of intervention and used random effects meta-analysis to combine mean differences between endpoint blood pressure in treatment and control groups in 105 trials randomizing 6805 participants. Robust statistically significant effects were found for improved diet, aerobic exercise, alcohol and sodium restriction, and fish oil supplements: mean reductions in systolic blood pressure of 5.0 mmHg [95% confidence interval (CI): 3.1–7.0], 4.6 mmHg (95% CI: 2.0–7.1), 3.8 mmHg (95% CI: 1.4–6.1), 3.6 mmHg (95% CI: 2.5–4.6) and 2.3 mmHg (95% CI: 0.2–4.3), respectively, with corresponding reductions in diastolic blood pressure. Relaxation significantly reduced blood pressure only when compared with non-intervention controls. We found no robust evidence of any important effect on blood pressure of potassium, magnesium or calcium supplements.

*Conclusions.*—Patients with elevated blood pressure should follow a weight-reducing diet, take regular exercise, and restrict alcohol and salt intake. Available evidence does not support relaxation therapies, calcium, magnesium or potassium supplements to reduce blood pressure.

▶ These authors used greater rigor and quantitative methods to arrive at the same conclusion as a recent American Heart Association Expert Panel.[1] In fact, the recommendations are not much different than those found in JNC 72 or a white paper from the National High Blood Pressure Education Program published a year earlier.[3] The challenge with these recommendations is not recognizing the dataset on which they are based, but the low proportion of patients in real-life clinical practice that follow these recommendations in the long term. Recidivism to less healthy lifestyles has been noted in research studies, but becomes a very large problem in everyday clinical practice.[4]

The second challenge with these recommendations in this era of evidence-based medicine is that these measures have not yet been shown to decrease cardiovascular morbidity and mortality. Such a study would have to enroll thousands of subjects and follow them for many years, and probably cannot be done for ethical and fiscal reasons. Nonetheless, the very effective lifestyle modifications used in the Treatment of Mild Hypertension Study (delivered by world-class experts in research clinics) were less effective in preventing cardiovascular events than the same measures plus antihypertensive drug therapy.[5] One can therefore argue that, at least in hypertensive patients, drug therapy plus lifestyle modifications are superior to lifestyle modifications alone. Similarly, in prehypertension, the Trial Of Preventing Hypertension (TROPHY) showed a trend toward fewer cardiovascular and all-cause hospitalizations in those given drug therapy plus lifestyle modification advice compared with those given placebo and lifestyle modification advice.[6] This leaves open the door for more randomized trials that may attempt to compare drug plus nondrug versus nondrug therapies for prevention of hypertension.

**W. J. Elliott, MD, PhD**

*References*

1. Appel LJ, Brands MW, Daniels SR, et al: Dietary approaches to prevent and treat hypertension: A scientific statement from the American Heart Association. *Hypertension* 47:296-308, 2006.
2. Chobanian AV, Bakris GL, Black HR, et al: Seventh Report of the Joint National Committee on Prevention, Detection, Evaluation and Treatment of High Blood Pressure. National High Blood Pressure Education Program Coordinating Committee. *Hypertension* 42:1206-1252, 2003.
3. Whelton PK, He J, Appel LJ, et al: Primary prevention of hypertension: Clinical and public health advisory from the National High Blood Pressure Education Program. *JAMA* 288:1882-1888, 2002.
4. Stamler R, Stamler J, Gosch FC, et al: Primary prevention of hypertension by nutritional-hygienic means: Final report of a randomized, controlled trial. *JAMA* 262:1801-1807, 1989.
5. Neaton JD, Grimm RH Jr, Prineas RJ, et al: Treatment of Mild Hypertension Study: Final results. *JAMA* 270:713-724, 1993.
6. Julius S, et al for the Trial of Preventing Hypertension (TROPHY) Study Investigators. Feasibility of treating prehypertension with an angiotensin-receptor blocker. *N Engl J Med* 354:1685-1697, 2006.

## Comparative Antihypertensive Effects of Hydrochlorothiazide and Chlorthalidone on Ambulatory and Office Blood Pressure

Ernst ME, Carter BL, Goerdt CJ, et al (Univ of Iowa, Iowa City)
*Hypertension* 47:352-358, 20006                1–38

Low-dose thiazide-type diuretics are recommended as initial therapy for most hypertensive patients. Chlorthalidone has significantly reduced stroke and cardiovascular end points in several landmark trials; however, hydrochlorothiazide remains favored in practice. Most clinicians assume that the drugs are interchangeable, but their antihypertensive effects at lower doses have not been directly compared. We conducted a randomized, single-blinded, 8-week active treatment, crossover study comparing chlorthalidone 12.5 mg/day (force-titrated to 25 mg/day) and hydrochlorothiazide 25 mg/day (force-titrated to 50 mg/day) in untreated hypertensive patients. The main outcome, 24-hour ambulatory blood pressure (BP) monitoring, was assessed at baseline and week 8, along with standard office BP readings every 2 weeks. Thirty patients completed the first active treatment period, whereas 24 patients completed both. An order–drug–time interaction was observed with chlorthalidone; therefore, data from only the first active treatment period was considered. Week 8 ambulatory BPs indicated a greater reduction from baseline in systolic BP with chlorthalidone 25 mg/day compared with hydrochlorothiazide 50 mg/day (24-hour mean = −12.41.8 mm Hg versus −7.41.7 mm Hg; $P=0.054$; nighttime mean = −13.51.9 mm Hg versus −6.41.8 mm Hg; $P=0.009$). Office systolic BP reduction was lower at week 2 for chlorthalidone 12.5 mg/day versus hydrochlorothiazide 25 mg/day (−15.72.2 mm Hg versus −4.52.1 mm Hg; $P=0.001$); however, by week 8, reductions were statistically similar (−17.13.7 versus −10.83.5; $P=0.84$). Within recommended doses, chlorthalidone is more effective in lowering systolic BPs than hydrochlorothiazide, as evidenced by 24-hour ambulatory BPs. These differences were not apparent with office BP measurements.

▶ Although relatively unknown to American physicians, chlorthalidone was the thiazide diuretic used in several NIH-sponsored clinical trials that demonstrated the benefits of antihypertensive drug therapy compared with usual care (Hypertension Detection and Follow-up Program [HDFP] and the Multiple Risk Factor Intervention Trial [MRFIT]),[1,2] placebo (Systolic Hypertension in the Elderly Program [SHEP] and the Treatment of Mild Hypertension Study [TOMHS]),[3,4] and other active antihypertensive agents (Antihypertensive and Lipid Lowering treatment to prevent Heart Attack Trial [ALLHAT]).[5,6] Hydrochlorothiazide was also a treatment option in MRFIT, but when interim morbidity and mortality data were reviewed by the study's data safety and monitoring board, all centers that used hydrochlorothiazide were told to switch all their subjects to chlorthalidone, after which the results improved.[2] A potential reason for the disparate results of ALLHAT and the Second Australian Blood Pressure Trial[7] was that the former used chlorthalidone and the latter used hydrochlorothiazide.[8]

The authors therefore attempted a head-to-head 8-week crossover study of the 2 drugs (chlorthalidone for 4 weeks each at 12.5 mg/d, then 25 mg/d, and hydrochlorothiazide at 25 mg/d, then 50 mg/d) in 30 hypertensive patients. The planned crossover design had to be abandoned because those who were randomized to receive chlorthalidone first had a significantly lower blood pressure at the beginning of the second treatment period, suggesting already that chlorthalidone had a bigger and longer-lasting effect on blood pressure than did hydrochlorothiazide. Analysis of the authors' ambulatory blood pressure monitoring data by a parallel-group comparison confirmed these observations, despite a nonsignificant difference in clinic readings (potentially due to a lack of study power). Unlike an indirect comparison of the 2 drugs in a network meta-analysis,[9] these data indicate that chlorthalidone is likely at least twice as potent in lowering blood pressure (milligram per milligram) than hydrochlorothiazide, and suggest that the drugs are likely to have different effects in hypertensive patients, with chlorthalidone being superior to hydrochlorothiazide.

**W. J. Elliott, MD, PhD**

*References*

1. Hypertension Detection and Follow-up Program Cooperative Group: Persistence of reduction in blood pressure and mortality of participants in the Hypertension Detection and Follow-up Program. *JAMA* 259:2113-2122, 1988.
2. Multiple Risk Factor Intervention Trial Research Group: Mortality after 10.5 years for hypertensive participants in the Multiple Risk Factor Intervention Trial. *JAMA* 282:1616-1628, 1990.
3. SHEP Cooperative Research Group: Prevention of stroke by antihypertensive drug treatment in older persons with isolated systolic hypertension: Final results of the Systolic Hypertension in the Elderly Program (SHEP). *JAMA* 265:3255-3264, 1991.
4. Neaton JD, Grimm RH, Prineas RJ, et al: Treatment of Mild Hypertension Study. Final Results. *JAMA* 270:713-724, 1993.
5. The ALLHAT Officers and Coordinators for the ALLHAT Collaborative Research Group: Major cardiovascular events in hypertensive patients randomized to doxazosin vs. chlorthalidone: The Antihypertensive and Lipid-Lowering Treatment to Prevent Heart Attack Trial (ALLHAT). *JAMA* 283:1967-1975, 2000.
6. The ALLHAT Officers and Coordinators for the ALLHAT Collaborative Research Group: Major outcomes in high-risk hypertensive patients randomized to angiotensin-converting enzyme inhibitor or calcium channel blocker vs. diuretic. The Antihypertensive and Lipid-Lowering Treatment to Prevent Heart Attack Trial (ALLHAT). *JAMA* 288:2981-2997, 2002.
7. Wing LMH, Reid CM, Ryan P, et al: A comparison of outcomes with angiotensin-converting enzyme inhibitors and diuretics for hypertension in the elderly. *N Engl J Med* 348:583-592, 2003.
8. Choi K, Chua D, Elliott WJ: Chlorthalidone vs. other low-dose diuretics [letter]. *JAMA* 292:1816-1817, 2004.
9. Psaty BM, Lumley T, Furberg CD: Meta-analysis of health outcomes of chlorthalidone-based vs nonchlorthalidone-based low dose diuretic therapies [letter]. *JAMA* 292:43-44, 2004.

### Clinical Events in High-Risk Hypertensive Patients Randomly Assigned to Calcium Channel Blocker Versus Angiotensin-Converting Enzyme Inhibitor in the Antihypertensive and Lipid-Lowering Treatment to Prevent Heart Attack Trial

Leenen FHH, for the Antihypertensive and Lipid-Lowering Treatment to Prevent Heart Attack Trial (ALLHAT) Collaborative Research Group (Univ of Ottawa Heart Inst, Ont, Canada; et al)
*Hypertension* 48:374-384, 2006                                    1–39

The Antihypertensive and Lipid-Lowering treatment to prevent Heart Attack Trial (ALLHAT) provides a unique opportunity to compare the long-term relative safety and efficacy of angiotensin-converting enzyme inhibitor and calcium channel blocker-initiated therapy in older hypertensive individuals. Patients were randomized to amlodipine (n=9048) or lisinopril (n=9054). The primary outcome was combined fatal coronary heart disease or nonfatal myocardial infarction, analyzed by intention-to-treat. Secondary outcomes included all-cause mortality, stroke, combined cardiovascular disease (CVD), end-stage renal disease (ESRD), cancer, and gastrointestinal bleeding. Mean follow-up was 4.9 years. Blood pressure control was similar in nonblacks, but not in blacks. No significant differences were found between treatment groups for the primary outcome, all-cause mortality, ESRD, or cancer. Stroke rates were higher on lisinopril in blacks (RR=1.51, 95% CI 1.22 to 1.86) but not in nonblacks (RR=1.07, 95% CI 0.89 to 1.28), and in women (RR=1.45, 95% CI 1.17 to 1.79), but not in men (RR=1.10, 95% CI 0.92 to 1.31). Rates of combined CVD were higher (RR=1.06, 95% CI 1.00 to 1.12) because of higher rates for strokes, peripheral arterial disease, and angina, which were partly offset by lower rates for heart failure (RR=0.87, 95% CI 0.78 to 0.96) on lisinopril compared with amlodipine. Gastrointestinal bleeds and angioedema were higher on lisinopril. Patients with and without baseline coronary heart disease showed similar outcome patterns. We conclude that in hypertensive patients, the risks for coronary events are similar, but for stroke, combined CVD, gastrointestinal bleeding, and angioedema are higher and for heart failure are lower for lisinopril-based compared with amlodipine-based therapy. Some, but not all, of these differences may be explained by less effective blood pressure control in the lisinopril arm.

▶ Although ALLHAT was designed to compare outcomes in hypertensive patients randomized to either chlorthalidone (the best-studied thiazide-like diuretic) or 1 of 3 "newer" antihypertensive agents (amlodipine, the most popular calcium antagonist), lisinopril (the most popular angiotensin-converting enzyme [ACE] inhibitor), or doxazosin (the most popular $\alpha_1$ blocker),[1,2] this post-hoc analysis was done to directly compare outcomes across the 2 classes of antihypertensive drugs that are currently most popular. Because of the excessive burden of hypertension and its sequelae in the black population, by design black subjects were recruited into ALLHAT at about 3 times their proportion in the US population. Since the ALLHAT protocol discouraged the use of thiazide-type or thiazide-like diuretics as second-line therapy, many blacks and nonblacks received atenolol as their second-line treatment when the initial therapy did not control blood pressure. This differentiates usual clinical practice from the treatment regimen in ALLHAT and (as suggested by these authors) may have accounted for the fact that blood pressure control was less well achieved in blacks who were randomized to lisinopril.[3] Unfortunately, it is not easy to tease out the consequences of worse blood pressure control according to randomized drug choice, as opposed to the results that are likely attributable to the drug class alone (eg, heart failure was diagnosed more commonly among patients randomized to calcium antagonists rather than an initial diuretic or β-blocker, or ACE inhibitor).[4-6]

In ALLHAT, the rates of angioedema with lisinopril (38 of 9054, or 0.42% overall, but 0.72% in blacks and 0.26% in nonblacks) were significantly lower ($P < .02$ by $\chi^2$) than those reported with enalapril in the OCTAVE trial (86 of 12634, or 0.68% overall, but 3.1 times more common among blacks).[7] Perhaps because nearly all patients in ALLHAT were "rolled over" from prior antihypertensive drug therapy to the randomized drug, there was a lower risk because of prior exposure to ACE inhibitors than was the case in OCTAVE. ALLHAT also observed a much higher rate of heart failure among those randomized to amlodipine than other studies that included a dihydropyridine calcium antagonist[8,9] The reasons for this are unclear.

These data further support the prior analyses and original conclusions of the ALLHAT Collaborative Research Group regarding the lower incidence of stroke and angioedema, but a higher incidence of heart failure, among those randomized to amlodipine.[10] These data also support the treatment recommendations of JNC 7 and (in part) the new British National Institute for health and Clinical Excellence (NICE) guidelines, which recommend the use of a dihydropyridine calcium antagonist as initial therapy for blacks and hypertensive people older than 55 years but an ACE inhibitor for young whites.[11]

**W. J. Elliott, MD, PhD**

*References*

1. Davis BR, Cutler JA, Gordon DJ, et al: Rationale and design for the Antihypertensive and Lipid Lowering Treatment to Prevent Heart Attack Trial (ALLHAT). *Am J Hypertens* 9:342-360, 1996.
2. Elliott WJ: ALLHAT: The largest and most important blood pressure trial ever in the USA [editorial]. *Am J Hypertens* 9:409-411, 1996.
3. Wright JT Jr et al for the ALLHAT Collaborative Research Group. Outcomes in hypertensive black and nonblack patients treated with chlorthalidone, amlodipine, and lisinopril. *JAMA* 293:1595-1608, 2005.
4. Turnbull F: Blood Pressure Lowering Treatment Trialists' Collaboration. Effects of different blood-pressure-lowering regimens on major cardiovascular events: Results of prospectively-designed overviews of randomised trials. *Lancet* 362:1527-1535, 2003.
5. Staessen JA, Wang J-G, Thijs L: Cardiovascular prevention and blood pressure reduction: A quantitative overview updated until 01 March 2003. *J Hypertension* 21:1005-1076, 2003.
6. Elliott WJ, Jonsson MC, Black HR: It's NOT beyond the blood pressure, It IS the blood pressure. *Circulation* 113:2763-2772, 2006.

7. Kostis JB, Kim HJ, Rusnak J, et al: Incidence and characteristics of angioedema associated with enalapril. *Arch Intern Med* 165:1637-1642, 2005.
8. Brown MJ, Palmer CR, Castaigne A, et al: Morbidity and mortality in patients randomised to double-blind treatment with a long-acting calcium-channel blocker or diuretic in the International Nifedipine GITS study: Intervention as a Goal in Hypertension Treatment (INSIGHT). *Lancet* 356:366-372, 2000.
9. Dahlöf B, Sever PS, Poulter NR, et al: Prevention of cardiovascular events with an antihypertensive regimen of amlodipine adding perindopril as required versus atenolol adding bendroflumethiazide as required, in the Anglo-Scandinavian Cardiac Outcomes Trial-Blood Pressure Lowering Arm (ASCOT-BPLA): A multicentre randomised controlled trial. *Lancet* 366:895-906, 2005.
10. Major outcomes in high-risk hypertensive patients randomized to angiotensin-converting enzyme inhibitor or calcium channel blocker vs. diuretic: The Antihypertensive and Lipid Lowering Treatment to Prevent Heart Attack Trial (ALLHAT). The ALLHAT Officers and Coordinators for the ALLHAT Collaborative Research Group. *JAMA* 288:2981-2997, 2002.
11. National Institute for Health and Clinical Excellence: *Hypertension: Management of hypertension in adults in primary care, a partial update of NICE clinical guideline 18*, www.nice.org.uk/page.aspx?o-cg034NICEguideline, accessed July 4, 2006.

## Fasting Glucose Levels and Incident Diabetes Mellitus in Older Nondiabetic Adults Randomized to Receive 3 Different Classes of Antihypertensive Treatment: A Report From the Antihypertensive and Lipid-Lowering Treatment to Prevent Heart Attack Trial (ALLHAT)

Barzilay JI, for the ALLHAT Collaborative Research Group (Emory Univ School of Medicine, Atlanta, Ga; et al)
*Arch Intern Med* 166:2191-2201, 2006
1–40

*Background.*—Elevated blood glucose levels are reported with thiazide-type diuretic treatment of hypertension. The significance of this finding is uncertain. Our objectives were to compare the effect of first-step antihypertensive drug therapy with thiazide-type diuretic, calcium-channel blocker, or angiotensin-converting enzyme inhibitor on fasting glucose (FG) levels and to determine cardiovascular and renal disease risks associated with elevated FG levels and incident diabetes mellitus (DM) in 3 treatment groups.

*Methods.*—We performed post hoc subgroup analyses from the Antihypertensive and Lipid-Lowering Treatment to Prevent Heart Attack Trial (ALLHAT) among nondiabetic participants who were randomized to receive treatment with chlorthalidone (n = 8419), amlodipine (n = 4958), or lisinopril (n = 5034) and observed for a mean of 4.9 years.

*Results.*—Mean FG levels increased during follow-up in all treatment groups. At year 2, those randomized to the chlorthalidone group had the greatest increase ($+8.5$ mg/dL [0.47 mmol/L] vs $+5.5$ mg/dL [0.31 mmol/L] for amlodipine and $+3.5$ mg/dL [0.19 mmol/L] for lisinopril). The odds ratios for developing DM with lisinopril (0.55 [95% confidence interval, 0.43-0.70]) or amlodipine (0.73 [95% confidence interval, 0.58-0.91]) vs chlorthalidone at 2 years were significantly lower than 1.0 ($P<.01$). There was no significant association of FG level change at 2 years with subsequent coronary heart disease, stroke, cardiovascular disease, total mortality, or end-stage renal disease. There was no significant association of incident DM at 2 years with clinical outcomes, except for coronary heart disease (risk ratio, 1.64; $P=.006$), but the risk ratio was lower and nonsignificant in the chlorthalidone group (risk ratio, 1.46; $P=.14$).

*Conclusions.*—Fasting glucose levels increase in older adults with hypertension regardless of treatment type. For those taking chlorthalidone vs other medications, the risk of developing FG levels higher than 125 mg/dL (6.9 mmol/L) is modestly greater, but there is no conclusive or consistent evidence that this diuretic-associated increase in DM risk increases the risk of clinical events.

▶ This report provides more details than the first ALLHAT final results report regarding the propensity of those randomized to chlorthalidone to be associated with more hyperglycemia compared with those given either lisinopril or amlodipine in ALLHAT.[1] The clinical importance of this hyperglycemia has been hotly debated. In their previous report, the ALLHAT investigators reported performing the appropriate analyses and claimed that there was no increased risk of cardiovascular events among those who developed hyperglycemia during ALLHAT's 4.9 years of mean follow-up. This study supports their point of view, which was also seen in patients randomized to chlorthalidone (vs placebo) in the Systolic Hypertension in the Elderly Program.[2] An alternative position has recently been adopted by guidelines promulgated by the British National Institute for Health and Clinical Excellence, which recommends avoiding diuretics (particularly with β-blockers) in those likely to develop diabetes because of the much higher cost of care for diabetics, given their lower blood pressure and lipid targets, which are likely to require more medications.[3]

Despite extensive training and methodologic rigor in the planning and execution of ALLHAT, only 53% of subjects who were not diabetic at randomization provided a blood sample for fasting glucose, upon which the presumptive diagnosis of diabetes is based in this study. Traditionally in clinical practice, 2 such values greater than 125 mg/dL are required for this diagnosis.[4] The authors performed extensive analyses of their data, adjusting the hazard ratios for development of diabetes and "hard cardiovascular end points" across the initial treatments for such interesting covariates as age, gender, race, fasting glucose level at the beginning of the interval, body mass index, and smoking as well as β-blocker treatment, hypokalemia, and statin treatment, which have been demonstrated in previous studies to affect fasting glucose levels. The subsequent results show that chlorthalidone was more likely to be associated with hyperglycemia, but that this did not translate to an increased risk of any of the hard cardiovascular end points studied in ALLHAT. This is surprisingly the same conclusion of Italian investigators who reported an increased risk of cardiovascular events among those who became diabetic after initiation of antihypertensive treatment, in which no significant increase in cardiovascular risk could be teased out that was associated with diuretic treatment.[5] Their analyses were based on 11 events in 43 new diabetics versus 39 events in 700 nondiabetics, after adjusting for age, left ventricular hypertrophy, and 24-hour ambulatory blood pressure at baseline.

Despite the publication of this important report describing the results in ALLHAT, the "largest and most important hypertension trial ever" in the United States,[6] the clinical importance of new-onset diabetes (and its relationship to antihypertensive drug therapy) is likely to remain controversial for some time.

**W. J. Elliott, MD, PhD**

*References*

1. Major outcomes in high-risk hypertensive patients randomized to angiotensin-converting enzyme inhibitor or calcium channel blocker vs. diuretic: The Antihypertensive and Lipid Lowering Treatment to Prevent Heart Attack Trial (ALLHAT). The ALLHAT Officers and Coordinators for the ALLHAT Collaborative Research Group. *JAMA* 288:2981-2997, 2002.
2. Kostis JB, Wilson AC, Freudenberger RS, et al: Long-term effect of diuretic-based therapy on fatal outcomes in subjects with isolated systolic hypertension with and without diabetes. *Am J Cardiol* 95:29-35, 2005.
3. National Institute for Health and Clinical Excellence: *Hypertension: Management of hypertension in adults in primary care, a partial update of NICE clinical guideline 18*, www.nice.org.uk/page.aspx?o-cg034NICEguideline, accessed July 4, 2006.
4. American Diabetes Association Position Statement: Diagnosis and classification of diabetes mellitus. *Diabetes Care* 27(suppl 1):S5-S10, 2004.
5. Verdecchia P, Reboldi G, Angeli F, et al: Adverse prognostic significance of new diabetes in treated hypertensive subjects. *Hypertension* 43:963-969, 2004.
6. Elliott WJ. ALLHAT: The largest and most important blood pressure trial ever in the USA [editorial]. *Am J Hypertension* 9:409-411, 1996.

### Effect of Ramipril on the Incidence of Diabetes

Gerstein HC, and the DREAM Trial Investigators (McMaster Univ, Hamilton, Canada; et al)
*N Engl J Med* 355:1551-1562, 2006                                    1–41

*Background.*—Previous studies have suggested that blockade of the renin–angiotensin system may prevent diabetes in people with cardiovascular disease or hypertension.

*Methods.*—In a double-blind, randomized clinical trial with a 2-by-2 factorial design, we randomly assigned 5269 participants without cardiovascular disease but with impaired fasting glucose levels (after an 8-hour fast) or impaired glucose tolerance to receive ramipril (up to 15 mg per day) or placebo (and rosiglitazone or placebo) and followed them for a median of 3 years. We studied the effects of ramipril on the development of diabetes or death, whichever came first (the primary outcome), and on secondary outcomes, including regression to normoglycemia.

*Results.*—The incidence of the primary outcome did not differ significantly between the ramipril group (18.1%) and the placebo group (19.5%; hazard ratio for the ramipril group, 0.91; 95% confidence interval [CI], 0.81 to 1.03; P=0.15). Participants receiving ramipril were more likely to have regression to normoglycemia than those receiving placebo (hazard ratio, 1.16;

95% CI, 1.07 to 1.27; P=0.001). At the end of the study, the median fasting plasma glucose level was not significantly lower in the ramipril group (102.7 mg per deciliter [5.70 mmol per liter]) than in the placebo group (103.4 mg per deciliter [5.74 mmol per liter], P=0.07), though plasma glucose levels 2 hours after an oral glucose load were significantly lower in the ramipril group (135.1 mg per deciliter [7.50 mmol per liter] vs. 140.5 mg per deciliter [7.80 mmol per liter], P=0.01).

*Conclusions.*—Among persons with impaired fasting glucose levels or impaired glucose tolerance, the use of ramipril for 3 years does not significantly reduce the incidence of diabetes or death but does significantly increase regression to normoglycemia. (ClinicalTrials.gov number, NCT00095654 [ClinicalTrials.gov].)

▶ After the Heart Outcomes Prevention Evaluation showed a 24% reduction of incident diabetes with ramipril 10 mg/d versus placebo in patients at high risk for cardiovascular events,[1] the Diabetes Reduction Assessment with Ramipril and Rosiglitazone Medications (DREAM) trial was organized by many of the same investigators to compare, in a 2 × 2 factorial design, these 2 medications in the prevention of diabetes in individuals at high risk for it. This was the first randomized, placebo-controlled, multicenter trial to report incident diabetes as a primary (or high secondary) end point, which many feel is required before believing the observations from studies that include it as a post-hoc or tertiary (or even lower) end point. Nonetheless, the somewhat disappointing and nonsignificant results (9% relative risk reduction, 95% confidence interval: −3% to 20%) from DREAM directly contradict several prior meta-analyses that had shown a significant prevention of incident diabetes with angiotensin-converting enzyme inhibitors, especially in hypertensive patients.[2-6]

The reasons for the disagreement are discussed in this study but are difficult to pinpoint. To their credit, the authors analyzed their data many ways, including adjustment for covariates that should have been equalized by randomization (e.g., use of diuretics or β-blockers). One possibility not addressed by the investigators is the presence of a intertrial interaction; the chances of seeing a significant decrease in new diabetes attributed to ramipril may have been attenuated when half of the subjects were given rosiglitazone, which was much more effective. This situation may also have caused the antihypertensive comparison in the Anglo-Scandinavian Cardiac Outcome Study to fail to reach statistical significance, since so many primary outcomes (fatal or nonfatal coronary disease) were prevented by the second randomization (atorvastatin).[7,8]

Nonetheless, DREAM was performed in a rigorous fashion, but perhaps would have found a significant result if it had followed its subjects for more than 3 years. The finding in the other randomized arm of DREAM of a protective effect of rosiglitazone on incident diabetes is reassuring.[9] There is a hint from the "regression to normoglycemia" data and the 2-hour postprandial glucose levels that ramipril at least did something positive to glucose tolerance in DREAM. It is unlikely that including death in the primary end point of DREAM confounded the data, since the deaths were about evenly split (31 vs 32), and the first secondary end point (development of diabetes but not death) didn't show a significant benefit of ramipril either. Perhaps the subjects in DREAM (average age 55 years) were at lower intrinsic risk of incident diabetes than those in HOPE (average age 65 years, many of whom were hypertensive, who appear to have an increased risk of incident diabetes compared with normotensive controls). Two ongoing trials may help decide of blockers of the renin-angiotensin system (angiotensin-converting enzyme inhibitors, angiotensin II receptor blockers, and perhaps even direct renin inhibitors) prevent incident diabetes in hypertensive patients. We therefore must await the results of the Nateglinide and Valsartan in Impaired Glucose Tolerance Outcomes Research (NAVIGATOR) trial as well as the much larger Ongoing Telmisartan Alone and in Combination with Ramipril Global Endpoint Trial (ONTARGET) and its companion, the Telmisartan Randomized Assessment Study in ACE-Intolerant Patients with Cardiovascular Disease (TRANSCEND).[10]

**W. J. Elliott, MD, PhD**

*References*

1. Yusuf S, Gerstein H, Hoogwerf B, et al: Ramipril and the development of diabetes. *JAMA* 286:1882-1885, 2001.
2. Opie LH, Schall R: Old antihypertensives and new diabetes. *J Hypertension* 22:1453-1458, 2004.
3. Scheen AJ: Renin-angiotensin system inhibition prevents type 2 diabetes mellitus. Part 1. A meta-analysis of randomised clinical trials. *Diabetes Metab* 30:487-496, 2004.
4. Elliott WJ: Differential effects of antihypertensive drugs on new-onset diabetes? *Curr Hypertens Rep* 7:249-256, 2005.
5. Abuissa H, Jones PG, Marso SP, et al: Angiotensin-converting enzyme inhibitors or angiotensin receptor blockers for prevention of type 2 diabetes: A meta-analysis of randomized clinical trials. *J Am Coll Cardiol* 46:821-826, 2005.
6. Gillespie EL, White CM, Kardas M, et al: The impact of ACE inhibitors or angiotensin II type 1 receptor blockers on the development of new-onset type 2 diabetes. *Diabetes Care* 28:2261-2266, 2005.
7. Dahlöf B, Sever PS, Poulter NR, et al: Prevention of cardiovascular events with an antihypertensive regimen of amlodipine adding perindopril as required versus atenolol adding bendroflumethiazide as required, in the Anglo-Scandinavian Cardiac Outcomes Trial-Blood Pressure Lowering Arm (ASCOT-BPLA): A multicentre randomised controlled trial. *Lancet* 366:895-906, 2005.
8. Sever PS, Dahlöf B, Poulter NR, et al: Prevention of coronary and stroke events with atorvastatin in hypertensive patients who have average or lower-than-average cholesterol concentrations, in the Anglo-Scandinavian Cardiac Outcomes Trial-Lipid Lowering Arm (ASCOT-LLA): A multicentre randomised controlled trial. *Lancet* 361:1149-1158, 2003.
9. Gerstein HC, et al for the DREAM Investigators: Effect of rosiglitazone on the frequency of diabetes in patients with impaired glucose tolerance or impaired fasting glucose: a randomised controlled trial. *Lancet* 368:1096-1105, 2006.
10. Teo K, Yusuf S, Anderson C, et al: Rationale, design, and baseline characteristics of 2 large, simple, randomized trials evaluating telmisartan, ramipril, and their combination in high-risk patients: The Ongoing Telmisartan Alone and in Combination with Ramipril Global Endpoint Trial/Telmisartan Randomized Assessment Study in ACE Intolerant Subjects with Cardiovascular Disease (ONTARGET/TRANSCEND) trials. *Am Heart J* 148:52-61, 2004.

### Differing Effects of Antihypertensive Drugs on the Incidence of Diabetes Mellitus Among Patients With Hypertensive Kidney Disease

Thornley-Brown D, for the African American Study of Kidney Disease and Hypertension Study Group (Univ of Alabama at Birmingham; et al)
*Arch Intern Med* 166:797-805, 2006                    1–42

*Background.*—The African American Study of Kidney Disease and Hypertension was a multicenter trial of African Americans with hypertensive kidney disease randomized to an angiotensin-converting enzyme inhibitor (ramipril), a β-blocker (metoprolol succinate), or a calcium channel blocker (amlodipine besylate). We compared the incidence of type 2 diabetes mellitus (DM) and the composite outcome of impaired fasting glucose or DM (IFG/DM) for the African American Study of Kidney Disease and Hypertension interventions.

*Methods.*—Cox regression models were used to evaluate (post hoc) the association of the randomized interventions and the relative risk (RR) of DM and IFG/DM and to assess the RR of DM and IFG/DM by several prerandomization characteristics.

*Results.*—Among 1017 participants, 147 (14.5%) developed DM; 333 (42.9%) of 776 participants developed IFG/DM. Respective DM event rates were 2.8%, 4.4%, and 4.5% per patient-year in the ramipril-, amlodipine-, and metoprolol-treated groups. The RRs of DM with ramipril treatment were 0.53 ($P$=.001) compared with metoprolol treatment and 0.49 ($P$=.003) compared with amlodipine treatment. Respective IFG/DM event rates were 11.3%, 13.3%, and 15.8% per patient-year in the ramipril-, amlodipine-, and metoprolol-treated groups. The RRs of IFG/DM with ramipril treatment were 0.64 ($P$<.001) compared with metoprolol treatment and 0.76 ($P$=.09) compared with amlodipine treatment. The RRs of DM and IFG/DM with amlodipine treatment compared with metoprolol treatment were 1.07 ($P$=.76) and 0.84 ($P$=.26), respectively.

*Conclusion.*—Ramipril treatment was associated with a significantly lower risk of DM in African Americans with hypertensive kidney disease than amlodipine or metoprolol treatment.

▶ These data, derived from only 1017 participants, confirm and extend the observations in many other studies that both angiotensin-converting enzyme inhibitors and angiotensin receptor blockers are associated with a decreased risk of new-onset type 2 diabetes mellitus.[1-4] These results were obtained in African American hypertensive patients with nondiabetic chronic kidney disease; similar results have been seen in heart failure patients,[5,6] hypertensive patients with baseline serum creatinine values less than 2.0 mg/dL,[7] hypertensive patients with coronary disease,[8] high-risk patients (usually with known vascular disease),[9,10] and newly diagnosed hypertensive patients.[11]

Like many other clinical trials, however, these results may have been confounded by differential use of thiazide-type diuretics (but not β-blockers, which was a randomized choice), across the arms of the African American Study of Kidney Disease. The percentages of visits at which a thiazide-type diuretic was used were 9.4% (ramipril), 13.9% (amlodipine), and 11.3% (metoprolol). Diuretic use was not included as a covariate in adjusted analyses, primarily because this difference did not exist at baseline, and it is difficult (but not impossible[12]) to include time-dependent variables in most commonly used adjusted analyses. To their credit, the authors did supplemental analyses that separated the subjects into those who were or were not taking a thiazide diuretic at the most recent follow-up visit, and they claim (but do not show the data) that their overall conclusions were unchanged. These data also do not address the current controversy as to whether diabetes that emerges during follow-up in a clinical trial has a different prognosis than diabetes that was present at randomization.

These data are therefore consistent with a growing amount of clinical trial evidence suggesting that angiotensin-converting enzyme inhibitors and angiotensin receptor blockers have a protective effect against new-onset diabetes. Several trials currently in progress are using incident diabetes as a primary or high secondary end point and will add greatly to our knowledge about this issue.[13,14]

**W. J. Elliott, MD, PhD**

*References*

1. Scheen AJ: Prevention of type 2 diabetes mellitus through inhibition of the renin-angiotensin system. *Drugs* 64:2537-2565, 2004.
2. Elliott WJ: Differential effects of antihypertensive drugs on new-onset diabetes? *Curr Hypertens Rep* 7:249-256, 2005.
3. Abuissa H, Jones PG, Marso SP, et al: Angiotensin-converting enzyme inhibitors or angiotensin receptor blockers for prevention of type 2 diabetes: A meta-analysis of randomized clinical trials. *J Am Coll Cardiol* 46:821-826, 2005.
4. Gillespie EL, White CM, Kardas M, et al: The impact of ACE inhibitors or angiotensin II type 1 receptor blockers on the development of new-onset type 2 diabetes. *Diabetes Care* 28:2261-2266, 2005.
5. Vermes E, Ducharme A, Bourassa MG, et al: Enalapril reduces the incidence of diabetes in patients with chronic heart failure: Insight from the Studies of Left Ventricular Dysfunction (SOLVD). Studies of Left Ventricular Dysfunction. *Circulation* 107:1291-1296, 2003.
6. Yusuf S, Ostergren JB, Gerstein HC, et al: Effects of candesartan on the development of a new diagnosis of diabetes in patients with heart failure. *Circulation* 112:48-53, 2005.
7. Major outcomes in high-risk hypertensive patients randomized to angiotensin-converting enzyme inhibitor or calcium channel blocker vs. diuretic: The Antihypertensive and Lipid Lowering Treatment to Prevent Heart Attack Trial (ALLHAT). The ALLHAT Officers and Coordinators for the ALLHAT Collaborative Research Group. *JAMA* 288:2981-2997, 2002.
8. Pepine CJ, Handberg EM, Cooper-DeHoff RM, et al: A calcium antagonist vs. a non-calcium antagonist hypertension treatment strategy for patients with coronary artery disease: The International Verapamil-Trandolapril Study (INVEST): A randomized controlled trial. The INVEST Investigators. *JAMA* 290:2805-2816, 2003.
9. Yusuf S, Gerstein H, Hoogwerf B, et al: Ramipril and the development of diabetes. *JAMA* 286:1882-1885, 2001.
10. Angiotensin-converting-enzyme inhibition in stable coronary artery disease. The PEACE Trial Investigators. *N Engl J Med* 351:2058-2068, 2004.

11. Lindholm LH, Persson M, Alaupovic P, et al: Metabolic outcome during 1 year in a newly-detected hypertensives: Results of the Antihypertensive Treatment and Lipid Profile in a North of Sweden Efficacy Evaluation (ALPINE Study). *J Hypertens* 21:1563-1574, 2003.

12. Elliott WJ, Hewkin AC, Kupfer S, et al: A drug dose model for predicting clinical outcomes in hypertensive coronary disease patients. *J Clin Hypertens (Greenwich)* 7:654-663, 2005.

13. Gerstein HC, Yusuf S, Holman R, et al: Rationale, design and recruitment characteristics of a large, simple international trial of diabetes prevention: The DREAM Trial Investigators. *Diabetologia* 47:1519-1527, 2004.

14. Teo K, Yusuf S, Anderson C, et al: Rationale, design, and baseline characteristics of 2 large, simple, randomized trials evaluating telmisartan, ramipril, and their combination in high-risk patients: The Ongoing Telmisartan Alone and in Combination with Ramipril Global Endpoint Trial/Telmisartan Randomized Assessment Study in ACE Intolerant Subjects with Cardiovascular Disease (ONTARGET/TRANSCEND) trials. *Am Heart J* 148:52-61, 2004.

## Dogma Disputed: Can Aggressively Lowering Blood Pressure in Hypertensive Patients with Coronary Artery Disease Be Dangerous?

Messerli FH, Mancia G, Conti CR, et al (St Luke's-Roosevelt Hosp, New York; Univ of Milan, Italy; Univ of Florida, Gainesville; et al)

*Ann Intern Med* 144:884-893, 2006

1–43

*Background.*—Because coronary perfusion occurs mainly during diastole, patients with coronary artery disease (CAD) could be at increased risk for coronary events if diastolic pressure falls below critical levels.

*Objective.*—To determine whether low blood pressure could be associated with excess mortality and morbidity in this population.

*Design.*—A secondary analysis of data from the International Verapamil-Trandolapril Study (INVEST), which was conducted from September 1997 to February 2003.

*Setting.*—862 sites in 14 countries.

*Patients.*—22 576 patients with hypertension and CAD. Interventions: Patients from INVEST were randomly assigned to a verapamil sustained-release– or atenolol-based strategy; blood pressure control and outcomes were equivalent.

*Measurements.*—An unadjusted quadratic proportional hazards model was used to evaluate the relationship between average on-treatment blood pressure and risk for the primary outcome (all-cause death, nonfatal stroke, and nonfatal myocardial infarction [MI]), all-cause death, total MI, and total stroke. A second model adjusted for differences in baseline covariates.

*Results.*—The relationship between blood pressure and the primary outcome, all-cause death, and total MI was J-shaped, particularly for diastolic pressure, with a nadir at 119/84 mm Hg. After adjustment, the J-shaped relationship persisted between diastolic pressure and primary outcome. The MI–stroke ratio remained constant over a wide blood pressure range, but at a lower diastolic blood pressure, there were substantially more MIs than strokes. An interaction between decreased diastolic pressure and history of revascularization was observed; low diastolic pressure was associated with a relatively lower risk for the primary outcome in patients with revascularization than in those without revascularization.

*Limitations.*—This is a post hoc analysis of hypertensive patients with CAD.

*Conclusions.*—The risk for the primary outcome, all-cause death, and MI, but not stroke, progressively increased with low diastolic blood pressure. Excessive reduction in diastolic pressure should be avoided in patients with CAD who are being treated for hypertension.

▶ The existence and importance of a J-curve (excessive risk associated with lower diastolic blood pressure) in patients with CAD has been hotly debated for nearly 2 decades.[1,2] Many epidemiological studies have noted that, even in untreated patients, a low diastolic blood pressure is a poor prognostic sign, suggesting that the phenomenon is not treatment related. The Hypertension Optimal Treatment (HOT) study was designed to prospectively answer the question: 18,790 hypertensive patients were randomized to diastolic blood pressures of 90, 85, and 80 mm Hg or less, with the primary end point of myocardial infarction, stroke, or cardiovascular death. After a mean of 3.8 years, no significant difference was found across groups, showing that the lowest diastolic blood pressure target was neither harmful nor helpful,[3] and validating the time-honored blood pressure target (for uncomplicated hypertensive patients) of less than 140/90 mm Hg that has been reaffirmed in JNC 7.[4]

The authors' dataset was the largest ever collected in which patients with hypertension and CAD were randomized to 1 of 2 antihypertensive drug regimens. Since the regimens were said to be equivalent for the prevention of the primary end point (the first occurrence of all-cause mortality, nonfatal stroke, or myocardial infarction),[5] the randomized data were pooled and these post-hoc analyses were done to see if those who achieved the lower diastolic blood pressures had a higher risk of the primary end point than those with higher on-treatment blood pressures.

The authors point out that the risk of MI, but not stroke, increased significantly with the lowest on-treatment diastolic blood pressures, suggesting (but not proving) the finding to be specific.

In the grand scope of things, these data (however impressive) can hardly overrule the conclusion of a large, well-conducted prospective clinical trial (designed expressly to answer the question and analyzed by intent-to-treat methods) that did not find a significantly higher risk with a lower diastolic blood pressure. These data do, however, suggest that hypertension treatment should be carefully monitored in patients with known coronary disease and that excessive blood pressure reduction should be avoided whenever possible.

**W. J. Elliott, MD, PhD**

*References*

1. Cruickshank JM, Thorp JM, Zacharias FJ: Benefits and potential harm of lowering high blood pressure. *Lancet* 1:581-583, 1987.
2. Farnett L, Mulrow CD, Linn WD, et al: The J-curve phenomenon and the treatment of hypertension: Is there a point beyond which pressure reduction is dangerous? *JAMA* 265:489-495, 1991.

3. Hansson L, Zanchetti A, Carruthers SG, et al: Effects of intensive blood-pressure lowering and low dose aspirin in patients with hypertension: Principal results of the Hypertension Optimal Treatment (HOT) randomised trial. *Lancet* 351:1755-1762, 1998.

4. Seventh Report of the Joint National Committee on Prevention, Detection, Evaluation and Treatment of High Blood Pressure: National High Blood Pressure Education Program Coordinating Committee. *Hypertension* 42:1206-1252, 2003.

5. Pepine CJ, Handberg EM, Cooper-DeHoff RM, et al: A calcium antagonist vs. a non-calcium antagonist hypertension treatment strategy for patients with coronary artery disease: The International Verapamil-Trandolapril Study (INVEST): A randomized controlled trial. The INVEST Investigators. *JAMA* 290:2805-2816, 2003.

---

### Predictors of Adverse Outcome Among Patients With Hypertension and Coronary Artery Disease

Pepine CJ, for the INVEST Investigators (Univ of Florida, Gainesville; et al)
*J Am Coll Cardiol* 47:547-551, 2006                                1–44

---

*Objectives.*—We sought to determine predictors for adverse outcomes in hypertensive patients with coronary artery disease (CAD).

*Background.*—Factors leading to adverse outcomes in hypertensive patients with CAD are poorly understood. The INternational VErapamil-trandolapril STudy (INVEST) compared outcomes in hypertensive patients with CAD that were assigned randomly to either a verapamil sustained-release (SR)- or an atenolol-based strategy for blood pressure (BP) control. Trandolapril and hydrochlorothiazide were used as added agents. During follow-up (61,835 patient-years), BP control and the primary outcome (death, nonfatal myocardial infarction, and nonfatal stroke) were not different between strategies.

*Methods.*—We investigated risk for adverse outcome associated with baseline factors, follow-up BP, and drug treatments using Cox modeling.

*Results.*—Previous heart failure (adjusted hazard ratio [HR] 1.96), as well as diabetes (HR 1.77), increased age (HR 1.63), U.S. residency (HR 1.61), renal impairment (HR 1.50), stroke/transient ischemic attack (HR 1.43), smoking (HR 1.41), myocardial infarction (HR 1.34), peripheral vascular disease (HR 1.27), and revascularization (HR 1.15) predicted increased risk. Follow-up systolic BP <140 mm Hg or diastolic BP <90 mm Hg (HRs 0.82 or 0.70, respectively) and trandolapril with verapamil SR (HRs 0.78 and 0.79) were associated with reduced risk.

*Conclusions.*—In hypertensive patients with CAD, increased risk for adverse outcomes was associated with conditions related to the severity of CAD and diminished left ventricular function. Lower follow-up BP and addition of trandolapril to verapamil SR each were associated with reduced risk.

▶ This report presents a prespecified analysis of the original INVEST trial, which showed little difference in the primary end point (death, nonfatal myocardial infarction, or nonfatal stroke) across the 2 randomized arms.[1] Although the randomization was between initial atenolol or verapamil extended release, only about 17% of patients ended up taking monotherapy; hydrochlorothiazide or trandolapril (respectively) was added as second-line treatment as necessary.

The predictors of adverse clinical outcomes in the INVEST trial were more similar to the important prognostic indicators for heart disease than is typical for most clinical trials in uncomplicated hypertension. Five of the strongest predictors were existing cardiovascular disease at randomization: prior heart failure, myocardial infarction, stroke, peripheral vascular disease, or revascularization procedure. The others, however, were those typical of any high-risk population: older age, diabetes, chronic kidney disease, cigarette smoking, and (perhaps surprisingly) residence in the United States.

Perhaps most importantly, however, was the finding that lower blood pressure was associated with an improved prognosis, as was the use of combination antihypertensive drug therapy (which was likely the proximal cause of the lowered blood pressure). These data can be viewed as a mild contradiction to the J-shaped curve hypothesis (lowering blood pressure too far in a patient with coronary disease may lead to hypoperfusion of the coronary vessels and increased risk),[2] although this hypothesis was not directly tested in INVEST. Similarly, the addition of trandolapril to verapamil extended release in INVEST did seem to be beneficial (perhaps because it lowered blood pressure further), which was not the result for trandolapril in the PEACE trial.[3] Perhaps the most interesting outcome was in the group given low-dose verapamil plus low-dose trandolapril, which had a significantly lowered risk of the primary end point compared with those who received only low-dose atenolol. In other analyses, it was not possible to tease out the use of the drugs and their effects on blood pressure.[4] Nonetheless, it appears that most patients require multiple drugs to achieve the recommended blood pressure targets; other data suggest that in patients with coronary disease and hypertension, an angiotensin-converting enzyme inhibitor can be recommended, particularly if their other risk factors are not well controlled.[5,6]

**W. J. Elliott, MD, PhD**

*References*

1. Pepine CJ, Handberg EM, Cooper-DeHoff RM, et al: A calcium antagonist vs. a non-calcium antagonist hypertension treatment strategy for patients with coronary artery disease: The International Verapamil-Trandolapril Study (INVEST): A randomized controlled trial. The INVEST Investigators. *JAMA* 290:2805-2816, 2003.
2. Boutitie F, Gueyffier F, Pocock S, et al: J-shaped relationship between blood pressure and mortality in hypertensive patients: New insights from a meta-analysis of individual-patient data. *Ann Intern Med* 136:438-448, 2002.
3. Angiotensin-converting-enzyme inhibition in stable coronary artery disease. The PEACE Trial Investigators. *N Engl J Med* 351:2058-2068, 2004.
4. Elliott WJ, Hewkin AC, Kupfer S, et al: A drug dose model for predicting clinical outcomes in hypertensive coronary disease patients. *J Clin Hypertens (Greenwich)* 7:654-663, 2005.
5. Effects of an angiotensin-converting-enzyme inhibitor, ramipril, on death from cardiovascular causes, myocardial infarction, and stroke in high-risk patients. The Heart Outcomes Prevention Evaluation (HOPE) Study Investigators. *N Engl J Med* 342:145-153, 2000.

6. Fox KM, and the EUROPA investigators: Efficacy of perindopril in reduction of cardiovascular events among patients with stable coronary artery disease: Randomised, double-blind, placebo-controlled, multicentre trial (The EUROPA study). *Lancet* 362:782-788, 2003.

**Stop Hypertension With the Acupuncture Research Program (SHARP): Results of a Randomized, Controlled Clinical Trial**
Macklin EA, Wayne PM, Kalish LA, et al (New England Research Institutes, Watertown, Mass; New England School of Acupuncture, Watertown, Mass; Children's Hosp Boston; et al)
*Hypertension* 48:838-845, 2006                                          1–45

Case studies and small trials suggest that acupuncture may effectively treat hypertension, but no large randomized trials have been reported. The Stop Hypertension with the Acupuncture Research Program pilot trial enrolled 192 participants with untreated blood pressure (BP) in the range of 140/90 to 179/109 mm Hg. The design of the trial combined rigorous methodology and adherence to principles of traditional Chinese medicine. Participants were weaned off antihypertensives before enrollment and were then randomly assigned to 3 treatments: individualized traditional Chinese acupuncture, standardized acupuncture at preselected points, or invasive sham acupuncture. Participants received ≤12 acupuncture treatments over 6 to 8 weeks. During the first 10 weeks after random assignment, BP was monitored every 14 days, and antihypertensives were prescribed if BP exceeded 180/110 mm Hg. The mean BP decrease from baseline to 10 weeks, the primary end point, did not differ significantly between participants randomly assigned to active (individualized and standardized) versus sham acupuncture (systolic BP: −3.56 versus −3.84 mm Hg, respectively; 95% CI for the difference: −4.0 to 4.6 mm Hg; $P=0.90$; diastolic BP: −4.32 versus −2.81 mm Hg, 95% CI for the difference: −3.6 to 0.6 mm Hg; $P=0.16$). Categorizing participants by age, race, gender, baseline BP, history of antihypertensive use, obesity, or primary traditional Chinese medicine diagnosis did not reveal any subgroups for which the benefits of active acupuncture differed significantly from sham acupuncture. Active acupuncture provided no greater benefit than invasive sham acupuncture in reducing systolic or diastolic BP.

▶ Ouch! Many would like to believe that complementary and/or alternative medicines are natural and time tested and therefore would be much more acceptable to broad populations than chemicals synthesized in the laboratory, compressed into pills, taken orally, and then circulated throughout the body with the intent of having an allegedly specific effect. This study was organized to rigorously test the hypothesis that acupuncture, which has been used for millennia in China to lower blood pressure, stop smoking, control pain, and generally improve health would be superior to sham acupuncture. Sadly, this result was not seen in this study.

Proponents of complementary and alternative medicine typically discredit these sorts of studies. They would point to the lowering in blood pressures seen for all 3 groups during the first 10 weeks of the study as clear and convincing evidence of the efficacy of acupuncture. In addition, about 45% of the subjects receiving acupuncture were able to avoid antihypertensive pills for 1 year. Advocates of acupuncture would emphasize that it is traditionally one of several modalities used by holistic practitioners, and the effects of the needles should not be studied independently of the entire good health program they offer. They might say that continued acupuncture treatment is more likely to be effective than 10 weeks of acupuncture. They would likely criticize the choice of the "control" intervention, which in fact, did involve placing needles into points that are not traditionally associated with therapeutic acupuncture in China. They might even criticize the ability of the principal attending acupuncturist to determine the appropriate points for needle placement in those randomized to individualized acupuncture, despite his or her Chinese training and more than 12 years of experience. They would certainly object to the placement of needles into points not traditionally recommended by Chinese acupuncture as being nonstandard and potentially unethical, since most acupuncturists encourage patients to take antihypertensive medications until they are no longer necessary during and after a course of acupuncture.[1] Blinding of the subject to the treatments was not particularly effective, as the comparison for those who guessed their treatment assignment was nearly significant.

There are nonetheless many reasons to consider this study in a positive light. The authors designed and executed an invasive control arm, which seems to be a reasonable strategy to compare 2 invasive treatments.[2] They also followed their subjects for 1 year after randomization to compare the incidence of antihypertensive drug therapy across arms in an effort to detect a significant latent effect of acupuncture, which was not found. They might have performed ambulatory blood pressure monitoring at baseline and after 10 weeks of treatment to increase statistical power, but at a rather large cost. Blood tests for glucose and lipid control, as well as quality of life questionnaires, were not different across the 3 randomized arms. All in all, it seems that the authors' conclusions that "active acupuncture provided no greater benefit than invasive sham acupuncture in reducing systolic or diastolic blood pressure" are well-supported by their data.

**W. J. Elliott, MD, PhD**

*References*

1. Yin CS, Seo BK, Park HJ, et al: Acupuncture, a promising adjunctive therapy for essential hypertension: A double-blind, randomized, controlled trial. *Neurol Res* 29(Suppl 1):98-103, 2007.
2. Kaptchuk TJ: The placebo effect in alternative medicine: Can the performance of a healing ritual have clinical significance? *Ann Intern Med* 136:817-826, 2002.

### Improving Blood Pressure Control through Provider Education, Provider Alerts, and Patient Education: A Cluster Randomized Trial

Roumie CL, Elasy TA, Greevy R, et al (Vanderbilt Univ, Nashville, Tenn; VA Med Ctr, Nashville, Tenn)
*Ann Intern Med* 145:165-175, 2006                                         1–46

*Background.*—Inadequate blood pressure control is a persistent gap in quality care.

*Objective.*—To evaluate provider and patient interventions to improve blood pressure control.

*Design.*—Cluster randomized, controlled trial.

*Setting.*—2 hospital-based and 8 community-based clinics in the Veterans Affairs Tennessee Valley Healthcare System.

*Patients.*—1341 veterans with essential hypertension cared for by 182 providers. Eligible patients had 2 or more blood pressure measurements greater than 140/90 mm Hg in a 6-month period and were taking a single antihypertensive agent.

*Intervention.*—Providers who cared for eligible patients were randomly assigned to receive an e-mail with a Web-based link to the Seventh Report of the Joint National Committee on the Prevention, Detection, Evaluation and Treatment of High Blood Pressure (JNC 7) guidelines (provider education); provider education and a patient-specific hypertension computerized alert (provider education and alert); or provider education, hypertension alert, and patient education, in which patients were sent a letter advocating drug adherence, lifestyle modification, and conversations with providers (patient education).

*Measurements.*—Proportion of patients with a systolic blood pressure less than 140 mm Hg at 6 months; intensification of antihypertensive medication.

*Results.*—Mean baseline blood pressure was 157/83 mm Hg with no differences between groups ($P = 0.105$). Six-month follow-up data were available for 975 patients (73%). Patients of providers who were randomly assigned to the patient education group had better blood pressure control (138/75 mm Hg) than those in the provider education and alert or provider education alone groups (146/76 mm Hg and 145/78 mm Hg, respectively). More patients in the patient education group had a systolic blood pressure of 140 mm Hg or less compared with those in the provider education or provider education and alert groups (adjusted relative risk for the patient education group compared with the provider education alone group, 1.31 [95% CI, 1.06 to 1.62]; $P = 0.012$).

*Limitations.*—Follow-up blood pressure measurements were missing for 27% of study patients. The study could not detect a mechanism by which patient education improved blood pressure control.

*Conclusions.*—A multifactorial intervention including patient education improved blood pressure control compared with provider education alone.

▶ Historically, the United States Department of Veterans Affairs (VA) has played a leading role in demonstrating the benefits of antihypertensive drug therapy[1-3] and was the largest provider of research subjects in the recent Antihypertensive and Lipid-Lowering treatment to prevent Heart Attack Trial (ALLHAT).[4,5] Improving blood pressure control has become an important priority in the VA since 1998.[6] Several datasets have now shown very high rates of blood pressure control in VA clinics, about 50% to 70% higher than those of the general US population.[7,8]

The findings of this report showing improved blood pressure control in the group randomized to patient education is somewhat surprising, given the fact that other studies have not shown much improvement with similar interventions.[9] The fact that the improvement was small in the group that received both provider education and an alert may result from the fact that awareness of the importance of blood pressure control was already at a very high level in the VA clinics that were studied. Other studies have shown significant and potentially important improvements in blood pressure control when an alert is provided to the provider at the point of service when blood pressure control was found to be suboptimal just moments before. A similar program of both provider and patient education will soon be reported from a much larger study also performed in the VA, which may provide more answers on how to best control blood pressure in large, at-risk populations.[10]

**W. J. Elliott, MD, PhD**

*References*

1. Veterans Administration Cooperative Study Group on Antihypertensive Agents: Effects of treatment on morbidity in hypertension: Results in patients with diastolic blood pressure averaging 115 through 129 mm Hg. *JAMA* 202:1028-1034, 1967.
2. Veterans Administration Cooperative Study Group on Antihypertensive Agents. Effects of treatment on morbidity in hypertension. II. Results in patients with diastolic blood pressure averaging 90 through 114 mm Hg. *JAMA* 213:1143-1152, 1970.
3. Materson BJ, et al for the Department of Veterans Affairs Cooperative Study Group on Antihypertensive Agents: Single-drug therapy for hypertension in men. *N Engl J Med* 328:914-921, 1993.
4. Pressel S, Davis BR, Louis GT, et al: Participant recruitment in the Antihypertensive and Lipid-Lowering Treatment to Prevent Heart Attack Trial (ALLHAT). The ALLHAT Collaborative Research Group. *Con Clin Trials* 22:674-686, 2001.
5. Grimm RH Jr, Margolis KL, Papademetriou V, et al: Baseline characteristics of participants in the Antihypertensive and Lipid-Lowering Treatment to Prevent Heart Attack Trial (ALLHAT). The ALLHAT Collaborative Research Group. *Hypertension* 37:19-27, 2001.
6. Berlowitz DR, Ash AS, Hickey C, et al: Inadequate management of blood pressure in a hypertensive population. *N Engl J Med* 339:1967-1963, 1998.
7. Rehman SU, Hutchison FN, Hendrix K, et al: Ethnic differences in blood pressure control among men at Veterans Affairs clinics and other health care sites. *Arch Intern Med* 165:1041-1047, 2005.
8. Cheung BMY, Ong KL, Man YB, et al: Prevalence, awareness, treatment and control of hypertension: United States National Health and Nutrition Examination Survey, 2001-2002. *J Clin Hypertens* 8:93-98, 2006.
9. Hibbard JH: Engaging healthcare consumers to improve the quality of care. *Med Care* 41:I61-I70, 2003.

10. Bosworth HB, Olsen MK, Goldstein MK, et al: The Veterans' study to improve the control of hypertension (V-STITCH). *Contemp Clin Trials* 26:155-168, 2005.

### Efficacy and Safety of Benazepril for Advanced Chronic Renal Insufficiency

Hou FF, Zhang X, Zhang GH, et al (Southern Med Univ, Guangzhou, China)
*N Engl J Med* 354:131-140, 2006                                    1–47

*Background.*—Angiotensin-converting–enzyme inhibitors provide renal protection in patients with mild-to-moderate renal insufficiency (serum creatinine level, 3.0 mg per deciliter or less). We assessed the efficacy and safety of benazepril in patients without diabetes who had advanced renal insufficiency.

*Methods.*—We enrolled 422 patients in a randomized, double-blind study. After an eight-week run-in period, 104 patients with serum creatinine levels of 1.5 to 3.0 mg per deciliter (group 1) received 20 mg of benazepril per day, whereas 224 patients with serum creatinine levels of 3.1 to 5.0 mg per deciliter (group 2) were randomly assigned to receive 20 mg of benazepril per day (112 patients) or placebo (112 patients) and then followed for a mean of 3.4 years. All patients received conventional antihypertensive therapy. The primary outcome was the composite of a doubling of the serum creatinine level, end-stage renal disease, or death. Secondary end points included changes in the level of proteinuria and the rate of progression of renal disease.

*Results.*—Of 102 patients in group 1, 22 (22 percent) reached the primary end point, as compared with 44 of 108 patients given benazepril in group 2 (41 percent) and 65 of 107 patients given placebo in group 2 (60 percent). As compared with placebo, benazepril was associated with a 43 percent reduction in the risk of the primary end point in group 2 (P=0.005). This benefit did not appear to be attributable to blood-pressure control. Benazepril therapy was associated with a 52 percent reduction in the level of proteinuria and a reduction of 23 percent in the rate of decline in renal function. The overall incidence of major adverse events in the benazepril and placebo subgroups of group 2 was similar.

*Conclusions.*—Benazepril conferred substantial renal benefits in patients without diabetes who had advanced renal insufficiency.

▶ These data confirm and extend a somewhat similar trial carried out in Europe and published in the same journal almost 10 years ago,[1] as well as patient-level meta-analyses of angiotensin-converting enzyme (ACE) inhibitors in non-diabetic patients with chronic kidney disease.[2,3] This study is important for several reasons: (1) These authors randomized 224 patients (in group 2) with serum creatinine levels between 3.1 and 5.0 mg/dL to either benazepril 10 mg twice daily or placebo, given in addition to other antihypertensive drugs required to achieve goal blood pressure (less than 130/80 mm Hg). Patients with such an advanced degree of renal impairment had not previously been studied;

many felt that ACE inhibitors are contraindicated in patients with advanced renal disease because of concerns about acute increases in serum creatinine immediately after beginning treatment. (2) These authors also continued giving the ACE inhibitor, even when the patient's serum creatinine level increased. The current recommendation is to consider discontinuation of a renin-angiotensin-aldosterone inhibitor if serum creatinine increases more than 25% to 30% over baseline[4]; sadly, many physicians have a much lower threshold for discontinuing these renoprotective drugs. These data therefore indicate benefits from initiating and continuing ACE inhibitor therapy for patients with stage 4 chronic kidney disease (estimated glomerular filtration rate between 15 and 29 mL/min/1.73 m$^2$). (3) The authors took great pains in the design and execution of the study to make and keep the blood pressures in the randomized groups similar. There was a 3-step run-in phase before randomization: 8 weeks of benazepril 10 mg/d, then 4 weeks of benazepril 10 mg twice daily (if tolerated), during which alternative antihypertensive drug therapy was optimized, followed by discontinuation of benazepril for 3 weeks, with further titration of alternative antihypertensive drug therapy. Blood pressure declined in both randomized groups (from approximately 152/86 to 130/75 mm Hg) and was not significantly different between the 2 groups ($P = 0.18$). The authors concluded, therefore, contrary to a recent systematic review and meta-analysis,[5] that the benefits of benazepril in advanced renal impairment were unrelated to its blood pressure–lowering effects. (4) The authors noted a surprisingly low frequency of hyperkalemia (only 5%, with 3 of the 112 subjects withdrawing from therapy because of it). This could perhaps be attributed to exclusion of about 5% of patients for incident hyperkalemia during the open-label benazepril run-in period, relatively low dietary potassium intake in Chinese versus Western populations, and/or high prevalence of diuretic treatment (about 80% versus only about 40% in the Modification of Diet in Renal Disease study[6]). (5) Fully 17% (72 of the 422) of the patients who entered the open-label benazepril treatment period had the drug discontinued because of dry cough. Many prior studies have shown a higher incidence of cough (and discontinuation because of it) in Asians[7,8] and African Americans[9] than in non-Hispanic whites. (6) As with most other studies, the improvement in the primary outcome in this study (doubling of serum creatinine, end-stage renal disease, or death) was paralleled by a reduction in urinary protein excretion (by about 50% compared with baseline in the benazepril group), which many have recommended as a useful surrogate for progressive renal impairment.[10]

The unusual aspects of this study include twice-daily benazepril with a total daily dose of only 20 mg (half the maximal dose), the avoidance of placebo in the 141 subjects with initial serum creatinine levels of 1.5 to 3.0 mg/dL (all of whom were treated with benazepril), and the low reported dietary protein intake at baseline (compared with Western populations).

These data do provide evidence that using ACE inhibitors in patients with advanced chronic kidney disease is beneficial and suggests that they should not be stopped because of apparent decline in estimated glomerular filtration rate.

**W. J. Elliott, MD, PhD**

*References*

1. Maschio G, Alberti D, Janin G, et al: Effect of the angiotensin-converting-enzyme inhibitor benazepril on the progression of chronic renal insufficiency. The Angiotensin-Converting-Enzyme Inhibition in Progressive Renal Insufficiency Study Group. *N Engl J Med* 334:939-945, 1996.
2. Jafar TH, Schmid CH, Landa M, et al: Angiotensin-converting enzyme inhibitors and progression of nondiabetic renal disease: A meta-analysis of patient-level data. *Ann Intern Med* 135:73-87, 2001.
3. Jafar TH, Stark PC, Schmid CH, et al: Progression of chronic kidney disease: The role of blood pressure control, proteinuria, and angiotensin-converting enzyme inhibition: A patient-level meta-analysis. *Ann Intern Med* 139:244-252, 2003.
4. Bakris GL, Weir MR: Angiotensin-converting enzyme inhibitor-associated elevations in serum creatinine: Is this a cause for concern? *Arch Intern Med* 160:685-693, 2000.
5. Casas JP, Chua W, Loukogeorgakis S, et al: Effect of inhibitors of the renin-angiotensin system and other antihypertensive drugs on renal outcomes: Systematic review and meta-analysis. *Lancet* 366:2026-2033, 2005.
6. Klahr S, Levey AS, Beck GJ, et al: The effects of dietary protein restriction and blood-pressure control on the progression of chronic renal disease. Modification of Diet in Renal Disease Study Group. *N Engl J Med* 330:877-884, 1994.
7. Sesoko S, Kaneko Y: Cough associated with the use of captopril. *Arch Intern Med* 145:1524, 1985.
8. Woo KS, Norris RM, Nicholls G: Racial difference in incidence of cough with angiotensin-converting enzyme inhibitors (a tale of two cities). *Am J Cardiol* 75:967-968, 1995.
9. Elliott WJ: Higher incidence of discontinuation of ACE-inhibitors due to cough in blacks. *Clin Pharmacol Ther* 60:582-588, 1996.
10. K/DOQI clinical practice guidelines on hypertension and antihypertensive agents in chronic kidney disease. *Am J Kidney Dis* 43(5 suppl 2):1-290, 2004.

---

**Cardiovascular Outcomes in High-Risk Hypertensive Patients Stratified by Baseline Glomerular Filtration Rate**

Rahman M, for the ALLHAT Collaborative Research Group (Case Western Reserve Univ, Cleveland, Ohio; et al)
*Ann Intern Med* 144:172-180, 2006                                          1–48

---

*Background.*—Chronic kidney disease is common in older patients with hypertension.

*Objective.*—To compare rates of coronary heart disease (CHD) and end-stage renal disease (ESRD) events; to determine whether glomerular filtration rate (GFR) independently predicts risk for CHD; and to report the efficacy of first-step treatment with a calcium-channel blocker (amlodipine) or an angiotensin-converting enzyme inhibitor (lisinopril), each compared with a diuretic (chlorthalidone), in modifying cardiovascular disease (CVD) outcomes in high-risk patients with hypertension stratified by GFR.

*Design.*—Post hoc subgroup analysis.

*Setting.*—Multicenter randomized, double-blind, controlled trial.

*Participants.*—Persons with hypertension who were 55 years of age or older with 1 or more risk factors for CHD and who were stratified into 3 baseline GFR groups: normal or increased ($\geq$ 90 mL/min per 1.73 m²; $n =$

8126 patients), mild reduction (60 to 89 mL/min per 1.73 m$^2$; $n = 18,109$ patients), and moderate or severe reduction (< 60 mL/min per 1.73 m$^2$; $n = 5662$ patients).

*Interventions.*—Random assignment to chlorthalidone, amlodipine, or lisinopril.

*Measurements.*—Rates of ESRD, CHD, stroke, and combined CVD (CHD, coronary revascularization, angina, stroke, heart failure, and peripheral arterial disease).

*Results.*—In participants with a moderate to severe reduction in GFR, 6-year rates were higher for CHD than for ESRD (15.4% vs. 6.0%, respectively). A baseline GFR of less than 53 mL/min per 1.73 m$^2$ (compared with > 104 mL/min per 1.73 m$^2$) was independently associated with a 32% higher risk for CHD. Amlodipine was similar to chlorthalidone in reducing CHD (16.0% vs. 15.2%, respectively; hazard ratio, 1.06 [95% CI, 0.89 to 1.27]), stroke, and combined CVD (CHD, coronary revascularization, angina, stroke, heart failure, and peripheral arterial disease), but less effective in preventing heart failure. Lisinopril was similar to chlorthalidone in preventing CHD (15.1% vs. 15.2%, respectively; hazard ratio, 1.00 [CI, 0.84 to 1.20]), but was less effective in reducing stroke, combined CVD events, and heart failure.

*Limitations.*—Proteinuria data were not available, and combination therapies were not tested.

*Conclusions.*—Older high-risk patients with hypertension and reduced GFR are more likely to develop CHD than to develop ESRD. A low GFR independently predicts increased risk for CHD. Neither amlodipine nor lisinopril is superior to chlorthalidone in preventing CHD, stroke, or combined CVD, and chlorthalidone is superior to both for preventing heart failure, independent of level of renal function.

▶ Although these analyses were performed post hoc, the first major conclusion was that, even in older hypertensive patients with moderate to severe reductions in estimated GFR calculated by the simplified Modification of Diet in Renal Disease equation,[1] the risk of cardiovascular events was higher than for dialysis or transplantation. This is important because prior trials had shown that angiotensin-converting enzyme inhibitors and/or angiotensin II receptor blockers were quite effective in preventing the progression of renal disease in non-diabetics[2] or type 1 diabetics[3] and type 2 diabetics,[4,5] respectively. Because ALLHAT excluded patients with baseline serum creatinine levels greater than 2.0 mg/dL, it provided no data about the relative risk of cardiovascular versus renal events in those with stage 4 or 5 chronic kidney disease (as defined by the Kidney Disease Outcomes Quality Initiative: estimated GFR less than 30 mL/min/1.73 m$^2$).[6] This situation contrasts with the results of the Irbesartan Diabetic Nephropathy Trial (IDNT), and the Reduction of Endpoints in Non-Insulin Dependent Diabetes Mellitus with the Angiotensin II Antagonist Losartan (RENAAL) trials,[4,5] in which the risk of end-stage renal disease was, on average, about 60% higher than the risk of myocardial infarction or stroke.

The second important message from these analyses corroborates many other studies. Chronic kidney disease is a significant and graded risk factor for cardiovascular events: the worse the renal excretory function, the higher the risk for cardiovascular events. The potential confounder here is age, but future analyses are likely to assess whether estimated GFR predicts prognosis in ALLHAT, independent of age.

The third important message is that the overall conclusion of ALLHAT ("superiority of the thiazide-like diuretic in preventing one or more major forms of cardiovascular disease") was not contradicted in any subgroup and is independent of baseline renal function.[7]

**W. J. Elliott, MD, PhD**

*References*

1. Levey AS, Greene T, Kusek J, et al: A simplified equation to predict glomerular filtration rate from serum creatinine [abstract]. *J Am Soc Nephrol 11:A0828, 2000.*
2. Jafar TH, Stark PC, Schmid CH, et al: Progression of chronic kidney disease: The role of blood pressure control, proteinuria, and angiotensin-converting enzyme inhibition: A patient-level meta-analysis. *Ann Intern Med* 139:244-252, 2003.
3. Lewis EJ, Hunsicker LG, Bain RP, et al: The effect of angiotensin-converting-enzyme inhibition on diabetic nephropathy. The Collaborative Study Group. *N Engl J Med* 329:1456-1462, 1993.
4. Lewis EJ, Hunsicker LG, Clarke WR, et al: Renoprotective effect of the angiotensin-receptor antagonist irbesartan in patients with nephropathy due to type 2 diabetes. Collaborative Study Group. *N Engl J Med* 345:851-860, 2001.
5. Brenner BM, Cooper ME, de Zeeuw D, et al: Effects of losartan on renal and cardiovascular outcomes in patients with type 2 diabetes and nephropathy. Reduction of Endpoints in Non-Insulin Dependent Diabetes Mellitus with the Angiotensin II Antagonist Losartan (RENAAL) Study Group. *N Engl J Med* 345:861-869, 2001.
6. National Kidney Foundation: K/DOQI Clinical practice guidelines on hypertension and antihypertensive agents in chronic kidney disease. *Am J Kidney Dis* 43(suppl 1):S1-S290, 2004.
7. Major outcomes in high-risk hypertensive patients randomized to angiotensin-converting enzyme inhibitor or calcium channel blocker vs. diuretic: The Antihypertensive and Lipid Lowering Treatment to Prevent Heart Attack Trial (ALLHAT). The ALLHAT Officers and Coordinators for the ALLHAT Collaborative Research Group. *JAMA* 288:2981-2997, 2002.

---

**Effect of inhibitors of the renin-angiotensin system and other antihypertensive drugs on renal outcomes: systematic review and meta-analysis**
Casas JP, Chua W, Loukogeorgakis S, et al (Univ College London; London School of Hygiene & Tropical Medicine)
*Lancet* 366:2026-2033, 2005                                                    1–49

---

*Background.*—A consensus has emerged that angiotensin-converting-enzyme (ACE) inhibitors and angiotensin-II receptor blockers (ARBs) have specific renoprotective effects. Guidelines specify that these are the drugs of choice for the treatment of hypertension in patients with renal disease. We sought to determine to what extent this consensus is supported by the available evidence.

*Methods.*—Electronic databases were searched up to January, 2005, for randomised trials assessing antihypertensive drugs and progression of renal disease. Effects on primary discrete endpoints (doubling of creatinine and end-stage renal disease) and secondary continuous markers of renal outcomes (creatinine, albuminuria, and glomerular filtration rate) were calculated with random-effect models. The effects of ACE inhibitors or ARBs in placebo-controlled trials were compared with the effects seen in trials that used an active comparator drug.

*Findings.*—Comparisons of ACE inhibitors or ARBs with other antihypertensive drugs yielded a relative risk of 0.71 (95% CI 0.49–1.04) for doubling of creatinine and a small benefit on end-stage renal disease (relative risk 0.87, 0.75–0.99). Analyses of the results by study size showed a smaller benefit in large studies. In patients with diabetic nephropathy, no benefit was seen in comparative trials of ACE inhibitors or ARBs on the doubling of creatinine (1.09, 0.55–2.15), end-stage renal disease (0.89, 0.74–1.07), glomerular filtration rate, or creatinine amounts. Placebo-controlled trials of ACE inhibitors or ARBs showed greater benefits than comparative trials on all renal outcomes, but were accompanied by substantial reductions in blood pressure in favour of ACE inhibitors or ARBs.

*Interpretation.*—The benefits of ACE inhibitors or ARBs on renal outcomes in placebo-controlled trials probably result from a blood-pressure-lowering effect. In patients with diabetes, additional renoprotective actions of these substances beyond lowering blood pressure remain unproven, and there is uncertainty about the greater renoprotection seen in non-diabetic renal disease.

▶ The authors of this study must have been skeptical of recent clinical trials[1-4] and meta-analyses[5,6] that were specifically designed to answer their question of whether the retardation of the progression of chronic kidney disease was significantly improved with blockers of the renin-angiotensin-aldosterone system, as opposed to other antihypertensive drugs, in a manner that was independent of the blood pressure lowering seen in the trials. One might argue that this question was most directly answered (in the affirmative) by the comparison of the irbesartan versus amlodipine groups in the Irbesartan Diabetic Nephropathy Trial.[1] In that study, despite a similar blood pressure reduction (from 160/87 mm Hg or 159/87 mm Hg to 140/77 mm Hg or 141/77 mm Hg, respectively), irbesartan was significantly better (by 23%, $P = .006$) than amlodipine in preventing the composite primary (renal) end point of doubling of serum creatinine, end-stage renal disease, or death. Similarly, in the African American Study of Kidney Diseases and Hypertension, ramipril was significantly better than either amlodipine or metoprolol in preventing the decline in glomerular filtration rate from months 3 to 36, despite very small differential blood pressure reduction across the arms of the trial.[2] A third randomized, clinical trial recently reported better renal outcomes with benazepril (vs placebo) that were allegedly independent of blood pressure control.[3] This study was not included in the authors' analyses, as it was published a month later. A randomized clinical trial showed no significant benefit to lowering blood pressure beyond about 140/90 mm Hg in ACE inhibitor–treated patients with chronic kidney disease.[4]

Recent patient-level meta-analyses of the several trials that compared an ACE inhibitor with placebo (each in combination with other antihypertensive agents) in patients with nondiabetic renal disease have also indicated a significant benefit of the ACE inhibitor, allegedly independently of the blood pressure reductions seen in each group.[5,6] Lastly, many were favorably impressed by the conclusions of the COOPERATE study, which showed additional benefits in nondiabetics with chronic kidney disease in both proteinuria and time to doubling of serum creatinine or end-stage renal disease when an ACE inhibitor was given with an ARB.[7] In this study, there were no differences in blood pressures across the 3 years of follow-up in these groups.

These authors have nonetheless pooled data from all the trials they could find and have concluded that blood pressure control is very important for retarding the progression of chronic kidney disease, which is not a very surprising finding. The most impressive evidence for this is found in a figure in their study that clearly shows that the degree of protection against end-stage renal disease across trials is related to the degree of blood pressure lowering observed across treatment arms. They claimed, however, that they were unable to identify a "blood pressure independent effect" of ACE inhibitors or ARBs in their analyses.

The authors did not perform any meta-regression analyses, as has been done by others trying to answer similar questions about cardiovascular event protection "beyond blood pressure control" due to specific types of antihypertensive drugs.[8-11] It is admittedly difficult to tease out small differences in the face of large differences in outcomes because of differential blood pressure lowering across randomized groups. It is likely that this report will spur others to perform these and more complex statistical calculations to reexamine the question about blood pressure–independent effects of ACE inhibitors and ARBs in protecting the kidney. Even before then, however, it is unlikely that any informed person, including these authors, should or would refuse an ACE inhibitor or an ARB if he or she were to develop chronic kidney disease.

**W. J. Elliott, MD, PhD**

*References*

1. Lewis EJ, Hunsicker LG, Clarke WR, et al: Renoprotective effect of the angiotensin-receptor antagonist irbesartan in patients with nephropathy due to type 2 diabetes. Collaborative Study Group. *N Engl J Med* 345:851-860, 2001.
2. Wright JT Jr, Bakris GL, Greene T, et al: Effect of blood pressure lowering and antihypertensive drug class on progression of hypertensive kidney disease: Results from the AASK Trial. *JAMA* 288:2421-2431, 2002.
3. Hou FF, Zhang X, Zhang GH, et al: Efficacy and safety of benazepril in advanced renal insufficiency. *N Engl J Med* 354:131-140, 2006.
4. Ruggenenti P, Perna A, Loriga G, et al: Blood-pressure control for renoprotection in patients with non-diabetic chronic renal disease (REIN-2): Multicentre, randomised controlled trial. *Lancet* 365:939-946, 2005.

5. Jafar TH, Schmid CH, Landa M, et al: Angiotensin-converting enzyme inhibitors and progression of nondiabetic renal disease: A meta-analysis of patient-level data. *Ann Intern Med* 135:73-87, 2001.
6. Jafar TH, Stark PC, Schmid CH, et al: Progression of chronic kidney disease: The role of blood pressure control, proteinuria, and angiotensin-converting enzyme inhibition: A patient-level meta-analysis. *Ann Intern Med* 139:244-252, 2003.
7. Nakao N, Yoshimura A, Morita H, et al: Combination treatment of angiotensin-II receptor blocker and angiotensin-converting-enzyme inhibitor in non-diabetic renal disease (COOPERATE): A randomised controlled trial. *Lancet* 361:117-124, 2003.
8. Staessen JA, Wang J-G, Thijs L: Cardiovascular prevention and blood pressure reduction: A quantitative overview updated until 01 March 2003. *J Hypertension* 21:1005-1076, 2003.
9. Turnbull F: Blood Pressure Lowering Treatment Trialists' Collaboration. Effects of different blood-pressure-lowering regimens on major cardiovascular events: Results of prospectively-designed overviews of randomised trials. *Lancet* 362:1527-1535, 2003.
10. Verdecchia P, Reboldi G, Angeli F, et al: Angiotensin-converting enzyme inhibitors and calcium channel blockers for coronary heart disease and stroke prevention. *Hypertension* 46:386-392, 2005.
11. Elliott WJ, Jonsson MC, Black HR: It's NOT beyond the blood pressure, it IS the blood pressure! *Circulation* 2006. In press.

## Long-Term Renoprotective Effects of Standard Versus High Doses of Telmisartan in Hypertensive Nondiabetic Nephropathies

Aranda P, Segura J, Ruilope LM, et al (Hosp Regional Universitario Carlos Haya, Málaga, Spain; Hosp Universitario 12 de Octubre, Madrid)
*Am J Kidney Dis* 46:1074-1079, 2005                    1–50

*Background.*—This report describes an open randomized study intended to evaluate the long-term renoprotective effects of "standard" (80 mg once daily) versus "high" (80 mg twice daily) doses of telmisartan in hypertensive patients without diabetes with biopsy-proven chronic proteinuric nephropathies.

*Methods.*—We included 78 patients (age, 43.5 ± 13.2 years; 71.8% men). After a 4-week wash-out period, patients were randomly assigned to telmisartan, 80 mg once daily (n = 40) or 80 mg twice daily (n = 38), during a mean follow-up of 24.6 ± 2.2 months.

*Results.*—Baseline characteristics were similar in both groups, including blood pressure, renal function, and proteinuria. Blood pressure control did not differ between groups during follow-up. In the group administered telmisartan, 80 mg once daily, serum creatinine level increased from 1.6 ± 0.6 to 2.7 ± 0.9 mg/dL (141 ± 52 to 239 ± 80 μmol/L), and estimated creatinine clearance declined from 68 ± 30 to 50 ± 34 mL/min (1.13 ± 0.50 to 0.83 ± 0.57 mL/s), whereas in those administered 80 mg twice daily, serum creatinine (1.6 ± 0.7 to 1.6 ± 0.8 mg/dL [141 ± 62 to 141 ± 71 μmol/L]) and estimated creatinine clearance values (67 ± 38 to 74 ± 38 mL/min [1.12 ± 0.63 to 1.23 ± 0.63 mL/s]) did not change during the study. The decrease in proteinuria was more pronounced ($P < 0.01$) in patients administered the high dose of telmisartan compared with those treated with the standard dose. Serum potassium levels and lipid profiles did not change significantly in either group.

*Conclusion.*—Long-term administration of high doses of telmisartan seems to improve the efficacy of the drug to decrease proteinuria and slow the progression to end-stage renal failure in nondiabetic hypertensive renal disease.

▶ This may be the first successful trial of a supratherapeutic (ie, higher than that typically used in treatment of hypertension) dose of an angiotensin II receptor blocker (ARB) on proteinuria and estimated renal function in nondiabetic hypertensive patients with chronic kidney disease. Prior studies have shown a major benefit of angiotensin converting enzyme (ACE) inhibitors in this condition (with or without hypertension),[1] and one Japanese study showed further benefit by adding a full-dose ARB to what is considered (in Japan) a full dose of an ACE inhibitor.[2] Although there are many high-dose ARB studies that have been planned and/or are in progress, this open-label, usual clinical experience randomized trial does suggest that the more rigorous studies may also be positive. Until now, the published experience with big versus small dose ARBs in nephropathy consisted of only 3 trials: one compared losartan 100 versus 150 mg once daily in diabetics,[3] a second compared candesartan 16 versus 32 mg once daily in diabetics,[4] and the third compared candesartan 64 versus 16 mg/d in nondiabetics.[5] Each study had its shortcomings: the short serum half-life and relatively low-doses of losartan, the smaller-than-desired doses of candesartan, and a short-term evaluation of only proteinuria in 32 patients, respectively.

We can expect to see more of these sorts of studies reported soon, but nearly all are or will be performed outside the United States. The US Food and Drug Administration has approved antihypertensive drugs to prevent progression of kidney disease only in trials that used doubling of serum creatinine, end-stage renal disease, or death as the primary end point.[6,7] The agency has yet to accept proteinuria or albuminuria as a useful marker of severity of kidney disease (despite the recent Kidney Disease Outcomes and Quality Initiative guidelines),[8] and this has limited the enthusiasm of most pharmaceutical companies for performing these sorts of studies. We await the publication of more studies of this type to see if ARBs in higher-than-usual doses really do have beneficial effects in preventing the progression of hypertensive nephropathy.

**W. J. Elliott, MD, PhD**

*References*

1. Jafar TH, Stark PC, Schmid CH, et al: Progression of chronic kidney disease: The role of blood pressure control, proteinuria, and angiotensin-converting enzyme inhibition: A patient-level meta-analysis. *Ann Intern Med* 139:244-252, 2003.
2. Nakao N, Yoshimura A, Morita H, et al: Combination treatment of angiotensin-II receptor blocker and angiotensin-converting-enzyme inhibitor in non-diabetic renal disease (COOPERATE): A randomised controlled trial. *Lancet* 361:117-124, 2003.
3. Andersen S, Rossing P, Juhl TR, et al: Optimal dose of losartan for renoprotection in diabetic nephropathy. *Nephrol Dial Transplant* 17:1413-1418, 2002.

4. Rossing K, Christensen PK, Hansen BV, et al: Optimal dose of candesartan for renoprotection in type 2 diabetic patients with nephropathy: A double-blind, randomised crossover study. *Diabetes Care* 26:150-155, 2003.

5. Schmeider RE, Klingbeil AU, Fleischmann EH, et al: Additional antiproteinuric effect of ultrahigh dose candesartan: A double-blind randomized prospective study. *J Am Soc Nephrol* 16:3038-3045, 2005.

6. Brenner BM, Cooper ME, de Zeeuw D, et al: Effects of losartan on renal and cardiovascular outcomes in patients with type 2 diabetes and nephropathy. Reduction of Endpoints in Non-Insulin Dependent Diabetes Mellitus with the Angiotensin II Antagonist Losartan (RENAAL) Study Group. *N Engl J Med* 345:861-869, 2001.

7. Lewis EJ, Hunsicker LG, Clarke WR, et al: Renoprotective effect of the angiotensin-receptor antagonist irbesartan in patients with nephropathy due to Type 2 diabetes. Collaborative Study Group. *N Engl J Med* 345:851-860, 2001.

8. Levey AS, Rocco MV, Anderson S, et al: K/DOQI Clinical Practice Guidelines on Hypertension and Antihypertensive Agents in Chronic Kidney Disease. *Am J Kidney Dis* 43(suppl 1):S1-S290, 2004.

# 2 Pediatric Cardiovascular Disease

## Introduction

Again, it was a banner year in advances in pediatric cardiovascular disease. There is continued interest in the long-term follow-up after surgery for complex conditions, such as tetralogy of Fallot, complete transposition of the great arteries, congenitally corrected transposition of the great arteries, hypoplastic left heart syndrome, and various single ventricle entities. Issues include late arrhythmias, ventricular function abnormalities, valvular lesions, aortic dilatation, conduit issues, and outflow or inflow obstruction. The extra cardiac Fontan continues to gain acceptance although the lateral tunnel procedure has served and continues to serve many patients quite well. Cardiac magnetic resonance imaging is playing a larger role in the preoperative and postoperative management of many patients with excellent images, 3-dimensional reconstruction of chambers and vessels , flow studies, and tissue characterization using delayed gadolinium enhancement.

A novel contribution from Toronto indicates that remote ischemic preconditioning using limb ischemia may promote improved myocardial protection during cardiac surgery—a potentially major new breakthrough.

Thomas P. Graham, MD

## Tetralogy of Fallot

**Outcomes After Late Reoperation in Patients With Repaired Tetralogy of Fallot: The Impact of Arrhythmia and Arrhythmia Surgery**
Karamlou T, Silber I, Lao R, et al (Hosp for Sick Children, Toronto; Toronto Congenital Cardiac Ctr for Adults)
*Ann Thorac Surg* 81:1786-1793, 2006                                          2–1

*Background.*—We evaluated outcomes in patients requiring late reoperation after tetralogy of Fallot (ToF) repair to identify risk factors for arrhythmia and determine whether arrhythmia surgery decreased the risk of subsequent death or recurrent arrhythmia.

*Methods.*—Review was performed of all ToF patients from 1969 to 2005 undergoing reoperation late (> 1 year) after repair. Patients with associated lesions, except pulmonary atresia, were included. A total of 249 patients had 278 reoperations. Procedures at initial reoperation included pulmonary valve replacement (PVR) in 217, ablation in 63, and tricuspid valve repair/replacement in 46. Pre-reoperative arrhythmias were present in 75, including supraventricular tachycardia (SVT) in 31, ventricular tachycardia (VT) in 34, and SVT+VT in 10 patients.

*Results.*—Median age at reoperation was 23 years (range, 1 to 63). Ten-year survival after reoperation was 93%, and was independent of arrhythmia status ($p = 0.86$). Arrhythmia patients were characterized by older age at initial repair and at late reoperation, tricuspid and pulmonary regurgitation, and longer QRS duration ($p < 0.001$ for all). Risk factors for post-reoperative recurrent arrhythmia were longer QRS duration and not having PVR. Longer QRS duration, with a cut-point of more than 160 msec, was associated with recurrent SVT ($p = 0.004$). Supraventricular tachycardia ablation improved arrhythmia-free survival (75% versus 33%, $p < 0.001$) but VT ablation did not (96% versus 95%, $p = 0.50$). However, recurrent VT occurred in only 3 patients (10%).

*Conclusions.*—Late mortality in patients undergoing reoperation after ToF repair is not impacted by pre-reoperative arrhythmia. Prolongation of QRS identifies patients at risk for recurrent VT and SVT, but recurrent VT is uncommon. Early PVR, and surgical ablation in patients with SVT, decreases arrhythmic risk.

▶ These authors have attempted to deal with the issues of late PVR in patients who have had ToF repair as pediatric patients. The question regarding preoperative arrhythmia and long-term outcome is one that comes up frequently. These authors showed an excellent positive effect on decreasing the incidence of SVT as well as decreasing VT whether or not ablation was performed. They currently advocate early PVR in patients with significant increases in right ventricular end-diastolic volume of 185 mL/m² or greater and end-systolic volume of 85 mL/m² or greater. In addition, symptoms and moderate/severe tricuspid regurgitation, as well as increasing QRS duration, would also push one toward surgery. When to proceed with just valve replacement and when to proceed with preoperative or surgical ablation are still questions to be considered individually in each patient.

**T. P. Graham, MD**

**Total Transatrial Correction of Tetralogy of Fallot: No Outflow Patch Technique**

Airan B, Choudhary SK, Kumar HVJ, et al (All India Inst of Med Sciences, New Delhi)

*Ann Thorac Surg* 82:1316-1321, 2006                                      2–2

*Background.*—The aim of this study was to analyze the feasibility and early results of transatrial total correction of tetralogy of Fallot (TOF).

*Methods.*—Of the 860 patients undergoing total correction for TOF between January 2000 and July 2005, 334 patients were considered morphologically suitable for transatrial total correction. The ventricular septal defect (VSD) closure, infundibular resection, and pulmonary valvotomy were performed through the right atrium without a right ventriculotomy. Age ranged from 6 months to 40 years (median, 2.8 years), and weight ranged from 5.5 to 70 kg (median, 14 kg).

*Results.*—Peroperatively, 34 patients required right ventriculotomy and transannular patch; hence, they were excluded from the study. In addition, pulmonary arteriotomy was required in 71 patients (22.9%). There were 4 hospital deaths. There were 4 early reoperations (residual/additional VSD in 3 and tricuspid regurgitation in 1). Two patients had complete heart block requiring permanent pacemaker. Echocardiography at discharge showed a peak right ventricular outflow tract gradient of 20 ± 5.2 mm Hg. Mean follow-up was 26.8 ± 4.2 months (range, 1 to 52 months). The right ventricular outflow tract gradients reduced to 13 ± 4.2 mm Hg after a mean interval of 18.8 ± 5.2 months. Follow-up New York Heart Association class was I in 240 cases (82%), II in 49 (16%), and III in 7 (2%). There were no late deaths or reoperations.

*Conclusions.*—Transatrial total correction of TOF can be accomplished in selected patients with good early results. In 300 cases (90%), the feasibility of transatrial total correction could be predicted accurately.

▶ These authors show excellent results in terms of morbidity and mortality with this technique, which is gaining increased favor worldwide. It should be pointed out that most of these patients were older and had so-called good tetralogy anatomy. The authors feel that this technique can be applied to patients in a younger age range, such as those aged 3 months and older and/or weighing 5 kg or more. There were 16 patients with right ventricular outflow gradients greater than 30 mm Hg at discharge, and the gradients appeared to decrease or stay the same with follow-up. These authors suggested that this technique can be used in patients with pulmonary annulus *z* scores of −3 or less. This transatrial approach was possible in the setting of anomalous coronary pattern in 20 patients in this rather large series. Patients with low-output syndrome did not have evidence of primary right ventricular dysfunction. Finally, the patients had a low incidence of right bundle branch block of only 35%, which may prove to be important, although we have no data that long-term right bundle branch block is harmful in this group of patients.

**T. P. Graham, MD**

### Long-Term Neurodevelopmental Outcome and Exercise Capacity After Corrective Surgery for Tetralogy of Fallot or Ventricular Septal Defect in Infancy

Hövels-Gürich HH, Konrad K, Skorzenski D, et al (Aachen Univ of Technology, Germany; Inst for Medical Research and Information Processing, Aachen, Germany)

*Ann Thorac Surg* 81:958-967, 2006                                        2–3

*Background.*—The purpose of this prospective study was to assess whether neurodevelopmental status and exercise capacity of children 5 to 10 years after corrective surgery for tetralogy of Fallot or ventricular septal defect in infancy was different compared with normal children and influenced by the preoperative condition of hypoxemia or cardiac insufficiency.

*Methods.*—Forty unselected children, 20 with tetralogy of Fallot and hypoxemia and 20 with ventricular septal defect and cardiac insufficiency, operated on with combined deep hypothermic circulatory arrest and low flow cardiopulmonary bypass at a mean age of $0.7 \pm 0.3$ years (mean $\pm$ SD), underwent, at mean age $7.4 \pm 1.6$ years, standardized evaluation of neurologic status, gross motor function, intelligence, academic achievement, language, and exercise capacity. Results were compared between the groups and related to preoperative, perioperative, and postoperative status and management.

*Results.*—Rate of mild neurologic dysfunction was increased compared with normal children, but not different between the groups. Exercise capacity and socioeconomic status were not different compared with normal children and between the groups. Compared with the normal population, motor function, formal intelligence, academic achievement, and expressive and receptive language were significantly reduced ($p < 0.01$ to $p < 0.001$) in the whole group and in the subgroups, except for normal intelligence in ventricular septal defect patients. Motor dysfunction was significantly higher in the Fallot group compared with the ventricular septal defect group ($p < 0.01$) and correlated with neurologic dysfunction, lower intelligence, and reduced expressive language ($p < 0.05$ each). Reduced New York Heart Association functional class was correlated with lower exercise capacity and longer duration of cardiopulmonary bypass ($p < 0.05$ each). Reduced socioeconomic status significantly influenced dysfunction in formal intelligence ($p < 0.01$) and academic achievement ($p < 0.05$). Preoperative risk factors such as prenatal hypoxia, perinatal asphyxia, and preterm birth, factors of perioperative management such as cardiac arrest, lowest nasopharyngeal temperature, and age at surgery, and postoperative risk factors as postoperative cardiocirculatory insufficiency and duration of mechanical ventilation were not different between the groups and had no influence on outcome. Degree of hypoxemia in Fallot patients and degree of cardiac insufficiency in ventricular septal defect patients did not influence the outcome within the subgroups.

*Conclusions.*—Children with preoperative hypoxemia in infancy are at higher risk for motor dysfunction than children with cardiac insufficiency. Corrective surgery in infancy for tetralogy of Fallot or ventricular septal defect with combined circulatory arrest and low flow bypass is associated with reduced neurodevelopmental outcome, but not with reduced exercise capacity in childhood. In our experience, the general risk of long-term neurodevelopmental impairment is related to unfavorable effects of the global perioperative management. Socioeconomic status influences cognitive capabilities.

▶ These authors show corrective surgery in infancy for tetralogy or VSD with combined circulatory arrest and low-flow bypass is associated with reduced neurodevelopmental outcome and normal exercise capacity in childhood. The commentary after this article by the group from Children's Hospital in Philadelphia is quite helpful. The use of deep hypothermia and circulatory arrest remains controversial, but most studies show short periods (<40-45 minutes) of arrest are associated with similar neurodevelopmental results as continuous bypass. There is a distinct neurodevelopmental signature after cardiac surgery consisting of mild cognitive impairment with decreased motor skills and language abnormalities. Fortunately, these are usually mild, but this does continue to support the need for further study into mechanisms of central nervous system injury and for factors that may improve long-term outcome.

**T. P. Graham, MD**

---

**Complete Repair of Conotruncal Defects With an Interatrial Communication: Oxygenation, Hemodynamic Status, and Early Outcome**
Laudito A, Graham EM, Stroud MR, et al (Med Univ of South Carolina, Charleston)
*Ann Thorac Surg* 82:1286-1291, 2006                                    2–4

---

*Background.*—Complete repair of conotruncal defects frequently uses maintenance of an interatrial communication. Postoperative right ventricular dysfunction may be characterized by elevated right atrial pressure and decreased systemic oxygen saturation owing to right-to-left shunting at the atrial level.

*Methods.*—From January 1996 to December 2005, 112 patients younger than 6 months of age underwent complete repair of tetralogy of Fallot or truncus arteriosus. An interatrial communication was used in 80 of 112 patients (71%). Hemodynamic data were determined during the first 48 hours after surgery.

*Results.*—In patients with an atrial communication, mean oxygen saturation reached a nadir of 94% ± 6%, and mean arterial $PO_2$ a nadir of 73 ± 25 mm Hg at 16 to 24 hours after surgery; both increased during the second 24 hours. At hospital discharge, median oxygen saturation was 98% (range, 86% to 100%). During the first 48 hours, mean oxygen saturation was less than 90% in 13 patients; the only multivariate risk factor was younger patient age. Mean right atrial pressure was greater than 10 mm Hg in 30 patients; multivariate risk factors were older patient age and repair with a transannular patch.

*Conclusions.*—After complete repair of conotruncal defects using an interatrial communication, systemic oxygenation reaches a nadir at 24 hours after surgery, and improves by the time of hospital discharge. Clinically significant desaturation occurs in a small minority of patients. Infants undergoing repair before 2 months of age are at higher risk for systemic desaturation. The effects of an interatrial communication on systemic oxygenation should not be considered a contraindication to complete repair in early infancy.

▶ Many times an atrial communication is left in patients with complex tetralogy or truncus arteriosus. It can result in desaturation early postoperatively along with improved systemic output. It is rarely a cause of severe early postoperative hypoxemia when the defect is 4 to 5 mm or less. We have occasionally seen such patients 20 years later who became significantly desaturated with walking and required closure of the atrial defect at that time. This is easily accomplished now with device closure, and thus there is not a contraindication to keeping the atrial septal defect open when one feels it may contribute to improved hemodynamics in the early postoperative period. It is still unclear as to which patients can have these defects closed in the operating room and avoid this possible need for late closure. Some type of control study in this regard would be useful.

**T. P. Graham, MD**

---

**Endovascular Stenting of Obstructed Right Ventricle–to–Pulmonary Artery Conduits: A 15-Year Experience**
Peng LF, McElhinney DB, Nugent AW, et al (Children's Hosp Boston; Harvard Med School, Boston)
*Circulation* 113:2598-2605, 2006                                            2–5

---

*Background.*—The optimal treatment for dysfunctional right ventricle–to–pulmonary artery (RV-PA) conduits is unknown. Limited follow-up data on stenting of RV-PA conduits have been reported.

*Method and Results.*—Between 1990 and 2004, deployment of balloon-expandable bare stents was attempted in 242 obstructed RV-PA conduits in 221 patients (median age, 6.7 years). Acute hemodynamic changes after stenting included significantly decreased RV systolic pressure (89±18 to 65±20 mm Hg, *P*<0.001) and peak RV-PA gradient (59±19 to 27±14 mm Hg, *P*<0.001). There were no deaths, and, aside from 5 malpositioned stents requiring surgical removal, there were no serious procedural complications. During follow-up of 4.0±3.2 years, 9 patients died and 2 underwent heart transplantation, none related to catheterization or stent malfunction. During 155 follow-up catheterizations in 126 patients, the stent was redilated in 83 patients and additional stents were placed in 41. Stent fractures were diagnosed in 56 patients (43%) and associated with stent compression and substernal location but did not cause acute hemodynamic consequences. By Kaplan-Meier analysis, median freedom from conduit surgery after stenting was 2.7 years (3.9 years in patients >5 years), with younger age, homograft conduit, conduit diameter ≤10 mm, diagnosis other than tetralogy of Fallot, Genesis stent, higher prestent RV:aortic pressure ratio, and stent malposition associated with shorter freedom from surgery. Tricuspid regurgitation and RV function did not change between stent implantation and subsequent surgery.

*Conclusions.*—Conduit stenting is an effective interim treatment for RV-PA conduit obstruction and prolongs conduit lifespan in most patients. Stent fractures were common but not associated with significant complications or earlier conduit reoperation.

▶ Conduits continue to be an issue with patient growth and with pseudointimal proliferation after use of these devices for treatment of complex congenital heart disease. Stents can provide some relief of severe obstruction as a temporizing measure in patients in whom reoperation may not be in their best interest at a certain point in time. These authors show excellent results for mild decreases in gradient and lack of complications of right ventricular dysfunction or tricuspid regurgitation between stent implantation and subsequent surgery, which occurred approximately 3 years later overall and 4 years later in patients older than 5 years at the time of stenting. The authors make the point that preliminary balloon dilatation to determine the exact areas of obstruction was useful. In addition, test balloon dilatation without stent placement can be useful to be sure one is not expanding in an area that may compromise coronary circulation.

**T. P. Graham, MD**

---

**Encouraging results for the Contegra conduit in the problematic right ventricle–to–pulmonary artery connection**
Morales DLS, Braud BE, Gunter KS, et al (Baylor College of Medicine, Houston; Texas Children's Hosp, Houston)
*J Thorac Cardiovasc Surg* 132:665-671, 2006                                     2–6

---

*Objective.*—The Contegra conduit was developed for right ventricular outflow tract reconstruction. This report evaluates the Contegra conduit, with focus on certain subpopulations in which conduits are known to perform poorly (ie, patients with previous homograft conduits and infants).

*Methods.*—A retrospective review of 76 patients who had 77 Contegra conduits placed for right ventricular outflow tract reconstruction (January 2001 through August 2005) was completed. Characteristics include the following: median age of 1.6 years (range, 17 days-15.1 years), weight of 9.8 kg (range, 2.5-64.0 kg), and conduit diameter of 16 mm (range, 12-22 mm). Operations performed include right ventricular outflow tract reconstruction for pulmonary atresia–stenosis (n = 33), conduit exchange (n = 28), truncus repair (n = 7), primary conduit placement (n = 6), and the Ross procedure (n = 3). Seventy-nine percent were reoperations.

*Results.*—There was no hospital mortality. Mean follow-up was 20 ± 14 months. One-, 2-, and 3- year freedom from severe conduit regurgitation was 97%, 86%, and 81%, respectively, and freedom from severe conduit stenosis was 100%. Freedom from reoperation for conduit failure at 1 and 3 years is 98.3% and 93.1%, respectively. All conduit failures (n = 3) were for asymptomatic conduit pseudoaneurysms in the setting of multiple-level pulmonary branch stenoses. Survival at 3 years is 96%. Infants (n = 26) had a freedom from Contegra conduit failure at 3 years of 100%. Patients with previous homograft conduits (n = 26) had a freedom from Contegra conduit failure at 3 years of 100%.

*Conclusion.*—At midterm follow-up, the Contegra conduit remains a reliable, accessible, and easily implantable conduit for right ventricular outflow tract reconstruction. It appears to be the most promising conduit option for patients with previous homograft conduits and for infants.

▶ The Contegra conduit has many theoretic advantages including availability, price, and size up to 22 mm. You can have a longer proximal and distal segment than with many homografts, and it has good pliability, suturing, and tailoring characteristics as noted by the surgeons in this report. Its usefulness is reasonable for patients in the younger age group, although those with severe distal stenosis or pulmonary hypertension postoperatively are prone to severe conduit regurgitation and pseudoaneurysm formation (see Fig 1 on page 668 of the original article). Other authors have found more significant regurgitation even without severe obstruction in younger infants. It is a useful conduit for selected patients and can be used to effectively treat a number of patients requiring right ventricular pulmonary artery connections.

**T. P. Graham, MD**

### Risk factors for arrhythmia and late death in patients with right ventricle to pulmonary artery conduit repair—Japanese multicenter study

Tateno S, Niwa K, Nakazawa M, et al (Chiba Cardiovascular Ctr, Japan; Heart Inst of Japan Tokyo Women's Med Univ; Yokohama City Univ, Japan; et al)
*Int J Cardiol* 106:373-381, 2006      2–7

*Background.*—Arrhythmia and late cardiac deaths are thought to be major complications in patients after right ventricle (RV) to pulmonary artery (PA) conduit repair, although the incidence and predictors of these complications remain unknown. The aim of this study was to clarify the incidence and risk factors for arrhythmia and late deaths in patients with the RV to PA conduit repair through a Japanese multicenter study.

*Methods.*—Three hundred fifty-one hospital survivors who underwent the RV to PA conduit repair before 1995 were studied.

*Results.*—Survival rate after repair was 92% at 10 years, 88% at 20 and 25 years, respectively. Late death was observed in 30 (8.5%) including 4 patients with sudden death (SD). Higher right ventricular pressure ($p = 0.02$), larger cardio-thoracic ratio after repair ($p = 0.02$) and higher incidence of brady- or tachy-arrhythmia and SD (9/30) were associated with late death. Six (1.7%) patients developed ventricular tachycardia or ventricular fibrillation (VT/Vf). There were 22 patients who had 23 new-onset supraventricular tachy-arrhythmia (SVT). Right ventricular hypertension ($p = 0.04$) was associated with VT/Vf or SD. Male sex ($p < 0.01$), absence of previously aorto-pulmonary shunt ($p < 0.05$), older age at repair ($p < 0.01$) or longer length of follow-up ($p < 0.01$) were associated with SVT.

*Conclusion.*—Arrhythmia and late sudden death are relatively common late after the RV to PA conduit repair. Our data support recent surgical strategies of earlier primary operation and timely reoperation for progressive right ventricular outflow stenosis that may reduce the incidence of late arrhythmias and SD.

▶ These authors found arrhythmia and late SD in a small group of patients after right ventricular conduit repair. Late death was associated with high right ventricular pressure, larger cardiothoracic ratio after repair, and higher incidence of bradyarrhythmia or tachyarrhythmia. These data support continuing careful follow-up of these patients with timely reoperation for progressive stenosis, particularly associated with ventricular dysfunction, to hopefully prevent this terrible complication.

**T. P. Graham, MD**

### Ventricular Fibrosis Suggested by Cardiovascular Magnetic Resonance in Adults With Repaired Tetralogy of Fallot and Its Relationship to Adverse Markers of Clinical Outcome

Babu-Narayan SV, Kilner PJ, Li W, et al (Royal Brompton Hosp, London; Imperial College, London)
*Circulation* 113:405-413, 2006                                                    2–8

*Background.*—Late morbidity and mortality remain problematic after repair of tetralogy of Fallot (TOF). We hypothesized that fibrosis detected by late gadolinium enhancement (LGE) cardiovascular magnetic resonance (CMR) would be present in adults with repaired TOF and would be related to adverse markers of outcome.

*Method and Results.*—LGE was scored in the right and left ventricles (RV and LV) of 92 adult patients who had undergone TOF repair. RV LGE was seen in all patients at surgical sites located in the outflow tract (99%) or the site of ventricular septal defect patching (98%) and in the inferior RV insertion point (79%) and trabeculated myocardium (24%). LV LGE (53%) was located at the apex consistent with apical vent insertion (49%), in the inferior or lateral wall consistent with infarction (5%), or in other areas (8%). Patients with supramedian RV LGE score were older (38 versus 27 years, $P<0.001$) and more symptomatic (38% versus 8% in New York Heart Association class II or greater, $P=0.001$), had increased levels of atrial natriuretic peptide (7.3 versus 4.9 pmol/L, $P=0.041$), and had a trend to higher brain natriuretic peptide (12.3 versus 7.2 pmol/L, $P=0.086$), exercise intolerance (maximum $VO_2$ 24 versus 28 mL · min$^{-1}$ · kg$^{-1}$, $P=0.021$), RV dysfunction (RV end-systolic volume 61 versus 55 mL/m$^2$, $P=0.018$; RV ejection fraction 50% versus 56%, $P=0.007$), and clinical arrhythmia (26% versus 10%, $P=0.039$). Non-apical vent LV LGE also correlated with markers of adverse outcome. In a multivariate model, RV LGE remained a predictor of arrhythmia.

*Conclusions.*—RV and LV LGE were common after TOF repair and were related to adverse clinical markers, including ventricular dysfunction, exercise intolerance, and neurohormonal activation. Furthermore, RV LGE was significantly associated with clinical arrhythmia.

▶ The increasing use of LGE to detect fibrosis in postoperative patients has provided us with further potential correlates of abnormal function and arrhythmias in patients late after repair of congenital defects (see Figs 3 and 4 of the original article). As the authors state in their article, this noninvasive demonstration of fibrosis, whether reflecting a single insult or a progressive change with time, could help in management decisions in regard to medical or surgical therapy.

**T. P. Graham, MD**

## Transposition of the Great Arteries

### Relation Between Right Ventricular Structural Alterations and Markers of Adverse Clinical Outcome in Adults With Systemic Right Ventricle and Either Congenital Complete (After Senning Operation) or Congenitally Corrected Transposition of the Great Arteries

Giardini A, Lovato L, Donti A, et al (Univ of Bologna, Italy)
*Am J Cardiol* 98:1277-1282, 2006                                                    2–9

This study sought to determine if areas of late gadolinium enhancement (LGE) would be present in adults with systemic right ventricles and if LGE would be associated with markers of adverse outcomes. Using gadolinium-enhanced magnetic resonance and cardiopulmonary exercise testing, 34 adults with systemic right ventricles (23 patients with atrial repair for transposition of the great arteries and 11 with congenitally corrected transposition) were studied at a mean age of 25 years. LGE was present in 14 patients (41%). The presence of LGE was associated with older age ($p = 0.037$), a lower right ventricular (RV) ejection fraction (34% vs 45%, $p = 0.006$), higher RV wall stress ($p = 0.0001$), reduced peak oxygen uptake (47% vs 56%, $p = 0.001$), and a history of arrhythmia ($p = 0.005$). The RV ejection fraction was correlated with RV wall stress ($r = -0.81$, $p < 0.0001$) and peak oxygen uptake ($r = 0.74$, $p < 0.0001$). Twelve patients experienced worsening of their clinical conditions. This was associated with decreases in biventricular function and increases in the prevalence and number of LGE areas. In conclusion, patients with systemic right ventricles have areas of abnormal myocardium, presumably due to fibrosis, that can be seen by contrast-enhanced magnetic resonance imaging. The presence of abnormal myocardial regions is associated with RV dysfunction, poor exercise tolerance, arrhythmia, and progressive clinical deterioration.

▶ This represents another use of gadolinium enhancement with MRI studies to detect fibrosis. This enhancement correlated with older age, lower RV ejection fraction, higher wall stress, reduced peak oxygen uptake, and a history of arrhythmia. Again, these data may help to explain the pathogenesis of clinical deterioration as well as provide help in decision making in regard to intervention in these patients.

**T. P. Graham, MD**

### Aortic Valve Regurgitation After Arterial Switch Operation for Transposition of the Great Arteries: Incidence, Risk Factors, and Outcome

Losay J, Touchot A, Capderou A, et al (Centre Chirurgical Marie-Lannelongue, Le Plessis-Robinson, France)
*J Am Coll Cardiol* 47:2057-2062, 2006                    2–10

*Objectives.*—The aims of this study were to assess the prevalence and incidence of aortic valve regurgitation (AR) after arterial switch operation (ASO), its outcome, and the risk factors.

*Background.*—After an ASO, the long-term fate of the aortic valve is a concern as follow-up lengthens.

*Methods.*—Operative and follow-up data on 1,156 hospital survivors after ASOs between 1982 and December 2000 were reviewed.

*Results.*—At last follow-up (mean duration 76.2 ± 60.5 months), 172 patients (14.9%) had an AR. Complex transposition of the great arteries, prior pulmonary banding done in 75 patients (21 with intact ventricular septum), aortic arch anomalies, AR at discharge, older age at ASO, and aortic/pulmonary size discrepancy were associated with AR. On multivariate analysis, the presence of a ventricular septal defect (VSD) or AR at discharge multiplied the risk by 2 and 4, respectively. Freedom from AR was 77.9% and 69.5% at 10 and 15 years, respectively; hazard function for AR declined rapidly and slowly increased thereafter. Reoperation from AR was done in 16 patients with one death, valvuloplasty being unsuccessful. Freedom from reoperation for AR was 97.7% and 96.8% at 10 and 15 years, respectively; hazard function slowly increased from 2 to 16 years. Higher late mortality was not associated with AR.

*Conclusions.*—After ASO, AR was observed and was related to VSD with attending high pressure and flow and AR at discharge. Progression of AR was slow, but incidence increased with follow-up. Reoperation for AR was rare. Late aortic valve function warrants long-term monitoring.

▶ This is the largest series to date of medium-term follow-up of patients with ASO. As with previous studies, AR was related to the presence of a VSD, dilatation of the pulmonary artery, or pulmonary artery banding. It was present in almost 15% of patients after a 17-month median follow-up and in 22% after 10 years, and can be observed late—up to 16 years. Surgery was needed in only 1.4% of survivors, which is exceedingly rare but may, unfortunately, be required in others with long-term follow-up.

**T. P. Graham, MD**

### Pathology of coronary narrowing after arterial switch operation: autopsy findings in two patients who died within 3 months of surgical treatment and review of the literature

Bartoloni G, Bianca S, Patanè L, et al (Università di Catania, Italy; Centro di Consulenza Genetica e di Teratologia della Riproduzione, Catania, Italy; Centro Cuore Morgagni, Pedara, Italy; et al)

*Cardiovasc Pathol* 15:49-54, 2006                                                   2–11

The arterial switch operation (ASO) has become the surgical treatment of choice for transposition of the great arteries (TGA). Myocardial ischemia owing to coronary complication remains the commonest cause of mortality and morbidity following ASO. The main clinical manifestations of coronary obstruction reported after a switch procedure are heart failure, arrhythmias, or sudden death. Coronary complications are responsible for about 50% of early death and for almost all late deaths.

We describe pathologic and anatomic findings in two cases of late sudden death after an ASO. Critical intimal thickening and acute take-off of coronary trunks were the main pathological substrates of death. Histological examination revealed an obstructive coronary proliferation characterised by a concentric stratum of intimal smooth muscle cell hyperplasia with preserved tunica media.

Pathogenetic assessment of intimal coronary lesions after an ASO should consider the role of endothelium and vascular parietal wall in the unavoidable response to injury caused by arterial reconstruction. Since a rapidly progressive proliferative disease is suspected, to explain coronary narrowing, understanding endothelial biology and improving surgical technique should help to prevent late coronary events.

▶ Although this report details coronary anatomy in only 2 patients after ASOs, there is a review of other cases of coronary death and autopsy or clinical findings from the literature. These authors describe what appears to be a rapidly progressive proliferative disease of the endocardium and vascular parietal wall, which suggests that it may be an unavoidable response to injury caused by arterial reconstruction in certain patients. Obviously it is a rare complication, fortunately, but any patient with unexplained symptoms that might represent ischemia should be investigated early after ASO.

**T. P. Graham, MD**

### Intermediate Results of the Double-Switch Operations for Atrioventricular Discordance

Koh M, Yagihara T, Uemura H, et al (Natl Cardiovascular Ctr, Osaka, Japan; Royal Brompton Hosp, London)

*Ann Thorac Surg* 81:671-677, 2006                                                   2–12

*Background.*—Since 1987, anatomic biventricular repair using the double-switch operations has been our principal choice for patients with atrioventricular discordance. These alternative procedures have the theoretical advantage of using the anatomic left ventricle to support the systemic circulation.

*Methods.*—A total of 45 patients underwent the double-switch operation. Their ages ranged from 6 months to 21 years. Associated malformations included pulmonary atresia in 27, pulmonary stenosis in 11, and Ebstein's malformation in 5. An atrial switch plus an arterial switch procedure was performed in 7, and an atrial switch plus a Rastelli-type ventriculoarterial switch procedure in 38. Follow-up ranged from 6 months to 15 years.

*Results.*—Early mortality was 8.9% (n = 4). In the latter half of the series (n = 23, since 1994), there was no early death. Six patients died late. Actuarial survival at 5 and 10 years was 83.6% and 77.6%, respectively. Six patients required conduit replacement, and 2 required revision of an intraatrial baffle for pulmonary venous channel obstruction and infection, respectively. Freedom from reoperation was 95.3% at 5 years and 76.2% at 10 years. Freedom from arrhythmia was 88.8% at 5 years and 78.4% at 10 years. The systemic ventricular ejection fraction was 0.568 ± 0.103 at 1 year (n = 39), 0.555 ± 0.105 at 5 years (n = 17), and 0.539 ± 0.098 at 10 years (n = 12).

*Conclusions.*—The surgical results of the double-switch operations have been improving. Intermediate follow-up suggests that these alternative procedures are a reasonable option for patients with atrioventricular discordance.

▶ This report of double-switch operations gives the whole story of the management issues both in the selection of patients for the procedure and the results in 62 patients with congenitally corrected transposition of the great arteries. Forty-five were deemed acceptable for a double-switch. Reasons for not performing the double-switch were older age, small ventricular septal defect (VSD), VSD unsuitable for rerouting, mitral regurgitation, criss-cross arrangement, tricuspid valve attachments not favorable for rerouting, and small left ventricular volume. The outcome was quite reasonable, with maintenance of systemic ventricular ejection fraction at a reasonable level of 54% over 10 years. There were significant problems with conduits as well as intra-atrial baffles, as might be expected. The early mortality rate was 9%, and the late mortality rate was 14% (6/41). Reintervention was relatively common, and freedom from arrhythmia was 78% at 10 years.

This is a difficult operation that requires a long cross-clamp time. These authors improved this time in the latter half of the series to 147 ± 34 minutes, which still is remarkably long. Those patients with anatomy in which an atrial and arterial switch is an option are the best candidates for this operation, and those with other subtypes should be considered carefully before embarking on this operation, particularly those who require considerable VSD enlargement, which can contribute to further ventricular dysfunction, as indicated by these investigators.

**T. P. Graham, MD**

## Hypoplastic Left Heart Syndrome

**Impact of preoperative treatment strategies on the early perioperative outcome in neonates with hypoplastic left heart syndrome**
Stieh J, Fischer G, Scheewe J, et al (Univ Hosp Schleswig Holstein–Campus Kiel, Germany; Ruhr-Univ Bochum, Germany)
*J Thorac Cardiovasc Surg* 131:1122-1129, 2006                              2–13

*Objective.*—This study was undertaken to determine the impact of specific intensive care procedures on preoperative hemodynamics, incidence of preoperative organ dysfunction, and in-hospital mortality among neonates with hypoplastic left heart syndrome with pulmonary overcirculation and to assess the influence of the change in preoperative management on early postoperative outcome.

*Methods.*—In this retrospective evaluation of 72 neonates with classic hypoplastic left heart syndrome and severe pulmonary overcirculation with different preoperative management strategies from 1992 to 1995 and from 1996 to 2000, univariate and multivariate analyses of risk factors were performed with stepwise logistic regression.

*Results.*—Among patients with ventilatory and inotropic support from admission until surgery, degree of metabolic acidosis (lowest recorded and prerepair pH values) was significantly higher than among patients who received systemic vasodilators without ventilation before surgery. Preoperative organ dysfunction occurred in 19 of 72 patients (26%), predominantly before 1996; the most significant was hepatic failure in 13 (68%). Lowest recorded and prerepair pH values did not predict the development of organ dysfunction, whereas inotropic medication, lack of afterload reduction, and especially ventilatory support correlated significantly with organ injury. In-hospital mortality decreased from 65% (13/20) to 13% (6/46) from the first to the second period. According to multivariate analysis, ventilatory support and organ dysfunction were significantly related to in-hospital mortality.

*Conclusion.*—In neonates with hypoplastic left heart syndrome, systemic afterload reduction can avoid preoperative artificial respiration, identified as a significant risk factor for the development of preoperative dysfunction of end organs and in-hospital mortality.

▶ These authors make the case for a change in preoperative management beginning at the referring hospital to account for the significantly improved outcome between 2 treatment periods. They indicate that systemic afterload reduction begun early can avoid artificial ventilation and the need for decreased inspired oxygen or increased inspired carbon dioxide to modulate pulmonary blood flow. The hypothesis is that such a strategy can prevent preoperative and/or postoperative dysfunction and improve hospital mortality. Many facets of care can change over an era as one begins to tackle such a difficult problem as hypoplastic left heart syndrome surgery. Among these would be the surgical skill as increasing numbers of patients are repaired, management in the postoperative and preoperative ICU, and earlier diagnosis, particularly prenatally. Despite those caveats, one should look seriously at the systemic afterload reduction therapy being used. Whether its use can eliminate the need for preoperative ventilation in the majority of patients is unclear, but hopefully this approach can improve overall morbidity and mortality.

**T. P. Graham, MD**

---

**Single-ventricle palliation for high-risk neonates: The emergence of an alternative hybrid stage I strategy**
Bacha EA, Daves S, Hardin J, et al (Univ of Chicago Children's Hosp)
*J Thorac Cardiovasc Surg* 131:163-171, 2006                    2–14

---

*Background.*—Survival after stage I palliation for hypoplastic left heart syndrome or related anomalies remains poor in high-risk neonates. We hypothesized that a less invasive hybrid approach would be beneficial in this patient population.

*Methods.*—The hybrid stage I procedure was performed in the catheterization laboratory. Via a median sternotomy, both branch pulmonary arteries were banded, and a ductal stent was delivered via a main pulmonary artery puncture and positioned under fluoroscopic guidance.

*Results.*—Between October 2003 and June 2005, 14 high-risk neonates underwent a hybrid stage I procedure. Eleven of 14 had hypoplastic left heart syndrome. Two also underwent atrial septal stenting, and 5 required percutaneous atrial stenting later. Two neonates with an intact or highly restrictive atrial septum had emergency percutaneous atrial stent placement. Hospital survival was 11 (78.5%) of 14. One patient required extracorporeal membrane oxygenation support for intraoperative cardiac arrest. He underwent cardiac transplantation but died later of sepsis. One patient died of ductal stent embolization, and a third died of progressive cardiac dysfunction. The first 4 patients required pulmonary artery band revisions. There were none after we modified our technique and added branch pulmonary artery angiograms. There were 2 interstage deaths from atrial stent occlusion and from preductal retrograde coarctation. Eight patients underwent stage II procedures, consisting of aortic arch reconstruction, atrial septectomy, and cavopulmonary shunt. Two patients died after stage II. One patient is awaiting stage II.

*Conclusions.*—The hybrid stage I palliation is a valid option in high-risk neonates. As experience is accrued, it may become the preferred alternative. However, in aortic atresia, the development of preductal retrograde coarctation is a significant problem.

▶ This approach has been applied to high-risk neonates, with a theoretically lower-risk stage I operation performed in the catheterization lab, with both pulmonary arteries banded and a ductal stent delivered by main pulmonary artery puncture with fluoroscopic guidance. In addition, atrial dilatation was performed if needed. Patients then have a stable situation theoretically until their stage II operation, which is a long operation and complicated by dealing with a ductal stent that is rock hard according to the authors. Nevertheless, this appears to be a valid option in high-risk neonates. Whether this strategy can be translated to other centers is still open to question.

**T. P. Graham, MD**

## Early Cavopulmonary Anastomosis After Norwood Procedure Results in Excellent Fontan Outcome

Jaquiss RDB, Siehr SL, Ghanayem NS, et al (Med College of Wisconsin, Milwaukee; Children's Hosp of Wisconsin, Milwaukee)
*Ann Thorac Surg* 82:1260-1266, 2006                                                    2–15

*Background.*—Children with univentricular hearts and aortic arch obstruction are treated sequentially with Norwood procedure, superior cavopulmonary anastomosis (SCPA), and Fontan operation. Early SCPA results in lower initial $O_2$ saturation and longer hospitalization, but not increased mortality. We sought to determine the impact of early SCPA on Fontan candidacy and outcomes.

*Methods.*—Eighty-five consecutive patients undergoing Norwood operation between January 1998 and February 2003 were divided into group 1 (SCPA at less than 4 months, n = 33) and group 2 (SCPA at more than 4 months, n = 52). Of the original cohort, 69 have undergone Fontan operation, 7 await Fontan, 1 was transplanted, 3 are not Fontan candidates, and 5 died late after SCPA. Group 1 (n = 25) and group 2 (n = 44) patients who have completed Fontan operation were compared for preoperative and perioperative variables: age, size, $O_2$ saturation, pulmonary artery pressure and size, prevalence of tricuspid regurgitation and ventricular dysfunction, extubation rate in operating room, duration of pleural drainage, hospital stay, and discharge $O_2$ saturation. Late functional status and ventricular function were also compared. Survival was compared for original groups 1 and 2.

*Results.*—There were no differences for any preoperative or perioperative variable, or late functional assessment. Actuarial survival at 6 years was also not different (88% ± 5% for group 1 and 94% ± 4% for group 2, $p = 0.72$).

*Conclusions.*—Although initially more cyanotic and hospitalized longer than older peers, younger SCPA patients achieve clinical equivalence by the time of Fontan operation and afterward. We conclude that both short- and long-term outcomes support performance of early SCPA.

▶ These superb results for hypoplastic left heart surgery indicate similar excellent outcomes in groups that had an early cavopulmonary anastomosis at a mean age of 94 days versus those who had a cavopulmonary shunt at a mean age of 165 days. Both had their Fontan completion at a mean age of 2.5 years, with no operative deaths and excellent current status. These data indicate that early cavopulmonary shunts can be carried out under optimal conditions at a relatively early age.

**T. P. Graham, MD**

### Validation and Re-Evaluation of a Discriminant Model Predicting Anatomic Suitability for Biventricular Repair in Neonates With Aortic Stenosis

Colan SD, McElhinney DB, Crawford EC, et al (Children's Hosp, Boston; Harvard Med School, Boston)
*J Am Coll Cardiol* 47:1858-1865, 2006                              2–16

*Objectives.*—The purpose of this study was to validate and re-evaluate our previously reported scoring systems for predicting optimal management in neonates with aortic stenosis (AS).

*Background.*—In 1991, we reported a multivariate discriminant equation and an ordinal scoring system for predicting which neonates with AS are suitable for biventricular repair and which are better served by single ventricle management.

*Methods.*—Retrospective analysis was performed to: 1) validate our scoring systems in 89 additional neonates with AS and normal mitral valve area, 2) assess the effects of 5% measurement variation on predictive scores, 3) evaluate our cohort with the Congenital Heart Surgeons' Society scoring system, and 4) repeat the discriminant analysis on the basis of all 126 patients.

*Results.*—The original scores each predicted outcome accurately in 68 patients (77%). Minor (5%) measurement variation changed the outcome predicted by the discriminant equation in 8 patients (9%) and by the threshold system in 13 patients (15%). The most accurate model for predicting survival with a biventricular circulation among the full cohort is: 10.98 (body surface area) $+0.56$ (aortic annulus $z$-score) $+5.89$ (left ventricular to heart long-axis ratio) $-0.79$ (grade 2 or 3 endocardial fibroelastosis) $-6.78$. With a cutoff of $-0.65$, outcome was predicted accurately in 90% of patients.

*Conclusions.*—Both of our original scoring systems are less accurate at predicting outcome than in our original analysis. Revised discriminant analysis yielded a model similar to our original equation that was 90% accurate at predicting survival with a biventricular circulation among neonates with AS and a mitral valve area $z$-score $>-2$.

▶ The ability to predict anatomic suitability for biventricular versus single ventricle repair on echocardiographic data in neonates with AS is frequently relatively easy to determine. However, in a small percentage of patients who obviously have borderline mitral valve size, aortic root size, subaortic area size, and left ventricular cavity volume, it becomes increasingly difficult. As these authors point out, these models can be useful when applying them in the context of the whole patient, including in clinical decision-making the direction of flow in the ascending aorta and transverse arch. In addition, these formulas should not be used in patients with coarctation, as has been pointed out by others. Patients who have borderline left ventricles with isolated coarctation will virtually always have adequate left ventricular output after surgery if there are no other limiting factors such as mitral valve or aortic hypoplasia.

**T. P. Graham, MD**

**Influence of surgical strategies on outcome after the Norwood procedure**
Griselli M, McGuirk SP, Stümper O, et al (Diana, Princess of Wales Children's Hosp, Birmingham, England)
*J Thorac Cardiovasc Surg* 131:418-426, 2006                2–17

*Objective.*—The study objective was to identify how the evolution of surgical strategies influenced the outcome after the Norwood procedure.

*Methods.*—From 1992 to 2004, 367 patients underwent the Norwood procedure (median age, 4 days). Three surgical strategies were identified on the basis of arch reconstruction and source of pulmonary blood flow. The arch was refashioned without extra material in group A (n = 148). The arch was reconstructed with a pulmonary artery homograft patch in groups B (n = 145) and C (n = 74). Pulmonary blood flow was supplied by a modified Blalock-Taussig shunt in groups A and B. Pulmonary blood flow was supplied by a right ventricle to pulmonary artery conduit in group C. Early mortality, actuarial survival, and freedom from arch reintervention or pulmonary artery patch augmentation were analyzed.

*Results.*—Early mortality was 28% (n = 102). Actuarial survival was 62% ± 3% at 6 months. Early mortality was lower in group C (15%) than group A (31%) or group B (31%; $P <.05$). Actuarial survival at 6 months was better in group C (78% ± 5%) than group A (59% ± 5%) or group B (58% ± 4%; $P <.05$). Fifty-three patients (14%) had arch reintervention. Freedom from arch reintervention was 76% ± 3% at 1 year, with univariable analysis showing no difference among groups A, B, and C ($P =.71$). One hundred patients (27%) required subsequent pulmonary artery patch augmentation. Freedom from patch augmentation was 61% ± 3% at 1 year, and was lower in group C (3% ± 3%) than group A (80% ± 4%) or group B (72% ± 5%; $P <.05$).

*Conclusions.*—Survival after the Norwood procedure improved after the introduction of a right ventricle to pulmonary artery conduit, but a greater proportion of patients required subsequent pulmonary artery patch augmentation. The type of arch reconstruction did not affect the incidence of arch reintervention.

▶ These authors show improved survival after going from the Norwood procedure with aortic-pulmonary shunt to the procedure with right ventricular pulmonary artery conduit. The results currently are quite good, with early mortality in the latest pulmonary artery conduit group at 15%. Since this is not a simultaneous comparison, the question comes up as to whether there were multiple factors associated with improved results after the change in the type of shunt used. The authors feel that there were improvements in postoperative care as well as getting patients in better shape before the operation. There appear to be no other risk factors that were different between the 2 groups.

A large number of groups currently selectively use one or the other procedure, feeling that certain patients are better off with one procedure versus the other. Excellent results are being obtained in a number of centers with both procedures, and only a randomized trial, which currently is being done, will answer the question as to which would be better in the long run.

**T. P. Graham, MD**

---

**Fetal Aortic Valve Stenosis and the Evolution of Hypoplastic Left Heart Syndrome: Patient Selection for Fetal Intervention**
Mäkikallio K, McElhinney DB, Levine JC, et al (Harvard Med School, Boston; Univ of Oulu, Finland)
*Circulation* 113:1401-1405, 2006                                          2–18

---

*Background.*—Fetal aortic valvuloplasty may prevent progression of aortic stenosis (AS) to hypoplastic left heart syndrome (HLHS). Predicting which fetuses with AS will develop HLHS is essential to optimize patient selection for fetal intervention. The aim of this study was to define echocardiographic features associated with progression of midgestation fetal AS to HLHS.

*Method and Results.*—Fetal echocardiograms were reviewed from 43 fetuses diagnosed with AS and normal left ventricular (LV) length at ≤30 weeks' gestation. Of 23 live-born patients with available follow-up data, 17 had HLHS and 6 had a biventricular circulation. At the time of diagnosis, LV length, mitral valve, aortic valve, and ascending aortic diameter Z-scores did not differ between fetuses that ultimately developed HLHS and those that maintained a biventricular circulation postnatally. However, all of the fetuses that progressed to HLHS had retrograde flow in the transverse aortic arch (TAA), 88% had left-to-right flow across the foramen ovale, 91% had monophasic mitral inflow, and 94% had significant LV dysfunction. In contrast, all 6 fetuses with a biventricular circulation postnatally had antegrade flow in the TAA, biphasic mitral inflow, and normal LV function. With advancing gestation, growth arrest of left heart structures became evident in fetuses developing HLHS.

*Conclusions.*—In midgestation fetuses with AS and normal LV length, reversed flow in the TAA and foramen ovale, monophasic mitral inflow, and LV dysfunction are predictive of progression to HLHS. These physiological features may help refine patient selection for fetal intervention to prevent the progression of AS to HLHS.

▶ With the advent of fetal intervention for AS, it has become critical to determine which patients are at risk for progressing to HLHS in utero. These authors have performed an intriguing study trying to answer this question. It appears that reverse flow in the TAA and foramen ovale, and LV dysfunction in midgestation are predictive features for progression to HLHS. If these data can be refined a little further, they will provide a very important advance in promoting this intervention for patients who are likely to progress to HLHS.

**T. P. Graham, MD**

# Fontan Operation

## Clinical Outcome of 193 Extracardiac Fontan Patients: The First 15 Years

Giannico S, Hammad F, Amodeo A, et al (Bambino Gesǔ Hosp, Rome)
*J Am Coll Cardiol* 47:2065-2073, 2006                                 2–19

*Objectives.*—We sought to evaluate the mid-term outcome of hospital survivors with extracardiac Fontan circulation.

*Background.*—Few data exist about the mid-term and long-term results of the extracardiac Fontan operation.

*Methods.*—From November 1988 to November 2003, 221 patients underwent an extracardiac Fontan procedure as primary (9 patients) or secondary (212 patients) palliation, at a mean age of 72.2 months (range 13.1 to 131.3 months). A total of 165 of 193 early survivors underwent programmed noninvasive follow-up evaluations and at least one cardiac catheterization.

*Results.*—The overall survival, including operative deaths, was 85% at 15 years. Freedom from late failure among hospital survivors is 92% at 15 years. A total of 127 of 165 survivors (77%) were in New York Heart Association functional class I. The incidence of late major problems was 24% (42 major problems in 36 of 165 patients): 19 patients had arrhythmias (11%), 5 patients had obstruction of the extracardiac conduit (3%) and 6 of the left pulmonary artery (3.5%), and 5 patients experienced ventricular failure (3%), leading to heart transplantation in 3 patients. Protein-losing enteropathy was found in two patients (1%). The incidence of late re-interventions was 12.7% (21 of 165 patients, including 15 epicardial pacemaker implantations). Four patients died (2.3%), two after heart transplantation.

*Conclusions.*—After 15 years of follow-up, the overall survival, the functional status, and the cardiopulmonary performance of survivors of the extracardiac Fontan procedure compare favorably with other series of patients who underwent the lateral tunnel approach. The incidence of late deaths, obstructions of the cavopulmonary pathway, re-interventions, and arrhythmias is lower than that reported late after other Fontan-type operations.

▶ These authors show good results for the extracardiac Fontan in 165 patients for up to 15 years. Late major problems occurred in 24%, with protein-losing enteropathy in only 2 patients or 1%. One of the most important aspects of this report is the longevity of the extracardiac conduit, which was excellent; conduit obstruction developed in only 5 patients, with 36 patients having follow-up for more than 10 years. The mechanism that the authors believe was responsible for late conduit obstruction was likely torsion during rapid growth, which could be treated by stent placement. They showed no internal diameter change of the conduit after the first 6 months by serial MRI studies. Conduit obstruction late still remains a potential problem. Conduit size was 16 to 24 mm, and the mean age of operation was 6 years in this study. Gore-Tex tubes were used since 1997 to minimize the risk of peel formation. The incidence of late arrhythmias was reduced in comparison with other studies of other types of Fontan operations, although the follow-up still is not long enough to be sure that the incidence of arrhythmias will be lower with this modification.

**T. P. Graham, MD**

---

### Fontan Completion in Infants

Pizarro C, Mroczek T, Gidding SS, et al (Alfred I duPont Hosp for Children, Wilmington, Del; St Christopher's Hosp for Children, Philadelphia)
*Ann Thorac Surg* 81:2243-2249, 2006                                                2–20

*Background.*—Since the implementation of the Fontan procedure, several clinical factors have been linked to outcome. A study of the outcome after Fontan completion was undertaken with particular attention to the influence of age and cardiac diagnosis.

*Methods.*—Review of all patients (n = 107) undergoing Fontan completion between January 1998 and July 2005 to identify predictors of outcome: early death, prolonged effusions, and prolonged hospital stay.

*Results.*—Median age was 13 months (range, 11 to 35) and median weight was 9.4 kgs (6.7 to 15.1). Hypoplastic left heart syndrome was present in 61 patients, and stage I Norwood was the initial palliation in 69. An interim superior cavopulmonary connection was performed in all. A lateral tunnel was used, and a deliberate right to left shunt was created in 99 patients. Mean transpulmonary gradient and pulmonary artery pressure were $5.7 \pm 1.5$ mm Hg and $11.6 \pm 2.2$ mm Hg, respectively. Median time to extubation was 5 hours (range, 2.5 to 184). Median duration of pleural effusion was 3 days (1 to 58) and was greater or equal to 14 days in 13 patients (12%). Overall mortality was 4.5% (5 of 107). Variables associated with poor outcome included associated noncardiac diagnosis ($p < 0.05$), elevated transpulmonary gradient ($p = 0.03$), and pulmonary artery pressure ($p < 0.02$). Hypoplastic left heart syndrome was the only variable associated with prolonged effusive complications.

*Conclusions.*—Fontan completion can be performed with good results in the first year of life independent of anatomic diagnosis. Significant noncardiac pathology, and a higher pulmonary artery pressure were predictive of worse outcome. Hypoplastic left heart syndrome was associated with prolonged effusions.

▶ These authors show successful Fontan completion early at a mean age of 13 months and a median weight of 9.4 kg with hypoplastic left heart syndrome in the majority of patients treated in this manner. All had interim superior cavopulmonary connection, and a lateral tunnel was used with a deliberate right-to-left shunt in most patients. Overall mortality was 4.5%, and patients did have prolonged effusions when compared with an older group. When required, it appears that the Fontan operation can be done successfully at a younger age, and hopefully growth of all connections will not be an issue.

**T. P. Graham, MD**

---

**Pulmonary artery growth fails to match the increase in body surface area after the Fontan operation**

Tatum GH, Sigfússon G, Ettedgui JA, et al (Univ of Pittsburgh, Pa; Pennsylvania State Univ, Hershey)
*Heart* 92:511-514, 2006                                    2–21

*Objective.*—To evaluate the growth of the pulmonary arteries after a Fontan procedure.

*Design.*—Retrospective review.

*Setting.*—Two paediatric cardiology tertiary care centres.

*Patients.*—61 children who underwent a modified Fontan operation and had angiography suitable for assessment of pulmonary artery size before the Fontan procedure and during long term follow up. An atriopulmonary connection (APC) was present in 23 patients (37.7%) and a total cavopulmonary connection (TCPC) was present in 38 (62.3%). Postoperative angiograms were performed 0.5–121 months (median 19 months) after the Fontan operation.

*Main Outcome Measure.*—Growth of each pulmonary artery measured just before the first branching point. The diameter was expressed as a z score with established nomograms used to standardise for body surface area.

*Results.*—The mean change in the preoperative to postoperative z scores of the right pulmonary artery was $-1.06$ (p = 0.004). The mean change in the preoperative to postoperative z scores of the left pulmonary artery was $-0.88$ (p = 0.003). Changes in the preoperative to postoperative z scores were more pronounced in the patients undergoing APC than TCPC, especially for the right pulmonary artery.

*Conclusion.*—After the Fontan operation, growth of the pulmonary arteries often fails to match the increase in body surface area.

▶ This intriguing study supports the concept that venous flow after the bidirectional Glenn procedure does not result in normal growth of pulmonary arteries after Fontan completion. Poor pulmonary artery growth may be a contributing factor to late Fontan failure. These data should be followed up in other patients who have had late failure of this operation. It is clear that patients with large pulmonary arteries at the time of their Fontan operation, because they had more pulmonary blood flow earlier, tend to sail through their operation and have at least very good intermediate results.

**T. P. Graham, MD**

**Effects of postural change on oxygen saturation and respiration in patients after the Fontan operation: Platypnea and orthodeoxia**
Suzuki H, Ohuchi H, Hiraumi Y, et al (Natl Cardiovascular Ctr, Osaka, Japan)
*Int J Cardiol* 106:211-217, 2006                                    2–22

The aim of this study was to assess whether platypnea and orthodeoxia occur in Fontan patients. We divided 14 Fontan patients into 2 groups: 8 patients who had pulmonary arteriovenous fistulas and/or intra-atrial shunts (group A) and 6 patients who had neither pulmonary arteriovenous fistulas nor intra-atrial shunts (group B). They were compared with 9 controls (group C). Arterial oxygen saturation, minute ventilation per body weight and ventilatory equivalent for carbon dioxide were measured in the supine and then sitting positions. In group A, 1 patient had platypnea and 3 patients had orthodeoxia (changes in the saturation from the supine position to the sitting position were $-4\%$ to $-7\%$) accompanied with slight hyperpnea, and all 4 patients had both pulmonary arteriovenous fistulas and intra-atrial shunts. Contrary, patients in group B had neither platypnea nor orthodeoxia. The saturation was significantly lower and the minute ventilation was significantly higher in the sitting position than in the supine position in group A ($p < 0.05$). The other groups showed no significant difference in the saturation or the minute ventilation between the 2 positions. All groups showed the ventilatory equivalent was significantly higher in the sitting position than in the supine position ($p < 0.05$ to $0.01$). We demonstrated platypnea and orthodeoxia in Fontan patients with pulmonary arteriovenous fistulas and intra-atrial shunts. We believe platypnea and orthodeoxia should be regarded as a complication in Fontan patients with pulmonary arteriovenous fistulas and/or intra-atrial shunts.

▶ Fontan patients frequently have residual or recurrent right-to-left shunts despite multiple attempts at closing them surgically or with interventional techniques. I have become more aware of this by obtaining oxygen saturations in patients at rest and after they have walked around the clinic area for a minute or two. It's amazing how many Fontan patients who seem to have an excellent repair show desaturation. These authors show changes with just the assumption of the upright position in a number of patients with pulmonary arteriovenous fistulas, intra-atrial shunts, or both. These simple oxygen saturation measurements should be made in all these patients at rest and with exercise so that desaturation can be addressed early before deterioration occurs due to cyanosis.

**T. P. Graham, MD**

## Conversion of the failed Fontan circulation

Backer CL, Deal BJ, Mavroudis C, et al (Northwestern Univ Feinberg School of Medicine, Chicago)
*Cardiol Young* 16:85-91, 2006                                    2–23

*Background.*—In the 1970s and 1980s, many patients with a functional univentricular heart were treated by using an atriopulmonary connection to create the Fontan circulation. This procedure was viewed initially as successful and provided arterial saturations of oxygen close to normal; however, some of these patients developed significant complications during follow-up. One of these complications is progressive right atrial dilatation, which leads to atrial arrhythmias such as atrial flutter or fibrillation. In recent years, most centers have abandoned the atriopulmonary connection as an approach to creating the Fontan circulation in favor of the lateral tunnel with cavopulmonary connections, or the extracardiac conduit. The strategy of conversion has been developed to address the anatomic and physiologic issues created in the patient with a failed atriopulmonary connection. The indications for conversion were reviewed, and the results of these procedures at Children's Memorial Hospital were presented and compared with those from other published series of conversion. In addition, the results of cardiac transplantation in this patient population were discussed.

*Methods.*—The computerized database for cardiac surgical procedures at an urban children's hospital was reviewed. Between 1994 and 2004, 78 patients underwent conversion of their Fontan circulation. Between 1990 and 2004, orthotopic cardiac transplantation was performed in 8 additional patients because of failure of the Fontan circuit. Of these, 4 patients had failed a previous attempt at conversion. The major operative steps of conversion were (1) placement of extracardiac Gore-Tex tubing (24-mm diameter) from the inferior caval vein to the pulmonary arteries; (2) excision of most of the dilated right atrium and atrial septectomy; (3) arrhythmic surgery consisting of right maze or third variant of Cox maze, both with cryoablation; (4) bidirectional superior cavopulmonary anastomosis; and (5) placement of an epicardial pacemaker.

*Results.*—A 15-year-old patient died at 2 months after conversion because of hepatic and renal failure and persistent low cardiac output. One patient underwent reoperation for bleeding. Significant sternal infections developed in 2 patients, 1 of whom was treated with vacuum-assisted closure, and the other with muscle flaps. Acute renal failure developed in 9 patients, with 5 requiring dialysis. One of these 5 patients required a renal transplant. The other 4 patients died, 1 while hospitalized and the other 3 at 5, 7, and 11 months after conversion.

*Conclusions.*—Cardiac transplantation for a patient with a failed Fontan circuit has a 6-month waiting list mortality of 14% and an operative mortality of 27%. These patients also face a lifetime risk of immunosuppression and the significant potential for noncompliance. In contrast, conversion to an extracardiac cavopulmonary connection with concomitant arrhythmic surgery and placement of a pacemaker has been shown to be excellent therapy for selected patients in whom an atriopulmonary Fontan circuit has failed.

▶ This review of conversion of failing atrial–pulmonary artery connections shows excellent results, as well as good details and figures as to how the operation is actually performed (see Fig 1 on p 86 and Fig 6 on p 88 of the original article). There was only 1 death in 78 patients early, and 3 deaths late after this procedure. The results are certainly better when surgical arrhythmia procedures are combined with the hemodynamic changes that are associated with the operation. Risk factors for death, transplant, or dialysis were more severe ventricular dysfunction, ischemic time greater than 100 minutes, age greater than 25 years, atrioventricular valve regurgitation of a more than mild degree, cardiopulmonary bypass time greater than 240 minutes, and right or indeterminate ventricular morphology. This operation can be very useful, and hopefully most of the atriopulmonary connection patients with poor quality of life and frequent arrhythmias will get this conversion done sooner rather than later.

The decision as to when to use a conversion procedure and when to go directly to transplant is a difficult one. Transplantation for Fontan patients is reviewed in this report and shows a 60-day mortality of 27% in 84 patients from a composite of 5 reports. Obviously, most of these patients were probably more severely compromised at the time of their procedure.

**T. P. Graham, MD**

## Pulmonary Atresia/Intact Ventricular Septum

**Successful Management of Patients With Pulmonary Atresia With Intact Ventricular Septum Using a Three Tier Grading System for Right Ventricular Hypoplasia**
Odim J, Laks H, Plunkett MD, et al (Univ of California-Los Angeles)
*Ann Thorac Surg* 81:678-684, 2006                                    2–24

*Background.*—We sought to validate a simple grading scheme for right ventricular hypoplasia in determining suitability for a biventricular repair.

*Methods.*—We reviewed the medical records for 106 patients with pulmonary atresia-intact ventricular septum (PA-IVS) treated between 1982 and 2001. Over this period, children were assigned to mild (>2/3 normal size, 23.7% of patients), moderate (1/3 to 2/3, 41.2%), or severe (1/3, 35.1%) right ventricular hypoplasia, and this grouping, along with severity of coronary anomalies (45% right ventricle to coronary fistulae, 16% with right ventricle dependent coronary circulation [RVDCC]), triaged children to eventual single ventricle (severe) or two-ventricle (mild or moderate) repair.

*Results.*—Actuarial 10-year survival was 86.3% with mortality predicted by severe hypoplasia (odds ratio [OR] 12.9, $p < 0.001$), RVDCC (OR 15.0, $p < 0.001$), and non-Caucasian race (OR 10.7, $p < 0.001$). Multivariate analysis with a Cox proportional hazards model confirmed only RVDCC (risk ratio [RR] 10.9, $p = 0.0009$) and non-Caucasian race (RR 6.9, $p = $

0.007) as significant. Although not an independent risk factor for survival, the degree of hypoplasia was the most important determinant for definitive repair. Severe hypoplasia virtually precluded two-ventricle repair (OR 33.1, $p < 0.001$ by $\chi^2$ analysis) and was the strongest risk factor for a one-ventricle system (OR 78.7, $p < 0.001$). Actuarial survival after either repair was 91%, and no biventricular repair later converted to a Fontan system.

*Conclusions.*—Surgical management of patients based on this three tier grade for right ventricular hypoplasia results in excellent survival and correctly predicts patients destined for eventual Fontan and biventricular repair.

▶ These overall excellent results with this difficult condition show how the use of appropriate triage can affect results significantly. An actuarial 10-year survival of 86% is encouraging. Mortality, as expected, was related to severe right ventricular hypoplasia and RVDCC—these usually go hand in hand. An additional finding was that non-Caucasian race was a significant risk factor for poor outcome. The reason for this was not forthcoming but warrants further study. This may be related to being able to get to the medical center on a timely basis for follow-up and subsequent operations. Hopefully, such discrepancies in outcome can be eliminated in the future.

**T. P. Graham, MD**

---

### Natural History of Pulmonary Atresia With Intact Ventricular Septum and Right-Ventricle–Dependent Coronary Circulation Managed by the Single-Ventricle Approach

Guleserian KJ, Armsby LB, Thiagarajan RR, et al (Harvard Med School, Boston)
*Ann Thorac Surg* 81:2250-2258, 2006                                     2–25

---

*Background.*—Long-term outcome of patients with pulmonary valvar atresia and intact ventricular septum with right-ventricle–dependent coronary circulation (PA/IVS-RVDCC) managed by staged palliation directed toward Fontan circulation is unknown, but should serve as a basis for comparison with management protocols that include initial systemic-to-pulmonary artery shunting followed by listing for cardiac transplantation.

*Methods.*—Retrospective review of patients admitted to our institution with the diagnosis of PA/IVS-RVDCC from 1989 to 2004. All angiographic imaging studies, operative reports, and follow-up information were reviewed. Right-ventricle–dependent coronary circulation was defined as situations in which ventriculocoronary fistulae with proximal coronary stenosis or atresia were present, putting significant left ventricle myocardium at risk for ischemia with right ventricle decompression.

*Results.*—Thirty-two patients were identified with PA/IVS-RVDCC. All underwent initial palliation with modified Blalock-Taussig shunt (BTS). Median tricuspid valve z-score was $-3.62$ ($-2.42$ to $-5.15$), and all had moderate (n = 13) or severe (n = 19) right ventricular hypoplasia. Median follow-up was 5.1 years (9 months to 14.8 years). Overall mortality was

18.8% (6 of 32), with all deaths occurring within 3 months of BTS. Aortocoronary atresia was associated with 100% mortality (3 of 3). Of the survivors (n = 26), 19 have undergone Fontan operation whereas 7, having undergone bidirectional Glenn shunt, currently await Fontan. Actuarial survival by the Kaplan-Meier method for all patients was 81.3% at 5, 10, and 15 years, whereas mean survival was 12.1 years (95% confidence interval: 10.04 to 14.05). No late mortality occurred among those surviving beyond 3 months of age.

*Conclusions.*—In patients with PA/IVS-RVDCC, early mortality appears related to coronary ischemia at the time of BTS. Single-ventricle palliation yields excellent long-term survival and should be the preferred management strategy for these patients. Those with aortocoronary atresia have a particularly poor prognosis and should undergo cardiac transplantation.

▶ This review of 32 patients represents excellent survival with good follow-up. As others have suggested, patients with complete coronary atresia are not going to be candidates for a single-ventricle approach and should go directly to transplantation as soon as possible. Once a patient gets over the initial infancy procedure and gets to the bidirectional Glenn at 3 to 6 months, the outcome has been quite good to date (see Fig 3 on page 2254 of the original article). The most difficult time for these patients is with the aortic-to-pulmonary shunt, at which time coronary ischemia occurs if hypotension ensues. In addition, the authors make the point that the right ventricle must be kept full during the bidirectional Glenn or the Fontan procedure. With these caveats, many of these patients can be nursed through to a good early outcome.

**T. P. Graham, MD**

---

**Determinants of Exercise Function Following Univentricular Versus Biventricular Repair for Pulmonary Atresia/Intact Ventricular Septum**
Sanghavi DM, Flanagan M, Powell AJ, et al (Univ of Massachusetts, Worcester; Dartmouth-Hitchcock Med Ctr, Hanover, NH; Harvard Med School, Boston)
*Am J Cardiol* 97:1638-1643, 2006                                                        2–26

---

This study aimed to determine whether the exercise capacity of patients with pulmonary atresia/intact ventricular septum (PA/IVS) who have undergone biventricular repair is superior to that of patients with single ventricle repairs and to account for any differences. PA/IVS is generally treated with either biventricular (outflow tract reconstruction) or univentricular (Fontan) palliation. Although biventricular repair is believed to result in superior exercise function, this theory is untested. Symptom-limited programmed bicycle ergometry with expiratory gas analysis was prospectively performed on all patients with PA/IVS >7 years old seen over 18 months. Nineteen biventricular and 10 Fontan patients (mean age 16.5 ± 6.5 vs 12.7 ± 5.0 years, p = 0.12) were enrolled. The exercise capacity of biventricular patients was not statistically superior to that of Fontan patients (predicted peak $VO_2$ 83.5 ± 21% vs 76.0 ± 17.5%, p = 0.34), although chronotropic function and ventilatory efficiency were significantly better in the former. The peak exercise capacity varied widely within each group, and there was considerable overlap between biventricular and Fontan patients. Within groups, imaging studies did not reliably predict exercise capacity. Most patients in each group had subnormal peak $VO_2$, and there was a trend toward impaired performance with increasing age regardless of type of repair. In conclusion, biventricular repair may not guarantee superior exercise performance over single-ventricle palliation in PA/IVS. Regardless of repair type, aerobic capacity may deteriorate with age and is not reliably predicted by noninvasive imaging. These findings underscore the need for a quantitative, proactive approach to the assessment and preservation of exercise function.

▶ This intriguing study shows quite significant overlap between exercise capacity and other variables between patients with pulmonary atresia who had biventricular versus Fontan repair (see Fig 1 in original article). It does indicate that regardless of repair, aerobic capacity may deteriorate with age and is not reliably predicted by noninvasive imaging. Exercise testing can be useful in long-term follow-up of patients with complex disease regardless of what type of repair they have.

**T. P. Graham, MD**

## Coarctation, Interrupted Arch

### Muscle Sparing Extrapleural Approach for the Repair of Aortic Coarctation

Dave HH, Buechel ERV, Prêtre R (Univ Children's Hosp Zurich, Switzerland)
*Ann Thorac Surg* 81:243-248, 2006                                       2–27

*Background.*—This paper describes a muscle-sparing, extrapleural approach to repair aortic coarctation, and evaluates the results with established standards.

*Methods.*—Forty consecutive patients with aortic coarctation (median age, 8 days; weight, 3.3 kg) were approached with a less invasive technique consisting of a short posterior thoracotomy, with only minimal (24 patients) or no (16 patients) division of thoracic wall muscles and a subperiosteal-extrapleural approach. Extended resection of the coarctation with enlargement of the distal aortic arch was performed in all patients. The median cross-clamp and operative times were 22 and 90 minutes, respectively.

*Results.*—The repair was possible in all patients without needing conversion. There was no intraoperative or postoperative related complication. Two patients died early of low cardiac output as a result of ventricular fibroelastosis and respiratory failure. One patient died late of unrelated cause. The perioperative mean gradients across the neoarch were less than 5 mm Hg in all but 3 patients with proximal (2 patients) or mid arch (1) stenosis. The median ventilation time, intensive care unit stay, and hospital stay in isolated coarctation repairs was 2, 4.5, and 11 days, respectively. One patient had a recurrent stenosis at the site of surgical repair. Two patients underwent successful balloon dilatation, and 2 had surgical enlargement of the proximal aortic arch at the time of intracardiac repair. None of the patients required chronic antihypertensive medication. At 29 months, freedom from reintervention on the isthmus and arch plus isthmus was 97.1% and 89.7%, respectively.

*Conclusions.*—A muscle-sparing, extrapleural approach for the repair of aortic coarctation is possible and provides results similar to conventional techniques. The approach reduces postoperative morbidity related to division of thoracic wall muscles and handling of the lung, restores a normal intercostal space, and produces superior cosmetic results, while at the same time leading to early and permanent relief of proximal hypertension.

▶ In keeping with a less invasive approach, these authors present excellent results for a muscle-sparing approach for repair of coarctation. It certainly has the potential for producing superior cosmetic results and less pain during recovery. Results were quite good in this infant group, with freedom of reoperation excellent. The authors were able to perform extended resection of the coarctation and simultaneous pulmonary banding when needed (see Fig 1 on page 244 of the original article). This certainly deserves consideration for maintaining excellent results while improving morbidity in this common operation.

**T. P. Graham, MD**

---

### Selective management of the left ventricular outflow tract for repair of interrupted aortic arch with ventricular septal defect: Management of left ventricular outflow tract obstruction

Suzuki T, Ohye RG, Devaney EJ, et al (Univ of Michigan, Ann Arbor)
*J Thorac Cardiovasc Surg* 131:779-784, 2006                          2–28

---

*Objective.*—Left ventricular outflow tract obstruction remains an early and late complication after repair of interrupted aortic arch and ventricular septal defect. We reviewed our experience with the selective management of the infundibular septum during primary repair to address left ventricular outflow tract obstruction.

*Methods.*—From 1991 through 2001, all 27 patients presenting with interrupted aortic arch/ventricular septal defect and posterior deviation of the infundibular septum were analyzed. Fifteen patients with the smallest subaortic areas underwent myectomy or myotomy of the infundibular septum concomitant with interrupted aortic arch/ventricular septal defect repair.

*Results.*—Patients undergoing myectomy-myotomy (Group I) had significantly smaller subaortic diameter indexes ($0.83 \pm 0.16$ cm/m$^2$) when compared with those who had only interrupted aortic arch/ventricular septal defect repair (group 2: $0.99 \pm 0.13$ cm/m$^2$, $P = .012$). Two hospital deaths occurred in group 1, and 1 occurred in group 2. No late deaths occurred. No patient in group 2 required reoperation. Six group 1 patients required 9 reoperations for left ventricular outflow tract obstruction. Five patients underwent resection of a new subaortic membrane. Only 1 patient had recurrent muscular left ventricular outflow tract obstruction. Three patients required a second reoperation, primarily related to aortic valve stenosis.

*Conclusions.*—Interrupted aortic arch/ventricular septal defect with posterior malalignment of the infundibular septum can be repaired with low mortality in the neonatal period. Tailored to the degree of subaortic narrowing, resection or incision of the infundibular septum at the time of primary repair was very effective in preventing or prolonging the interval to recurrent left ventricular outflow tract obstruction compared with the published data. However, reoperation for left ventricular outflow tract obstruction, often related to the development of a new and discrete subaortic membrane or valvar stenosis, is still required in a subset of patients.

▶ These authors present excellent results in this very difficult-to-treat group of patients. A small outflow tract and annulus are always associated with many preoperative measurements by echocardiogram, and then a difficult decision regarding whether to proceed with definitive repair, with or without myectomy. These authors have some overlap in subaortic and aortic annulus diameters between those who had myectomy and those who did not. Their current management is to proceed with the primary repair with concomitant resection or incision of the infundibular septum if the subaortic area is less than 4 mm. The smallest aortic annulus in this series was 3.7 mm, or $-7.5$ in $z$ value. From their experience, they suggest that if the aortic annulus is more than $-6.5$ in $z$ value, the valve leaflets are normal, and deviation of the infundibular septum is the main cause of subaortic stenosis, then transatrial excision or incision of the septum is the procedure of choice to relieve left ventricular outflow obstruction. Otherwise a Damus-Kaye-Stansel anastomosis/Rastelli or Ross/Konno procedure is required.

Some groups may be more likely to get good results in patients with borderline subaortic/annulus sizes with the latter approach. Interestingly, some of these patients developed subaortic membranes after myectomy. In addition, the majority do have bicuspid valves that will require therapy, obviously, in the future. This is an important article in this complex group of patients.

**T. P. Graham, MD**

---

**Covered Cheatham-Platinum Stents for Aortic Coarctation: Early and Intermediate-Term Results**
Tzifa A, Ewert P, Brzezinska-Rajszys G, et al (Guy's and St Thomas's Hosp, London; German Heart Inst, Berlin; Children's Mem Hosp, Warsaw)
*J Am Coll Cardiol* 47:457-463, 2006                                         2–29

---

*Objectives.*—This study sought to evaluate the use of covered Cheatham-platinum (CP) stents in the treatment of aortic coarctation (CoA).

*Background.*—Aortic aneurysms and stent fractures have been encountered after surgical and transcatheter treatment for CoA. Covered stents have previously been used in the treatment of abdominal and thoracic aneurysms in adults. We implanted covered CP stents as a rescue treatment in patients with CoA aneurysms or previous stent-related complications and in patients at risk of developing complications because of complex CoA anatomy or advanced age.

*Methods.*—Thirty-three covered CP stents were implanted in 30 patients; 16 patients had had previous procedures. The remaining patients had complex or near-atretic CoA.

*Results.*—The mean patient age and weight were 28 (±17.5) years (range 8 to 65 years), and 62 (13) kg (range 28 to 86 kg), respectively. The systolic gradient across the CoA decreased from a mean (±SD) of 36 ± 20 mm Hg before to a mean of 4 ± 4 mm Hg after the procedure ($p < 0.0001$), and the diameter of the CoA increased from 6.4 ± 3.8 mm to 17.1 ± 3.1 mm ($p < 0.0001$). The follow-up period was up to 40 months (mean, 11 months). All stents were patent and in good position on computed tomography or magnetic resonance imaging performed three to six months later. In 43% of the patients antihypertensive medication was either decreased or stopped.

*Conclusions.*—Covered CP stents may be used as the therapy of choice in patients with complications after CoA repairs, whereas they provide a safe alternative to conventional stenting in patients with severe and complex CoA lesions or advanced age.

▶ These covered stents have been used quite effectively for patients with complex coarctation, particularly older patients with aneurysm or potential aneurysms. Follow-up was a mean of 11 months with a range of up to 40 months, and all stents were in good position. Hypertensive medications were either decreased or stopped in 43% of patients. Surgery can be quite difficult in these patients, with issues in terms of getting to the coarctation and resecting aneurysmal tissue without significant bleeding and/or compromise of vital organs with potential neurologic damage.

**T. P. Graham, MD**

---

### Noninvasive diagnosis of aortic coarctation in neonates with patent ductus arteriosus

Lu C-W, Wang J-K, Chang C-I, et al (Shin Kong Wu Ho-Su Mem Hosp, Taipei, Taiwan; Natl Taiwan Univ, Taipei)
*J Pediatr* 148:217-221, 2006                                                    2–30

---

*Objectives.*—To find a noninvasive method to detect coarctation of the aorta (CoA) in the presence of a patent ductus arteriosus (PDA) in neonates.

*Study Design.*—From 1994 to 1998, 36 neonates with CoA and PDA confirmed by surgery or cardiac catheterization were studied; another 19 neonates with isolated PDA served as control patients. The prospective study was conducted from 2001 to 2002 on 162 neonates.

*Results.*—Among the 36 neonates in the CoA group, 14 patients (39%) had blood pressure discrepancy, 26 patients (72%) had a visualized posterior shelf by echocardiogram, and the ratio of isthmus/descending aorta diameters (I/D ratio) was below 0.64 in 32 patients (89%). None of the control patients had these features. A diagnostic approach was subsequently proposed, according to which a neonate with PDA who fulfilled any of the above features was diagnosed as CoA plus PDA. In the prospective study, the sensitivity and positive predictive values of this method were both 91.7%, whereas the specificity and negative predictive values were both 99.3%.

*Conclusions.*—Echocardiographic measurements of I/D ratio along with the delineation of posterior shelf and a BP discrepancy can satisfactorily identify CoA in the presence of PDA in neonates.

▶ It frequently is the source of discussion and multiple echocardiograms in terms of whether one is dealing with simple PDA or PDA with CoA, which will need to be addressed at the time of surgery. Obviously these 2 operations are different enough that the surgeon will need to know precisely what the diagnosis is before surgery for optimal outcome. Echocardiographic measurements of I/D ratio, definition of posterior shelf, and arm-leg blood pressure discrepancy are used by all of us but not to the rigorous extent characterized by these authors. These detailed measurements should put you in the right ballpark 90% or more of the time.

**T. P. Graham, MD**

## Atrial Septal Defect/Ventricular Septal Defect

### Caval Division Technique for Sinus Venosus Atrial Septal Defect With Partial Anomalous Pulmonary Venous Connection

Shahriari A, Rodefeld MD, Turrentine MW, et al (Indiana Univ, Indianapolis)
*Ann Thorac Surg* 81:224-230, 2006                                    2–31

*Background.*—Repair of sinus venosus atrial septal defect (ASD) with high partial anomalous pulmonary venous connection (PAPVC) using an internal patch may be complicated by obstruction of the superior vena cava (SVC) or pulmonary veins, or both, and sinus node dysfunction. In cases in which the anomalous veins insert more than 2 cm above the cavoatrial junction, we have adopted the technique of caval division in which the SVC is divided and the proximal end is anastomosed to the right atrial appendage, and the distal SVC serves as a conduit for pulmonary venous drainage to the left atrium through the ASD. We retrospectively compare the results of the internal patch repair versus the Warden technique.

*Methods.*—Between 1991 and 2004, 54 patients diagnosed with sinus venosus ASD and PAPVC have undergone repair at our institution. Mean age was 13.4 years (range, 1.5 to 58). Thirteen patients (24%) had high insertion of anomalous veins and underwent the Warden technique. Follow-up averages 4.3 years (range, 1 to 13).

*Results.*—There were no early or late deaths. All patients remain in normal sinus rhythm. Twelve of the 13 patients with Warden procedure have had postoperative echocardiograms, and 11 of these patients showed no evidence of SVC or pulmonary venous obstruction. In 1 patient, symptomatic pulmonary venous obstruction developed and required revision of a contracted intra-atrial pericardial baffle.

*Conclusions.*—Caval division for treatment of high PAPVC appears to be safe and is associated with low morbidity and mortality. The Warden procedure is an effective surgical option for patients undergoing correction of high PAPVC.

▶ This type of repair of sinus venosus ASD appears to have the best possibility, at least theoretically, for avoiding obstruction to caval flow when high insertion of anomalous veins is present. In addition, one avoids suturing in the area of the sinoatrial (SA) node and the SA nodal artery, and thus the likelihood for rhythm disorders should be reduced. These authors show excellent results in a small series of patients (see Figs 3-6 on pages 226-227 of the original article).

**T. P. Graham, MD**

---

**Percutaneous versus surgical closure of secundum atrial septal defect: Comparison of early results and complications**
Butera G, Carminati M, Chessa M, et al (Istituto Policlinico San Donato, San Donato Milanese, Italy)
*Am Heart J* 151:228-234, 2006                                                    2–32

---

*Background.*—Surgical closure of atrial septal defect (ASD) provides excellent results. Given the increasing popularity of percutaneous techniques, a comparison between the 2 methods is needed.

*Methods.*—Between December 1988 and June 2003, we performed 1284 procedures in 1268 consecutive patients with isolated secundum ASD. Five hundred and thirty-three patients underwent surgical repair of ostium secundum ASD (group A). Seven hundred and fifty-one consecutive patients underwent percutaneous ASD closure (group B). The following outcomes were studied: mortality, morbidity, hospital stay, and efficacy.

*Results.*—There were no postoperative deaths. The overall rate of complications was higher in group A than in group B: 44% (95% CI 39.8%-48.2%) versus 6.9% (95% CI 5%-8.7%) ($P < .0001$). Major complications were also more frequent in group A: 16% (95% CI 13%-19%) versus 3.6% (95% CI 2.2%-5.0%) ($P = .002$). Multiple logistic regression analysis showed that surgery was independently strongly related to the occurrence of total complication (odds ratio [OR] 8.13, 95% CI 5.75-12.20) and of major complications (OR 4.03, 95% CI 2.38-7.35). The occurrence of minor complications was independently related to surgery (OR 7.33, 95% CI 4.75-11.02), childhood (OR 1.52, 95% CI 1.01-2.34), and presence of systemic hypertension (OR 1.35, 95% CI 1.01-4.41). Hospital stay was shorter in group B ($3.2 \pm 0.9$ vs $8.0 \pm 2.8$ days, $P < .0001$).

*Conclusions.*—Percutaneous ASD closure provides, in experienced hands and in highly specialized centers, excellent results with a lower complication rate and requires a shorter stay in hospital.

▶ There continues to be some controversy regarding short- and long-term results of surgical versus percutaneous ASD closure. It usually depends on whether the surgeon or interventionalist does a study as to which outcome appears better in certain ways. This study shows excellent results in both groups in a large cohort. There were more complications in the surgical group, but these in general were minor. Certainly, percutaneous closure of secundum ASDs in experienced hands is getting to be standard therapy in most centers around the world. Surgical treatment remains an excellent option. The most important aspect is to choose the correct procedure for each patient. If there is a complicated ASD with small rims with the possibility for implanting a large defect that may have the potential for erosion, then these patients should go to the surgeon and not to the catheterization lab.

**T. P. Graham, MD**

---

**Paradoxical Emboli in Children and Young Adults: Role of Atrial Septal Defect and Patent Foramen Ovale Device Closure**
Bartz PJ, Cetta F, Cabalka AK, et al (Mayo Clinic, Rochester, Minn; Loyola Univ, Maywood, Ill; Univ of Parma, Italy; et al)
*Mayo Clin Proc* 81:615-618, 2006                                    2–33

---

*Objective.*—To describe a multicenter experience with patent foramen ovale (PFO) and atrial septal defect (ASD) device closure for presumed paradoxical emboli in children and young adults (<35 years old).

*Patients and Methods.*—Medical records were reviewed of patients who had device closure of an ASD or PFO, who were younger than 35 years, and who had a history of presumed paradoxical embolus between January 1999 and August 2005 at Mayo Clinic, Rochester, Minn, University of Parma, Parma, Italy, and Loyola University Medical Center, Maywood, Ill.

*Results.*—Forty-five patients fulfilled the inclusion criteria. Median patient age was 29.0 years (range, 5.0-34.9 years), and 23 patients (51%) were male. Clinical diagnoses included the following: stroke, 30 (67%); transient ischemic attack, 13 (29%); myocardial infarction, 1 (2%); and renal infarct, 1 (2%). Overall, 42 patients (93%) had a PFO, and 3 (7%) had an ASD. Seventeen patients had known cardiovascular disease risk factors: tobacco use (10 patients), hypercoagulable states (7 patients), systemic hypertension (3 patients), and hyperilpidemia (2 patients). No major procedural complications occurred. Median follow-up evaluation was performed at 5.3 months (range, 2.5-40.0 months). Forty-four patients (98%) had no recurrent neurologic events and no residual atrial shunt by contrast transthoracic echocardiography.

*Conclusions.*—Cryptogenic ischemic events occur in young patients and have serious sequelae. The potential for paradoxical embolization through a PFO or an ASD should be assessed in all such patients. In our short-term follow-up, device closure was a safe alternative therapeutic option for children and young adults with presumed paradoxical emboli.

▶ There has been considerable literature about what to do with the child or young adult with a PFO or an ASD and paradoxical emboli. This is a particularly difficult therapeutic discussion, with an annual recurrence of transient ischemia attacks or cerebral infarctions reported to be 3% to 4% in some studies. These authors show very good results in terms of catheter closure and median follow-up; 90% of patients had no recurrent neurologic events and no residual atrial shunt. Most were able to discontinue warfarin administration after 6 months, which is certainly a laudable goal. This is one reference that should be considered when a young patient is referred to you with presumed paradoxical embolism.

**T. P. Graham, MD**

---

**Transcatheter closure of atrial septal defects improves right ventricular volume, mass, function, pulmonary pressure, and functional class: a magnetic resonance imaging study**
Schoen SP, Kittner T, Bohl S, et al (Univ of Dresden, Germany)
*Heart* 92:821-826, 2006                                    2–34

---

*Objective.*—To characterise prospectively by magnetic resonance imaging (MRI) changes in right ventricular (RV) volume, function, and mass after transcatheter closure of atrial septal defects (ASDs) and to evaluate the course of pulmonary pressure and functional class criteria.

*Methods.*—In 20 patients with secundum-type ASD and dilated RV diameter, MRI was performed to quantify RV end diastolic (RVEDV) and end systolic volumes (RVESV), RV mass, tricuspid annular diameter, and RV ejection fraction before and 6 and 12 months after transcatheter closure of the ASD. RV systolic pressure was measured during follow up by transthoracic echocardiography.

*Results.*—Functional class improved in the majority of patients after ASD closure. RVESV (from 81 (18) ml/m² to 53 (15) ml/m², p < 0.001), RVEDV (from 127 (17) ml/m² to 99 (18) ml/m², p < 0.001), and RV mass (from 79 (10) g to 63 (8) g, p < 0.01) decreased significantly during follow up, although tricuspid annular diameter did not. RV ejection fraction improved (by 9% compared with baseline, p < 0.05) and RV systolic pressure decreased significantly (from 33 (8) mm Hg to 24 (6) mm Hg, p < 0.001) after closure.

*Conclusion.*—MRI studies showed significant improvement of RV volumes, mass, and function after transcatheter closure of ASDs. Restoration of the RV leads to decreased pulmonary pressure resulting in a better functional class in the majority of patients.

▶ Although it is clear that in most patients the heart gets smaller as detected by simple chest x-ray after ASD closure, this rather elegant study quantifies these changes in RV volume, function, and RV mass after percutaneous ASD closure. The results are gratifying (see Figs 3 and 4 of original article). The authors suggest in their discussion that these studies may show a faster recovery of RV function than in adults after surgery. They would have to do these MRI studies in the same manner after surgery to be certain about this.

**T. P. Graham, MD**

---

**Isolated ventricular septal defects detected by color Doppler imaging: evolution during fetal and first year of postnatal life**
Axt-Fliedner R, Schwarze A, Smrcek J, et al (Univ of Schleswig-Holstein, Campus Lübeck, Germany; Univ of Regensburg, Germany; Univ of Bonn, Germany)
*Ultrasound Obstet Gynecol* 27:266-273, 2006                     2–35

*Objective.*—To evaluate the development during gestation and up to 1 year postnatally of isolated small ventricular septal defects (VSDs) not visible by gray-scale imaging and detected only on color Doppler fetal echocardiography.

*Methods.*—This was a retrospective analysis of 146 fetuses with isolated VSDs detectable only on color Doppler echocardiography. Complete sequential gray-scale, color Doppler and spectral Doppler examination of the fetal heart were performed. The following variables were documented: site of the VSD, presence of extracardiac or chromosomal anomalies, outcome of the pregnancy and evolution of the defect up to 1 year postnatally.

*Results.*—A total of 113 fetuses reached their first year of postnatal life, 23 pregnancies were terminated, there were three stillbirths/neonatal deaths, and seven were lost to follow-up. It was observed that 32.7% ($n = 37$) of all defects in neonates alive after 1 year closed in utero, 44.3% ($n = 50$) of defects closed spontaneously within the first postnatal year, and 23.0% ($n = 26$) of defects did not close. In all, a comparable number of perimembranous and muscular septal defects closed spontaneously in utero and during the first year of postnatal life. Among 35 fetuses with extracardiac anomalies 51.4% ($n = 18$) were euploid.

*Conclusion.*—Small VSDs, detectable only by color Doppler echocardiography, show a high spontaneous intrauterine and postnatal closure rate. These findings might be of value for prenatal parental counseling.

▶ This study shows a high prevalence of small VSDs in fetuses, particularly those with extracardiac anomalies. The good news is that there is a high rate of spontaneous closure during intrauterine life as well as during the first postnatal year. These data are useful in counseling parents prenatally and postnatally about the nature of small VSDs, even when detected in utero.

**T. P. Graham, MD**

## Pulmonary Hypertension

### Pulmonary Artery Hypertension: Is It Really a Contraindicating Factor for Early Extubation in Children After Cardiac Surgery?

Vida VL, Leon-Wyss J, Rojas M, et al (Pediatric Cardiac Surgery Unit of Guatemala (UNICARP), Guatemala Ciudad)

*Ann Thorac Surg* 81:1460-1465, 2006      2–36

*Background.*—One of the perceived major contraindications to early extubation after pediatric cardiac surgery is preoperative pulmonary arterial hypertension (PAH). The objective of this study is to present the results of early extubation (within 6 hours after open heart surgery) in children who had varying degrees of preoperative pulmonary arterial hypertension.

*Methods.*—We reviewed the charts of 100 consecutive children who underwent subaortic ventricular septal defect closure and also had preoperative PAH. Outcomes measured included early extubation rate, clinical status of patients, and hospital costs.

*Results.*—The median age at surgery was 2.5 years (range, 0.4 to 30). Sixty-five patients were extubated successfully in the operating room; 25 additional patients were extubated in the intensive care unit within 6 hours from surgery, increasing the early extubation rate from 65% to 90%. Postoperative complications were present in 12 patients; 10 of these patients required mechanical ventilation for more than 6 hours, and 1 of them died postoperatively in septic shock. Two patients required reintubation 25 and 26 hours, respectively, after initial extubation in the operating room, for causes unrelated to pulmonary hypertensive crises or ventilatory failure. The mean cost of procedures in patients who had successful early extubation was US $3,786.50 ± 302.45. Every additional day in the intensive care unit, in case of delayed extubation, increased the overall cost of the procedure by 10%.

*Conclusions.*—Pulmonary artery hypertension does not seem to be a contraindicating factor to early extubation in patients who underwent ventricular septal defect closure, and may be considered a feasible way to decrease postoperative intensive care unit stay and hospital costs.

▶ These authors show interesting results in the early extubation of patients with ventricular septal defects who had significant PAH preoperatively. They are able to extubate in the operating room in the majority of patients and within 6 hours after surgery in another sizeable group. Only 2 patients required reintubation, 25 and 36 hours, respectively, after extubation for causes related to pulmonary hypertensive crisis. This strategy can significantly decrease the cost of surgery, which continues to be an issue in providing care for infants with significant cardiac pathology.

**T. P. Graham, MD**

## Inhaled Nitric Oxide Use in Bidirectional Glenn Anastomosis for Elevated Glenn Pressures

Agarwal HS, Churchwell KB, Doyle TP, et al (Vanderbilt Univ, Nashville, Tenn)
*Ann Thorac Surg* 81:1429-1435, 2006                                                     2–37

*Background.*—Children frequently undergo bidirectional Glenn anastomosis in the staged surgical management of single ventricle physiology. The purpose of our study was to investigate the role of inhaled nitric oxide therapy in children with marked elevations in Glenn pressures after this surgery.

*Methods.*—A retrospective study over a 30-month period was performed. The effect of inhaled nitric oxide therapy was analyzed in children with marked elevations of Glenn pressures resulting in decreased systemic perfusion. Effects on Glenn pressures, respiratory indices, and systemic perfusion were evaluated after initiation of nitric oxide therapy and compared with baseline parameters.

*Results.*—Sixteen patients were placed on nitric oxide therapy for marked elevations of Glenn pressures ($22.4 \pm 3.9$ mm Hg). In the 11 responsive patients, there were significant reductions in Glenn pressures (from 22.4 mm Hg to 17.1 mm Hg, $p < 0.001$) and significant improvement in partial pressure of oxygen to fraction of inspired oxygen ratio (from 49 to 74.3, $p = 0.001$) and oxygenation index (from 17 to 12, $p = 0.005$). There was simultaneous significant reduction in inotrope score (from 14.9 to 11.4, $p < 0.001$) and fluid volume support (from 11.4 mL/kg to 2.3 mL/kg, $p < 0.001$) in the responsive patients. Five patients that failed to show any response were found, subsequently, to have an anatomic lesion.

*Conclusions.*—Inhaled nitric oxide produces significant reduction in Glenn pressures and improvement in systemic perfusion and pulmonary gas exchange in patients with marked elevations of Glenn pressures after bidirectional Glenn anastomosis. Patients who fail to respond should be investigated for an anatomic lesion.

▶ The use of inhaled nitric oxide can be a lifesaving procedure in certain postoperative patients, including those identified here. The cost of this therapy remains prohibitively high for routine use, but it can mean the difference between successful and unsuccessful surgical outcomes in selected patients, as these investigators show.

**T. P. Graham, MD**

## Phosphodiesterase-5 Inhibitor in Eisenmenger Syndrome: A Preliminary Observational Study

Mukhopadhyay S, Sharma M, Ramakrishnan S, et al (GB Pant Hosp and Maulana Azad Med College, New Delhi, India)
*Circulation* 114:1807-1810, 2006                                                     2–38

*Background.*—Phosphodiesterase-5 inhibitors produce a significant decrease in pulmonary vascular resistance in patients with idiopathic pulmonary arterial hypertension. We studied the effects of tadalafil, a phosphodiesterase-5 inhibitor, on short-term hemodynamics, tolerability, and efficacy over a 12-week period in patients of Eisenmenger syndrome having a pulmonary vascular pathology similar to idiopathic pulmonary arterial hypertension.

*Method and Results.*—Sixteen symptomatic Eisenmenger syndrome patients (mean age, 25±8.9 years) were assessed hemodynamically at baseline and 90 minutes after a single dose of tadalafil (1 mg/kg body weight up to a maximum of 40 mg). The same dose was then continued daily for 12 weeks, and the patients were restudied. There was a significant decrease in mean pulmonary vascular resistance immediately (24.75±8.49 to 19.22±8.23 Woods units; $P<0.005$) and at 12 weeks (19.22±8.23 to 17.02±6.19 Woods units; $P=0.03$ versus 90 minutes). Thirteen of 16 patients (81.25%) showed a ≥20% decrease in pulmonary vascular resistance and were defined as responders. The mean systemic oxygen saturation improved significantly both immediately (84.34±5.47% to 87.39±4.34%; $P<0.005$) and at 12 weeks (87.39±4.34% to 89.16±3.8%; $P<0.02$ versus 90 minutes) without a significant change in systemic vascular resistance. None of the patients had a fall in systemic arterial pressure, worsening of systemic oxygen saturation, or any adverse reactions to the drug. The mean World Health Organization functional class improved from 2.31±0.47 to 1.25±0.44 ($P<0.0001$), and the 6-minute walk distance improved from 344.56±119.06 to 387.56±117.18 m ($P<0.001$).

*Conclusions.*—Preliminary evaluation of tadalafil has shown efficacy and safety in selected patients with Eisenmenger syndrome, warranting further investigation in this subgroup of patients.

▶ It seems like forever that we have been without anything useful that we could do in the way of drug therapy for Eisenmenger syndrome. Slowly, data are accumulating that some vasodilators that we thought would lower systemic resistance and cause worsening right-to-left shunting can be useful in these patients. This small study indicates that tadalafil can result in improved quality of life and help in deciding when a patient is a candidate for lung transplantation.

**T. P. Graham, MD**

---

**Usefulness of Cutting Balloon Angioplasty for Pulmonary Vein In-Stent Stenosis**

Cook AL, Prieto LR, Delaney JW, et al (Duke Univ, Durham, NC; Cleveland Clinic Found, Ohio)
*Am J Cardiol* 98:407-410, 2006                                                  2–39

---

After radiofrequency ablation for atrial fibrillation, patients may develop pulmonary vein stenoses requiring stent angioplasty. The treatment options for when such patients develop in-stent stenoses are poorly defined. The investigators retrospectively reviewed their initial experience with cutting balloon angioplasty for pulmonary vein in-stent stenosis. Ten patients with 21 previously stented pulmonary veins returned to the catheterization laboratory for in-stent stenoses. Angioplasty of individual in-stent stenotic vessels were grouped into standard angioplasty alone (n = 6) and a combination of cutting balloon followed by standard angioplasty (n = 15). Although final mean lesion diameter was increased significantly in the 2 groups, restenosis occurred in 4 of 6 vessels in the group with angioplasty alone and 2 of 15 vessels in the cutting balloon group. In conclusion, cutting balloon angioplasty for pulmonary vein in-stent stenosis appears to improve the intermediate results of repeat angioplasty.

▶ Any successful treatment for pulmonary vein stenosis, whether of the iatrogonic type or the more common congenital or postoperative type, is potentially a breakthrough in this difficult disease. The authors speculate that controlled tears by the 4 blades weakens the intimal proliferation within the previous placed stent, and then, when the standard balloon slowly dilates, it opens the vessel to the appropriate diameter without as much disruption as with an oversized standard balloon. Hopefully this can add to the means of treating this difficult disease, both after radiofrequency ablation and in those congenital or postoperative cases.

**T. P. Graham, MD**

---

### Role of atrial septostomy in the treatment of children with pulmonary arterial hypertension

Micheletti A, Hislop AA, Lammers A, et al (Great Ormond Street Hosp for Children and Inst of Child Health, London)
*Heart* 92:969-972, 2006 2–40

---

*Objectives.*—To assess in retrospect the safety and effectiveness of atrial septostomy in children with severe pulmonary arterial hypertension without an intracardiac communication.

*Methods.*—20 patients were reviewed retrospectively, 19 with idiopathic pulmonary arterial hypertension. The mean age at septostomy was 8.4 years (range 3 months to 17 years). Graded balloon septostomy alone was carried out in eight patients, a blade septostomy was done in two, a blade septostomy plus graded balloon septostomy was done in three, and a fenestrated device was inserted in seven.

*Results.*—There were no fatalities. Four children suffered complications during the procedure. None had further syncope and all improved symptomatically with a significant ($p < 0.01$) decrease in World Health Organization functional class (mean shift $-0.6$) and a significant improvement in the semiquantitative echocardiographic assessment of right ventricular function ($p < 0.03$). The mean oxygen saturation decreased by 7.8 percentage points. The atrial communication closed in two children, necessitating a repeat procedure. After a mean follow up of 2.1 years (range one month to 6.7 years), 18 of 20 children are still alive.

*Conclusion.*—Atrial septostomy improved symptoms and quality of life in a group of children deteriorating with severe pulmonary arterial hypertension. This procedure is to be recommended for severely symptomatic children, before they become critically ill. Fenestrated devices may help ensure indefinite patency of the atrial communication.

▶ The creation of a relatively small to moderate-sized atrial septal defect in patients with severe pulmonary hypertension to increase systemic output and decrease symptomatology is useful in rare cases in symptomatic children. Creation of a large atrial septal defect results in severe hypoxemia and usually a downward spiral in the catheterization lab that cannot be changed. Therefore, this is a procedure to be undertaken with caution, but which can be useful in improving symptomatology in carefully selected patients.

**T. P. Graham, MD**

## Miscellaneous

**Randomized Controlled Trial of the Effects of Remote Ischemic Preconditioning on Children Undergoing Cardiac Surgery: First Clinical Application in Humans**
Cheung MMH, Kharbanda RK, Konstantinov IE, et al (Hosp for Sick Children, Toronto)
*J Am Coll Cardiol* 47:2277-2282, 2006                                     2–41

*Objectives.*—We conducted a randomized controlled trial of the effects of remote ischemic preconditioning (RIPC) in children undergoing repair of congenital heart defects.

*Background.*—Remote ischemic preconditioning reduces injury caused by ischemia-reperfusion in distant organs. Cardiopulmonary bypass (CPB) is associated with multi-system injury. We hypothesized that RIPC would modulate injury induced by CPB.

*Methods.*—Children undergoing repair of congenital heart defects were randomized to RIPC or control treatment. Remote ischemic preconditioning was induced by four 5-min cycles of lower limb ischemia and reperfusion using a blood pressure cuff. Measurements of lung mechanics, cytokines, and troponin I were made pre- and postoperatively.

*Results.*—Thirty-seven patients were studied. There were 20 control patients and 17 patients in the RIPC group. The mean age and weight of the RIPC and control patients were not different ($0.9 \pm 0.9$ years vs. $2.2 \pm 3.4$ years, $p = 0.4$; and $6.9 \pm 2.9$ kg vs. $11.5 \pm 10$ kg, $p = 0.06$). Bypass and cross-clamp times were not different ($80 \pm 24$ min vs. $88 \pm 25$ min, $p = 0.3$; and $55 \pm 13$ min vs. $59 \pm 13$ min, $p = 0.4$). Levels of troponin I postoperatively were greater in the control patients compared with the RIPC group ($p = 0.04$), indicating greater myocardial injury in control patients. Postoperative inotropic requirement was greater in the control patients compared with RIPC patients at both 3 and 6 h ($7.9 \pm 4.7$ vs. $10.9 \pm 3.2$, $p = 0.04$; and $7.3 \pm 4.9$ vs. $10.8 \pm 3.9$, $p = 0.03$, respectively). The RIPC group had significantly lower airway resistance at 6 h postoperatively ($p = 0.009$).

*Conclusions.*—This study demonstrates the myocardial protective effects of RIPC using a simple noninvasive technique of four 5-min cycles of lower limb ischemia and reperfusion. These novel data support the need for a larger study of RIPC in patients undergoing cardiac surgery.

▶ This trial of RIPC represents a novel attempt at ameliorating the effects of induced ischemia during cardiac surgery on cardiac function. The results suggest that this may be quite useful for improving outcome, with no known risk for the 4- or 5-minute cycle of lower limb ischemia and reperfusion. This obviously deserves support for a larger study, as indicated by the authors.

**T. P. Graham, MD**

---

**Current Assessment of Mortality Rates in Congenital Cardiac Surgery**
Welke KF, Shen I, Ungerleider RM (Oregon Health and Science Univ, Portland)
*Ann Thorac Surg* 82:164-171, 2006                                            2–42

---

*Background.*—The purpose of this study is to evaluate whether published and widely quoted mortality rates for pediatric cardiac surgery accurately reflect current expectations. Our hypotheses are that (1) mortality rates at high-quality pediatric cardiac programs are lower than published national results despite (2) a change in case mix with a shift away from low complexity operations.

*Methods.*—We requested data for all pediatric cardiac surgical procedures performed between 2001 and 2004 at 29 Congenital Heart Surgeon's Society (CHSS) member institutions (using CHSS as a surrogate for recognized high quality). Procedures were categorized by Risk Adjustment for Congenital Heart Surgery, version 1 (RACHS-1) category. In-hospital mortality rates for each category were calculated and compared with those in the 2002 manuscript of Jenkins and colleagues.

*Results.*—We received data for 16,805 procedures from 11 institutions. In all, 12,672 operations (76%) could be placed into RACHS-1 categories. Overall in-hospital mortality for categorized operations was 2.9% and was most related to case mix. There was a significant decrease in the percentage of category 1 operations, and there were significant increases in category 2, 4, and 6 operations. There were significant decreases in category 2, 3, 4, and 6 mortality rates (Jenkins 2002 [CHSS]): (1) 0.4% [0.7%], (2) 3.8% [0.9%], (3) 8.5% [2.7%], (4) 19.4% [7.7%], (5) not applicable, and (6) 47.7% [17.2%]. There was no significant association between hospital surgical volume and mortality.

*Conclusions.*—This outcomes "footprint" suggests that we could hold ourselves accountable to higher benchmarks than those reflected by some published standards. Mortality rates declined, despite an increase in case mix complexity. The lack of association between hospital surgical volume and mortality suggests that other factors determine outcomes at high-quality institutions. In addition to continually validating our expectations for treatment, future research needs to identify these factors by understanding the system of care and identifying process measures that influence outcomes.

▶ These authors attempt to modernize the acceptable mortality rates for patients with simple as well as complex congenital heart disease by using current data that are risk adjusted as to severity of condition and difficulty of operation. Lower surgical mortality rates in 11 institutions were found when compared with data that were previously reported in 2002. There was a lack of association between hospital surgical volume and mortality, although most institutions had a reasonable surgical volume. An association between volume and mortality is probably still an issue; there must be a certain threshold of operations that are required to ensure acceptable results for a given procedure, although the data indicate that there may not be a continuum of improved morbidity and mortality over a certain volume.

**T. P. Graham, MD**

---

**A multicenter prospective randomized trial of corticosteroids in primary therapy for Kawasaki disease: Clinical course and coronary artery outcome**
Inoue Y, for the Gunma Kawasaki Disease Study Group (Gunma Univ, Japan; et al)
*J Pediatr* 149:336-341, 2006                                        2–43

---

*Objective.*—To investigate the role of corticosteroids in the initial treatment of Kawasaki disease (KD).

*Study Design.*—Between September 2000 and March 2005, we randomly assigned 178 KD patients from 12 hospitals to either an intravenous immunoglobulin (IVIG) group (n = 88; 1 g/kg for 2 consecutive days) or an IVIG plus corticosteroid (IVIG+PSL) group (n = 90). The primary endpoint was coronary artery abnormality (CAA) before a 1-month echocardiographic assessment. Secondary endpoints included duration of fever, time to normalization of serum C-reactive protein (CRP), and initial treatment failure requiring additional therapy. Analyses were based on intention to treat.

*Results.*—Baseline characteristics of groups were similar. Fewer IVIG+PSL patients than IVIG patients had a CAA before 1 month (2.2% vs 11.4%; $P$ = .017). The duration of fever was shorter ($P$ < .001) and CRP decreased more rapidly in the IVIG+PSL group than in the IVIG group ($P$ = .001). Moreover, initial treatment failure was less frequent (5.6% vs 18.2%; $P$ = .010) in the IVIG+PSL group. All patients assigned to the IVIG+PSL group completed treatment without major side effects.

*Conclusions.*—A combination of corticosteroids and IVIG improved clinical course and coronary artery outcome without causing untoward effects in children with acute KD.

▶ This randomized trial does show improved outcome in terms of clinical course and coronary artery outcome in a group of 178 patients with KD who were randomly assigned to standard treatment with or without the addition of corticosteroids. There were no complications resulting from this short course of steroid therapy. These findings will certainly generate some controversy as to what should be done with all patients with KD. Corticosteroids may be useful in patients with refractory disease, but this treatment is not yet ready for prime time for all patients with KD.

**T. P. Graham, MD**

---

### Exposure to repeat doses of antenatal glucocorticoids is associated with altered cardiovascular status after birth

Mildenhall LFJ, Battin MR, Morton SMB, et al (Kidz First Middlemore Hosp, Auckland, New Zealand; Univ of Auckland, New Zealand; Auckland District Health Board, New Zealand)
*Arch Dis Child Fetal Neonatal Ed* 91:F56-F60, 2006                     2–44

---

*Objective.*—To determine if exposure to more than one course of antenatal glucocorticoids is associated with changes in infant blood pressure and myocardial wall thickness in the first month after birth.

*Design.*—Prospective cohort study.

*Setting.*—Tertiary neonatal intensive care unit.

*Participants.*—Mothers who were eligible for but declined to enter a randomised trial of repeated doses of antenatal glucocorticoids (ACTORDS)— that is, who had a singleton, twin, or triplet pregnancy at <32 weeks gestation, had received an initial course of glucocorticoids seven or more days previously, and were considered to be at continued risk of preterm birth.

*Main Outcome Measures.*—Blood pressure daily for the first week then weekly until 4 weeks of age. End diastolic interventricular septal and left ventricular posterior wall (EDIVS and EDLVPW) thickness at 48–72 hours after birth.

*Results.*—Thirty seven women were enrolled and delivered 50 infants. Thirty mothers (39 infants) were exposed to one course of glucocorticoids, and seven mothers (11 infants) to more than one course. Blood pressures were higher in the first week after birth in infants exposed to multiple courses of glucocorticoids, and in infants with a latency between last exposure and delivery of less than seven days. Systolic blood pressure on day 1 was >2 SD above published normal ranges in 67% of babies exposed to multiple courses and 24% of babies exposed to a single course of glucocorticoids (p = 0.04). There was no difference between groups in thickness of the EDIVS or EDLVPW. However, 44/50 (88%) babies had EDIVS and 49/50 (98%) babies had EDLVPW thickness >2 SD above the expected mean for birth weight and gestation. EDIVS but not EDLVPW thickness increased with increasing latency (mean 0.02 mm/day, p = 0.03).

*Conclusion.*—Future randomised trials should assess the long term effects of exposure to antenatal glucocorticoids, particularly multiple courses, on the cardiovascular status of the infant.

▶ It is intriguing to me that in looking at echocardiograms in babies who either prenatally or postnatally have been on large doses of glucocorticoids, that left ventricular hypertrophy is common as is hypertension. This study quantifies that relationship and suggests that with time, these findings hopefully will go away. In using these medications, one always has to be cognizant of the potential side effects. Hopefully, these doses of steroids when needed for lung maturity or treatment of lung disease will not result in lasting cardiovascular abnormalities.

**T. P. Graham, MD**

---

**Venoarterial Extracorporeal Membrane Oxygenation (VA-ECMO) in Pediatric Cardiac Support**
Thourani VH, Kirshbom PM, Kanter KR, et al (Emory Univ, Atlanta, Ga; Children's Healthcare of Atlanta at Egleston, Ga)
*Ann Thorac Surg* 82:138-145, 2006                                            2–45

---

*Background.*—Resuscitation extracorporeal membrane oxygenation (R-ECMO) was introduced at our institution in July 2002. We reviewed the use of venoarterial (VA)-ECMO for cardiac diagnoses at our institution.

*Methods.*—Retrospective analysis of patients on VA-ECMO for cardiac failure was performed. Survival was defined as discharge from hospital.

*Results.*—Twenty-seven patients were supported with VA-ECMO (median age, 27 days; range, 1 to 640 days; median weight, 3.8 kg; range, 1.8 to 11.3 kg). Diagnoses were cardiomyopathy-myocarditis (CMM) in 8 (30%), systemic-to-pulmonary artery shunt-dependent single ventricle (SV) in 12 (44%), postcardiotomy for biventricular repair (BiV) in 6 (22%), and arrhythmia in 1 (4%). Sixteen of 27 patients survived (59%). Seven of 8 CMM patients survived (88%); 6 (75%) bridged to cardiac recovery, 1 to transplant (13%), and 1 death (13%). Seven of 12 SV patients survived (58%). The SV ECMO indications: post-Norwood ventricular dysfunction (n = 3, 2 deaths), postoperative cardiac failure (n = 6, 2 deaths), respiratory failure (n = 1, 1 death), and acute shunt occlusion (n = 2, 0 deaths). One of 6 BiV patients survived (17%). The BiV ECMO indications: failure to wean from CPB (n = 3, 3 deaths), postoperative cardiac failure (n = 2, 2 deaths), and pulmonary hypertension (n = 1, 0 deaths). Fifteen patients (56%) underwent cardiopulmonary resuscitation during ECMO cannulation. Eleven of 15 R-ECMO patients (73%) survived versus 5 of 12 non-R-ECMO patients (42%, $p = 0.13$). Median duration of R-ECMO: 66 hours (range, 18 to 179) versus 145 hours (range, 43 to 986, $p = 0.01$) for non-R-ECMO.

*Conclusions.*—Resuscitation extracorporeal membrane oxygenation is an appropriate application in pediatric patients with cardiac disease. Single ventricle patients experiencing cardiopulmonary collapse and CMM patients have favorable outcomes. Failure to wean from CPB and postoperative ventricular failure are higher risk indications.

▶ As one wanders through the ICU, I am amazed by the number of patients who have had ECMO and survived with a reasonable long-term outcome. This has to be associated with the ability to apply this technique in a rapid fashion. The decisions about when to go on and when to wean are difficult ones. Long-term outcome in terms of neurologic status will be an important aspect of follow-up in these particular patient groups.

**T. P. Graham, MD**

---

**Tricuspid Valve Repair for Ebstein's Anomaly in Young Children: A 30-Year Experience**
Boston US, Dearani JA, O'Leary PW, et al (Mayo Clinic and Found, Rochester, Minn)
*Ann Thorac Surg* 81:690-696, 2006                                              2–46

---

*Background.*—The purpose of this study was to examine early and late outcome of tricuspid valve repair for Ebstein's anomaly in young children.

*Methods.*—Between October 1974 and November 2003, 52 children (25 boys) underwent tricuspid valve repair and annuloplasty for Ebstein's anomaly. Mean age was 7.1 ± 3.9 years (range, 5 months to 12 years). Concomitant procedures included atrial septal defect closure (n = 46), division of accessory conduction pathways (n = 4), ventricular septal defect closure (n = 3), and other (n = 7).

*Results.*—Early mortality was 5.8% (3 of 52 patients; no mortality since 1984, n = 31). Risk factors were age younger than 2.5 years ($p = 0.03$) and weight less than 10.7 kg ($p = 0.03$). Morbidity included transient atrial (n = 11) and ventricular arrhythmias (n = 5), and early reoperation in 3 patients. There was no need for a permanent pacemaker. Mean follow-up was 12.2 ± 7.4 years (maximum, 24.3 years). Actuarial survival at 5, 10, and 15 years was 92.3% ± 3.7%, 89.9% ± 4.3%, and 89.9% ± 4.3%, respectively. Freedom from all reoperations at 5, 10, and 15 years was 91.0% ± 4.3%, 76.9% ± 6.8%, and 61.4% ± 8.8%, respectively. Moderate (grade II) or more tricuspid regurgitation on dismissal echocardiogram was the only risk factor for reoperation ($p = 0.04$). Tricuspid stenosis did not occur in any patient. At late follow-up, 89% of patients were in New York Heart Association class I or II.

*Conclusions.*—Ebstein's anomaly in young children can now be repaired with low mortality and good tricuspid valve durability. Tricuspid regurgitation at the completion of operation should be mild or less to minimize need for reoperation. Tricuspid valve repair and annuloplasty did not result in stenosis despite somatic growth. Most patients enjoy an excellent quality of life.

▶ This outstanding report for children with a mean age of 7 years shows excellent results. It should be noted that this report does not include those infants with severe cardiac enlargement in whom there is a difficult decision regarding possible valve repair versus a single ventricle/Fontan pathway. These authors were able to repair the valve in patients who had considerable mobility of the anterior leaflet, usually at least 50% of the anterior leaflet delaminated, and the leading edge not adherent to the endocardium, as discussed in the question-and-answer period after this presentation. In addition, plication of the thinned out, atrialized part of the ventricle is done selectively and much less than in the past. It was felt to be a source of ventricular arrhythmias when plicated, and is only plicated now if it is very thin, transparent, and scarred.

**T. P. Graham, MD**

---

### Outcome of newborns with asymptomatic monomorphic ventricular arrhythmia

De Rosa G, Butera G, Chessa M, et al (Catholic Univ, Rome; Istituto Policlinico San Donato, Milan, Italy)
*Arch Dis Child Fetal Neonatal Ed* 91:F419-F422, 2006                    2–47

---

*Background.*—Frequent premature ventricular contractions (PVCs), couplets (CPLTs) and episodes of ventricular tachycardia are extremely rare in the neonatal population. Limited information is available with regard to clinical relevance and outcome.

*Objectives.*—To evaluate the clinical characteristics and outcomes of a group of newborns with ventricular arrhythmias without heart disease. Patients and design: Between January 2000 and January 2003, 16 newborns with ventricular arrhythmias in the absence of heart disease were studied. The newborns were divided into three groups: PVC group (n = 8), CPLT group (n = 4) and ventricular tachycardia group (n = 4). All patients underwent physical examination, electrocardiography, Holter monitoring and echocardiography at diagnosis and at follow-up (1, 3, 6 and 12 months, and yearly thereafter).

*Results.*—Mean (standard deviation, SD) age of the patients was 3 (1.19) days in the PVC group, 3.25 (0.95) days in the CPLT group and 6.5 (9.1) days in the ventricular tachycardia group. Median follow-up was 36 months (range 24–48 months). PVCs disappeared during follow-up in all the neonates, in the PVC group, at a mean (SD) age of 2.1 (1.24) months; in the CPLT group, couplets disappeared at a mean (SD) age of 6.5 (1) months. All patients with ventricular tachycardia were treated; ventricular tachycardia disappeared at a mean (SD) age of 1.7 (0.9) months. Neither death nor complications occurred.

*Conclusions.*—Ventricular arrhythmias in newborns without heart disease have a good long-term prognosis. Frequent PVCs and CPLTs do not require treatment. Sustained ventricular tachycardia or high-rate ventricular tachycardia must be treated, but the prognosis is generally favourable.

▶ This article is an excellent reminder that PVCs with a normal heart are almost always benign. It is always worrisome when we see these abnormal ECGs in young infants. This study helps to keep this in proper perspective. Frequent single PVCs rarely, if ever, require treatment and usually disappear within a few months. The 4 patients with ventricular tachycardia were treated with amiodarone, propanolol, or both, and ventricular tachycardia disappeared at a mean age of 1.7 months. No complications occurred.

**T. P. Graham, MD**

---

**Right to left shunt through interatrial septal defects in patients with congenital heart disease: results of interventional closure**
Agnoletti G, Boudjemline Y, Ou P, et al (Necker Enfants Malades, Paris)
*Heart* 92:827-831, 2006                                                    2–48

---

*Objective.*—To study the effects of closure of interatrial communications associated with a right to left shunt in patients with congenital heart disease (CHD) who had a biventricular repair.

*Design.*—Retrospective study.

*Setting.*—Tertiary referral centre.

*Patients.*—15 patients with CHD with right to left shunt through an interatrial communication: three had repaired tetralogy of Fallot, five had repaired pulmonary atresia with intact ventricular septum, four had Ebstein's disease, and three had other CHDs. Two patients had had a stroke before closure of the interatrial communication.

*Interventions.*—Percutaneous atrial septal defect (n = 6) or persistent foramen ovale (n = 9) closure. All patients underwent an exercise test before and after interatrial communication closure.

*Results.*—Five patients were cyanotic at rest. During exercise, mean (SD) oxygen saturation diminished from 93.9 (3.8)% to 84.3 (4.8)% (p < 0.05). Interatrial communication closure led to an immediate increase of oxygen saturation from 93.9 (3.8)% to 98.6 (1.6)% (p < 0.05). At a median follow up of three years (range 0.5–5) all but one patient with a residual atrial septal defect had normal oxygen saturation at rest and during exercise. Maximum workload increased from 7.2 (1.9) to 9.0 (2.2) metabolic equivalents (p < 0.001).

*Conclusions.*—Percutaneous closure of interatrial communications associated with a right to left shunt allows restoration of normal oxygen saturation at rest, avoidance of desaturation during exercise, and improvement of exercise performance in patients with CHD.

▶ This therapy is useful not only in patients after Fontan repair but also in those with biventricular repairs who have developed desaturation either at rest or with exercise. There were no complications during the percutaneous closure, and results show improved exercise performance in all but one patient.

**T. P. Graham, MD**

---

**Trends in Sudden Cardiovascular Death in Young Competitive Athletes After Implementation of a Preparticipation Screening Program**
Corrado D, Basso C, Pavei A, et al (Univ of Padua, Italy; Ctr for Sports Medicine and Physical Activity, Padua, Italy)
*JAMA* 296:1593-1601, 2006                                                        2–49

---

*Context.*—A nationwide systematic preparticipation athletic screening was introduced in Italy in 1982. The impact of such a program on prevention of sudden cardiovascular death in the athlete remains to be determined.

*Objective.*—To analyze trends in incidence rates and cardiovascular causes of sudden death in young competitive athletes in relation to preparticipation screening.

*Design, Setting, and Participants.*—A population-based study of trends in sudden cardiovascular death in athletic and nonathletic populations aged 12 to 35 years in the Veneto region of Italy between 1979 and 2004. A parallel study examined trends in cardiovascular causes of disqualification from competitive sports in 42,386 athletes undergoing preparticipation screening at the Center for Sports Medicine in Padua (22 312 in the early screening period [1982-1992] and 20 074 in the late screening period [1993-2004]).

*Main Outcome Measures.*—Incidence trends of total cardiovascular and cause-specific sudden death in screened athletes and unscreened nonathletes of the same age range over a 26-year period.

*Results.*—During the study period, 55 sudden cardiovascular deaths occurred in screened athletes (1.9 deaths/100 000 person-years) and 265 sudden deaths in unscreened nonathletes (0.79 deaths/100 000 person-years). The annual incidence of sudden cardiovascular death in athletes decreased by 89% (from 3.6/100 000 person-years in 1979-1980 to 0.4/100 000 person-years in 2003-2004; $P$ for trend <.001), whereas the incidence of sudden death among the unscreened nonathletic population did not change significantly. The mortality decline started after mandatory screening was implemented and persisted to the late screening period. Compared with the prescreening period (1979-1981), the relative risk of sudden cardiovascular death in athletes was 0.56 in the early screening period (95% CI, 0.29-1.15; $P$ = .04) and 0.21 in the late screening period (95% CI, 0.09-0.48; $P$ = .001). Most of the reduced mortality was due to fewer cases of sudden death from cardiomyopathies (from 1.50/100 000 person-years in the prescreening period to 0.15/100 000 person-years in the late screening period; $P$ for trend = .002). During the study period, 879 athletes (2.0%) were disqualified from competition due to cardiovascular causes at the Center for Sports Medicine: 455 (2.0%) in the early screening period and 424 (2.1%) in the late screening period. The proportion of athletes who were disqualified for cardiomyopathies increased from 20 (4.4%) of 455 in the early screening period to 40 (9.4%) of 424 in the late screening period ($P = .005$).

*Conclusions.*—The incidence of sudden cardiovascular death in young competitive athletes has substantially declined in the Veneto region of Italy since the introduction of a nationwide systematic screening. Mortality reduction was predominantly due to a lower incidence of sudden death from cardiomyopathies that paralleled the increasing identification of athletes with cardiomyopathies at preparticipation screening.

▶ The Italian medical and sports medicine community has been progressive in trying to provide programs that prevent the tragic occurrence of sudden death in competitive athletes who appear to be in the prime of life. The question about preparticipation screening comes up frequently. Going ahead with a significantly detailed personal history, physical examination, and ECG in all athletes was associated with a decreasing incidence of sudden cardiovascular death in this region of Italy. They did this without the use of echocardiography in the screening. Whether or not such a program could be used in the United States is difficult to determine, as it would require additional personnel, time, and financing for this service. The Italian group was able to do it with a minimum charge of only approximately $50 for an ECG and workup as outlined. It is a laudable goal to strive for in the future.

**T. P. Graham, MD**

---

**The Congenital Long QT Syndrome and Implications for Young Athletes**
Kapetanopoulos A, Kluger J, Maron BJ, et al (Univ of Connecticut School of Medicine, Farmington; Minneapolis Heart Inst Found)
*Med Sci Sports Exerc* 38:816-825, 2006                                    2–50

---

*Background.*—The congenital long QT syndrome (LQTS) may manifest as syncope and/or sudden cardiac death in young persons and is often associated with exercise. The exact prevalence is unknown, but it is recognized with increasing frequency. In recent years, several high-visibility athletes and situations have highlighted the issue of LQTS and athletic participation, and have raised the question of whether young athletes should be screened for LQTS. The genetic basis, pathophysiology, and clinical characteristics of the congenital LQTS were reviewed, and recommendations for its management in the physically active and athletic population were provided.

*Overview.*—There are 2 distinct clinical phenotypes involved in congenital LQTS, based on the type of inheritance and the presence of deafness. Romano-Ward syndrome is the most common type and is transmitted as an autosomal dominant disorder causing QT prolongation without deafness. Jervell and Lange–Nielsen syndrome is the less common but more severe phenotype of LQTS. It is transmitted as an autosomal recessive trait associated with congenital sensorineural deafness. Congenital LQTS is caused by more than 150 different mutations in 7 currently defined genes. Symptomatic patients with LQTS may present with palpitations, presyncope, syncope, seizures, or cardiac arrest. The diagnostic criteria for LQTS include clinical and ECG parameters. Asymptomatic mutation carriers are identified by ECG testing for an unrelated reason or during screening because of an affected family member. The QT interval is typically measured in lead II of a 12-lead ECG and corrected for rate by using Bazett's formula. A QTc interval of greater than 440 milliseconds in men or greater than 460 milliseconds in women is considered prolonged. However, Bazett's formula has been criticized as inaccurate. QT interval adjustment programs may be more accurate, but most of the available data for the congenital LQTS are derived from studies using Bazett's formula. It has become evident that the triggers of cardiac events in LQTS are genotype specific. There are also differences in the specific triggers of arrhythmic events among LQTS variants. β-Blocker therapy has become the standard first-line prophylactic therapy for patients with diagnosed LQTS. A variety of novel pharmacotherapies have been attempted on the basis of the concept of gene-specific treatment, but none have any currently established clinical role.

*Conclusions.*—The association of life-threatening cardiac events with exercise in LQTS has created concerns in regard to young athletes and young active persons in general. However, LQTS-related sudden cardiac death in young athletes is rare, and routine ECG screening is impractical and not recommended in the United States. However, persons with a personal or family history suggestive of LQTS should be further evaluated, at least with an ECG. Genetic testing is commercially available and will probably play a larger role in the diagnosis, risk stratification, and management of patients with LQTS.

▶ The decision about what to do with patients with a borderline or definite prolonged QT interval on an ECG has been a source of concern for cardiologists and sports medicine officials for many years. These authors give a detailed review of the issues involved and provide very nice examples of ECGs they consider to be classic for LQTS (see Figs 2 and 3 from the original article). The data in this article and the proposed risk groups for stratification are shown in Figure 4 from the original article and should be quite useful as one deals with a very complex problem.

**T. P. Graham, MD**

# 3  Cardiac Surgery

## Introduction

Cardiac surgery remains, in many regards, "the canary in the mine shaft" in terms of the public evaluation of outcomes and "quality." There have been several important contributions to the literature in this regard this year. They should be of importance to individuals participating in local quality assessment programs as well as those engaged in the public debate. This year's selections also include studies addressing some of the more common questions surrounding adult cardiac surgery, including the use of lipid-lowering agents, the clinical significance of perioperative enzyme release, and the treatment of perioperative atrial fibrillation. Finally, an intriguing study of the use of stress testing following coronary revascularization represents just the first step in a very worthwhile series of studies assessing the cost effectiveness of current practice patterns. A landmark study concerning complete arterial revascularization is included again this year, reflecting the critical importance of this issue in evaluating modern surgical revascularization techniques. The issue of PCI versus CABG is again addressed with an analysis of outcomes when bilateral ITA grafts are used.

In the area of valvular heart disease, there has been renewed interest in the subject of patient/prosthesis mismatch. An intriguing analysis from Washington University suggests that simplistic analyses will not suffice, but rather that the patients themselves should be stratified with important differences in outcomes assessed according to specific patient profiles. Surprisingly, perhaps, this approach has not been commonly adopted in addressing this subject. In addition, we have included analyses of valvular prosthesis choice comparing results with mechanical and biological prosthesis in several settings. Interest in valve repair remains high, and an important analysis of the midterm results of valve-sparing root repair is provided by the procedure's originator. Progress continues to be made in our understanding of the results of mitral valve repair in both degenerative and ischemic disease.

The field of transplantation continues to be vexed by the limitation in donor supply, and important studies evaluating the impact of strategies to expand that donor pool have been forthcoming in the year past.

Finally, there has been great excitement surrounding the endovascular treatment of thoracic aortic aneurysmal disease. Complementary studies, both industry-sponsored and population-based, provide a balanced view of the status of the field.

Thoralf M. Sundt III, MD

## Coronary Artery Disease

### How many arterial grafts are enough? A population-based study of mid-term outcomes

Guru V, Fremes SE, Tu JV (Univ of Toronto)
*J Thorac Cardiovasc Surg* 131:1021-1028, 2006                    3–1

*Objective.*—Current evidence suggests arterial grafting improves freedom from cardiac events after coronary artery bypass graft surgery. It has been shown that 2 arterial grafts provide improved outcome compared with 1 arterial graft. This population study seeks to understand trends in arterial graft use and midterm outcomes of patients receiving 1, 2, or 3 arterial grafts.

*Methods.*—This study is a retrospective population-based cohort of 53,727 patients (47,214 with 1 arterial graft, 5466 with 2 arterial grafts, and 1047 with 3 arterial grafts) undergoing isolated coronary artery bypass graft surgery in Ontario (1991-2001). The patients were followed by using linked clinical and administrative data, with complete follow-up until December 31, 2003 (average patient years of follow-up: 6 years for those with 1 arterial graft, 5 years for those with 2 arterial grafts, and 4 years for those with 3 arterial grafts). Propensity matching was used to compare outcomes between patients receiving 1 versus 2 arterial grafts, 2 versus 3 arterial grafts, and 1 versus 2 or 3 arterial grafts. The outcomes included death, repeat revascularization (angioplasty or coronary artery bypass grafting), cardiac readmission (readmission for angina, heart failure, and myocardial infarction), and a composite comprising all of these outcomes. Cox proportional hazards models were used to compare outcomes for propensity-matched patients. Subgroup analyses of various patient risk categories defined by the tercile of predicted 30-day mortality risk were conducted between propensity-matched individuals.

*Results.*—The use of multiple arterial grafts (defined as >1 arterial graft) increased mainly in the latter part of the study, from 4% in 1991 to 27% in 2001. Four thousand nine hundred sixty-eight patients were propensity matched (91% of patients receiving 2 arterial grafts) to compare outcomes with those of patients receiving 1 arterial graft. One thousand twenty-eight patients were propensity matched (98% of those receiving 3 arterial grafts) to compare outcomes with those of patients receiving 2 arterial grafts. Five thousand four hundred ninety-one patients were propensity matched (84% of those receiving 2 or 3 arterial grafts) to compare outcomes with those of patients receiving 1 arterial graft. Two arterial grafts were shown to be protective for cardiac readmission (0.8; 95% confidence interval, 0.76-0.92) and a composite outcome (0.9; 95% confidence interval, 0.72-0.95) compared with 1 arterial graft. Two or 3 arterial grafts were further found to im-

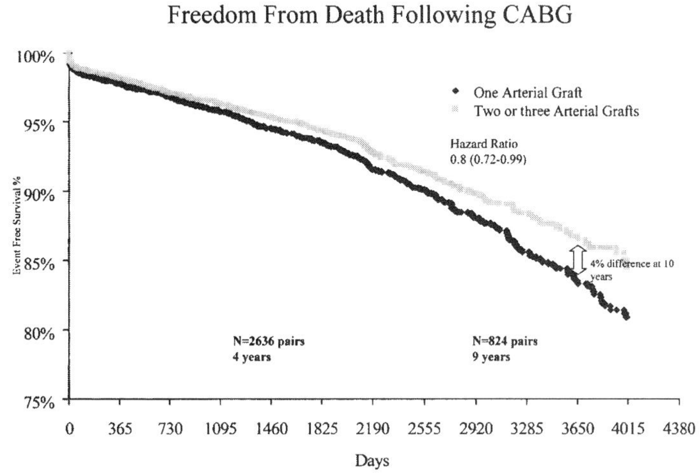

## Freedom From Death Following CABG

FIGURE 2.—Freedom from death after coronary artery bypass grafting (*CABG*) for those with 2 or 3 arterial grafts versus propensity-matched patients with 1 arterial graft in Ontario (1991-2001). (Reprinted from Guru V, Fremes SE, Tu JV: How many arterial grafts are enough? A population-based study of midterm outcomes. *J Thorac Cardiovasc Surg* 131:1021-1028, 2006. Copyright 2006 Elsevier.)

prove survival (0.8; 95% confidence interval, 0.72-0.99). In all patient operative risk categories, 2 or 3 arterial grafts were protective for cardiac readmission (hazard ratio, 0.7-0.8) and the composite outcome (hazard ratio, 0.8). There was no difference in the Cox hazard ratios of propensity-matched patients in the comparison of the groups receiving 3 versus 2 arterial grafts.

*Conclusions.*—Few patients received more that 1 arterial graft in our region. There was a survival benefit in receiving 2 or 3 arterial grafts. Patients with low, moderate, and high operative risk receiving 2 or 3 arterial grafts had lower rates of cardiac readmission compared with patients receiving only 1 arterial graft. This suggests that the standard of care should include the use of at least 2 arterial bypasses in all categories of operative risk to allow for optimal midterm outcomes (Fig 2).

▶ This large population-based study demonstrates a benefit of multiple arterial grafts in conferring improved freedom from death after coronary artery bypass grafting. A 4% difference was apparent at 10 years, as demonstrated in the accompanying figure. As a retrospective study, this work certainly suffers some limitations, particularly with respect to unmeasured covariates. Still, the power of this very large study with propensity matching is impressive.

The current reluctance of surgeons to use multiple arterial grafting is principally driven by concerns over sternal dehiscence and infection with bilateral internal thoracic artery (ITA) use, as well as the increased complexity of the procedure. Recent studies suggest that bilateral ITAs can be harvested without significant increased risk of sternal complications if the graft is harvested in a skeletonized manner; however, this has still been an uncommon practice, both in Canada and the United States. It is appropriate, however, to continue to ask ourselves whether we are doing enough with using only one ITA graft.

**T. M. Sundt III, MD**

---

**Indications for angiography subsequent to coronary artery bypass grafting**
Alter P, Vogt S, Herzum M, et al (Philipps Univ of Marburg/Lahn, Germany)
*Am Heart J* 149:1082-1090, 2005                                    3–2

---

*Background.*—Postoperative myocardial infarction is a rare, but potentially severe complication after coronary artery bypass grafting (CABG). Early markers for coronary bypass graft failure or native vessel occlusion are required, because immediate intervention could prevent major myocardial damage.

*Methods.*—One thousand patients with coronary artery disease consecutively underwent CABG. Postoperative coronary angiography was performed in 40 patients with suspected myocardial ischemia. Creatine kinase (CK), CK-MB, leukocyte count, C-reactive protein (CRP), lactate dehydrogenase (LDH), and glutamate-oxalacetate transaminase (GOT) were assessed at 0, 6, 12, 24, 48, and 72 hours after CABG as well as 12-lead standard electrocardiography (ECG).

*Results.*—Postoperative angiography of 40 patients with suspected myocardial infarction revealed graft failure or occluded native vessels in 13 (32.5%) individuals. Patients with graft or vessel occlusion presented elevated ($P < .005$) leukocyte counts (17,215 ± 6632 vs 10,773 ± 3902 G/L) immediately after CABG. CK-MB concentrations differed ($P < .05$) at 6 hours after CABG (54 ± 48 vs 30 ± 18 U/L). CK, CRP, LDH, and GOT did not show any differences between both groups. Frequency of ECG ST-segment elevation was increased ($P < .05$) in ischemic patients (69.2% vs 29.6%).

*Conclusions.*—Common signs of myocardial ischemia usually allow to diagnose unstable angina or myocardial infarction under native conditions. In contrast, these criteria frequently fail after CABG. Combined diagnostic criteria of elevated leukocytes (14,000 G/L, at hour 0) and either ST elevation or CK-MB concentrations >35 U/L (at hour 6) at least seem to be very useful in detecting myocardial infarction after bypass grafting. In parallel, CK-MB elevation (>70 U/L, at hour 6) alone seems to predict ischemia. Both criteria should indicate angiography and potential revascularization. If these conditions were not fulfilled, the risk of perioperative myocardial infarction appears to be moderate.

▶ Postoperative myocardial infarction resulting from graft occlusion is, fortunately, a very rare occurrence. Accordingly, there is a need for guidelines for angiography after coronary revascularization. The results of this study suggest that a combination of ST elevation and CKMB leak may be useful. In addition, marked CKMB elevation alone should also trigger angiography. In one third of the cases in this study, graft failure or an occluded native vessel was identified.

Unfortunately, missing from this study is any information about hemodynamics. In my own practice, I have found unexpected hemodynamic compromise to be a more useful indicator that one should proceed to coronary arteriography. One's threshold for coronary imaging should surely be low because the opportunity to correct the ischemia with additional interventional techniques presents itself only in a very narrow window.

**T. M. Sundt III, MD**

---

**Use of Stress Testing Early After Coronary Artery Bypass Graft Surgery**
Eisenberg MJ, for the ROSETTA-CABG Investigators (Jewish Gen Hosp, Montreal; et al)
*Am J Cardiol* 97:810-816, 2006                                                 3–3

---

The American College of Cardiology/American Heart Association guidelines for exercise testing do not take a position regarding the utility of routine stress testing after coronary artery bypass grafting (CABG). Our purposes were (1) to document the patterns of use of stress testing after CABG and (2) to establish whether the choice of stress testing strategy is associated with clinical characteristics of patients. The Routine versus Selective Exercise Treadmill Testing after Coronary Artery Bypass Graft Surgery (ROSETTA-CABG) Registry is a prospective multicenter study that examined the use of stress testing after CABG among 395 patients at 16 clinical centers in 6 countries. During the 12 months after CABG, 37% of patients underwent stress testing (range across centers 0% to 100%). Among patients who underwent stress testing, 24% had a clinical indication and 76% had it as a routine follow-up. A total of 65% of stress tests involved exercise treadmill testing alone, 17% involved stress nuclear perfusion imaging, 13% involved stress echocardiographic imaging, and 5% involved other types of stress tests, such as positron emission tomographic scans. The first stress test was performed at a median of 13 weeks after CABG, with 20% of patients having second tests at a median of 28 weeks and 6% having additional tests at a median of 34 weeks. Univariate and multivariate analyses demonstrated that the chief determinant of using routine stress testing was the clinical center. In conclusion, these results suggest that there is little consensus on the appropriate use of stress testing soon after CABG. Practice patterns vary widely; poorly diagnostic tests are used routinely; and the clinical center at which the procedure is performed, rather than the clinical characteristics of the patient, determines the use of stress testing after CABG.

▶ Heath care costs are skyrocketing. Surely this must be in significant measure due to the expense of diagnostic tests. In this study, the authors ask the very practical question "How should the postoperative coronary bypass patient be evaluated?" Stress testing after coronary artery bypass surgery is notoriously poorly diagnostic unless combined with ventricular imaging. Even with such additional imaging, its utility is unclear as evidenced by the wide variation in use of stress testing across centers. In this study, the variation could not have been wider: the use of stress testing varied from 0% to 100%. And what of the subset that underwent testing? Sixty-five percent of the patients undergoing testing in this study were asymptomatic, with 76% undergoing the testing as a "routine follow-up" rather than on the basis of clinical indications. The authors suggest that there are significant savings to be had simply by applying more rational clinical protocols. The results of the test are not included in this study, so we cannot determine the clinical yield; however, given the variation in practice, this looks to be an appealing target for cost reduction.

**T. M. Sundt III, MD**

---

**Preoperative statin therapy is associated with reduced cardiac mortality after coronary artery bypass graft surgery**
Collard CD, for the Multicenter Study of Perioperative Ischemia (MCSPI) Research Group, Inc, and the Ischemia Research and Education Found (IREF) Investigators (Baylor College of Medicine; et al)
*J Thorac Cardiovasc Surg* 132:392-400, 2006                    3–4

---

*Objective.*—Statin therapy in ambulatory populations is associated with a significant reduction in adverse cardiovascular events, including death and myocardial infarction. Much less is known about the beneficial effects of statins on acute perioperative cardiovascular events. The purpose of this study was to determine whether preoperative statin therapy is associated with a reduced risk of early cardiac death or nonfatal, in-hospital postoperative myocardial infarction after primary, elective coronary artery bypass graft surgery requiring cardiopulmonary bypass.

*Methods.*—The Multicenter Study of Perioperative Ischemia (*McSPI*) Epidemiology II Study was a prospective, longitudinal study of 5436 patients undergoing coronary artery bypass graft surgery between November 1996 and June 2000 at 70 centers in 17 countries. The present study consisted of a pre-specified subset of these subjects divided into patients receiving (n = 1352) and not receiving (n = 1314) preoperative statin therapy. To control for potential bias related to use of statin therapy, the study estimated propensity scores by logistic regression to determine the predicted probability of inclusion in the "statin" group. Multivariate, stepwise logistic regression was then performed, controlling for patient demographics, medical history, operative characteristics, and propensity score to determine whether preoperative statin therapy was independently associated with a reduction in the risk of early (DOS-POD3) cardiac death and/or nonfatal, in-hospital postoperative myocardial infarction.

*Results.*—Preoperative statin therapy was independently associated with a significant reduction (adjusted odds ratio [OR] 0.25; 95% confidence intervals [CI] 0.07-0.87) in the risk of early cardiac death after primary, elective coronary bypass surgery (0.3% vs 1.4%; $P < .03$), but was not associated with a reduced risk of postoperative nonfatal, in-hospital myocardial infarction (7.9% vs 6.2%; $P$ = not significant). Discontinuation of statin therapy after surgery was independently associated with a significant increase in late (POD4-discharge) all-cause mortality (adjusted OR 2.64; 95% CI 1.32-5.26) compared with continuation of statin therapy (2.64% vs 0.60%; $P < .01$). This was true even when controlling for the postoperative discontinuation of aspirin, beta-blocker, or angiotensin-converting enzyme inhibitor therapy. Discontinuation of statin therapy after surgery was also independently associated with a significant increase in late cardiac mortality (adjusted OR 2.95; 95% CI 1.31-6.66) compared with continuation of statin therapy (1.91% vs 0.45%; $P < 0.01$).

*Conclusions.*—Preoperative statin use is associated with reduced cardiac mortality after primary, elective coronary artery bypass grafting. Postoperative statin discontinuation is associated with increased in-hospital mortality. Although further randomized trials are needed to confirm these findings, these data suggest the importance of perioperative statin administration.

▶ This study demonstrates the importance of pharmacologic adjuncts in reducing the risk of perioperative death at the time of coronary artery bypass surgery. There is increasing recognition of the importance of statins among both physicians and surgeons. This large study demonstrates the value of preoperative statin therapy. It further demonstrates the importance of continuation of statin therapy after surgery. The mechanism of this effect remains incompletely understood despite recognition of their impact on platelet function, endothelial cell function, and vascular remodeling. Regardless, the clinical message is clear: administration of statins is an appropriate process variable and targets for quality improvement. Moreover, we should do our best to initiate therapy before operative intervention.

**T. M. Sundt III, MD**

---

### Limitations of Hospital Volume as a Measure of Quality of Care for Coronary Artery Bypass Graft Surgery

Welke KF, Barnett MJ, Sarrazin MSV, et al (Oregon Health and Science Univ, Portland; Univ of Iowa Carver College of Medicine, Iowa City)
*Ann Thorac Surg* 80:2114-2120, 2005                                    3–5

---

*Background.*—While prior research has found an inverse relationship between hospital volume and mortality after coronary artery bypass graft surgery (CABG), the use of volume as a proxy for quality and a means for selecting hospitals is controversial. The objective of this study is to quantify the relationship between hospital volume alone and CABG mortality.

*Methods.*—A retrospective cohort of 948,093 Medicare patients undergoing CABG in 870 US hospitals from 1996 to 2001 was categorized into quintiles, based on hospital CABG volume. Hospitals were also classified by volume criterion proposed by the Leapfrog Group. Logistic regression was used to adjust hospital mortality rates (in-hospital or within 30 days after

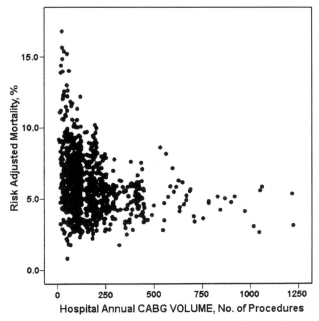

**FIGURE 1.**—*Risk-adjusted hospital mortality rates by coronary artery bypass graft* (CABG) *procedural volume.* (Courtesy of Welke KF, Barnett MJ, Sarrazin MSV, et al: Limitations of hospital volume as a measure of quality of care for coronary artrey bypass graft surgery. *Ann Thorac Surg* 80:2114-2120. Copyright 2005 Elsevier.)

CABG) for patient characteristics; discrimination of the volume categories was assessed by the $c$ statistic.

*Results.*—The range in risk-adjusted mortality for hospitals within the quintiles was substantial: 1% to 17% at very low, 2% to 12% at low, 2% to 10% at medium, 2% to 9% at high, and 3% to 11% at very high volume hospitals. Moreover, volume alone was a poor discriminator of mortality ($c$ statistic = 0.52). Similar variation in adjusted mortality was seen within the Leapfrog low-volume (1% to 17%) and high-volume groups (2% to 11%), and the Leapfrog criterion was a poor discriminator of mortality ($c$ statistic = 0.51). Of the 660 low-volume Leapfrog hospitals, 253 (38%) had risk-adjusted mortality rates that were similar to or lower than the overall risk-adjusted mortality of high-volume hospitals (5.2%).

*Conclusions.*—Volume alone, as a discriminator of mortality, is only slightly better than a coin flip ($c$ statistic of 0.50) (Fig 1).

▶ Case volume is commonly used as a surrogate for quality of care, not so much becasaue we are convinced of its accuracy as we are of its ease of definition. This study, like many others, demonstrates that, although volume data are easy numbers to obtain, they are in truth inadequate. As shown in Fig 1, although there is a general relationship between volume and the risk-adjusted mortality rate, the variation within each annual volume category is so wide as to make selection of an individual providing hospital on this basis alone as intellectually flawed as looking for your keys underneath the lamppost where the light is good even though you dropped them halfway down the street. Statistics do indeed tell you about the group, but they tell you precious little about the individual. Unfortunately, volume as a surrogate is supported by such organizations as the *U.S. News & World Report* magazine and the Leapfrog Group. It is important for us to make it clear to the public that this is an inadequate assessment. If one wants to look at quality, one should look at quality.

**T. M. Sundt III, MD**

## Valve Disease

### Valve Replacement Surgery in End-Stage Renal Failure: Mechanical Prostheses Versus Bioprostheses

Chan V, Jamieson WRE, Fleischer AG, et al (Univ of British Columbia, Vancouver, Canada; Westchester Med Ctr, Valhalla, NY)
*Ann Thorac Surg* 81:857-862, 2006            3–6

*Background.*—The 1998 American College of Cardiology/American Heart Association Guidelines recommend mechanical prostheses for valve replacement in patients with end-stage renal disease requiring dialysis. The aim of the study is to evaluate the combined experience at two academic centers.

*Methods.*—Sixty-nine valve replacements (aortic 40; mitral 22; multiple 7; 47 bioprostheses, 22 mechanical prostheses) were performed. Total follow-up was 128.7 patient-years (bioprostheses, 68.4; mechanical prostheses, 60.4).

*Results.*—Patient populations were homogeneous, except for age (bioprostheses greater than mechanical prostheses, $p = 0.012$), previous myocardial infarction (bioprostheses greater than mechanical prostheses, $p = 0.040$), and concomitant CABG (bioprostheses greater than mechanical prostheses, $p = 0.019$). A survival advantage was observed in favor of mechanical prostheses ($p = 0.0299$) at 5 years. Freedom from valve-related complications at 5 years was calculated for thromboembolism plus thrombosis plus hemorrhage (bioprostheses, 93.0% ± 3.9%; mechanical prostheses, 76.4% ± 12.7%), thromboembolism excluding thrombosis (bioprostheses, 93.0% ± 3.9%; mechanical prostheses, 88.9% ± 10.5%), and hemorrhage (bioprostheses, 100%; mechanical prostheses, 95.2% ± 4.7%). One case of structural valve deterioration occurred in the bioprostheses group at 95 months after surgery. Five-year freedom from all valve-related complications was 82.8% ± 8.1% for bioprostheses and 76.4% ± 12.7% for mechanical prostheses.

*Conclusions.*—Overall survival was poor. Differences between populations were related to age at operation and coronary artery disease. Structural valve deterioration was not accentuated with bioprostheses. Considering lack of homogeneity between prostheses groups there was no superiority of mechanical prostheses over bioprostheses in terms of freedom from composites of complications. Bioprostheses should be considered in the management of valvular disease in end-state renal disease patients.

▶ Valve replacement in the setting of renal failure: what prosthesis to use? Is a biological valve preferred in the interest of avoiding coumadin or to be avoided out of concern for accelerated calcification? The issue remains largely unresolved. Indeed, concern over the use of bioprosthetic valves in patients with end-stage renal disease drove the ACC/AHA Guidelines Committee to recommend mechanical prostheses for patients with end-stage renal disease. To be sure, we all have anecdotal experience with individual patients with accelerated calcification of a bioprosthetic valve in the setting of dialysis, but how solid is the evidence?

In this study, Jamieson et al in Vancouver in association with the West Chester Medical Center in Valhalla attempt to bring some hard data to bear on this important question. Interestingly, in their study, a survival advantage was observed in favor of mechanical valves, reminiscent of the findings of the 2 existent randomized studies of bioprosthetic versus mechanical valves.[1,2] To be sure, overall survival was remarkably poor. Early mortality was 29%, with a 36% mortality in the bioprosthetic group and a 13% mortality rate in the mechanical group. At 5 years, survival overall was only 30%, with 50% of those undergoing mechanical valve replacement alive and only 21% of those with bioprosthetic valves surviving. Outcome was particularly and uniformly poor among patients with significant coronary artery disease requiring bypass grafting, with all of the observed survival advantage of mechanical prostheses in the nonbypass patients. The data appear to support the guidelines.

Is there more to the story than this, however? In any retrospective surgical series, one must be wary of systematic selection bias, with unmeasured covariates accounting for uneven distribution of patients between groups (the application of "clinical judgment" to put, in this case, mechanical prostheses in the "healthier" patients). Short of a randomized study, there is no amount of statistical manipulation that can correct for such bias—because unmeasured variables cannot be entered into a model! So I would suggest that the findings be taken with a grain of salt. And there is more here to consider as well. I see that among those patients with bioprosthetic valves there was only one instance of structural valve deterioration! In other words, although we all remember the few patients with early calcification of such a prosthesis, it is in fact, uncommon. This leads to the important conclusion of the study: that bioprosthetic valves remain a very reasonable choice between 2 less-than-ideal options.

**T. M. Sundt III, MD**

*References*

1. Hammermeister K, Sethi GK, Henderson WG, et al: Outcomes 15 years after valve replacement with a mechanical versus a bioprosthetic valve: Final report of the Veterans Affairs randomized trial. *J Am Coll Cardiol* 36:1152-1158, 2000.
2. Oxenham H, Bloomfield P, Wheatley DJ, et al. Twenty year comparison of a Bjork-Shiley mechanical heart valve with porcine bioprostheses. *Heart* 89:715-721, 2003.

## Mitral Valve Surgery in the Adult Marfan Syndrome Patient

Bhudia SK, Troughton R, Lam B-K, et al (Cleveland Clinic Found, Ohio)
*Ann Thorac Surg* 81:843-848, 2006                                   3–7

*Background.*—Because mitral valve dysfunction in adults with Marfan syndrome is poorly characterized, this study compares mitral valve pathophysiology and morphology with that of myxomatous mitral disease, documents types of mitral valve operations, and assesses long-term survival and durability of mitral valve surgery in Marfan patients.

*Methods.*—From May 1975 to June 2000, 27 adults with Marfan syndrome underwent mitral valve surgery. Their valve pathophysiology and morphology was compared with that of 119 patients with myxomatous mitral disease undergoing surgery from September 1995 to March 1999. Survival and repair durability were assessed at follow-up.

*Results.*—Compared with myxomatous disease patients, Marfan patients had less posterior leaflet prolapse (44% versus 70%, $p = 0.01$), more bileaflet (44% versus 28%, $p = 0.09$) and anterior leaflet prolapse (11% versus 3%, $p = 0.07$), and presented earlier for surgery (age $41 \pm 12$ years versus $57 \pm 13$, $p < 0.0001$). Marfan patients had longer and thinner leaflets. Mitral valve repair was performed less frequently in Marfan (16 of 27, 59%) than myxomatous disease patients (112 of 119, 94%). There were no hospital deaths; at 10 years, survival was 80% and freedom from reoperation 96%, with only 1 reoperation among the 16 repairs.

*Conclusions.*—Mitral valve pathophysiology and morphology differ between Marfan and myxomatous mitral valve diseases. Valve repair in Marfan patients is durable and gives acceptable long-term results, even in adults who present with advanced mitral valve pathology. With increasing use of the modified David reimplantation operation and sparing of the aortic valve, mitral valve repair is a greater imperative, particularly since we have not had to reoperate on any Marfan patients with reimplantations.

▶ This article is included in the YEAR BOOK selections more because of the importance of the question asked than because of the value of the data presented. It is remarkable that in an institution with such an enormous experience in mitral valve repair, relatively few patients with Marfan syndrome have come to mitral surgery. This is not to cast aspersions on the institution, which is beyond reproach in this regard, but rather to highlight the low frequency with which mitral valve disease brings Marfan patients to intervention. Furthermore, these data give us some insights into the practicability of mitral repair in the setting of Marfan syndrome.

Despite the authors' conclusion that mitral valve repair is durable, close inspection of their data tables demonstrate that since 1985 only about half of their patients have undergone repair. Although only 1 patient underwent reoperation, only 2 patients underwent mitral surgery between 1975 and 1985 and overall only 59% of patients had repair! The reason for this is obscure, although there may have been a lower threshold for mechanical valve replacement if simultaneous mechanical composite root replacement was being performed. This may well change now that valve-sparing root repair as described by David et al[1] is becoming more widespread, as suggested by the authors. The apparent durability of both procedures is an exciting development for this interesting group of patients who often come to surgical intervention at a relatively young age.

**T. M. Sundt III, MD**

*Reference*

1. David TE, Feindel CM, Webb GD, et al: Long-term results of aortic valve-sparing operations for aortic root aneurysm. *J Thorac Cardiovasc Surg* 132:347-354, 2006.

**Prosthesis–patient mismatch after aortic valve replacement predominately affects patients with preexisting left ventricular dysfunction: Effect on survival, freedom from heart failure, and left ventricular mass regression**

Ruel M, Al-Faleh H, Kulik A, et al (Univ of Ottawa, Ont, Canada)
*J Thorac Cardiovasc Surg* 131:1036-1044, 2006                    3–8

*Objective.*—The effect of prosthesis–patient mismatch on clinical outcome and left ventricular mass regression after aortic valve replacement remains controversial. Data on whether the clinical effect of prosthesis–patient mismatch depends on left ventricular function at the time of aortic valve replacement are lacking. This study examined the long-term clinical and echocardiographic effects of prosthesis–patient mismatch in patients with and without left ventricular systolic dysfunction at the time of aortic valve replacement.

*Methods.*—Preoperative and serial postoperative echocardiograms were performed in 805 adults who underwent aortic valve replacement between 1990 and 2003 and who were subsequently followed up in a dedicated valve clinic (follow-up, mean ± SD, 5.5 ± 3.5 years; maximum, 14.2 years). Preoperative left ventricular function was defined as normal (ejection fraction ≥50%) in 548 patients and impaired (ejection fraction <50%) in 257 patients.

*Results.*—Patients with impaired preoperative left ventricular function and prosthesis-patient mismatch (indexed effective orifice area ≤0.85 cm²/m²) had a decreased overall late survival (hazard ratio, 2.8; $P = .03$), decreased freedom from heart failure symptoms or heart failure death (odds ratio of 5.1 at 3 years after aortic valve replacement; $P = .009$), and diminished left ventricular mass regression compared with patients with impaired preoperative left ventricular function and no prosthesis–patient mismatch. These effects of prosthesis–patient mismatch were not observed in patients with normal preoperative left ventricular function.

*Conclusions.*—Prosthesis–patient mismatch at an indexed effective orifice area of 0.85 cm²/m² or less after aortic valve replacement primarily affects patients with impaired preoperative left ventricular function and re-

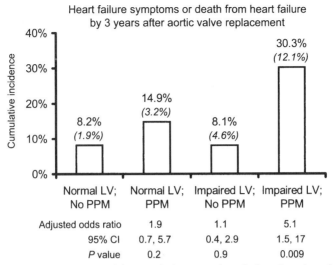

Heart failure symptoms or death from heart failure by 3 years after aortic valve replacement

| | Normal LV; No PPM | Normal LV; PPM | Impaired LV; No PPM | Impaired LV; PPM |
|---|---|---|---|---|
| Adjusted odds ratio | | 1.9 | 1.1 | 5.1 |
| 95% CI | | 0.7, 5.7 | 0.4, 2.9 | 1.5, 17 |
| *P* value | | 0.2 | 0.9 | 0.009 |

FIGURE 2.—Effect of preoperative left ventricular function and prosthesis–patient mismatch on the cumulative incidence of heart failure symptoms or death related to heart failure at 3 years after aortic valve replacement. Nonitalic percentages, bars, and odds ratios refer to the occurrence of either heart failure symptoms or death. Italic percentages in parentheses indicate heart failure death. Odds ratios are in comparison to the "Normal LV: No PPM" group and are adjusted for risk factors of decreased freedom from heart failure after AVR[2] and for baseline patient characteristics. Patients with the combination of impaired preoperative left ventricular function and postoperative prosthesis–patient mismatch had a lower freedom from heart failure despite adjustment for confounding factors. *CI,* Confidence interval; *LV,* left ventricle; *PPM,* prosthesis–patient mismatch. (Reprinted from Ruel M, Al-Faleh H, Kulik A, et al: Prosthesis–patient mismatch after aortic valve replacement predominately affects patients with preexisting left ventricular dysfunction: Effect on survival, freedom from heart failure, and left ventricular regression. *J Thorac Cardiovasc Surg* 131:1036-1044, 2006. Copyright 2006 Elsevier.)

sults in decreased survival, lower freedom from heart failure, and incomplete left ventricular mass regression. Patients with impaired left ventricular function represent a critical population in whom prosthesis–patient mismatch should be avoided at the time of aortic valve replacement (Fig 2).

▶ A debate over the clinical significance of "patient-prosthesis mismatch" rages on among surgeons and cardiologists. Although it makes no logical sense to replace a stenotic native valve with a stenotic prosthesis, the data on impact of patient-prosthesis mismatch on outcome has been quite mixed. The debate is complicated by varying definitions of patient-prosthesis mismatch, including both the critical ratio of orifice area to body surface area and the very definition of orifice area, be it geometric or effective.

Several investigators have attempted to look at this question more closely. Ruel et al have tried to refine their question, seeking to stratify patients by left ventricular function. Importantly, their data demonstrate, as shown in the accompanying figure, an impact of patient-prosthesis mismatch in both populations, although those with normal left ventricular function demonstrate a relatively smaller increased incidence of congestive failure.

I take 2 points away from this study. First, clearly patient-prosthesis mismatch is to be avoided among patients with congestive failure and left ventricular dysfunction. Every effort should be made to optimize the valve orifice area in these individuals. Second, even in those with normal left ventricular function, there is an impact. Although it may not demonstrate statistical significance in the numbers of patients available in such a study, there is no question that I want the largest possible valve in my aortic outflow tract if I am the patient. It is also clear, however, that in an otherwise high-risk patient with a good ventricle, one can slip by with some degree of patient-prosthesis mismatch without impairing long-term survival excessively. From a surgical standpoint, it will be important in any individual patient to do the mental calculation as to whether the increased operative risk associated with a more complex procedure to implant a larger orifice valve is worthwhile in terms of long-term survival and freedom from congestive failure. There will be no substitute for an individualized approach.

**T. M. Sundt III, MD**

### A comparison of outcomes of mitral valve repair for degenerative disease with posterior, anterior, and bileaflet prolapse

David TE, Ivanov J, Armstrong S, et al (Toronto Gen Hosp; Univ of Toronto)
*J Thorac Cardiovasc Surg* 130:1242-1249, 2005                     3–9

*Objective.*—We sought to compare the clinical and echocardiographic outcomes of mitral valve repair for mitral regurgitation in patients with degenerative disease of the mitral valve with posterior, anterior, or bileaflet prolapse.

*Methods.*—Patients underwent operations from 1981 through 2001: 359 had posterior (mean age, 60.4 years), 92 had anterior (mean age, 53.3 years), and 250 had bileaflet (means age, 56.4 years) prolapse. Patients with anterior prolapse were younger ($P = .04$) and had more associated aortic valve disease ($P = .02$), particularly bicuspid aortic valve disease ($P < .001$). Anterior prolapse was corrected by using chordal replacement with Gore-Tex sutures in most patients, but early on in this series, leaflet resection, chordal shortening, and chordal transfer were also used. Echocardiograms were done annually, and clinical follow-up was complete at a mean of 6.9 ± 4.0 years (range, 0-23 years).

*Results.*—The overall survival at 12 years was 75% ± 5%, with no difference among the posterior, anterior, and bileaflet prolapse groups ($P = .3$). The freedom from reoperation at 12 years was 96% ± 2% for posterior, 88% ± 4% for anterior, and 94% ± 2% for bileaflet prolapse ($P = .019$). Anterior prolapse was the only independent predictor of reoperation. The freedom from moderate or severe mitral regurgitation at 12 years was 80% ± 4% for posterior, 65% ± 8% for anterior, and 67% ± 6% for bileaflet prolapse ($P = .001$). Anterior and bileaflet prolapse, age, ejection fraction of less than 40%, and aortic valve disease were independent predictors of recurrent moderate or severe mitral regurgitation.

*Conclusions.*—The pathophysiology of mitral regurgitation affects the durability of mitral valve repair for degenerative disease, and the results of

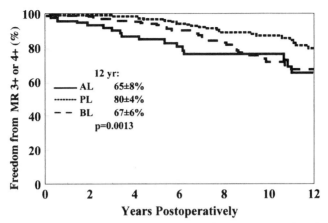

FIGURE 4.—Freedom from recurrent moderate or severe mitral regurgitation (*MR*) in patients with posterior (*PL*), anterior (*AL*), and bileaflet (*BL*) prolapse. (Reprinted from David TE, Ivanov J, Armstrong S, et al: A comparison of outcomes of mitral valve repair for degenerative disease with posterior, anterior, and bileaflet prolapse. *J Thorac Cardiovasc Surg* 130:1242-1249, 2006. Copyright 2006 Elsevier.)

posterior prolapse are better than those of anterior and bileaflet prolapse. This study indicates that rates of reoperation underscore the rates of failure of mitral valve repair (Fig 4).

▶ This important article from the Toronto group reviews their experience with mitral valve repair. The results are important from several perspectives. First, as has been shown previously, the durability of mitral valve repair for anterior leaflet prolapse falls below that for posterior leaflet prolapse. The authors conclude that this is due to inherent differences in the patient population and the pathophysiology of anterior leaflet prolapse. This is easy for a surgeon familiar with mitral valve repair to understand. One would certainly expect the long-term durability of an otherwise normal mitral valve with isolated rupture of a chord to P2 undergoing resection or repair of that individual segment to have much better long-term durability than an inherently abnormal valve with myxomatous degeneration, bileaflet prolapse, and chordal abnormalities. These data then simply support the clinical impression.

What of the more extensively diseased valve? As the authors point out in their discussion, mitral valve repair does not alter the underlying degenerative changes. They have, however, attempted to mitigate some of the abnormality, more recently using large numbers of artificial chordae tendineae constructed of PTFE suture. They have hopes that this will improve the results of anterior leaflet repairs. This too is logical because data from the Mayo Clinic have demonstrated that approximately half of all redo operations after mitral valve repair are for new pathology including, quite commonly, a newly ruptured chord.[1]

Additionally, and perhaps of even broader importance, is the demonstration that freedom from reoperation does not parallel freedom from recurrent mitral regurgitation. One should not confuse one outcome for the other. There are many reasons why one might not reoperate on a patient with valvular heart disease, only one of which is the degree of valvular dysfunction. This same caveat must be applied to all data concerning freedom from reoperation after valve repair or replacement.

**T. M. Sundt III, MD**

*Reference*

1. Suri RM, Schaff HV, Dearani JA, et al: Recurrent mitral regurgitation after repair: Should the mitral valve be re-repaired? *J Thorac Cardiovasc Surg* 132:1390-1397, 2006.

---

**Is a good perioperative echocardiographic result predictive of durability in ischemic mitral valve repair?**
Serri K, Bouchard D, Demers P, et al (Univ of Montreal)
*J Thorac Cardiovasc Surg* 131:565-573, 2006                          3–10

---

*Background.*—Chronic ischemic mitral regurgitation is associated with poor long-term survival. Despite the increasing popularity of valve repair, its durability and long-term outcome for ischemic mitral regurgitation have recently been questioned.

*Methods.*—Seventy-eight patients underwent repair for ischemic mitral regurgitation between 1996 and 2002 at our institution. Of these patients, 73 had complete clinical and echocardiographic follow-up. Preoperative, intraoperative, and postoperative clinical data were obtained, and the results of echocardiograms were reviewed to assess the rate of recurrence of regurgitation after repair and to identify predictive factors.

*Results.*—The mean preoperative mitral regurgitation grade, New York Heart Association class, and left ventricular ejection fraction were 2.72, 2.65, and 39.4%, respectively. Mortality was 12.3% at 30 days and 30.1% at a mean follow-up of $39 \pm 25$ months. Immediate postoperative echocardiography showed absent or mild mitral regurgitation in 89.4% of patients and showed moderate mitral regurgitation in 10.6%. Freedom from reoperation was 93.2%. Recurrent moderate mitral regurgitation (2+) was present in 36.7% of patients, and severe mitral regurgitation (3+ to 4+) was present in 20.0% at mean follow-up of $28.1 \pm 22.5$ months. Only age ($P = .0130$) and less marked preoperative posterior tethering ($P = .0362$) were predictive of recurrent mitral regurgitation. Patients with a preoperative New York Heart Association class greater than II and recurrent mitral regurgitation greater than 2+ had decreased survival ($P = .0152$ and $P = .0450$, respectively).

*Conclusions.*—Significant recurrent mitral regurgitation occurs following repair for ischemic mitral regurgitation, despite good early results. This finding raises questions about the need for improved repair techniques, better patient selection, or eventual mitral valve replacement in selected patients.

▶ There is increasing attention paid to the impact of mitral regurgitation in the setting of ischemic heart disease. Although the trend among surgeons has been very strongly toward mitral repair over replacement, the problem of ischemic cardiomyopathy is a particularly vexing one. A number of studies have demonstrated a significant incidence of recurrent or residual ischemic mitral regurgitation after repair in this setting, stimulating the development of a number of new procedures and some remarkably unusual appearing prosthetic rings. I would note that much of the discussion of this article when it was presented focused around the technical aspects for repair of ischemic mitral regurgitation, including the use of downsizing and remodeling rings. The authors' own data demonstrate a very high incidence of recurrent mitral regurgitation. More than half had recurrent mitral regurgitation grade 2 or more at midterm follow-up. This is similar to results reported previously by others and should not be dismissed as a center-specific finding (or failing). Quite appropriately the authors question if there is more of a role for replacement in this setting than has been previously thought. I agree and personally have a low threshold to replace the valve in the setting of ischemic disease.

Perhaps on an even more fundamental level, there is debate over whether repair of the mitral valve in the setting of ischemic cardiomyopathy has any impact on long-term outcome. The unreliability of repair only complicates this argument because advocates of intervention on the mitral valve suggest that recurrent or residual regurgitation may be the reason for poor late survival.

**T. M. Sundt III, MD**

---

### Determinants of operative mortality in valvular heart surgery

Rankin JS, Hammill BG, Ferguson TB, et al (Vanderbilt Univ, Nashville, Tenn; Duke Univ Med Ctr, Durham, NC; Society of Thoracic Surgeons Adult Cardiac Surgery Database, Durham, NC; et al)
*J Thorac Cardiovasc Surg* 131:547-557, 2006                                    3–11

---

*Objective.*—In some respects, outcome reporting in valvular surgery has been hampered by focusing on specific populations, reluctance to publish high-risk subgroups, and possibly skewed or inadequate samples. The goal of this study was to evaluate risk factors for operative mortality comprehensively across the entire spectrum of cardiac valvular procedures over the past decade.

*Methods.*—All 409,904 valve procedures in the Society of Thoracic Surgeons database performed between 1994 and 2003 were assessed, and Society of Thoracic Surgeons preoperative and operative variables were related to operative mortality by using a multivariable logistic regression model. Data were greater than 95% complete, and the relative importance of relevant risk factors was determined by ranking odds ratios. The analysis had a high predictive power, with a C statistic of 0.735.

*Results.*—In the model, 19 variables independently influenced operative mortality (all $P < .01$). The most significant was nonelective (acute) presentation (odds ratios, 2.11), followed by advanced age (odds ratios, 1.88), reoperation (odds ratios, 1.61), endocarditis (odds ratios, 1.59), and coronary disease (odds ratios, 1.58). Generally, valve replacement was associated

**TABLE 4.—Effects of Baseline Variables on Outcome**

| Variable | Unadjusted Mortality (%) | Unadjusted Mortality Difference | Adjusted Mortality (%) | Adjusted Mortality Difference | Adjusted Odds Ratio | $\chi^2$ | Parameter Estimate | P Value |
|---|---|---|---|---|---|---|---|---|
| Acute presentation | 12.9 | — | 10.7 | — | 2.11 | 3244 | 0.7445 | <.001 |
| Elective | 5.1 | 7.8 | 5.5 | 5.2 | | | | |
| Age ≥70 y | 9.4 | — | 9.1 | — | 1.88 | 2150 | 0.6322 | <.001 |
| Age <70 y | 5.0 | 4.4 | 5.2 | 3.9 | | | | |
| Reoperation, yes | 11.3 | — | 9.7 | — | 1.61 | 1123 | 0.4762 | <.001 |
| Reoperation, no | 6.2 | 5.1 | 6.4 | 3.3 | | | | |
| Endocarditis, yes | 10.6 | — | 10.3 | — | 1.59 | 338 | 0.4614 | <.001 |
| Endocarditis, no | 6.9 | 3.7 | 7.0 | 3.3 | | | | |
| CAD, yes | 9.3 | — | 8.4 | — | 1.58 | 1024 | 0.4552 | <.001 |
| CAD, no | 5.0 | 4.3 | 5.6 | 2.8 | | | | |
| Valve replacement | 7.2 | — | 7.4 | — | 1.52 | 408 | 0.4158 | <.001 |
| Valve repair | 6.8 | 0.4 | 5.1 | 2.3 | | | | |
| CHF, yes | 10.5 | — | 8.3 | — | 1.39 | 605 | 0.3262 | <.001 |
| CHF, no | 5.4 | 5.1 | 6.3 | 2.0 | | | | |
| Female gender | 8.4 | — | 8.3 | — | 1.37 | 590 | 0.3139 | <.001 |
| Male gender | 6.2 | 2.2 | 6.3 | 1.9 | | | | |
| EF ≥0.35 | 6.6 | — | 6.9 | — | 1.34 | 280 | 0.2944 | <.001 |
| EF <0.35 | 11.1 | 4.5 | 8.9 | -2.0 | | | | |
| Year ≥1999 | 6.9 | — | 6.4 | — | 1.34 | 511 | 0.2945 | <.001 |
| Year <1999 | 7.5 | -0.6 | 8.3 | -1.9 | | | | |
| 0 Comorbidities | 4.5 | — | 5.0 | — | 1.19 | 1586 | 0.1716 | <.001 |
| 1 Comorbidity | 5.5 | 1.0 | 5.8 | 0.8 | (Average per comorbidity) | | | |
| 2 Comorbidities | 6.4 | 1.9 | 6.8 | 1.8 | | | | |
| 3 Comorbidities | 8.1 | 3.6 | 7.9 | 2.9 | | | | |
| 4 Comorbidities | 10.5 | 6.0 | 9.1 | 4.1 | | | | |
| Severe Lesion, yes | 6.8 | — | 6.9 | — | 0.83 | 151 | -0.1880 | <.001 |
| Severe Lesion, no | 8.4 | -1.6 | 8.1 | -1.2 | | | | |
| Overall | 7.1 | — | 7.1 | — | | | | |
| Procedures (referenced to AVR) | | | | | | | | |
| Aortic root | 11.1 | 5.4 | 13.5 | 7.9 | 2.78 | 650 | 1.0227 | <.001 |
| Isolated tricuspid | 10.7 | 5.0 | 11.4 | 5.8 | 2.26 | 199 | 0.8173 | <.001 |
| Multiple valve | 11.2 | 5.5 | 10.5 | 4.9 | 2.06 | 1440 | 0.7203 | <.001 |
| Isolated mitral | 7.7 | 2.0 | 7.9 | 2.3 | 1.47 | 578 | 0.3880 | <.001 |
| Isolated pulmonic | 4.4 | -1.3 | 7.1 | 1.5 | 1.29 | 2 | 0.2556 | .141 |
| Isolated aortic | 5.7 | — | 5.6 | — | 1.00 | — | — | — |
| Concurrent operation, yes | 10.0 | — | 9.9 | — | 1.58 | 736 | 0.4568 | <.001 |
| Concurrent operation, no (referenced to valve-only procedure) | 6.7 | 3.3 | 6.7 | 3.2 | | | | |

The regression intercept was −4.3817. CAD, Coronary artery disease; CHF, congestive heart failure; EF, ejection fraction; AVR, aortic valve replacement.
(Reprinted from Rankin JS, Hammill BG, Ferguson TB, et al: Determinants of operative mortality in valvular heart surgery. J Thorac Cardiovasc Surg 131:547-557, 2006. Copyright 2006 Elsevier.)

with higher mortality than repair (odds ratios, 1.52). Overall, female gender was very important (odds ratios, 1.37), and earlier year of operation increased risk (odds ratios, 1.34), implying improving outcomes over time. Although any single comorbidity, on average, was only moderately contributory (odds ratios, 1.19), specific comorbidities, such as renal failure, or multiple comorbidities in a given patient could be very significant. Aortic root reconstruction carried the highest risk (odds ratios, 2.78), followed by tricuspid valve surgery (odds ratios, 2.26), multiple valve procedures (odds ratios, 2.06), and then isolated mitral (odds ratios, 1.47), pulmonic (odds ratios, 1.29), and aortic (reference procedure) operations. Reduced ejection fraction and severity of valve lesion were relatively less important (odds ratios, 1.34 and 0.83, respectively).

*Conclusions.*—These data illustrate the significance of acute presentation in determining operative risk, and earlier surgical intervention under elective conditions might be emphasized for all types of significant valve lesions. Because aortic root reconstruction doubles mortality compared with simple aortic valve procedures, root replacement should be reserved for specific root pathology. Finally, issues related to reoperation, endocarditis, valve repair, gender, and the various procedures deserve more detailed examination (Table 4).

▶ This is an important article from the Society of Thoracic Surgeons' database. This is a voluntary database that is maintained by the Society of Thoracic Surgeons that includes currently almost three fourths of all patients undergoing cardiac surgery in the United States. As such, it provides information that cannot be gleaned from other literature. Most authors publish only their best results, and therefore the view of operative risk may be significantly skewed. In addition, complex valvular procedures are uncommon in most hospitals, and therefore it is difficult to perform a comprehensive analysis at a single center. These authors have leveraged the power of the STS database to answer some important questions about valve surgery in the world of clinical practice.

By using data from more than 400,000 procedures, the authors were able to analyze a number of risk factors for operative deaths. The most useful information from the article is summarized in Table 4. Among patient variables, the most powerful predictor of increased risk was acute presentation, with an adjusted odds ratio of 2.11. Age greater than 70 years was the next most powerful predictor, with an odds ratio of 1.88; reoperation, endocarditis, and the presence of coronary artery disease all fell behind these parameters, with odds ratios of approximately 1.6. These data emphasize the importance of referral before these individuals are in extremis. Earlier referral and elective operations will produce the best outcomes.

Among the procedure variables, performing aortic root replacement was associated with an almost threefold increase in operative risk. The raw mortality rate for root reconstruction for aortic aneurysms is 10.5%, whereas that for aortic dissection was 23.7% and root replacement without root pathology was 9.5%. This has important implications for the debate over appropriate management of the bicuspid aortic valve, a pathology some surgeons suggest should always be treated with root replacement. If the STS data are correct, this approach would significantly increase operative mortality for this common condition. These data may also give pause to advocates of the pulmonary autograft and stentless xenograft procedures.

**T. M. Sundt III, MD**

---

### Surgical Correction of Mitral Regurgitation in the Elderly: Outcomes and Recent Improvements
Detaint D, Sundt TM, Nkomo VT, et al (Mayo Clinic, Rochester, Minn)
*Circulation* 114:265-272, 2006                                                    3–12

---

*Background.*—In the elderly, mitral regurgitation (MR) is frequent, but surgery risks are considered high. Benefits and indications of MR surgery are uncertain in the elderly.

*Method and Results.*—Baseline characteristics, outcome, and trends for surgical results improvement were analyzed in elderly patients ($\geq$75 years of age; n=284) operated on for MR in 1980 to 1995 compared with younger patients (65 to 74 years of age, n=504; and <65 years of age, n=556). Preoperatively, class III to IV symptoms, atrial fibrillation, coronary disease, creatinine, and comorbidity index were more severe in elderly patients (all $P<0.002$). In the long term after surgery, observed survival stratified by age ($\geq$75, 65 to 74, <65 years) was lower in elderly than in younger patients (at 5 years, 57±3%, 73±2%, and 85±2%, respectively; $P<0.001$), but ratios of observed to expected survival were similar (83%, 85%, and 88%, respectively). In multivariate analysis adjusted to expected survival, elderly patients showed no difference in life expectancy restoration compared with younger patients (adjusted hazard ratio, 0.89; 95% confidence interval, 0.73 to 1.30; $P=0.54$). Temporal trends showed that risk of operative mortality, although higher in elderly patients ($P<0.001$), declined markedly for all ages (27% to 5% in those $\geq$75 years of age, $P<0.01$; 21% to 4% in those 65 to 74 years of age, $P<0.01$; and 7% to 2% in those <65 years of age, $P=0.06$), with a parallel decline in low cardiac output and length of hospital stay. Over time, valve repair feasibility increased in all age groups (30% to 84% overall and 31% to 93% in degenerative MR; $P<0.0001$).

*Conclusions.*—Elderly patients undergoing MR surgery display more severe preoperative characteristics and incur higher operative risks than younger patients. However, restoration of life expectancy after surgery is similar in elderly and younger patients, and outstanding recent surgical improvements particularly benefited elderly patients. Thus, elderly patients with MR can now carefully be considered for surgery before refractory heart failure is present.

▶ Because we are confronted increasingly with elderly patients facing valve surgery, studies such as this gain heightened importance. It is no longer a rare event to discuss the option of mitral valve surgery in the octogenarian. An important aspect of this study is the demonstrated reduction in operative mortality over time, such that in the current era the operative mortality rate for patients over 75 years of age was only 5% in this institution. Importantly, the improvement in long-term survival is equivalent for the elderly as it is for younger patients. A surprising detail in the body of the article is the low stroke rate. Rather surprisingly, there was no significant difference in ischemic stroke among age groups, with a rate of only 1.8% for those greater than 75 years of age. All in all, these data support the application of mitral repair to the elderly population.

**T. M. Sundt III, MD**

## Aortic Disease

### Drug-Eluting Stents Versus Bilateral Internal Thoracic Grafting for Multivessel Coronary Disease

Herz I, Moshkovitz Y, Loberman D, et al (Tel Aviv Univ, Israel; Assuta Med Ctr, Tel Aviv, Israel; Hadassah Hebrew Univ Hosp, Ein Karem, Jerusalem)
*Ann Thorac Surg* 80:2086-2090, 2005                    3–13

*Background.*—Reduction of restenosis and reinterventions was recently reported with percutaneous interventions (PCI), including drug-eluting stents (Cypher; Cordis, Miami Lakes, FL). This study compares results of multivessel Cypher stenting with those of bilateral internal thoracic artery (BITA) grafting.

*Methods.*—From January 2002 to June 2004, 768 consecutive patients underwent multivessel myocardial revascularization; 138 by PCI including Cyphers and 630 by BITA. After matching for age, sex, ejection fraction, extent of coronary disease, and congestive heart failure, two groups (113 patients each) were used to compare the two revascularization modalities.

*Results.*—Both groups were similar; however, left main and intraaortic balloon were more prevalent in the BITA group. The number of coronary vessels treated per patient was higher in the BITA group (2.87 vs 2.22, $p <$ 0.001). Follow-up ranged between 6 and 34 months. Thirty-day mortality was 0.9% in the BITA and zero in the PCI group ($p = 0.32$). There were no late deaths in the BITA and three (2.7%) in the Cypher group ($p = 0.08$). Angina returned in 28.3% of the Cypher and 12.4% of the BITA group, $p =$ 0.003. A Cox proportional hazard model revealed assignment to the Cypher group to be the only predictor of angina recurrence (odds ratio 2.78, 95% confidence interval 1.46-2.56). There were 16 (14.2%) reinterventions in the Cypher group compared with six (5.3%) in the BITA group. One-year reintervention-free survival (Kaplan-Meier) of the BITA was 96% compared with 86.6% in the Cypher group ($p = 0.005$, log-rank test).

*Conclusions.*—Despite improved results of PCI with Cyphers, midterm clinical outcome of multivessel patients treated with BITA is still better.

▶ The principal strength of this study is the use of contemporary techniques—drug-eluting stents in the PCI group and bilateral internal thoracic arteries in the surgical group. Although the numbers are small, this study is one of very few that truly reflect current clinical practice. The results demonstrate a small but statistically significant difference in angina-free survival and intervention-free survival between groups with bilateral internal thoracic arteries being favored in both regards. The question remains whether the degree of this difference is sufficient to drive one's clinical decision making back toward surgical intervention when PCI is so remarkably successful in a large number of patients. A larger comparative analysis, particularly with economic outcomes, is warranted.

**T. M. Sundt III, MD**

---

### Thoracic Stent Grafting for Acute Aortic Pathology

Kaya A, Heijmen RH, Overtoom TT, et al (St Antonius Hosp, Nieuwegein, The Netherlands)

*Ann Thorac Surg* 82:560-566, 2006                                          3–14

---

*Background.*—Elective endovascular repair of the thoracic aorta has shown reduced morbidity and mortality when compared with open surgery. The number of studies describing the use of thoracic endovascular stent grafts for acute pathology is limited, however. The purpose of this study was to describe our increasing experience with stent grafting for acute thoracic aortic pathology.

*Methods.*—Since January 2002, 28 patients underwent endovascular stent graft treatment for various types of acute thoracic aorta diseases, including complicated Stanford type B dissection (n = 12), ruptured descending aorta aneurysms (n = 7), intramural hematoma (n = 4), traumatic rupture of the thoracic aorta (n = 2), aortopulmonary fistula (n = 2), and penetrating aortic ulcer (n = 1). These acute thoracic aortic syndromes were predominantly localized in the proximal descending thoracic aorta (75%). Talent stent grafts were used in 26 patients and Excluder stent grafts in 2 patients.

*Results.*—Stent graft deployment at the intended position was successful in all patients. There was 1 intraoperative death (3.6%), due to acute myocardial infarction, after successful exclusion of the lesion with a stent graft. Hospital mortality was 21.4% (n = 6). Four of 6 hospital deaths, however, were directly related to the severely compromised clinical status preoperatively, including extensive bowel ischemia and irreversible cerebral damage after resuscitation. New neurologic symptoms were seen in 4 patients. The majority of the neurologic symptoms improved and faded away during hospital stay. Mean follow-up was 11 months (range, 1 to 31), and all the hospital survivors (n = 22) were alive. There was 1 nonrelated stroke 4 months postoperatively. During follow-up, 2 patients required transposition of the left subclavian artery for malperfusion, and 2 patients required a second stent graft procedure for endoleak. Additionally, 2 patients with early type II endoleaks were treated conservatively, and 1 of them sealed spontaneously at 6 months.

*Conclusions.*—Thoracic stent grafting for acute aortic pathology is feasible in critically ill patients. Postoperative morbidity and mortality is predominantly related to the compromised preoperative clinical status, illustrating its use as salvage strategy.

▶ One of the most exciting applications of stent graft technology is in the treatment of acute aortic syndromes. This relatively small series of patients demonstrates enticing results. Although the in-hospital mortality rate was 21%, this is probably an acceptable rate in comparison with open surgical procedures in these extremely high-risk patients, including those with ruptured aneurysms and complicated dissections. The authors of this study are well recognized as outstanding aortic surgeons and I suspect that this contributes to their excellent results. It is critical that individuals performing these procedures understand aortic disease and these outstanding results argue in favor of such an approach. Thoracic aortic diseases are complex and there is much more to this than the technical aspects of deploying the stent graft.

**T. M. Sundt III, MD**

### Extended Applications of Thoracic Aortic Stent Grafts
Dagenais F, Shetty R, Normand J-P, et al (Laval Hosp, Québec City)
*Ann Thorac Surg* 82:567-572, 2006                                    3–15

*Background.*—Thoracic stent-grafts (TSG) show excellent early and mid-term results for localized diseases of the descending aorta. Extending TSG applications for arch pathologies or to other yet unproven indications remains to be established. We herein report our experience in 18 patients with extended applications of TSG.

*Methods.*—Ten patients with inadequate proximal aortic neck length required coverage of at least one arch vessel with or without extra-anatomic bypass. One patient required an extra-anatomic visceral bypass to extend the distal aortic neck, 6 patients were treated with TSG for yet unproven indications, and 1 patient required an unusual vascular access.

*Results.*—A mean of $2.4 \pm 1.0$ stents per patient were inserted. Primary or secondary success rate was 100%. Hospital mortality occurred in one patient (5.5%). Mean follow-up was $24.1 \pm 13.7$ months. Four endoleaks were diagnosed: two of type 1, one of type 2, and one that remains undetermined. Two patients died during follow-up; both deaths were linked to the presence of a type 1 endoleak. Actuarial survival at 3 years was 79.0%. Freedom from endoleak and stent-graft-related death at 3 years were, respectively, 71.0% and 83.7%. No stent-graft migration was observed.

*Conclusions.*—Early and mid-term results of extended applications of TSG are acceptable in well-selected high-risk patients. Endoleak at follow-up remains a concern and may impede long-term outcome of TSG in complex procedures.

▶ This article from Quebec City is included in this year's YEAR BOOK to heighten awareness of broadened applications of thoracic aortic stent grafts. In particular, surgeons are exploring debranching procedures to deal with inadequate proximal and distal landing zones. Such patients represent a significant proportion of the patients in the study population, although notably not all. The authors report a quite good in-hospital mortality rate of only 1 death. Unfortunately, 4 endoleaks were identified, 2 of which led to death. The occurrence of type I endoleaks, those caused by inadequate seating of the stent graft either proximally or distally, are of particular note. Despite efforts to construct extra-anatomic bypasses to render necks adequate, the authors were unsuccessful in a significant percentage of patients, particularly if one eliminates from this series the individuals with traumatic disruption.

The results of these extended applications will again need to be held against the surgical standard. With significant questions about even the standard indications for stent grafting, is it really appropriate to extend indications at this point in time?

**T. M. Sundt III, MD**

---

**Results of endovascular repair of the thoracic aorta with the Talent Thoracic stent graft: The Talent Thoracic Retrospective Registry**
Fattori R, Nienaber CA, Rousseau H, et al (Univ Hosp S Orsola, Bologna, Italy; Univ Hosp Rostock, Germany; Hôpital de Rangueil, Toulouse, France; et al)
*J Thorac Cardiovasc Surg* 132:332-339, 2006                    3–16

---

*Background.*—Endovascular treatment of thoracic aortic diseases demonstrated low perioperative morbidity and mortality when compared with conventional open repair. Long-term effectiveness of this minimally invasive technique remains to be proven. The Talent Thoracic Retrospective Registry was designed to evaluate the impact of this therapy on patients treated in 7 major European referral centers over an 8-year period.

*Methods.*—Data from 457 consecutive patients (113 emergency and 344 elective cases) who underwent endovascular thoracic aortic repair with the Medtronic Talent Thoracic stent graft (Medtronic/AVE, Santa Rosa, Calif) were collected. Follow-up analysis ($24 \pm 19.4$ months, range 1-85.1 months) was based on clinical and imaging findings, including all adverse events. To ensure consistency of data interpretation and event reporting, one physician reviewed all adverse events and deaths for the whole cohort of patients. In the case of discrepancies, the treating physicians were queried.

*Findings.*—Among 422 patients who survived the interventional procedure (in-hospital mortality 5%, 23 patients), mortality during follow-up was 8.5% (36 patients), and in 11 of them the death was related to the aortic disease. Persistent endoleak was reported at imaging follow-up in 64 cases: 44 were primary (9.6%) and 21 occurred during follow-up (4.9%). Seven patients with persistent endoleak had aortic rupture during follow-up, at a variable time from 40 days to 35 months, and all subsequently died. A minor incidence of migration of the stent graft (7 cases), graft fabric alteration (2 cases), and modular disconnection (3 cases) was observed at imaging. Kaplan-Meier overall survival estimate at 1 year was 90.97%, at 3 years was 85.36%, and at 5 years was 77.49%. At the same intervals, freedom from a

less invasive? If so, this would arguably be in error. The mortality rate observed in this study for aortic aneurysms smaller than 50 mm in diameter was still 4.7%. This likely exceeds the mortality rate expected for the natural history of these aneurysms.

In addition, stent grafts were used for the treatment of chronic type B aortic dissection in 20% of cases. This is an extremely controversial indication. It is unclear that stent grafts have any role at all to play in this condition. It should be noted that the mortality rate in this subset was 15%. Overall morbidity was significant. Despite the authors' stated conclusion that stent grafting can be performed with "acceptable" postoperative morbidity, a 10% mortality rate within 3 months, 16% endoleak rate, 6 instances of paraplegia, and other catastrophic complications such as aortoesophageal fistula in cerebral embolization occurred at nontrivial rates. This is in the face of a condition the natural history of which (in uncomplicated dissection) is an expected acute mortality rate of approximately 10%.[1]

This is not to condemn stent grafting. Surely it is here to stay. We must be very cautious in its application, however, and objective when analyzing the results. We should not mistake this for a simple solution to a very complex problem.

**T. M. Sundt III, MD**

*Reference*

1. Hagan PG, Nienaber CA, Isselbacher EM, et al: The International Registry of Acute Aortic Dissection (IRAD): New insights into an old disease. *JAMA* 283:897-903, 2000.

---

### Risk-corrected impact of mechanical versus bioprosthetic valves on long-term mortality after aortic valve replacement

Lund O, Bland M (Univ of York, England)
*J Thorac Cardiovasc Surg* 132:20-26, 2006                              3–18

---

*Objective.*—Choice of a mechanical or biologic valve in aortic valve replacement remains controversial and rotates around different complications with different time-related incidence rates. Because serious complications will always "spill over" into mortality, our aim was to perform a meta-analysis on overall mortality after aortic valve replacement from series with a maximum follow-up of at least 10 years to determine the age- and risk factor-corrected impact of currently available mechanical versus stented bioprosthetic valves.

*Methods.*—Following a formal study protocol, we performed a dedicated literature search of publications during 1989 to 2004 and included articles on adult aortic valve replacement with a mechanical or stented bioprosthetic valve if age, mortality statistics, and prevalences of well-known risk factors could be extracted. We used standard and robust regression analyses of the case series data with valve type as a fixed variable.

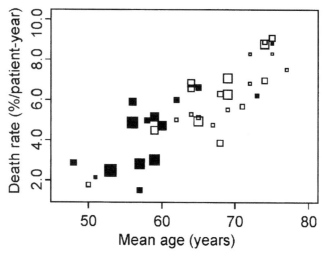

FIGURE 2.—Total death rate of the 15 mechanical (■) and 23 bioprosthetic (□) valve series in relation to mean age of each series. Areas of the squares are proportional to the total follow-up (patient-y) in each valve series. (Reprinted from Lund O, Bland M: Risk-corrected impact of mechanical versus bioprosthetic valves on long-term mortality after aortic valve replacement. *J Thorac Cardiovasc Surg* 132:20-26, 2006. Copyright 2006 Elsevier.)

*Results.*—We could include 32 articles with 15 mechanical and 23 biologic valve series totaling 17,439 patients and 101,819 patient-years. The mechanical and biologic valve series differed in regard to mean age (58 vs 69 years), mean follow-up (6.4 vs 5.3 years), coronary artery bypass grafting (16% vs 34%), endocarditis (7% vs 2%), and overall death rate (3.99 vs 6.33 %/patient-year). Mean age of the valve series was directly related to death rate with no interaction with valve type. Death rate corrected for age, New York Heart Association classes III and IV, aortic regurgitation, and coronary artery bypass grafting left valve type with no effect. Included articles that abided by current guidelines and compared a mechanical and biologic valve found no differences in rates of thromboembolism.

*Conclusion.*—There was no difference in risk factor-corrected overall death rate between mechanical or bioprosthetic aortic valves irrespective of age. Choice of prosthetic valve should therefore not be rigorously based on age alone. Risk of bioprosthetic valve degeneration in young and middle-aged patients and in the elderly and old with a long life expectancy would be an important factor because risk of stroke may primarily be related to patient factors (Fig 2).

▶ This comprehensive meta-analysis performed by a cardiac surgeon with a remarkable background in statistics provides an important insight into the debate over a mechanical versus bioprosthetic valves. As a surgeon, he brings a very practical clinical perspective to a sophisticated statistical analysis. Many studies have been performed over the course of the years attempting to aid in the choice between mechanical and bioprosthetic valves. Each study aims in some statistical way to determine the best choice for an individual patient. In the end, I have always felt, and this study just reinforces that the differences between valves are primarily qualitative and not quantitative, and accordingly the decision between options is entirely subjective. It is the patient who accepts the risks and must choose between these qualitatively distinct courses of action and resulting consequences. We cannot make the decisions for the patients; they must make them for themselves. The choice of valve is the quintessential patient-centered decision.

**T. M. Sundt III, MD**

## Long-term results of aortic valve-sparing operations for aortic root aneurysm

David TE, Feindel CM, Webb GD, et al (Univ of Toronto)
*J Thorac Cardiovasc Surg* 132:347-354, 2006                    3–19

*Objectives.*—To examine the results of aortic valve sparing for aortic root aneurysm.

*Methods.*—Two hundred twenty consecutive patients who had aortic valve sparing for aortic root aneurysm were prospectively studied with annual clinical assessments and echocardiography. Their mean age was $46 \pm 15$ years, 40% had Marfan syndrome, 17% had aortic dissection, and 7% had bicuspid aortic valve. Reimplantation of the aortic valve was performed in 167 patients and remodeling of the aortic root in 53. Aortic cusp repair was performed in 80 patients, and reinforcement of the free margin of one of the cusps with a fine polytetrafluoroethylene (Gore-Tex) suture in 48. The mean follow-up was $5.2 \pm 3.7$ years and it was complete.

*Results.*—There were 3 operative and 13 late deaths. Patients' survival at 10 years was $88\% \pm 3\%$. Age older than 65 years, advanced functional class, and ejection fraction less than 40% were independent predictors of death. Moderate aortic insufficiency developed in 7 patients and severe insufficiency in 6. Freedom from moderate or severe aortic insufficiency at 10 years was $85\% \pm 5\%$ for all patients, but it was $94\% \pm 4\%$ after reimplantation and $75\% \pm 10\%$ after remodeling ($P = .04$). Five patients required aortic valve replacement; the freedom from valve replacement at 10 years was $95\% \pm 3\%$. One case of endocarditis developed 11 years postoperatively. At the latest follow-up, 88% of the patients were in functional class I, and 10% were in class II.

*Conclusions.*—Aortic valve-sparing operation is associated with low rates of valve-related complications. The probability of late aortic insufficiency was lower after the reimplantation procedure than after remodeling in our experience.

▶ This is truly a landmark study of the "David" valve-sparing operation for aortic root aneurysm. Dr David is an innovative pioneer in valve surgery, and the procedure he describes here has captured the interest of the cardiac surgical community even if it is not familiar to many readers of the YEAR BOOK OF CARDIOLOGY. The procedure itself permits repair of aortic root aneurysm while preserving the native valve leaflets. Two competing techniques have been described, the first devised by Sir Magdi Yacoub and termed a "remodeling" procedure, whereas that devised by David involves "reimplantation" or resuspension of the valve leaflets within a Dacron graft. Both approaches replace the aortic sinuses. Yacoub's operation has been criticized because it does not stabilize the diameter of the aortoventricular junction. On the other hand, it has the advantage of creating neosinuses of Valsalva. The David operation is somewhat more extensive in that it fixes the aortoventricular junction. Several modifications have been made to the reimplantation procedure in the interest of creating neosinuses of Valsalva, but in any event they are somewhat less prominent than those observed in the Yacoub operation.

In general, the David operation has enjoyed increasing acceptance over the Yacoub procedure, with a number of groups reporting superior results with the reimplantation technique. Indeed, although we began with the Yacoub, in our own institution we have shifted to the David approach. In addition to stabilizing the annulus, this method is in fact a somewhat more straightforward and reproducible operation to perform than the Yacoub operation. The question remains, however, what will be the fate of the native aortic valve cusps suspended in a Dacron environment? Will the leaflets themselves abrade against the Dacron grafts? Will the hemodynamic forces present in a nondistensible root overstress the leaflets? Furthermore, specifically in the case of Marfan syndrome, will abnormality of the leaflets themselves lead to eventual leaflet prolapse and aortic regurgitation?

Dr David's data suggest that the answer to these questions is "no." The long-term durability of his operation appears quite satisfactory although the mean follow-up is only about 5 years. With 27 patients out at 10 years, the freedom from reoperation is 95%, but this is only a little over 1 of 10 of the total number of patients having undergone the procedure. Still, these data are encouraging and most surgeons with expertise in aortic root surgery are adopting this procedure. It is encouraging us to intervene somewhat earlier. This is an important development, particularly with the recognition of the risks of aortic dissection among patients with aortic roots in the 5- to 6-cm range. I should also note that this procedure is applicable to patients with bicuspid aortic valve and indeed this may prove to be the population in which its greatest application will be found.

**T. M. Sundt III, MD**

---

**Long-Term Outcome of Surgically Treated Aortic Regurgitation: Influence of Guideline Adherence Toward Early Surgery**
Tornos P, Sambola A, Permanyer-Miralda G, et al (Hosp Universitari Vall d'Hebron, Barcelona)
*J Am Coll Cardiol* 47:1012-1017, 2006                                              3–20

---

*Objectives.*—The purpose of this study was to compare postoperative outcome in two groups of patients with chronic severe aortic regurgitation (AR): those operated on early and those operated on late according to the guidelines.

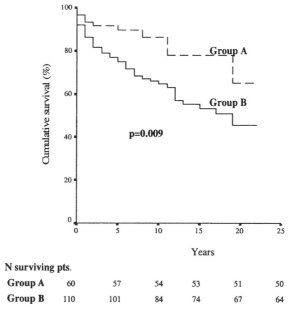

N surviving pts.

| | | | | | |
|---|---|---|---|---|---|
| **Group A** | 60 | 57 | 54 | 53 | 51 | 50 |
| **Group B** | 110 | 101 | 84 | 74 | 67 | 64 |

FIGURE 1.—Overall survival in study groups. pts. = patients. (Reprinted with permission from the American College of Cardiology from Tornos P, Sambola A, Permanyer-Miralda G, et al: Long-term outcome of surgically treated aortic regurgitation: Influence of guideline adherence toward early surgery. *J Am Coll Cardiol* 47:1012-1017. Copyright 2006 Elsevier.)

*Background.*—The impact of earlier surgery for chronic severe AR as defined in guidelines has not been evaluated.

*Methods.*—A total of 170 patients with chronic severe AR submitted to aortic valve replacement were prospectively followed up. Patients were divided in two groups depending on the clinical situation at the time of surgery. Group A were 60 patients who were operated on following guidelines advice of earlier surgery, and group B were 110 patients who were operated on late with regard to guideline recommendations.

*Results.*—Follow-up was 10 ± 6 years (1 to 22 years). During follow-up 44 patients died, 7 patients (12%) from group A and 37 (37%) from group B (p = 0.001). The cause of death was non-cardiac in 11 patients, 2 (3%) in group A and 9 (8%) in group B. Cardiac deaths occurred in 33 patients, 5 (9%) from group A and 28 (28%) from group B (p = 0.002). Causes of death differed between groups A and B: heart failure or sudden death were significantly more frequent in group B (20 patients vs. 1 patient, p = 0.001). Overall survival in groups A and B was 90 ± 4% vs. 75 ± 8% at 5 years, 86 ± 5% vs. 64 ± 5% at 10 years, and 78 ± 7% vs. 53 ± 6% at 15 years, respectively (p = 0.009).

*Conclusions.*—Early operation as defined in the guidelines improves long-term survival in patients with chronic AR (Fig 1).

▶ Surgeons may be rightly accused of encouraging earlier and earlier referral for operative intervention in a number of conditions, including aortic valve disease. Although it is true that one cannot make an asymptomatic patient feel better, is there nonetheless a role for surgery in the asymptomatic patient? The ACC/AHA guidelines committee thinks so, and these data support their recommendations. Patients undergoing aortic valve replacement in accordance with the ACC/AHA guidelines have superior survival. These guidelines establish a class I recommendation for aortic valve surgery in all symptomatic patients and in asymptomatic patients with a left ventricular ejection fraction at rest lower than 49%. An end-systolic diameter >55 mm is considered a class II indication. These parameters are quite similar to those adopted by the European Society of Cardiology, whose guidelines recommend surgery in asymptomatic patients with severe aortic regurgitation and resting left ventricular ejection fraction less than 50% or enlarged ventricles with an end-diastolic diameter greater than 70 mm or end-systolic diameter greater than 50 mm.

In the current study, the difference in survival between those patients operated on according to these guidelines and those in whom surgery was delayed was both statistically and clinically significant. Furthermore, as shown in the accompanying figure, this difference in survival appeared to increase progressively over time.

The trend toward recommendation of surgery among asymptomatic patients on the basis of echocardiographic criteria seems only a reasonable step. Although the importance of clinical assessment of the patient cannot be underestimated, at the same time we should certainly use the data we obtain from these sophisticated tests to foresee problems and prevent their development rather than reacting only once patients become symptomatic. Although it is difficult for some patients, and physicians, to accept the notion of surgery in the asymptomatic patient, the data such as those presented in this article make it clear that the evidence-based practice is to proceed with surgery in settings such as these. After all, it is unlikely that such a patient with severe aortic regurgitation will survive long without surgical intervention. Why should they take both the ultimate risk of surgery and the interval risk of ventricular decompensation when earlier surgery subjects them only to the former?

**T. M. Sundt III, MD**

---

**Prosthesis-Patient Mismatch After Aortic Valve Replacement: Impact of Age and Body Size on Late Survival**
Moon MR, Pasque MK, Munfakh NA, et al (Washington Univ School of Medicine, St Louis)
*Ann Thorac Surg* 81:481-489, 2006                                                    3–21

---

*Background.*—The purpose of this study was to identify patient subgroups in which prosthesis-patient mismatch most influenced late survival.

*Methods.*—Over a 12-year period, 1,400 consecutive patients underwent bioprosthetic (933 patients) or mechanical (467) aortic valve replacement.

Prosthesis-patient mismatch was defined as prosthetic effective orifice area/ body surface area less than 0.75 cm²/m² and was present with 11% mechanical and 51% bioprosthetic valves.

*Results.*—With bioprosthetic valves, prosthesis-patient mismatch was associated with impaired survival for patients less than 60 years old (10-year: 68% ± 7% mismatch versus 75% ± 7% no mismatch, $p < 0.02$) but not older patients ($p = 0.47$). Similarly, with mechanical valves, prosthesis-patient mismatch was associated with impaired survival for patients less than 60 years old (10-year: 62% ± 11% versus 79% ± 4%, $p < 0.005$) but not older patients ($p = 0.26$). For small patients (body surface area less than 1.7 m²), prosthesis-patient mismatch did not impact survival with bioprosthetic ($p = 0.32$) or mechanical ($p = 0.71$) valves. For average-size patients (body surface area 1.7 to 2.1 m²), prosthesis-patient mismatch was associated with impaired survival with both bioprosthetic ($p < 0.05$) and mechanical ($p < 0.005$) valves. For large patients (body surface area greater than 2.1 m²), prosthesis-patient mismatch was associated with impaired survival with mechanical ($p < 0.04$) but not bioprosthetic ($p = 0.40$) valves.

*Conclusions.*—Prosthesis-patient mismatch had a negative impact on survival for young patients, but its impact on older patients was minimal. In addition, although prosthesis-patient mismatch was not important in small patients, prosthesis-patient mismatch negatively impacted survival for average-size patients and for large patients with mechanical valves.

▶ The issue of patient-prosthesis mismatch (PPM) remains of importance to surgeons and cardiologists alike. Should a surgeon perform an aortic root enlargement—a more complex procedure that many would argue increases operative risk—or accept a smaller valve in a small root? And what of the patient noted postoperatively to have what seems a high gradient? Should reoperation be considered? Moon et al from Washington University have attempted to further our understanding of PPM by refining the question a bit. In this very original look at the problem, they have attempted to stratify patients into clinically relevant subgroups: young and old, large and small. But before we look at their results, an important aspect of their methods must be highlighted. The literature on this subject is muddied by various definitions of PPM, including variation in the orifice area used to calculate it and the particular ratio of orifice area to body surface area used to define it. So a word of caution to the reader of this literature: take note of the definitions applied. In this study the authors have defined patient PPM rather conservatively as an effective orifice area of 0.75 cm²/m². Despite this conservative definition, more than half of the patients in their series receiving biologic valves were identified as having PPM.

The results of this study are reassuring. Mismatch was clinically significant in younger patients but not older patients (over 60 years of age), encouraging surgeons to be more aggressive in the very subgroup in whom one would expect any added risk to be minimized. Furthermore, although one might have dismissed this finding among patients with bioprosthetic valves as simply patient selection, with young patients receiving bioprosthetic valves being those in whom the surgeons thought life expectancy was short, the same was true for mechanical valves. In addition, when patients were stratified by body surface area, the effect was no longer apparent among small patients while it persisted among those of average or large size.

This article provides clinically useful guidelines for the practicing surgeon. It is likely that one need not lose a lot of sleep over the size of the valve implanted into a very small patient (body surface area <1.7). Likewise in the elderly patient, extreme efforts to enlarge the aortic annulus may be unwarranted. In the younger patient, however, we should continue to strive to optimize the orifice area for the patient.

**T. M. Sundt III, MD**

---

**Outcome of 622 Adults With Asymptomatic, Hemodynamically Significant Aortic Stenosis During Prolonged Follow-Up**
Pellikka PA, Sarano ME, Nishimura RA, et al (Mayo Clinic and Mayo Found, Rochester, Minn)
*Circulation* 111:3290-3295, 2005                                           3–22

---

*Background.*—This study assessed the long-term outcome of a large, asymptomatic population with hemodynamically significant aortic stenosis (AS).

*Method and Results.*—We identified 622 patients with isolated, asymptomatic AS and peak systolic velocity ≥4 m/s by Doppler echocardiography who did not undergo surgery at the initial evaluation and obtained follow-up (5.4±4.0 years) in all. Mean age (±SD) was 72±11 years; there were 384 (62%) men. The probability of remaining free of cardiac symptoms while unoperated was 82%, 67%, and 33% at 1, 2, and 5 years, respectively. Aortic valve area and left ventricular hypertrophy predicted symptom development. During follow-up, 352 (57%) patients were referred for aortic valve surgery and 265 (43%) patients died, including cardiac death in 117 (19%). The 1-, 2-, and 5-year probabilities of remaining free of surgery or cardiac death were 80%, 63%, and 25%, respectively. Multivariate predictors of all-cause mortality were age (hazard ratio [HR], 1.05; $P<0.0001$), chronic renal failure (HR, 2.41; $P=0.004$), inactivity (HR, 2.00; $P=0.001$), and aortic valve velocity (HR, 1.46; $P=0.03$). Sudden death without preceding symptoms occurred in 11 (4.1%) of 270 unoperated patients. Patients with peak velocity ≥4.5 m/s had a higher likelihood of developing symptoms (relative risk, 1.34) or having surgery or cardiac death (relative risk, 1.48).

*Conclusions.*—Most patients with asymptomatic, hemodynamically significant AS will develop symptoms within 5 years. Sudden death occurs in approximately 1%/y. Age, chronic renal failure, inactivity, and aortic valve velocity are independently predictive of all-cause mortality.

▶ This is an important follow-up article from a prior study published by these investigators asking, "Should asymptomatic patients with severe aortic stenosis be followed up or operated on?" Their prior work supported the nonoperative approach. They suggested that one can get away with closely monitoring these patients and waiting for symptoms to appear. But how does this play out in real clinical practice? What of the patients lost to follow-up?

Several points are worthy of note from a surgeon's perspective. First, the majority of patients had symptoms within 5 years. With a mean follow-up of only 5.4 years, 57% of patients were referred for aortic valve replacement. With a mean age of 72 years in the study group, given the improved durability of current generation bioprostheses resulting in an estimated 95% or better freedom from structural valve deterioration among patients over the age of 65 years, patients such as those in this study may be referred for tissue aortic valve replacement with little risk for reoperation in the future. What was really gained by waiting?

Second, it has been said that the common cause of sudden death in the asymptomatic patient with aortic stenosis is surgical mortality. That is clearly no longer the case. The mortality rate due to sudden death in this series was approximately 1% per year. In experienced hands, the mortality rate for aortic valve replacement now approaches this number under elective circumstances, such that within a very short period of time postoperatively the patient has gained back the risk they accepted at surgery. Why should patients be subjected to the risk of sudden death as well as that of valve replacement?

The data presented here should encourage referral of patients with asymptomatic hemodynamically significant aortic stenosis for surgery, particularly if they are over the age of 65 years, in which case a tissue prosthesis may be implanted at low operative risk with low risk of reoperation. For those much younger, the risk of operation is so low as to make it more dangerous to the patient to monitor the valve than to proceed with surgical intervention. It is time for us to change our practice.

**T. M. Sundt III, MD**

## Miscellaneous

### HLA-DR Matching Improves Survival After Heart Transplantation: Is it Time to Change Allocation Policies?

Kaczmarek I, Deutsch M-A, Rohrer M-E, et al (Grosshadern Univ Hosp, Munich)
*J Heart Lung Transplant* 25:1057-1062, 2006                                      3–23

*Background.*—HLA matching has improved outcome in kidney transplantation but is not considered in current allocation policies in heart transplantation. The aim of this single-center study was to assess the impact of HLA matching on long- term outcome after heart transplantation.

*Methods.*—The records of 240 consecutive heart transplant recipients (time period 1995 to 2002; mean age 51.8 ± 11.7 years; mean follow-up 5.9 ± 1.8 years) were analyzed retrospectively. According to the renal allocation policy, HLA mismatches (MM) on the major antigen loci HLA-A, HLA-B and HLA-DR were calculated, demonstrating 0 to 6 MM. Patients with primary graft failure were excluded from statistical analysis.

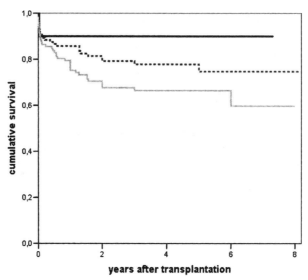

**years after transplantation**

FIGURE 2.—Kaplan–Meier survival analysis according to number of HLA-DR mismatches. Solid line: 0 HLA-DR mismatch; dotted line: 1 HLA-DR mismatch; shaded line: 2 HLA-DR mismatches. (Courtesy of Kaczmarek I, Deutsch M-A, Rohrer M-E, et al: HLA-DR matching improves survival after heart transplantation: Is it time to change allocation policies? *J Heart Lung Transplant* 25:1057-1062. Copyright 2006 Elsevier.)

*Results.*—Survival analysis revealed a statistically significant impact of HLA-DR MM on survival. Five-year survival was 90% in patients without HLA-DR MM ($n = 10$), 79% in patients with 1 HLA-DR MM ($n = 113$), and 68.1% in patients with 2 HLA-DR MM ($n = 117$) (1 MM vs 2 MM: $p < 0.05$). Freedom from cardiac allograft vasculopathy after 5 years was 89% in HLA-DR-identical recipients ($n = 10$), 61% in patients with 1 HLA-DR MM ($n = 102$), 54% in patients with 2 HLA-DR MM ($n = 104$). Conventional matching with 6 mismatches over the three major HLA antigen loci revealed a trend toward a higher relative risk for adverse outcome in patients with increased MM.

*Conclusions.*—HLA-DR matching had a significant impact on survival after heart transplantation (HTx) at our center. In the effort to achieve the best comparative use of scarce donor organs the inclusion of HLA-DR matching into allocation policies might improve long-term outcome after HTx (Fig 2).

▶ This important contribution from the Department of Cardiac Surgery in Munich documents the impact of HLA class II matching on cardiac allograft survival. This effect has been long hypothesized and it is gratifying to see it play out in practice. As shown in Fig 2, survival is superior for those with HLA matching. In fact absent, apart from the perioperative risk, the survival looks darn near perfect. In an accompanying figure demonstrating freedom from graft coronary artery disease, the lines are quite similar to those shown here.

The fly in the ointment here, unfortunately, is not an issue of immunology but of logistics. The individuals performing this study are fortunate to have a system in which HLA matching is possible. Unfortunately, in the United States, given its size and relatively low population density, only a few centers in very populous areas would be able to carry out a similar policy. Furthermore, we are already committed to organ distribution according to the clinical status of the recipient and not the HLA match. Could this change? There is exciting progress being made in modalities for organ preservation that might extend the safe travel time. Such a breakthrough might make HLA matching a possibility. Until this occurs, however, reports such as this are scientifically important but still not clinically terribly relevant.

**T. M. Sundt III, MD**

---

**Analysis of the Complex Effect of Donor's Age on Survival of Subjects Who Underwent Heart Transplantation**
Pedotti P, Mattucci DA, Gabbrielli F, et al (Ospedale Policlinico–IRCCS, Milan, Italy; Natl Transplant Ctr, Milan, Italy)
*Transplantation* 80:1026-1032, 2005                                        3–24

---

*Background.*—Only half of the patients waiting for a heart transplant undergo surgery, whereas several patients continue to die while on the waiting list. Donor organ availability still represents a major problem with respect to reducing the length of the cardiac transplant waiting list. One option to improve donor availability is the use of so called "marginal donors." The aims of the present study are to analyze the short-mid term survival of cardiac transplanted patients in Italy, and investigate the effect of donor age on prognosis.

*Methods.*—A prospective cohort study including all adult patients who underwent heart transplantations in Italy was used to analyze the main factors contributing to organ survival.

*Results.*—From 1995–2002, 2,504 adult subjects underwent a cardiac transplant, and were followed up for a period of 540.9 days. Overall, 1-year graft survival was 83.1%. Organs from donors older than 55 years had a lower survival than organs from younger donors. By multivariate analysis, both donor's and recipient's age seem to be important determinants of graft survival. A more sophisticated analysis shows that the trend of the risk of graft failure according to donor's age is not linear, with a peak at age 47.3 years, and differs according to sex.

*Conclusions.*—Results from the present analysis suggest that the association between heart transplant survival and donor's age is not a linear one, but follows a complex mathematical model, with influences of sex, at least in our sample.

▶ This study of transplantation in Italy addresses the complex effect of donor age on patient survival. The findings are intriguing, and in some cases at first glance counterintuitive. As one might guess, 1-year graft survival was higher for recipients less than 55 years of age (84.7%) than for those recipients greater than 55 years of age (80.9%). Similarly, recipients of organs from donors greater than 55 years of age had poorer survival than those receiving organs from younger donors (76.5% vs 83.5%, respectively). Risk increases approximately 20% for each decade of donor age and for each decade of recipient age. This relationship is nonlinear, however, with regard to donor age. Although the risk of graft failure increases most rapidly with increasing recipient age between 35 and 55 years, in all decades it increases somewhat. The relationship with donor age, however, is more complex; there is a decrease in risk with increasing age up to 32 years and then a steep increase from 32 to 47 years. Risk then decreases again after donor age 47 years (see figure). The curve is of similar shape regardless of donor sex, although in general the risk is higher with female organs.

How does one interpret these data? The recipient age effect is intuitive. The donor effect is also intuitive, with a reduction in risk as donors enter the ideal range of the late 20s to early 30s. The young adult heart is better able to cope with the increased pulmonary vascular resistance common among transplant recipients than the adolescent. The risk then rises again as donors advance to their late 30s and 40s. The curious decrease in risk after age 47 years is no doubt simply due to increasingly stringent acceptance criteria for donors in this age range.

The bottom line is that risk continues to rise with recipient and donor age. Although we increasingly are compelled to use organs from donors in their 40s and even 50s, the incremental risk is significant. Despite the pressure to transplant more patients with marginal organs, we have to remain cognizant of the increased risks.

**T. M. Sundt III, MD**

---

**A Decade Experience of Cardiac Retransplantation in Adult Recipients**
Topkara VK, Dang NC, John R, et al (Columbia Univ College of Physicians and Surgeons, New York)
*J Heart Lung Transplant* 24:1745-1750, 2005                                3–25

---

*Background.*—Cardiac retransplantation is considered to be the best therapeutic option for a failing cardiac allograft. However, poor outcomes with retransplantation have previously been reported, a factor that raises important ethical, logistic and financial issues given the limited organ donor supply.

*Methods.*—Seven hundred sixty-six adult patients underwent cardiac transplantation for end-stage heart failure at our institution from 1992 to 2002. Of these, 41 (5.4%) were retransplants. Variables examined included recipient and donor demographics, indications for retransplant, comorbidities, cytomegalovirus (CMV) serology status, left ventricular assist device use before transplant, donor ischemic time, rate of early mortality (within 30 days), and post-transplantation survival rate.

*Results.*—Indications for cardiac retransplant were transplant-related coronary artery disease in 37, acute rejection in 3, and other causes in 1. The mean interval between transplantation and retransplantation was $5.9 \pm 3.4$ years. Baseline characteristics such as recipient age, gender, CMV serology status, and donor age were similar in the primary transplant and retransplant groups. Early mortality after transplantation was comparable between the 2 groups, but post-transplant survival was significantly lower in retransplant patients compared with primary transplants with 1-, 3-, 5-, and 7-year actuarial survival rates of 72.2%, 66.3%, 47.5%, and 40.7% vs. 85.1%, 79.2%, 72.9%, and 66.8%, respectively ($p < 0.001$).

*Conclusions.*—Cardiac retransplantation offers short-term outcomes similar to primary transplantation but lower long-term survival rates. Non-retransplant surgical options should also be considered in these patients. Careful patient selection and risk-assessment is necessary to govern appropriate allocation of limited donor organs.

▶ The issue of cardiac retransplantation has been highly debated in the literature. We are indebted to our colleagues at Columbia University for readdressing this matter in such an honest manner as their own institutional data have fed some of the arguments. A number of studies have documented lower posttransplant survival rates among patients undergoing retransplantation. These include single-center results and those derived from the Registry of the International Society of Heart and Lung Transplantation. A prior study from Columbia, however, called this into question. More recently, however, the group at Columbia has refined their selection criteria for retransplantation and since 1993 have excluded patients with intractable acute rejection within 6 months after prior transplant and those with primary allograft dysfunction. With these refined criteria for retransplantation, which are consonant with those of most other centers today, the authors have now accumulated 10-year follow-up on twice the number of patients previously reported. Their findings have now changed. These more comprehensive results demonstrate an important difference in survival. Given the shortage of donor organs, this is an important finding that will influence practice in many centers around the world. The difficulty, of course, is that it is hard to say no to patients who have been within one's transplant center for years. Still, our responsibility to other patients on the list demands that we pay attention to these data. I cannot emphasize enough how important it is that these investigators have so forthrightly reassessed their results. Not all of us can admit that our initial findings were wrong. We should take our hats off to these honest investigators.

**T. M. Sundt III, MD**

## Outcomes With an Alternate List Strategy for Heart Transplantation

Felker GM, Milano CA, Yager JEE, et al (Duke Univ School of Medicine, Durham, NC)

*J Heart Lung Transplant* 24:1781-1786, 2005                    3–26

*Background.*—Heart transplantation (HT) is an effective therapy for end-stage heart failure, but its impact is limited by the scarcity of donor organs and stringent selection criteria for both donors and recipients. The creation of an alternate list to match recipients with contraindications to traditional HT with sub-optimal donor organs has been implemented at some centers, but outcomes using this approach are uncertain.

*Methods.*—We created an alternate list that matched recipients in whom standard HT was contraindicated with donor organs that had been rejected for use in standard transplantation. Data on patient characteristics and outcomes were compared with a control group of patients transplanted on the standard list over the same time period.

*Results.*—Fifty patients received HT on the alternate list, compared with 195 on the standard list. The most common reasons for recipient listing on the alternate list were age >65 years ($n = 28$) and diabetes with end-organ dysfunction ($n = 9$). Alternate-list patients were older and more likely to have an ischemic etiology and diabetes mellitus. The most common reasons for allocation of donor organs to alternate-list patients were coronary artery disease ($n = 12$), positive hepatitis serology ($n = 12$) or left ventricular (LV) dysfunction ($n = 8$). Two-year survival was 70% for alternate-list patients

TABLE 2.—Recipient and Donor Criteria for Assignment to the Alternate List

| Characteristic | N | Mortality |
|---|---|---|
| Recipient | | |
| Age >65 years | 28 | 6/28 (21%) |
| Diabetes mellitus with end-organ dysfunction | 9 | 2/9 (22%) |
| Hepatitis C antibody positive | 5 | 1/5 (20%) |
| Peripheral vascular disease | 5 | 2/5 (40%) |
| Chronic renal insufficiency (serum creatinine >2 mg/dl) | 4 | 1/4 (25%) |
| Other systemic illness (rheumatoid arthritis, multiple sclerosis, COPD) | 3 | 0/3 (0%) |
| Hepatitis B core Ab-positive with negative hepatitis B surface Ag | 2 | 0/2 (0%) |
| Critically ill, no other donor available | 2 | 1/2 (50%) |
| History of CVA with residual deficit | 1 | 0/1 (0%) |
| Donor | | |
| Donor single-vessel CAD | 12 | 1/12 (8%) |
| Donor LV dysfunction without apparent etiology | 8 | 3/8 (38%) |
| Hepatitis B core Ab-positive with negative hepatitis B surface Ag | 7 | 2/7 (29%) |
| High-risk donor behavior with negative serology | 6 | 1/6 (17%) |
| Hepatitis C antibody positive | 5 | 4/5 (80%) |
| LV hypertrophy (wall thickness >1.5 cm) | 5 | 0/5 (0%) |
| Smaller donor, open offer | 5 | 0/5 (0%) |
| Older donor, no catheter available | 3 | 0/3 (0%) |
| High inotrope requirement | 2 | 0/2 (0%) |

More than one characteristic may be present in the same donor/recipient. Ab, antibody; Ag, antigen; CAD, coronary artery disease; CVA, cerebrovascular accident; COPD, chronic obstructive pulmonary disease.

compared with 88% for standard-list patients ($p = 0.02$). Post-transplant morbidity did not differ significantly between the 2 groups except that alternate-list patients were hospitalized more frequently.

*Conclusions.*—The use of an alternate list can expand the applicability of HT to patients who would otherwise be denied this therapy. Although associated with greater morbidity and mortality than standard-list HT, alternate-list HT resulted in clinical outcomes that were significantly better than the natural history of end-stage heart failure (Table 2).

▶ This is another important article addressing the issue of so-called "alternate list" strategies to increase the number of organs used in transplantation. The authors compared their results with the alternate-list patients with those observed on their standard list. Importantly, patients on the alternate list were both themselves marginal candidates and (appropriately) received marginal organs.

The most important information in this study in my view is available in Table 2, which we have included that for the reader. Note that the mortality rate associated with age greater than 65 years was 20% and that associated with critical illness with no other donor available was 50%. Forty percent of those with significant peripheral vascular disease died. With regard to donor characteristics, the mortality rate associated with left ventricular dysfunction of uncertain etiology was almost 40% and that associated with positive hepatitis C serology was 80%.

Although when taken together the 2-year survival rate was not statistically significantly different for those on the alternate list versus the standard list, it is difficult to say that these differences are not clinically significant. Is a 2-year survival rate of 70% acceptable? Of course, it depends on whether one is measuring that against the natural history of the disease or against that expected for transplantation under optimal circumstances. In the end, I believe that this is the most important issue. If results are going to be measured against those expected for standard-list patients, there is no question an alternate-list strategy results in a higher mortality rate. If public reporting will hold transplant centers to the standard of results expected with standard lists, this strategy will not survive. We need to be reasonable in our expectations of transplant centers.

**T. M. Sundt III, MD**

---

**Optimal Surgical Management of Severe Tricuspid Regurgitation in Cardiac Transplant Patients**

Filsoufi F, Salzberg SP, Anderson CA, et al (Mount Sinai Med Ctr, New York; Harvard Med School)
*J Heart Lung Transplant* 25:289-293, 2006                                    3–27

---

*Background.*—Severe tricuspid regurgitation (TR) with signs of right-sided heart failure is rare after orthotopic heart transplantation (OHT). In some instances, this condition will require surgical correction using reconstructive surgery or prosthetic valve replacement. Repair techniques of atrioventricular valves are now well described. However, the results of the different surgical procedures in this setting have not been widely reported and may depend on the type of valvular dysfunction and lesions present. Herein we report our experience in a group of patients requiring surgical correction of symptomatic severe TR after OHT.

*Methods.*—We reviewed our transplant experience during the period from July 1992 to July 1999 ($n = 138$ cardiac transplants). Eight patients (5.8%) developed symptomatic severe TR requiring surgical correction after a mean duration of 21 months after OHT. Patients were divided into 2 groups based on the mechanism of regurgitation using Carpentier's functional classification. In Group 1 ($n = 4$), the mechanism of tricuspid regurgitation was Carpentier's Type I, secondary to annular dilation. In Group 2 ($n = 4$) the mechanism of TR was leaflet prolapse (Type II), due to chordal rupture after biopsy injury. Initially, tricuspid valve integrity was surgically restored in all 8 patients with either valve repair ($n = 6$) or replacement ($n = 2$). In Group 1, 2 patients underwent valve repair using a ring annuloplasty and 2 patients underwent valve replacement with a bioprosthetic valve ($n = 1$) or pulmonary allograft ($n = 1$). In Group 2, all patients underwent valve repair using a variety of techniques in combination with tricuspid annuloplasty.

*Results.*—During the follow-up period, 3 of the 6 (50%) primary repairs (1 patient in Group 1 and 2 in Group 2) failed and required replacement with a bioprosthesis at 8 days, 14 days and 4 years, respectively. The pulmonary allograft failed secondary to valvular stenosis and was replaced with a bioprosthesis after 10 months. Overall, no failures occurred in any of the 5 bioprosthetic valves placed at the primary operation ($n = 1$) or after failed tricuspid repair/pulmonary allograft ($n = 4$), after a mean follow-up of 55 months.

*Conclusions.*—TR requiring surgical correction after OHT is a rare condition and requires a tailored surgical strategy. This strategy should take into account the mechanism of valve dysfunction and specific valvular lesions. In patients with Type I dysfunction secondary to annular dilation, valve repair with a remodeling annuloplasty should be performed; however, in the presence of any residual TR on transesophageal echocardiography (TEE) at the completion of cardiopulmonary bypass (CPB), a valve replacement with a bioprosthesis is warranted during the same procedure. In patients with Type II dysfunction with leaflet prolapse and biopsy-induced chordal injury, a bioprosthetic valve replacement seems a reliable surgical option.

▶ The authors of this article address a clinically important problem, that of tricuspid regurgitation after cardiac transplantation. Although the authors find it infrequently in their center, sadly it is not so uncommonly identified in our own! Accordingly, I find that results of their study most interesting, and I appreciate their decision to share the results with us.

The authors argue that a tailored approach to this entity should be undertaken, with valve repair seriously considered in patients with annular dilation while replacement is the preferred option for chordal rupture. Quite frankly, this is counter to my personal experience and admittedly counter to my bias. More important, I think that their own data argue the opposite.

Of 4 patients with annular dilation, 2 underwent valve repair and 2 replacement with a bioprosthetic valve. The latter had an excellent result; however, 1 of the 2 repaired valves failed within 3 years. Admittedly, this is only 1 patient, but it is a 50% failure rate nonetheless. It is certainly not data in support of repair. Among patients with chordal rupture, all 4 had an attempted repair. Of these, 2 failed within 3 years—yielding the same durability as that of repair of annular dilatation. How then can one argue for differential treatment? One may well argue that replacement is preferred in all cases if one finds a 50% failure rate unacceptable (which one might well argue).

I actually happen to agree that bioprosthetic valves are quite reasonable. Bioprosthetic valves in the tricuspid position are remarkably durable and certainly, given the expected outcome with transplantation, can be anticipated to last as long as the patient may need them. I suspect the authors' conclusions, however, are somewhat dictated by their own prestudy bias. I conclude from these data that one should have a low threshold for bioprosthetic replacement in this setting.

**T. M. Sundt III, MD**

---

### Influence of Pre-Existing Donor Atherosclerosis on the Development of Cardiac Allograft Vasculopathy and Outcomes in Heart Transplant Recipients

Li H, Tanaka K, Anzai H, et al (Peking Univ Third Hosp, Beijing, China; Univ of Calif Los Angeles)
*J Am Coll Cardiol* 47:2470-2476, 2006                                    3–28

---

*Objectives.*—This study sought to evaluate the influence of donor lesions on the development of cardiac allograft vasculopathy and outcomes in heart transplant recipients.

*Background.*—After orthotopic heart transplantation (OHT), coronary artery narrowing occurs as a combination of pre-existing donor lesions and new lesions that develop as a result of cardiac allograft vasculopathy.

*Methods.*—Intravascular ultrasound (IVUS) studies were performed in 301 recipients at $1.3 \pm 0.6$ months and again at $12.2 \pm 0.8$ months after OHT. Additional IVUS studies were performed in 90 patients at two and three years of follow-up. Sites at baseline with maximum intimal thickness $\geq 0.5$ mm were defined as pre-existing donor lesions. The angiographic diagnosis of transplant coronary artery disease (TCAD) was defined as a new $\geq 50\%$ diameter narrowing of a major epicardial vessel.

*Results.*—Donor lesions were present in 30% of the hearts. By IVUS, sites with donor lesions did not have a greater increase in intimal area compared with sites without donor lesions. Angiographically, the incidence of TCAD up to three years after transplantation was higher in recipients with donor lesions than in recipients without donor lesions (25% vs. 4%, $p < 0.001$).

However, the three-year mortality rate was similar between recipients with or without donor lesions (4.5% vs. 5.2%, p = 1.0).

*Conclusions.*—Pre-existing donor lesions do not act as a nidus for accelerating the progression of intimal hyperplasia. However, patients with donor lesions have a higher incidence of angiographic TCAD. Donor lesions do not affect the long-term survival of patients with OHT up to three years.

▶ The challenge of dealing with the shortage of donor organs continues to grow worse. If anything, organ donation is on the decline. Unfortunately, recipient lists are on the rise. Transplant surgeons are therefore challenged to use increasingly "marginal" donors. One of the criteria for acceptable organs a decade ago was freedom from atherosclerotic coronary artery disease. This has been called into question, most conspicuously by Hill Laks and his colleagues at UCLA, who have pioneered performing coronary artery bypass grafts on donor hearts at the time of transplant into their "marginal donor" list.

Even more challenging, however, is the decision making regarding use of an organ with only moderate disease. The study by Li et al at UCLA addresses this group of potential donors. Their data demonstrate that in fact hearts with preexisting atherosclerotic disease do have a higher incidence of transplant coronary artery disease. This is a somewhat disappointing, if not surprising, result. The authors argue on the brighter side that there was no difference in the 3-year mortality rate of recipients whether they received hearts with or without donor lesions. The trouble, of course, is that cardiac transplantation is, in most people's minds, a 10-year therapy, not a 3-year therapy. Are data at 3 years really good enough to answer the question? I personally do not think so, and so I do not find these data to be particularly comforting. I think that most of us will still regard organs with preexisting atherosclerotic disease as marginal and will be reluctant to transplant them into young patients with an otherwise good long-term prognosis.

**T. M. Sundt III, MD**

---

**Surgical ventricular restoration in patients with ischemic dilated cardiomyopathy: Evaluation of systolic and diastolic ventricular function, wall stress, dyssynchrony, and mechanical efficiency by pressure-volume loops**
Tulner SAF, Steendijk P, Klautz RJM, et al (Leiden Univ Med Ctr, The Netherlands)
*J Thorac Cardiovasc Surg* 132:610-620, 2006                    3–29

---

*Objectives.*—Surgical ventricular restoration aims at improving cardiac function by normalization of left ventricular shape and size. Recent studies indicate that surgical ventricular restoration is highly effective with an excellent 5-year outcome in patients with ischemic dilated cardiomyopathy. We used pressure-volume analysis to investigate acute changes in systolic and diastolic left ventricular function, mechanical dyssynchrony and efficiency, and wall stress.

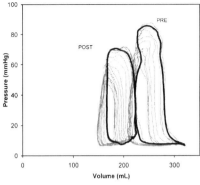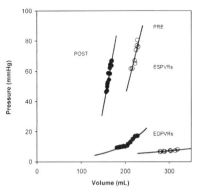

FIGURE 2.—Typical example of pressure-volume relations in a patient with ischemic dilated cardiomyopathy before *(PRE)* and after *(POST)* surgical ventricular restoration. The steady-state pressure-volume loops show a significant reduction in end-diastolic and end-systolic volumes with unchanged stroke volume indicating improved LV ejection fraction. Before surgery, LV volume decreased during the presystolic contraction phase, reflecting severe mitral regurgitation. This effect disappeared in the postsurgery loops as mitral regurgitation was treated by restrictive mitral annuloplasty. The load-independent end-systolic pressure-volume relationship *(ESPVR)* showed a leftward shift with increased slope, indicating improved systolic function. The end-diastolic pressure-volume relationship *(EDPVR)* also showed a leftward shift with increased slope, indicating increased diastolic chamber stiffness postsurgery. (Reprinted from Tulner SAF, Steendijk P, Klautz RJM, et al: Surgical ventricular restoration in patients with ischemic dilated cardiomyopathy: Evaluation of systolic and diastolic ventricular function, wall stress, dyssynchrony, and mechanical efficiency by pressure-volume loops. *J Thorac Cardiovasc Surg* 132:610-620, 2006. Copyright 2006 Elsevier.)

*Methods.*—In 3 patient groups (total, n = 33), pressure-volume loops were measured by conductance catheter before and after surgery. The main study group consisted of 10 patients with ischemic dilated cardiomyopathy (New York Heart Association class III/IV, left ventricular ejection fraction <30%) who had surgical ventricular restoration and coronary artery bypass grafting. In this group, 7 patients had additional restrictive mitral annuloplasty. To assess potential confounding effects of restrictive mitral annuloplasty and cardiopulmonary bypass, we included a group of 10 patients (New York Heart Association class III/IV, left ventricular ejection fraction <30%) who had isolated restrictive mitral annuloplasty and a group of 13 patients with preserved left ventricular function who had isolated coronary artery bypass grafting.

*Results.*—After surgical ventricular restoration, end-diastolic and end-systolic volumes were reduced from 211 ± 54 to 169 ± 34 mL ($P = .03$) and from 147 ± 41 to 110 ± 59 mL ($P = .04$), respectively. Left ventricular ejection fraction (from 27% ± 7% to 37% ± 13%, $P = .04$) and end-systolic elastance (from 1.12 ± 0.71 to 1.57 ± 0.63 mm Hg/mL, $P = .03$) improved. Peak wall stress (from 358 ± 108 to 244 ± 79 mm Hg, $P < .01$) and mechanical dyssynchrony (from 26% ± 4% to 19% ± 6%, $P < .01$) were reduced, whereas mechanical efficiency improved (from 0.34 ± 13 to 0.49 ± 0.14, $P = .03$). End-diastolic pressure increased (from 13 ± 6 to 20 ± 5 mm Hg, $P < .01$), whereas the diastolic chamber stiffness constant tended to be increased (from 0.021 ± 0.009 to 0.037 ± 0.021 mL$^{-1}$, NS).

*Conclusions.*—Surgical ventricular restoration achieves normalization of left ventricular volumes and improves systolic function and mechanical efficiency by reducing left ventricular wall stress and mechanical dyssynchrony (Fig 2).

▶ The Dor procedure for surgical ventricular restoration was first described almost 2 decades ago now, but only in the last 5 years has interest peaked in its application to patients with dilated ischemic cardiomyopathic processes. Its virtues as an alternative to traditional linear closures of discreet anteroseptal aneurysms are clear, with the latter approach neglecting to address the septal component of the infarct. What is less clear is its application to patients with diffuse, global scar and generalized left ventricular dysfunction. Defining the role of this procedure is one of the aims of the STICH trial.

In most studies, the mortality rate associated with this procedure is approximately twice that for coronary artery bypass alone. Considering the high-risk subset of patients in whom it is applied, this seems quite acceptable. The critical issue, of course, is what one gains in return for this. The authors of this study have looked carefully at ventricular function after the Dor procedure and demonstrated normalization of left ventricular function volumes and improved efficiency of the ventricle. Most of the patients in this study have true aneurysms and, in this regard, such an improvement is not surprising. The real question is the applicability of this approach when no discrete aneurysm is present. The jury is still out on that score.

**T. M. Sundt III, MD**

---

**Relationship Between Postoperative Cardiac Troponin I Levels and Outcome of Cardiac Surgery**
Croal BL, Hillis GS, Gibson PH, et al (Univ of Aberdeen, Scotland)
*Circulation* 114:1468-1475, 2006                                              3–30

---

*Background.*—Cardiac surgery may be associated with significant perioperative and postoperative morbidity and mortality. Underlying pathology, surgical technique, and postoperative complications may all influence outcome. These factors may be reflected as a rise in postoperative troponin levels. Interpretation of troponin levels in this setting may therefore be complex. This study assessed the prognostic significance of such measurements, taking into account potential confounding variables.

*Method and Results.*—One-thousand three hundred sixty-five patients undergoing cardiac surgery underwent measurement of cardiac troponin I (cTnI) at 2 and 24 hours after surgery. The relationship of these measurements to subsequent mortality was established. After taking into account all other variables, cTnI levels measured at 24 hours were independently predictive of mortality at 30 days (odds ratio [OR] 1.14 per 10 μg/L, 95% confidence interval [CI] 1.05 to 1.24, $P=0.002$), 1 year (OR 1.10 per 10 μg/L, 95% CI 1.03 to 1.18, $P=0.006$), and 3 years (OR 1.07 per 10 μg/L, 95% CI 1.00 to 1.15, $P=0.04$). Cardiac TnI levels in the highest quartile at 24 hours were associated with a particularly poor outcome.

*Conclusions.*—cTnI levels measured 24 hours after cardiac surgery predict short-, medium-, and long-term mortality and remain independently predictive when adjusted for all other potentially confounding variables, including operation complexity.

▶ This large study addresses the relationship between postoperative enzyme release and long-term outcome after cardiac surgery. Troponin release after cardiac surgery is commonplace. The majority of individuals undergoing on-pump surgery will have at least some release of enzymes detectable within the first several hours after surgery. This has complicated previous attempts to assess the value of troponin levels in this clinical setting. The important observation in this study is that the predictive value of troponin increases at 24 hours. In this study of more than 1300 patients, the majority of whom (more than 1000) underwent isolated coronary bypass, there was a relationship between troponin release and outcome both early and late after surgery, as shown in the accompanying figure. In this analysis, patients were divided into quartiles. Although the authors were unable to identify a universally acceptable cutoff value or threshold for troponins, it is clear that as the troponin level increases cumulative survival diminishes.

What is the utility of this observation? There may be some utility in using troponin release as a surrogate outcome in the comparison of on-pump versus off-pump coronary bypass. More broadly, however, it is likely useful in identifying a group of patients at increased risk of late death who, therefore, warrant special attention. Of course, the unknown is how one might intervene on these individuals. Perhaps some more intensive postoperative medical regimen would be indicated. It is also of interest parenthetically that when other analyses were performed looking at predictors of outcome, only the postoperative use of statins was predictive. This is consonant with other studies, and statins have become standard practice for surgeons after coronary revascularization.

**T. M. Sundt III, MD**

---

**Public versus private institutional performance reporting: What is mandatory for quality improvement?**
Guru V, and the Cardiac Care Network (CCN) of Ontario (Inst for Clinical Evaluative Sciences, Toronto; et al)
*Am Heart J* 152:573-578, 2006                                    3–31

---

*Background.*—In the past 11 years, Ontario has generated institution-level performance report cards on outcomes of coronary artery bypass graft (CABG) surgery. The objective of this study was to evaluate the differences in patient characteristics and outcomes observed during the transition from no reporting to confidential, and ultimately public performance report cards for CABG surgery in a public health system.

*Methods.*—We used clinical and administrative data to assess crude, expected, and risk-adjusted 30-day mortality rates after isolated CABG surgery in Ontario for 67693 patients from September 1, 1991, to March 31, 2002. Confidence intervals on relative mortality reductions were determined by bootstrapping. We compared 30-day mortality trends to a control outcome (risk-adjusted 30-day all-cause readmission). We analyzed in-hospital mortality trends for Ontario compared with the rest of Canada for the period from 1992 to 1998.

*Results.*—The risk-adjusted 30-day mortality rate decreased 29% (95% CI 21-39) from the era of no reporting (1991-1993) to confidential reporting (1994-1998). There was no further decrease with public reporting (1999-2001). The control outcome of 30-day readmission did not decrease across reporting eras. Inhospital mortality fell significantly faster in Ontario during the period of confidential reporting than in other parts of Canada.

*Conclusion.*—Ontario CABG mortality outcomes improved sharply after provider results were confidentially disclosed at an institutional level. No such changes were seen for nondisclosed outcomes or regions outside Ontario. Further public reporting of outcomes had no discernible impact on performance. These results are consistent with the hypothesis that confidential disclosure of outcomes was sufficient to accelerate quality improvement in a public system with little competition for patients between hospitals.

▶ The results of this study should, in theory, serve to disarm arguments by policymakers for public disclosure of outcomes on the grounds that such serves to assure quality improvement. Unfortunately, given that public reporting of outcomes is here to stay, it would be easy to dismiss the findings of this study as irrelevant. In fact, regardless of the results of such studies, the demand by society for "transparency" can only be satisfied by the public provision of information. The important point, however, is that we must ensure that the data provided are fair and accurate. It is also worthwhile remembering that ultimately the most important aim of such public reporting is to improve the quality of care for all patients and improve the performance of all providers. In the end, this will provide the greatest good for the greatest number. Insofar as this is the case, results of this study are reassuring. In point of fact, it demonstrates quite convincingly that confidential monitoring of outcomes does indeed provide for quality improvement. The institution of confidential report card did in fact improve the quality of care. In that regard, there is no question that the institution of these programs has met its objective. The further step of public reporting, however, had no positive impact on quality of care. This reinforces the importance that we ensure no negative consequences.

Our patients are justified in asking for the data. It is our responsibility to provide it in an understandable and appropriate manner.

**T. M. Sundt III, MD**

### Massachusetts Cardiac Surgery Report Card: Implications of Statistical Methodology

Shahian DM, Torchiana DF, Shemin RJ, et al (Caritas St Elizabeth's Med Ctr, Boston; Massachusetts Gen Hosp, Boston; Boston Univ Med Ctr; et al)
*Ann Thorac Surg* 80:2106-2113, 2005                                   3–32

*Background.*—Choice of statistical methodology may significantly impact the results of provider profiling, including cardiac surgery report cards. Because of sample size and clustering issues, logistic regression may overestimate systematic interprovider variability, leading to false outlier classification. Theoretically, the use of hierarchical models should result in more accurate representation of provider performance.

*Methods.*—Extensively validated and audited data were available for all 4,603 isolated coronary artery bypass grafting procedures performed at 13 Massachusetts hospitals during 2002. To produce the official Massachusetts cardiac surgery report card, a 19-variable predictor set and a hierarchical generalized linear model were employed. For the current study, this same analysis was repeated with the 14 predictors used in the New York Cardiac Surgery Reporting System. Two additional analyses were conducted using each set of predictor variables and applying standard logistic regression. For each of the four combinations of predictors and models, the point estimates of risk-adjusted 30-day mortality, 95% confidence or probability intervals, and outlier status were determined for each hospital.

*Results.*—Overall unadjusted mortality for coronary bypass operations was 2.19%. For most hospitals, there was wide variability in the point estimates and confidence or probability intervals of risk-adjusted mortality depending on statistical model, but little variability relative to the choice of predictors. There were no hospital outliers using hierarchical models, but there was one outlier using logistic regression with either predictor set.

*Conclusions.*—When used to compare provider performance, logistic regression increases the possibility of false outlier classification. The use of hierarchical models is recommended.

▶ Report cards have become a fact of life for cardiovascular surgical practitioners in many states and work environments in the United States and Europe. Although they are intended to serve a just need—the right of patients to assess the quality of the care provider before committing to surgical intervention—they are powerful instruments that can also create unintended consequences. Errors in the rankings may unjustly stigmatize a provider, having a profound impact on his or her personal professional satisfaction and, indeed, livelihood. Equally they may have an unintended impact on patients themselves, making physicians unwilling to perform high-risk surgical procedures and thereby denying patients potentially life-prolonging interventions.

This important contribution from practitioners in the state of Massachusetts demonstrates the critical importance of decisions made concerning statistical methods on the results and interpretation of such rankings. The majority of rankings in public reporting are based on logistic regression rather than on hierarchical models. This creates potential problems on several fronts. As the authors point out in the text of their manuscript, "logistic regression neglects clustering of observations among providers such as heart failure patients at transplant centers." The hierarchical approach accepts the notion that there are unmeasured factors that may lead to systematic differences. The hierarchical model is also likely more accurate in assessing the quality of low-volume providers because small sample size is particularly an issue in the use of logistic regression. Errors generated as a result of small sample size may overestimate systemic intraprovider variability while underestimating random variability, thereby increasing the risk the provider will be falsely classified as an outliner. Hierarchical methods permit "shrinking" of the observed variables representing a weighted average. They also mitigate against problems arising from multiple comparisons. Accordingly, many statisticians endorse the use of hierarchical models. Several studies have been previously performed using both the New York State database and the Pennsylvania database supporting this notion.

Admittedly there is a tradeoff between sensitivity and specificity in these models, just as there are in any statistical analysis. Where that bar is set is a matter of public policy. What is important is that the consumer appreciates the impact of these statistical methodologic decisions on the resulting ranking.

It is also worth noting that the data use in this analysis were collected according to the Society of Thoracic Surgeons National Cardiac Database and therefore represent what surgeons themselves would feel is the most accurate set of variables and definitions. In addition, the Massachusetts database is an audited database, representing a significant strength.

These sorts of analyses are heavy sledding from a statistical standpoint for those of us principally focused on clinical practice; however, given the likely abuse of such data sets and their reporting on the Internet to the public, they very rapidly become a matter of importance to all of us.

**T. M. Sundt III, MD**

# 4 Coronary Heart Disease

## Introduction

This has been another interesting year with major developments in the number of fields, and in particular, ST-elevation, myocardial infarction (STEMI), percutaneous coronary intervention (PCI), and epidemiology. I have tried to select not only important papers but other articles that reflect the diversity of clinical research in the field of coronary artery disease.

Reperfusion therapy for STEMI continues to attract interest and controversy but also produces excellent randomized control trials. The negative results of the large ASSENT-IV trial of Facilitated PCI have certainly dampened enthusiasm for this initially promising approach. The issue should be settled one way or another by 2 other smaller trials due to be presented in 2007, but it is doubtful whether this approach will stand the test of time. The momentum has certainly shifted away from Facilitated PCI to what is being called "the Pharmacoinvasive strategy," which was the basis for 2 studies from the city of Vienna, Austria, and a Canadian trial that have been selected. As shown in a trial from the United Kingdom, crucial to the success of a thrombolytic or Pharmacoinvasive strategy is the availability of immediate "rescue PCI." On the other hand, the Open Artery Trial of patients 3 to 28 days post infarction certainly suggests that routine angiography to detect a closed artery is of no value unless this is being done very early as an emergency prior to "rescue". I believe that we are at a stage in regard to reperfusion therapy where we know what to do. The challenge, however, is one of implementation, and in this respect one size does not fit all, and networks will vary according to geography, weather, types of health system, resources, and coordination of resources, etc. Several papers which focus upon strategies for delivering care have been selected.

The other controversial and evolving area in patients with acute and chronic coronary disease is the use of cell repair therapy. Several trials have been published, and for the first time we are seeing discordant results whereas prior studies, both clinical and experimental, demonstrated an almost "universality" of benefits. This remains an area of intense interest and an unusual situation in that as although the mechanisms of benefit are not at all completely understood, clinical trials are proceeding. The ultimate success or lack thereof of cell repair therapy will depend upon basic science and clinical researchers and trialers working in tandem. There are many clinical questions to be asked in regard to cell therapy, and trials should be focused such as to answer these. In my opinion, large randomized trials with death and mortality as an end point are premature at this time.

The world of non-ST segment elevation acute coronary syndrome is focused largely upon antithrombotic and antiplatelet strategies as has largely been the case in prior years.

The manuscripts on chronic coronary artery disease reflect a variety of topics including the neutral trials of homocysteine lowering with folic acid, several biomarker studies, a meta-analysis of angiotensin converting enzyme inhibitors, and a fascinating paper from a Brazilian randomized control trial on the impact of clinical judgment on treatment options in coronary artery disease.

The field of PCI has been dominated by trials and registries of drug-eluting stents and their association with increased late events in some studies. The controversy continues and is likely to be the subject of numerous additional analyses in the coming year or two. Moreover, more data are sorely needed, particularly in regard to duration of Clopidogrel use and event rates and relative benefits versus risk in patients with non-FDA-labeled indications. Several papers deal with various adjunctive therapies in patients undergoing coronary bypass surgery; one comparative trial of PCI, CABG, and medical therapy is included, and a paper on the role of PCI versus coronary bypass surgery in left main disease has been selected as well as studies of off pump versus conventional coronary bypass.

There are 2 important studies on nonsteroidal anti-inflammatory drugs, and aspirin/Plavix have been included in the clinical pharmacology section.

As is always the case, I have included epidemiologic studies covering a diverse spectrum of topics including seasonality and daily weather conditions and sudden cardiac death, coffee and genotypes in myocardial infarction, diabetes, selenium supplementation, the risk of myocardial infarction in patients with psoriasis, obesity, diet, and the impact of citywide ordinances banning smoking on rates of myocardial infarction.

The psychosocial aspects of cardiac disease are a critically important determinate of outcomes. I wish that space would allow more papers in this area. Irrespective of country or region, the concept of the socioeconomic gradient in relationship to the development and prognosis of coronary disease persists.

Finally, the topics of stress testing in patients undergoing vascular surgery and the impact of the new definition of myocardial infarction upon outcomes are addressed. A widespread adoption of the troponins is certainly going to result in marked changes in our perceived incidence and prevalence of myocardial infarction and perhaps on prognosis.

The final paper is from a biostatistician and illustrates a very useful and simple test to check for a difference between treatments and a randomized controlled trial. I have personally found this to be extremely useful when discussing trial design and outcomes. It requires neither an advanced knowledge of biostatistics nor the use of a calculator and enables one to assess rapidly whether or not an apparent difference is statistically significant.

Bernard Gersh, MB, ChB, DPhil, FRCP

## Acute ST-Segment Elevation Myocardial Infarction

**Coronary Intervention for Persistent Occlusion after Myocardial Infarction**
Hochman JS, for the Occluded Artery Trial Investigators (New York Univ School of Medicine; et al)
*N Engl J Med* 355:2395-2407, 2006                                          4–1

*Background.*—It is unclear whether stable, high-risk patients with persistent total occlusion of the infarct-related coronary artery identified after the currently accepted period for myocardial salvage has passed should undergo percutaneous coronary intervention (PCI) in addition to receiving optimal medical therapy to reduce the risk of subsequent events.

*Methods.*—We conducted a randomized study involving 2166 stable patients who had total occlusion of the infarct-related artery 3 to 28 days after myocardial infarction and who met a high-risk criterion (an ejection fraction of <50% or proximal occlusion). Of these patients, 1082 were assigned to routine PCI and stenting with optimal medical therapy, and 1084 were as-

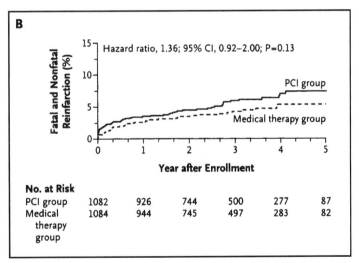

FIGURE 2.—The estimated cumulative event rates for fatal and nonfatal reinfarction in the two groups, respectively, were 5.9% and 4.3% in 3 years, 7.0% and 5.3% in 4 years, and 7.4% and 5.3% at 5 years. (Reprinted by permission of *The New England Journal of Medicine* from Hochman JS, for the Occluded Artery Trial Investigators: Coronary intervention for persistent occlusion after myocardial infarction. *N Engl J Med* 355:2395-2407, 2006. Copyright 2006, Massachusetts Medical Society. All rights reserved.)

signed to optimal medical therapy alone. The primary end point was a composite of death, myocardial reinfarction, or New York Heart Association (NYHA) class IV heart failure.

*Results.*—The 4-year cumulative primary event rate was 17.2% in the PCI group and 15.6% in the medical therapy group (hazard ratio for death, reinfarction, or heart failure in the PCI group as compared with the medical therapy group, 1.16; 95% confidence interval [CI], 0.92 to 1.45; P=0.20). Rates of myocardial reinfarction (fatal and nonfatal) were 7.0% and 5.3% in the two groups, respectively (hazard ratio, 1.36; 95% CI, 0.92 to 2.00; P=0.13) (Fig 2). Rates of nonfatal reinfarction were 6.9% and 5.0%, respectively (hazard ratio, 1.44; 95% CI, 0.96 to 2.16; P=0.08); only six reinfarctions (0.6%) were related to assigned PCI procedures. Rates of NYHA class IV heart failure (4.4% vs. 4.5%) and death (9.1% vs. 9.4%) were similar. There was no interaction between treatment effect and any subgroup variable (age, sex, race or ethnic group, infarct-related artery, ejection fraction, diabetes, Killip class, and the time from myocardial infarction to randomization).

*Conclusions.*—PCI did not reduce the occurrence of death, reinfarction, or heart failure, and there was a trend toward excess reinfarction during 4 years of follow-up in stable patients with occlusion of the infarct-related artery 3 to 28 days after myocardial infarction.

▶ The "open-artery conflict" first promulgated approximately 20 years ago is intriguing, but proof has been long awaited.[1,2] This trial, the largest and the most representative of contemporary practice including stents, which were widely utilized, not only demonstrates a lack of benefit but an unexpected trend toward excess reinfarction.

The open-artery concept suggested that late reperfusion of an included infarct-related artery resulted in a number of beneficial effects independent of myocardial salvage.[2] Potential mechanisms include the provision of collaterals, the elimination of silent ischemia, an improvement in left ventricular remodeling by a scaffolding effect, and an unexplained impact on electrical stability. Multiple nonrandomized retrospective studies and a few small randomized trials provided some suggestive but also contradictory evidence that opening an included infarct-related artery would be beneficial. Nonetheless, as is often the case, these attractive hypotheses have to withstand the rigorous scrutiny of a randomized controlled trial. One explanation for the trend toward excess reinfarction in this trial could be the loss of recruitable collateral flow after PCI of a total occlusion, and the high rate would be the blocker use in the medically treated group.

Irrespective of the explanations or the lack thereof, this trial would suggest that the common clinical practice of performing angiography in asymptomatic postinfarct survivors with the sole objective of identifying an occluded infarct related artery is not warranted.

**B. J. Gersh, MB, ChB, DPhil, FRCP**

*References*

1. Kim CB, Braunwald E: Potential benefits of late reperfusion of infarcted myocardium. The open artery hypothesis. *Circulation* 88:2426-2436, 1993.
2. Califf RM, Topol EJ, Gersh BJ: From myocardial salvage to patient salvage in acute myocardial infarction: the role of reperfusion therapy. *J Am Coll Cardiol* 14:1382-1388, 1989.

---

**Driving Times and Distances to Hospitals With Percutaneous Coronary Intervention in the United States: Implications for Prehospital Triage of Patients With ST-Elevation Myocardial Infarction**
Nallamothu BK, Bates ER, Wang Y, et al (Ann Arbor VA Med Ctr, Mich; Univ of Michigan Med School, Ann Arbor; Yale Univ School of Medicine, New Haven, Conn; et al)
*Circulation* 113:1189-1195, 2006                                                    4–2

---

*Background.*—The success of prehospital triage protocols for patients with ST-elevation myocardial infarction (STEMI) will depend, in part, on how patients are geographically distributed around hospitals that perform percutaneous coronary intervention (PCI). Accordingly, we determined the proportion of the adult population in the United States with timely access to PCI hospitals using driving times and distances.

*Method and Results.*—We performed a cross-sectional study using hospital-level data from the American Hospital Association Annual Survey and Census tract-level data on adults 18 years of age or older from the 2000 United States Census. Our aims were to determine the proportion of the adult population who (1) lived within 60 minutes of a PCI hospital and (2) had additional transport times within 30 minutes if directly referred to a PCI hospital as opposed to a closer, non-PCI hospital. Median times and distances to the closest PCI hospital were 11.3 (interquartile range [IQR] 5.7 to 28.5) minutes and 7.9 (IQR 3.5 to 22.4) miles, respectively. A total of 79.0% of the adult population lived within 60 minutes of a PCI hospital. Among those with a non-PCI hospital as their closest facility, 74.0% required additional transport times of <30 minutes if directly referred to a PCI hospital as opposed to the non-PCI hospital. These estimates varied substantially across regions and urban, suburban, and rural Census tracts.

*Conclusions.*—Nearly 80% of the adult population in the United States lived within 60 minutes of a PCI hospital in 2000. Even among those living closer to non-PCI hospitals, almost three fourths would experience <30 minutes of additional delay with direct referral to a PCI hospital, which suggests that such a strategy might be feasible for these individuals.

▶ This rather unique study has important policy implications for strategies aimed at improving timely access for primary percutaneous coronary intervention (PPCI). It would appear that in a high proportion of urban and suburban areas, facilities for PPCI are abundant and distances between non-PCI hospitals and referral PCI-capable hospitals are short. This varies from region to region and there are, as expected, major differences between rural and urban areas.

Because PPCI is acknowledged to be the optimal reperfusion strategy, these data suggest that in many parts of the country a strategy of triaging patients to a PCI-capable hospital could be effective. Such programs are already being established.[1] Nonetheless, although we know what to do, the devil is in the details and the logistics are complex.

There are limitations to this study, as the authors recognize, and the numbers quoted should be considered as estimates only. Driving times may be modified by factors such as weather or traffic. Nonetheless, it would appear that strategies aimed at preferentially transferring patients to PCI-capable hospitals is certainly feasible in many parts of the United States. In areas where this is not possible, particularly many rural communities, the prompt administration of fibrinolytics remains the cornerstone of care.

**B. J. Gersh, MB, ChB, DPhil, FRCP**

*Reference*

1. Williams DO: Treatment delayed is treatment denied. *Circulation* 109:1806-1808, 2004.

---

**Primary versus tenecteplase-facilitated percutaneous coronary intervention in patients with ST-segment elevation acute myocardial infarction (ASSENT-4 PCI): randomised trial**

Assessment of the Safety and Efficacy of a New Treatment Strategy with Percutaneous Coronary Intervention (ASSENT-4 PCI) Investigators (Leuven, Belgium; et al)

*Lancet* 367:569-578, 2006                                                          4–3

---

*Background.*—Primary percutaneous coronary intervention (PCI) is more effective than fibrinolytic therapy for ST-segment elevation acute myocardial infarction (STEMI), but time to intervention can be considerable. Our aim was to investigate whether the administration of full-dose tenecteplase before a delayed PCI could mitigate the negative effect of this delay.

*Methods.*—We did a randomised study in which we assigned patients with STEMI of less than 6 h duration (scheduled to undergo primary PCI with an anticipated delay of 1–3 h) to standard PCI (n=838) or PCI preceded by administration of full-dose tenecteplase (n=829). All patients received aspirin and a bolus, without an infusion, of unfractionated heparin. Our primary endpoint was death or congestive heart failure or shock within 90 days. Analyses were by intention to treat. This study is registered with ClinicalTrials.gov, number NCT00168792.

*Findings.*—We planned to enroll 4000 patients, but early cessation of enrollment was recommended by the data and safety monitoring board because of a higher in-hospital mortality in the facilitated than in the standard PCI group (6% [43 of 664] vs 3% [22 of 656], p=0.0105). Of those en-

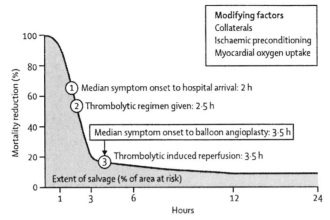

FIGURE.—Myocardial salvage and mortality reduction after reperfusion therapy is greatest in first 2–3 hours after onset of acute myocardial infarction. This period could be prolonged by presence of functioning coronary collateral vessels, ischaemic preconditioning, and reduced myocardial oxygen demand. Potential for myocardial salvage is greatly diminished after this early period, though late restoration of infarct artery patency can increase survival through time-independent mechanisms. Average patient presents with acute myocardial infarction at about 2 h after symptom onset (point 1). As part of facilitated angioplasty strategy, pharmacological regimen is administered within 30 min (point 2). Thrombolysis then needs on average 60 min for arterial recanalisation (point 3), perhaps slightly faster if administered with glycoprotein IIb/IIa inhibitor. Thus about 90 min is needed for lytic-induced reperfusion, the current benchmark for primary angioplasty. Moreover, many arteries will be reperfused at a time (point 3) when opportunity for myocardial salvage has largely passed. Thus unless patients present very early (within 60–90 min of symptom onset), and great delay to angioplasty occurs—eg, more than 2–3 h— little benefit of preangioplasty administration of fibrinolytic therapy would be anticipated. Figure adapted from reference 23 with permission. (Courtesy of Stone GW, Gersh BJ: Facilitated angioplasty: paradise lost [editorial]. *Lancet* 367:543-546. Copyright 2006 Elsevier.)

rolled, six were lost to follow-up in the facilitated PCI group and seven in the other group. Median time from randomisation to first balloon inflation was similar in both groups. The median time from bolus tenecteplase to first balloon inflation was 104 min. We noted the primary endpoint in 19% (151 of 810) of patients assigned facilitated PCI versus 13% (110 of 819) of those randomised to primary PCI (relative risk 1.39, 95% CI 1.11–1.74; p=0.0045). During hospital stay, significantly more strokes (1.8% [15 of 829] vs 0, p<0.0001), but not major non-cerebral bleeding complications (6% [46 of 829] vs 4% [37 of 838], p=0.3118), were reported in patients assigned facilitated rather than standard PCI. We also noted more ischaemic cardiac complications, such as reinfarction (6% [49 of 805] vs 4% [30 of 820], p=0.0279) or repeat target vessel revascularisation (7% [53 of 805] vs 3% [28 of 818], p=0.0041) within 90 days in this study group.

*Interpretation.*—A strategy of full-dose tenecteplase with antithrombotic co-therapy, as used in this study and preceding PCI by 1–3 h, was associated with more major adverse events than PCI alone in STEMI and cannot be recommended (Figure).

► The results of this trial have been eagerly awaited, and the increase in adverse events in patients undergoing facilitated angioplasty with full-dose tenecteplase is somewhat of a disappointment, and in some quarters probably came as a surprise. Potential explanations include the prespecified lack of heparin use so as to minimize the risks of bleeding, a higher rate of stroke (not unexpectedly), and the relatively short time to primary percutaneous coronary intervention (PPCI). In addition, fibrinolytic drugs were given relatively late after symptom onset—at a time when recanalization of the infarct-related artery by fibrinolytic drugs alone is attenuated.

A recent meta-analysis in the same issue of the journal of 17 trials of facilitated angioplasty demonstrated no benefit over PPCI in the management of ST-segment elevation acute myocardial infarction.[1] Thus facilitation with full-dose fibrinolytic therapy is associated with an increase in adverse events and should be avoided. In trials that included IIb/IIIa platelet inhibitors alone or platelet inhibitor drugs in combination with low-dose lytics, the results have been neutral but with no suggestion of a benefit.

The accompanying editorial by Stone and Gersh points out that in routine clinical practice times to treatment are such that facilitation is likely to exert its impact on the "flat" part of the curve during which the benefits of earlier opening of the infarct-related artery are likely to be small.[2] This is illustrated in the accompanying figure that is based on a hypothetical construct, but the superimposition of times to treatment on the basis of large registry studies in the United States emphasize the relatively time-independent situation once the patient is on the "flat" part of the slope of the curve.[3]

Currently, I would recommend that patients who present within 2 to 3 hours of symptom onset with a large myocardial infarction in which a significant transfer delay for angioplasty is anticipated should still receive fibrinolytic therapy in the presenting community hospital. For patients presenting after 3 hours who are on the flat part of the curve, probably the best therapy is immediate transfer for PPCI preceded by aspirin, a clopidogrel loading dose, intravenous β-blockade in the absence of contraindications, and probably unfractionated heparin, although there is little evidence to support the latter. Such decisions, however, need to be modified by clinical common sense, such as the risk of bleeding from fibrinolytics, a realistic appreciation of the anticipated delay, and the hemodynamic stability of the patient.

B. J. Gersh, MB, ChB, DPhil, FRCP

*References*

1. Keeley EC, Bourn JA, Grines CL: Comparison of primary and facilitated percutaneous coronary interventions for ST-elevation myocardial infarction: Quantitative review of randomized trials. *Lancet* 367:579-588, 2006.
2. Stone GW, Gersh BJ: Facilitated angioplasty: Paradise lost. *Lancet* 367:543-546, 2006.
3. Gersh BJ, Stone GW, White HD, et al: Pharmacological facilitation of primary percutaneous coronary intervention for acute myocardial infarction: Is the slope of the curve the shape of the future? *JAMA* 293:979-986, 2005.

### Rescue Angioplasty after Failed Thrombolytic Therapy for Acute Myocardial Infarction

Gershlick AH, for the REACT Trial Investigators (Univ Hospitals of Leicester, England; et al)

*N Engl J Med* 353:2758-2768, 2005                                                          4–4

*Background.*—The appropriate treatment for patients in whom reperfusion fails to occur after thrombolytic therapy for acute myocardial infarction remains unclear. There are few data comparing emergency percutaneous coronary intervention (rescue PCI) with conservative care in such patients, and none comparing rescue PCI with repeated thrombolysis.

*Methods.*—We conducted a multicenter trial in the United Kingdom involving 427 patients with ST-segment elevation myocardial infarction in whom reperfusion failed to occur (less than 50 percent ST-segment resolution) within 90 minutes after thrombolytic treatment. The patients were randomly assigned to repeated thrombolysis (142 patients), conservative treatment (141 patients), or rescue PCI (144 patients). The primary end point was a composite of death, reinfarction, stroke, or severe heart failure within six months.

*Results.*—The rate of event-free survival among patients treated with rescue PCI was 84.6 percent, as compared with 70.1 percent among those receiving conservative therapy and 68.7 percent among those undergoing repeated thrombolysis (overall P=0.004). The adjusted hazard ratio for the occurrence of the primary end point for repeated thrombolysis versus conservative therapy was 1.09 (95 percent confidence interval, 0.71 to 1.67; P=0.69), as compared with adjusted hazard ratios of 0.43 (95 percent confidence interval, 0.26 to 0.72; P=0.001) for rescue PCI versus repeated thrombolysis and 0.47 (95 percent confidence interval, 0.28 to 0.79;

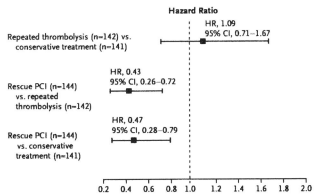

FIGURE 2.—Adjusted Hazard Ratios for the Occurrence of the Composite Primary End Point (Death, Recurrent Myocardial Infarction, Severe Heart Failure, or Cerebrovascular Accident) among the Trial Groups. HR denotes hazard ratio, CI confidence interval, and PCI percutaneous coronary intervention. (Reprinted by permission of *The New England Journal of Medicine* from Gershlick AH, for the REACT Trial Investigators: Rescue angioplasty after failed thrombolytic therapy for acute myocardial infarction. *N Engl J Med* 353:2758-2768, 2005. Copyright © 2005, Massachusetts Medical Society. All rights reserved.)

P=0.004) for rescue PCI versus conservative therapy. There were no significant differences in mortality from all causes. Nonfatal bleeding, mostly at the sheath-insertion site, was more common with rescue PCI. At six months, 86.2 percent of the rescue-PCI group were free from revascularization, as compared with 77.6 percent of the conservative-therapy group and 74.4 percent of the repeated-thrombolysis group (overall P=0.05).

*Conclusions.*—Event-free survival after failed thrombolytic therapy was significantly higher with rescue PCI than with repeated thrombolysis or conservative treatment. Rescue PCI should be considered for patients in whom reperfusion fails to occur after thrombolytic therapy (Fig 2).

▶ Rescue angioplasty after failed percutaneous coronary intervention (PCI) is a logical concept that has been around for a considerable period of time. Because in approximately 40% of patients receiving thrombolytics TIMI grade 3 flow is not achieved, the potential for "rescue" by transferring for PCI is an important issue, but clinical trial proof has been somewhat elusive. This trial was terminated prematurely because of declining enrollment and funding constraints. Fortunately however, sufficient patients were enrolled so as to provide some persuasive answers. Rescue PCI is better than repeat thrombolysis or conservative management for patients in whom fibrinolytic drugs appear to have failed.

Virtually every prior trial has struggled with enrollment.[1] This may be in part related to connotations implicit in the word "rescue," which may well have contributed to concerns about not referring such patients to catheterization labs in centers with the available facilities.

For" rescue" PCI to achieve its full potential, referrals need to be prompt. It is often difficult to assess the efficacy of thrombolytics on the basis of clinical findings alone, but far too many "thrombolytic failures" are recognized as the result of hemodynamic complications and at a time when the benefits of mechanical refusion may be diminished. The decision to refer for "rescue" should be made at about 60 to 90 minutes after the administration of thrombolytic therapy and the persistence of symptoms or failure of ST-segment resolution on the electrocardiogram are strong indications for prompt referral.[2]

Another increasingly used approach is to transfer all patients after thrombolysis to a referral hospital for further assessment and either rescue PCI or deferred "elective" angiography, depending on the clinical situation. This may work in some regions but not in others and costs may be an issue, but the approach is certainly a logical one and perhaps the most effective.

**B. J. Gersh, MB, ChB, DPhil, FRCP**

*References*

1. Ellis SG, da Silva ER, Spaulding CM, et al: Review of immediate angioplasty after fibrinolytic therapy for acute myocardial infarction: Insights from the RESCUE I, RESCUE II, and other contemporary clinical experiences. *Am Heart J* 139:1046-1053, 2000.

2. Zeymer U, Schroder R, Tebbe U, et al: Non-invasive detection of early infarct vessel patency by resolution of ST-segment elevation in patients with thrombolysis for acute myocardial infarction: Results of the angiographic substudy of the Hirudin for Improvement (HIT)-4 trial. *Eur Heart J* 22:768-775, 2001.

**Autologous bone marrow-derived stem-cell transfer in patients with ST-segment elevation myocardial infarction: double-blind, randomised controlled trial**

Janssens S, Dubois C, Bogaert J, et al (Univ of Leuven, Belgium; Stem Cell Inst, Leuven, Belgium)
*Lancet* 367:113-121, 2006                                                          4–5

*Background.*—The benefit of reperfusion therapies for ST-elevation acute myocardial infarction (STEMI) is limited by post-infarction left-ventricular (LV) dysfunction. Our aim was to investigate the effect of autologous bone marrow-derived stem cell (BMSC) transfer in the infarct-related artery on LV function and structure.

*Methods.*—We did a randomised, double-blind, placebo-controlled study in 67 patients from whom we harvested bone marrow 1 day after successful percutaneous coronary intervention for STEMI. We assigned patients optimum medical treatment and infusion of placebo (n=34) or BMSC (n=33). Our primary endpoint was the increase in LV ejection fraction and our secondary endpoints were change in infarct size and regional LV function at 4 months' follow-up, all assessed by MRI. We assessed changes in myocardial perfusion and oxidative metabolism with serial 1-[$^{11}$C]acetate PET. Analyses were per protocol. This study is registered with clinicaltrials.gov, number NCT00264316.

*Findings.*—Mean global LV ejection fraction 4 days after percutaneous coronary intervention was 46.9% (SD 8.2) in controls and 48.5% (7.2) in

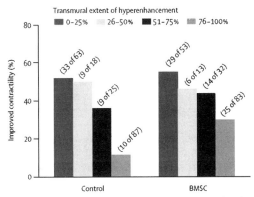

FIGURE 4.—Relation between transmural extent of hyperenhancement at baseline and the likelihood of increased contractility in all dysfunctional segments at months' follow-up. (Courtesy of Janssens S, Dubois C, Bogaert J, et al: Autologous bone marrow-derived stem-cell transfer in patients with ST-segment elevation myocardial infarction: double-blind, randomised controlled trial. *Lancet* 367, 113-121. Copyright 2006 Elsevier.)

BMSC patients, and increased after 4 months to 49.1% (10.7) and 51.8% (8.8; OR for treatment effect 1.036, 95% CI 0.961-1.118, p=0.36). Compared with placebo infusion, BMSC transfer was associated with a significant reduction in myocardial infarct size (BMSC treatment effect 28%, p=0.036) and a better recovery of regional systolic function. Myocardial perfusion and metabolism increased similarly in both groups. We noted no complications associated with BMSC transfer and all but one patient in the BMSC group completed the 4 months' follow-up.

*Interpretation.*—Intracoronary transfer of autologous bone marrow cells within 24 h of optimum reperfusion therapy does not augment recovery of global LV function after myocardial infarction, but could favourably affect infarct remodelling (Fig 4).

▶ This meticulously designed trial is the first published double-blind randomized controlled trial of stem cell transfer in patients with acute myocardial infarction, although data from another trial have been presented.

At first glance, the results are disappointing in that they demonstrate no change in overall ejection fraction nor in left ventricular remodeling. Nonetheless, over 4 months the treated group had a greater decline in infarct size, and among those segments with the greatest extent of transmurality, subsequent improvements in regional contractility were greater in the stem cell treatment group (see Fig 4).

This is an area of enormous excitement but it is also associated with a considerable degree of hype and unrealistic expectations. Small, carefully executed double-blind trials such as this one are exactly what is needed to move the field onward. There are a myriad of clinical questions that need to be answered: What is the best cellular phenotype? What dose? Methods of administration? Which patients, the timing of cell transfer and safety issues? The process of myocardial infarction is an evolving one and at each stage of the process homing signals and the local environment may change. If a specific cell works at one stage in the process, this does not necessarily guarantee efficacy at other times.

Perhaps the most important unresolved issues are the mechanisms of apparent benefits. Are these due to stem cell transdifferentiation, and even if this occurs, are the numbers of cell sufficient to account for the somewhat striking improvements in ventricular function noted in animal and early unblinded clinical studies?[1] It is becoming increasingly apparent that the process of cell transfer may result in the production of cytokines and other paracrine effects that could in themselves modify repair or regeneration or cellular protection.

This is an area in which clinicians and trialists need to work in tandem with basic scientists, perhaps in a consortial arrangement. The attraction of this form of therapy is intuitively obvious that the rigorous scrutiny of randomized controlled trials is sorely needed. The authors of this trial have taken an important first step.

**B. J. Gersh, MB, ChB, DPhil, FRCP**

*Reference*

1. Wollert KC, Drexler H: Clinical applications of stem cells for the heart. *Circ Res* 96:151-163, 2005.

**Stem Cell Mobilization Induced by Subcutaneous Granulocyte-Colony Stimulating Factor to Improve Cardiac Regeneration After Acute ST-Elevation Myocardial Infarction: Result of the Double-Blind, Randomized, Placebo-Controlled Stem Cells in Myocardial Infarction (STEMMI) Trial**

Ripa RS, Jørgensen E, Wang Y, et al (Univ Hosp Rigshospitalet, Copenhagen; Univ Hosp Hvidovre, Denmark; Aalborg Univ Hosp, Denmark)
*Circulation* 113:1983-1992, 2006                                                    4–6

*Background.*—Phase 1 clinical trials of granulocyte-colony stimulating factor (G-CSF) treatment after myocardial infarction have indicated that G-CSF treatment is safe and may improve left ventricular function. This randomized, double-blind, placebo-controlled trial aimed to assess the efficacy of subcutaneous G-CSF injections on left ventricular function in patients with ST-elevation myocardial infarction.

*Method and Results.*—Seventy-eight patients (62 men; average age, 56 years) with ST-elevation myocardial infarction were included after successful primary percutaneous coronary stent intervention <12 hours after symptom onset. Patients were randomized to double-blind treatment with G-CSF (10 µg/kg of body weight) or placebo for 6 days. The primary end point was change in systolic wall thickening from baseline to 6 months determined by cardiac magnetic resonance imaging (MRI). An independent core laboratory analyzed all MRI examinations. Systolic wall thickening improved 17% in the infarct area in the G-CSF group and 17% in the placebo group ($P=1.0$). Comparable results were found in infarct border and noninfarcted myocardium. Left ventricular ejection fraction improved similarly in the 2 groups measured by both MRI (8.5 versus 8.0; $P=0.9$) and echocardiography (5.7 versus 3.7; $P=0.7$). The risk of severe clinical adverse events was not increased by G-CSF. In addition, in-stent late lumen loss and target vessel revascularization rate in the follow-up period were similar in the 2 groups.

*Conclusions.*—Bone marrow stem cell mobilization with subcutaneous G-CSF is safe but did not lead to further improvement in ventricular function after acute myocardial infarction compared with the recovery observed in the placebo group.

▶ This is one of 2 randomized, double-blind, placebo-controlled trials that probably signals the end of subcutaneous G-CSF as sole therapy for acute myocardial infarction.[1] This comes as a disappointment given the encouraging results from an earlier study, which, however, did not include a control population.[2] As has been the case with other modalities of sole repair therapy in acute myocardial infarction, randomization and double-blinding have resulted in a number of recent trials that have been neutral, and introduce a healthy dose of reality into an area brimming with great expectations. Since left ventricular function frequently improves spontaneously after successful revascularization in acute myocardial infarction, a control group and double-blinding are essential components with any study.

An accompanying editorial points out that G-CSF could still find a place as adjunct to therapy for peripheral blood cell mobilization and harvesting for the purposes of ex vivo manipulation and direct delivery.[3]

Cell repair therapy is an intuitively attractive therapeutic option, and there is certainly a compelling clinical need. Nonetheless, enormous hurdles need to be overcome before cell repair therapy becomes a clinical reality. The basic mechanisms of potential benefit, whether due to sole regeneration or paracrine effects, remain a source of vigorous debate. What cells, the timing and site of administration, the optimal dose, the method of delivery, and to which patients are still critical questions waiting for answers.[4] For this field to progress, basic scientists, clinical cardiologists, and the trialists need to work in tandem.

**B. J. Gersh, MB, ChB, DPhil, FRCP**

*References*

1. Zohlnhofer D, Ott I, Mehilli J, et al: Stem cell mobilization by granulocyte colony-stimulating factor in patients with acute myocardial infarction: A randomized controlled trial. *JAMA* 295:1003-1010, 2006.
2. Ince HP, Petzch M, Kleine HD, et al: Preservation from left ventricular remodeling by front-integrated revascularization and stem cell liberation in evolving acute myocardial infarction by use of granulocyte colony-stimulating factor (FIRSTLINE-AMR). *Circulation* 112:3097-3106, 2005.
3. Hill JM, Bartunek J: The end of granulocyte colony-stimulating factor in acute myocardial infarction? Reaping the benefits beyond cytokine mobilization. *Circulation* 113:1926-1928, 2006.
4. Gersh BJ, Simari RD: Cardiac-cell repair therapy: Clinical issues. *Nat Clin Pract Cardiovasc Med* 3:S105-S109, 2006.

---

### Implementation of Guidelines Improves the Standard of Care: The Viennese Registry on Reperfusion Strategies in ST-Elevation Myocardial Infarction (Vienna STEMI Registry)

Huber K, for the Vienna STEMI Registry Group (Wilhelminenhospital, Vienna; et al)

*Circulation* 113:2398-2405, 2006                                                       4–7

---

*Background.*—The purpose of this study was to determine whether implementation of recent guidelines improves in-hospital mortality from acute ST-elevation myocardial infarction (STEMI) in a metropolitan area.

*Method and Results.*—We organized a network that consisted of the Viennese Ambulance Systems, which is responsible for diagnosis and triage of patients with acute STEMI, and 5 high-volume interventional cardiology departments to expand the performance of primary percutaneous catheter intervention (PPCI) and to use the fastest available reperfusion strategy in STEMI of short duration (2 to 3 hours from onset of symptoms), either PPCI or thrombolytic therapy (TT; prehospital or in-hospital), respectively. Implementation of guidelines resulted in increased numbers of patients receiving 1 of the 2 reperfusion strategies (from 66% to 86.6%). Accordingly, the proportion of patients not receiving reperfusion therapy dropped from 34% to 13.4%, respectively. PPCI usage increased from 16% to almost 60%, whereas the use of TT decreased from 50.5% to 26.7% in the participating centers. As a consequence, in-hospital mortality decreased from 16% before establishment of the network to 9.5%, including patients not receiving reperfusion therapy. Whereas PPCI and TT demonstrated comparable in-hospital mortality rates when initiated within 2 to 3 hours from onset of symptoms, PPCI was more effective in acute STEMI of >3 but <12 hours' duration.

*Conclusions.*—Implementation of recent guidelines for the treatment of acute STEMI by the organization of a cooperating network within a large metropolitan area was associated with a significant improvement in clinical outcomes.

▶ This is a rather gratifying article that shows what can be achieved in the field of reperfusion therapy by developing a city-wide network of central triage. The participants in this network in Vienna, Austria, were able to make radical changes to the system between 2002 and 2004, resulting in improvements in the delivery of care on multiple fronts. The proportion of patients not receiving any reperfusion therapy decreased from approximately 30% to 13.4%, the use of fibrinolytic drugs declined, and the use of PPCI increased substantially. Over the years during which the system was activated, the investigators found that the implementation of guidelines for early reperfusion therapy of acute STEMI was substantially increased, resulting in a decrease in mortality, though one has to remember that this is a registry study and not a randomized trial. Nonetheless, the apparent decline in mortality is impressive.

What is interesting is the comparison of in-hospital mortality rates stratified by the nature of the therapy and the duration of ischemia. This makes sense given the slope of the curve describing the relationship between the duration of ischemia, mortality reduction, and the extent of salvage after reperfusion therapy.[1] In the first 2 to 3 hours, there is a narrow window of substantial opportunity. At this juncture, time to treatment is critical, and delays incurred by transfer for PPCI may have an adverse effect. Subsequently on the "flat" part of the curve, time dependence is less of an issue, and the major objective is to open the infarct-related artery. In this setting, PPCI will be superior to lytics. In the Viennese experience, the mortality in the first 2 hours was actually slightly lower with TT, followed by a clear and increasing advantage for PPCI with longer periods of ischemia before reperfusion. This is entirely consistent with what one would expect from the "slope of the curve."

In regard to the current era of reperfusion therapy, we know what to do—it is now a matter of logistics, as stated in the accompanying editorial by Dr Verheugt.[2] Nonetheless, the logistical constraints are highly variable depending upon country, region, systems of health care delivery, distance, and weather, to name but a few of the factors. It is not just the nature of the therapy that is important but the efficacy of its delivery.

**B. J. Gersh, MB, ChB, DPhil, FRCP**

*References*

1. Gersh BJ, Stone GW, White HD, et al: Pharmacological facilitation of primary percutaneous coronary intervention for acute myocardial infarction: Is the slope of the curve the shape of the future? *JAMA* 293:979-986, 2005.
2. Verheugt FWA: Reperfusion therapy starts in the ambulance (editorial). *Circulation* 113:2377-2379, 2006.

---

**Intracoronary Bone Marrow Cell Transfer After Myocardial Infarction: Eighteen Months' Follow-Up Data From the Randomized, Controlled BOOST (BOne marrOw transfer to enhance ST-elevation infarct regeneration) Trial**
Meyer GP, Wollert KC, Lotz J, et al (Hannover Med School, Germany)
*Circulation* 113:1287-1294, 2006                                          4–8

---

*Background.*—Intracoronary transfer of autologous bone marrow cells (BMCs) may enhance recovery of left ventricular (LV) function in patients after acute myocardial infarction (AMI). However, clinical studies addressing the effects of BMCs after AMI have covered only limited time frames ranging from 3 to 6 months. The critical question of whether BMC transfer can have a sustained impact on LV function remains unanswered.

*Method and Results.*—After percutaneous coronary intervention with stent implantation (PCI) of the infarct-related artery, 60 patients were randomized 1:1 to a control group with optimal postinfarction therapy and a BMC transfer group that also received an intracoronary BMC infusion 4.8±1.3 days after PCI. Cardiac MRI was performed 3.5±1.5 days, 6±1 months, and 18±6 months after PCI. BMC transfer was not associated with adverse clinical events. In the control group, mean global LV ejection fraction increased by 0.7 and 3.1 percentage points after 6 and 18 months, respectively. LV ejection fraction in the BMC transfer group increased by 6.7 and 5.9 percentage points. The difference in LVEF improvement between groups was significant after 6 months but not after 18 months ($P=0.27$). The speed of LV ejection fraction recovery over the course of 18 months was significantly higher in the BMC transfer group ($P=0.001$).

*Conclusions.*—In this study, a single dose of intracoronary BMCs did not provide long-term benefit on LV systolic function after AMI compared with a randomized control group; however, the study suggests an acceleration of LV ejection fraction recovery after AMI by BMC therapy.

▶ The 6-month results of this trial of the intracoronary infusion of autologous BMCs within 5 days after successful stenting in patients with ST-elevation AMI demonstrated a significant improvement in regional LV function and global LV ejection fraction at 6 months.[1] The current analysis of the 18-month follow-up provides further support for the safety of the procedure, as their was no excess in adverse clinical events. Nonetheless, these results strongly suggest that a single dose of BMCs is unlikely to promote sustained improvement in LV function. Some of the lack of apparent benefit may be due to spontaneous improvements in LV function in the control group as a result of successful PCI and long-term pharmacologic therapy.

This and other studies raise many questions about the clinical efficacy of this increasingly exciting field. Is the initial improvement in LV function a paracrine effect without any accompanying regenerative process?[2] Which patients may need a second infusion of cells? What type of cells and in what number? What is the optimal site and method of delivery, and to which patient and at what time after myocardial infarction? These are all leading questions that will take time to be answered.

I do not feel that this is the time to be performing large-scale trials with death and congestive heart failure as an end point. Nonetheless, many of the basic scientific questions about cell repair therapy may not be answered for years or decades. From this perspective, relatively small, focused clinical trials such as the one featured in this article, can play an important role as we try and translate from the bench to the bedside. Close collaboration between basic scientists and the clinical community is essential if we are to move forward.[3]

**B. J. Gersh, MB, ChB, DPhil, FRCP**

*References*

1. Wollert KC, Mayer GP, Lotz J, et al: Intracoronary autologous bone-marrow cell transfer after myocardial infraction: The BOOST randomized, controlled, clinical trial. *Lancet* 364:1411-1418, 2004.
2. Gersh BJ, Simari RD: Cardiac-cell repair therapy; Clinical issues and the nature of clinical practice. *Cardiovasc Med* 3:S1-S6, 2006.
3. Welt FGP, Losordo W: Cell therapy for acute myocardial infarction: Curb your enthusiasm? *Circulation* 113:1272-1274, 2006.

---

**Routine Thrombectomy in Percutaneous Coronary Intervention for Acute ST-Segment–Elevation Myocardial Infarction: A Randomized, Controlled Trial**

Kaltoft A, Bøttcher M, Nielsen SS, et al (Aarhus Univ Hosp, Skejby, Denmark; Aarhus Univ Hosp, Aalborg, Denmark)
*Circulation* 114:40-47, 2006                                    4–9

---

*Background.*—Distal embolization during primary percutaneous coronary intervention (PCI) for ST-elevation myocardial infarction may result in reduced myocardial perfusion, infarct extension, and impaired prognosis.

*Method and Results.*—In a prospective randomized trial, we studied the effect of routine thrombectomy in 215 patients with ST-segment-elevation myocardial infarction lasting <12 hours undergoing primary PCI. Patients were randomized to thrombectomy pretreatment or standard PCI. The primary end point was myocardial salvage measured by sestamibi SPECT, calculated as the difference between area at risk and final infarct size determined after 30 days (percent). Secondary end points included final infarct size, ST-segment resolution, and troponin T release. Baseline variables, including ST-segment elevation and area at risk, were similar. Salvage was not statistically different in the thrombectomy and control groups (median, 13% [interquartile range, 9% to 21%] and 18% [interquartile range, 7% to 25%]; $P=0.12$), but 24 patients in the thrombectomy group and 12 patients in the control group did not have an early SPECT scan, mainly because of poor general or cardiac condition ($P=0.04$). In the thrombectomy group, final infarct size was increased (median, 15%; [interquartile range, 4% to 25%] versus 8% [interquartile range, 2% to 18%]; $P=0.004$).

*Conclusions.*—Thrombectomy performed as routine therapy in primary PCI for ST-elevation myocardial infarction does not increase myocardial salvage. The study suggests a possible deleterious effect of thrombectomy, resulting in an increased final infarct size, and does not support the use of thrombectomy in unselected primary PCI patients.

▶ Despite great success in the achievement of TIMI grade III flow in the infarct-related artery, particularly with primary percutaneous coronary intervention, optimal myocardial perfusion remains an elusive goal and one of the major unconquered frontiers of reperfusion therapy. Myocardial perfusion can be assessed by a variety of techniques, with ST-segment resolution and myocardial blush grade being probably the 2 most frequently utilized. Irrespective of the method, there appears to be a strong correlation with myocardial malperfusion and mortality.[1]

In the animal model, multiple pharmacologic agents have shown to be effective, leading to a large agenda of clinical trials and very disappointing results. No trial of pharmacologic therapy has achieved its primary end point, although strategies including cooling, aqueous oxygen, adenosine, and nicorandil show some promise. The failure of the pharmacologic approach then set the stage for mechanical strategies, with great interest focused on distal protection to prevent the embolization of atherosclerotic debris. The largest trial published so far in this area was emphatically negative, as have been other smaller trials.[2]

This randomized trial from Denmark strongly suggests that thrombectomy performed as routine therapy does not increase myocardial salvage and may be deleterious. It is a familiar refrain akin to "another one bites the dust." So, it is back to the drawing board. Perhaps one major difference between experimental models and the clinical situation is the lack of underlying atherosclerosis and inflammation in the animal. Could it be that the microvascular dysfunction caused by atherosclerosis and inflammation is preexisting and antedates the processes of achieving reperfusion of the epicardial infarct-related artery? Could it be that all that we do is too late to achieve optimal myocardial perfusion? In that event, if we were able to treat patients at the very onset of myocardial infarction, would we ever be able to demonstrate a difference, since in this setting mortality is extremely low and infarct size is minimal? This has certainly been a difficult area in which to demonstrate progress, and it will likely continue as an area of challenge but also frustration.

**B. J. Gersh, MB, ChB, DPhil, FRCP**

*References*

1. Sorajja P, Gersh BJ, Costantini C, et al: Combined prognostic utility of ST-Segment recovery and myocardial blush after primary percutaneous coronary intervention in acute myocardial infarction. *Eur Heart J* 26:667-674, 2005.
2. Stone GW, Webb, J, Cox DA, et al: Distal microcirculatory protection during percutaneous coronary intervention in acute ST-segment elevation myocardial infarction: A randomized controlled trial. *JAMA* 239:1063-1072, 2005.

**Intracoronary Bone Marrow–Derived Progenitor Cells in Acute Myocardial Infarction**
Schächinger V, for the REPAIR-AMI Investigators (Johann Wolfgang Goethe Univ, Frankfurt, Germany; et al)
*N Engl J Med* 355:1210-1221, 2006                                                   4–10

*Background.*—Pilot trials suggest that the intracoronary administration of autologous progenitor cells may improve left ventricular function after acute myocardial infarction.

*Methods.*—In a multicenter trial, we randomly assigned 204 patients with acute myocardial infarction to receive an intracoronary infusion of progenitor cells derived from bone marrow (BMC) or placebo medium into the infarct artery 3 to 7 days after successful reperfusion therapy.

*Results.*—At 4 months, the absolute improvement in the global left ventricular ejection fraction (LVEF) was significantly greater in the BMC group than in the placebo group (mean [±SD] increase, 5.5±7.3% vs. 3.0±6.5%; $P=0.01$). Patients with a baseline LVEF at or below the median value of 48.9% derived the most benefit (absolute improvement in LVEF, 5.0%; 95% confidence interval, 2.0 to 8.1). At 1 year, intracoronary infusion of BMC was associated with a reduction in the prespecified combined clinical end point of death, recurrence of myocardial infarction, and any revascularization procedure ($P=0.01$).

*Conclusions.*—Intracoronary administration of BMC is associated with improved recovery of left ventricular contractile function in patients with acute myocardial infarction. Large-scale studies are warranted to examine the potential effects of progenitor-cell administration on morbidity and mortality (Fig 3).

▶ It is not surprising that the tantalizing prospect of regenerating necrotic myocardium by the administration of stem cells has generated extraordinary excitement. There is a compelling clinical need, preclinical studies have been positive, and the concept is intuitively appealing.

A major unresolved question hinges on the mechanisms of benefit, since there is little evidence that adult stem cells can dedifferentiate into cardiac myocytes and, if so, whether they can in meaningful numbers. The weight of opinion is shifting toward a paracrine effect, which results in the secretion of cytokines or growth factors that may promote cardiac myocyte survival, repair, regeneration, or angiogenesis.

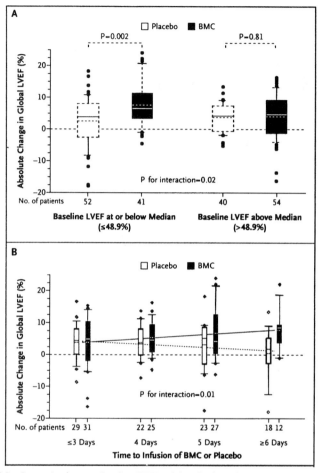

FIGURE 3.—Interaction between Baseline LVEF and the Absolute Change in LVEF (Panel A) and between the Timing of Intracoronary Infusion of BMC or Placebo after Reperfusion Therapy and the Absolute
Change in LVEF (Panel B). In Panel A, the P values for interaction was determined by analysis of variance. In
both panels, the upper and lower edges of each box plot indicate the 25th and 75th percentiles, the "whis-
kers" the 10th and 90th percentiles, the solid horizontal line the median, and the dotted line the mean. All
outliers are shown as individual data points. In Panel B, the P value for interaction was calculated with the use
of a general linear model. The solid line in Panel B shows the regression curve for the BMC group, and the
dotted line shows the regression curve for the placebo group. (Reprinted by permission of *The New England
Journal of Medicine* from Schächinger V, for the REPAIR-AMI Investigators: Intracoronary bone marrow–
derived progenitor cells in acute myocardial infarction. *N Engl J Med* 355:1210-1221, 2006. Copyright 2006
Massachusetts Medical Society. All rights reserved.)

Given these fundamental unresolved issues, are clinical trials premature?
Although some argue that this is the case, I personally believe that well-
designed focus studies can help answer the multiplicity of questions arising
from animal studies, but only if these are performed in collaboration with basic
science. After all, drugs such as aspirin and aldosterone antagonists were subjected to clinical trials long before we really understood their mechanisms of

benefits. Nonetheless, I agree that it is premature to design large trials with mortality in congestive heart failure end points.

The REPAIR-AMI Trial is encouraging in regard to the improvements in LVEF and the trend toward a reduction in clinical events. Nonetheless, we need to realize that other well-designed, randomized, controlled trials with intracoronary bone marrow cells have been negative, including those trials that utilized the most sophisticated approaches to measuring left ventricular function.[1,2] There are many burning questions to be answered. Are the small changes in left ventricular function clinically relevant? Which cells, in what number, in which patients, and when? What are the best methods and sites of delivery? What will be the clinical impact both early and late? What are the mechanisms of benefit?

The hype should not disguise the major technological strides being made in stem cell research. Well-designed clinical trials have their role to play, but we need to be cautious about unrealistic expectations. Stem cell therapy is not a clinical tool, and the unanswered question is whether it will be so in the future. It remains an exciting and fascinating area of research in which well-designed clinical trials will play their part.

**B. J. Gersh, MB, ChB, DPhil, FRCP**

*References*

1. Lunde K, Solheim S, Aakhus S, et al: Intracoronary injection of mononuclear bone marrow cells in acute myocardial infarction. *N Engl J Med* 355:1199-1209, 2006.
2. Janssens S, Dubois C, Bogaert J, et al: Autologous bone marrow-derived stem cell transfer in patients with ST-segment elevation myocardial infarction: Double-blind randomized control trial. *Lancet* 367:113-121, 2006.

---

**Broken bodies, broken hearts? Limitations of the trauma system as a model for regionalizing care for ST-Elevation Myocardial Infarction in the United States**

Nallamothu BK, Taheri PA, Barsan WG, et al (VA Med Ctr, Ann Arbor, Mich; Univ of Michigan Med School, Ann Arbor)
*Am Heart J* 152:613-618, 2006

4–11

Many cardiovascular experts have called for the creation of specialized myocardial infarction centers and networks in the United States analogous to the current model for major trauma. Patients suffering ST-elevation myocardial infarction (STEMI) and trauma share an essential feature that makes the argument for regionalization persuasive: rapid triage and treatment by highly trained personnel improve survival in both conditions. Despite this similarity, however, the trauma system may be limited as a model for regionalizing STEMI care. First, the development of trauma systems has been hindered by the struggle for sufficient and stable funding, competing interests among individual stakeholders, and the overall lack of desire for state-sponsored healthcare planning in the United States. These same obstacles would need to be overcome if STEMI care is regionalized. Second, unique characteristics related to STEMI care, such as its varied clinical presentation and more lucrative reimbursement, will create new challenges. In this article, we briefly review the current status of trauma systems in the United States and describe why the regionalization of STEMI care may require different methods of healthcare organization.

▶ At first glance, a strong case can be made for the regionalization of STEMI care and the establishment of myocardial infarction centers analogous to the development of trauma centers.[1] These could maximize the utilization of technology for primary percutaneous coronary intervention, potentially improve institutional and operative volumes, and be more amenable to quality improvement initiatives. In some parts of the world in which health care is administered at a national level, implementation of such as policy will be much easier than in the environment currently existing in the United States.

In this excellent review by Nallamothu et al, the challenges, diagnostic, and economic implications of regionalizing care for STEMI in the United States are discussed. Similar concerns apply to the regionalization of care for all forms of acute coronary syndromes.[2] Unlike trauma centers, which are often costly, the care of myocardial infarction may be a source of profit for an institution; in our competitive environment, this will be an issue. For a myocardial infarction center to succeed, this will require very close collaboration between cardiologists and emergency medical services. The possibility that large numbers of patients without ST-elevation myocardial infarction could end up being transferred to myocardial infarction centers is another cause for concern. In addition, whereas trauma is centered around densely populated areas, the distribution of myocardial infarction is diffuse, incorporating many rural communities. Finally, although primary percutaneous coronary intervention may be the optimal reperfusion strategy, in many situations, fibrinolytic drugs are highly effective. This is an interesting area of providing opportunities to improve patient outcomes but also challenges in the regard to implementation of such centers.

**B. J. Gersh, MB, ChB, DPhil, FRCP**

*References*

1. Weaver WD: All hospitals are not equal for treatment of patients with acute myocardial infarction. *Circulation* 108:1809-1814, 2003.
2. Rathore SS, Epstein AJ, Volpp, K, et al: Regionalization of care for acute coronary syndromes: More evidence is needed. *JAMA* 293:1383-1387, 2005.

### Long-term Outcome of Primary Percutaneous Coronary Intervention vs Prehospital and In-Hospital Thrombolysis for Patients With ST-Elevation Myocardial Infarction

Stenestrand U, for the RIKS-HIA Registry (Univ Hosp, Linköpking, Sweden; Uppsala Univ, Sweden)
*JAMA* 296:1749-1756, 2006                                                4–12

*Context.*—Whether the superior results of percutaneous coronary intervention (PCI) reported in clinical trials in which patients with ST-segment elevation myocardial infarction (STEMI) received reperfusion treatment can be replicated in daily practice has been questioned, especially whether it is superior to prehospital thrombolysis (PHT).

*Objective.*—To evaluate the outcome of different reperfusion strategies in consecutive STEMI patients.

*Design, Setting, and Patients.*—A prospective observational cohort study of 26 205 consecutive STEMI patients in the Register of Information and Knowledge about Swedish Heart Intensive Care Admissions (RIKS-HIA) who received reperfusion therapy within 15 hours of symptom onset. The registry includes more than 95% of all Swedish patients, of all ages, who were treated in a coronary intensive care unit between 1999 and 2004.

*Interventions.*—Seven thousand eighty-four patients underwent primary PCI; 3078, PHT; and 16 043, in-hospital thrombolysis (IHT).

*Main Outcome Measures.*—Mortality, reinfarction, and readmissions as reported in the National Health Registries through December 31, 2005.

*Results.*—After adjusting for younger age and less comorbidity, primary PCI was associated with lower mortality than IHT at 30 days (344 [4.9%] vs 1834 [11.4%]; hazard ratio [HR], 0.61; 95% confidence interval [CI], 0.53-0.71) and at 1 year (541 [7.6%] vs 2555 [15.9%]; HR, 0.68; 95% CI, 0.60-0.76). Also primary PCI correlated with lower mortality than PHT at 30 days (344 [4.9%] vs 234 [7.6%]; HR, 0.70; 95% CI, 0.58-0.85) and 1 year (541 [7.6%] vs 317 [10.3%]; HR, 0.81; 95% CI, 0.69-0.94). Prehospital thrombolysis predicted a lower mortality than IHT at 30 days (HR, 0.87; 95% CI, 0.76-1.01) and at 1 year (HR, 0.84; CI 0.74-0.95). Beyond 2 hours' treatment delay, the observed mortality reductions with PHT tended to decrease while the benefits with primary PCI seemed to remain regardless of time delay. Primary PCI was also associated with shorter hospital stay and less reinfarction than either PHT or IHT.

*Conclusions.*—In unselected patients with STEMI, primary PCI, which compared favorably with IHT and PHT, was associated with reduced duration of hospital stay, readmission, reinfarction, and mortality.

▶ This is an important report describing the results of different reperfusion strategies in a large nationwide database from Sweden. The results are somewhat surprising given prior (albeit, much smaller) studies emphasizing the benefits of very early reperfusion, including PHT.[1,2] An integral aspect of such a strategy is a low threshold for rescue PCI and early angiography, suggesting that the administration of lytics should be followed by transfer to a center with cardiac catheterization facilities.

The data from this large set registry will add fuel to the debate over the establishment of specialized myocardial infarction centers analogous of trauma centers. Whereas this may be feasible in Sweden, such an approach is unlikely to be widely accepted in the United States for multiple reasons.[3] The fact is that for most countries, resource constraints, availability, access, and the logistics of patient transfer will result in many patients who can receive primary percutaneous coronary intervention, particularly within the 19-minute window recommended by the current guidelines.

One problem with this registry study is the marked baseline differences between treatment groups, which may have favored the approach of primary PCI. Propensity analyses can adjust to some extent the differences in measured baseline variables but cannot eliminate these or account for unmeasured variables that can exert a substantial impact on prognosis. Indeed a prior study from this Registry implied a magnitude of benefit from statins way beyond that seen from the randomized controlled trial.

To my mind, within the first 2 to 3 hours of an acute STEMI, time to treatment is critical and for many patients in community hospitals without cardiac catheterization facilities, fibrinolytics followed by transfer to a catheterization-capable facility is the optimal therapy.[4] Later, after symptom onset, time is less of a critical factor and transfer for PCI without preceding lytics is preferred. This recipe or algorithm needs a healthy garnish of common sense, including an assessment of bleeding risk, transport delays, and so forth, but it is consistent with current guidelines. In hospitals with the requisite facilities, primary PCI is the preferred modality providing it can be performed well and expeditiously.

**B. J. Gersh, MB, ChB, DPhil, FRCP**

*References*

1. Steg PG, Bonnefoy E, Chabaud S, et al: Impact of time to treatment on mortality after prehospital fibrinolysis or primary angioplasty: Data from the CAPTIM Randomized Clinical Trial. *Circulation* 108:2851-2856, 2003.
2. Danchin N, Blanchard D, Steg PG, et al: Impact of prehospital thrombolysis for acute myocardial infarction on 1-year outcome: Results from the French Nationwide USIC 2006 Registry. *Circulation* 110:1909-1915, 2004.
3. Nallamothu BK, Taheri PA, Barsan WD, et al: Broken bodies, broken hearts? Limitations of the trauma system as a model for regionalizing care for ST-elevation myocardial infarction in the United States. *Am Heart J* 152:613-618, 2006.
4. Gersh BJ, Stone GW, White HD, Holmes DR Jr: Pharmacological facilitation of primary percutaneous coronary intervention for acute myocardial infarction: Is the slope of the curve the shape of the future? *JAMA* 293:979-986, 2005.

**A comparison of pharmacologic therapy with/without timely coronary intervention vs. primary percutaneous intervention early after ST-elevation myocardial infarction: the WEST (Which Early ST-elevation myocardial infarction Therapy) study**

Armstrong PW, and the WEST Steering Committee (Univ of Alberta Edmonton, Canada)

*Eur Heart J* 27:1530-1538, 2006                                         4–13

*Aims.*—Uncertainty exists as to which reperfusion strategy for ST-elevation myocardial infarction (MI) is optimal. We evaluated whether optimal pharmacologic therapy at the earliest point of care, emphasizing pre-hospital randomization and treatment was non-inferior to expeditious primary percutaneous coronary intervention (PCI).

*Method and Results.*—Which Early ST-elevation myocardial infarction Therapy (WEST) was a four-city Canadian, open-label, randomized, feasibility study of 304 STEMI patients (>4 mm ST-elevation/deviation) within 6 h of symptom onset, emphasizing pre-hospital ambulance treatment and participation of community and tertiary care centres. All received aspirin, subcutaneous enoxaparin (1 mg/kg), and were randomized to one of three groups: (A) tenecteplase (TNK) and usual care, (B) TNK and mandatory invasive study ≤24 h, including rescue PCI for reperfusion failure, and (C) primary PCI with 300 mg loading dose of clopidogrel. Time from symptom onset to treatment was rapid (to TNK for A = 113 and B = 130 min and for PCI in C = 176 min). The primary outcome, a composite of 30-day death, reinfarction, refractory ischaemia, congestive heart failure, cardiogenic shock, and major ventricular arrhythmia, was 25% (Group A), 24% (Group B), and 23% (Group C), respectively. However, there was a higher frequency of the combination of death and recurrent MI in Group A vs. Group C (13.0 vs. 4.0%, respectively, *P*-logrank = 0.021), yet no difference between Group B (6.7%, *P*-logrank = 0.378) and C.

*Conclusion.*—These data suggest that a contemporary pharmacologic regimen rapidly delivered, coupled with a strategy of regimented rescue and routine coronary intervention within 24 h of initial treatment, may not be different from timely expert PCI.

▶ This pilot study provides promising and needed data on the benefits of a pharmacoinvasive approach to reperfusion therapy. The latter is defined by fibrinolytic therapy followed by a mandatory invasive study of at least 2 hours, including protocol-specified rescue PCI. The major reasons why such data are welcome include recent evidence that the strategy of facilitated PCI is ineffective.[1] In addition, the time delays incurred in transporting patients presenting with STEMI in community hospitals without catheterization laboratories to tertiary care hospitals for primary PCI provide another incentive for alternative strategies.

The trend toward higher BNP levels and increased rates of congestive heart failure and shock in the PPCI group in this study may simply be a function of small numbers, although given the relatively short time to the administration of thrombolytic drugs, these findings are similar to those noted in the CAPTIM Trial and reinforce the benefits of early thrombolytic therapy within the first 2 hours of symptoms.[2]

These data also emphasize the benefits of a strategy of reperfusion therapy followed by transfer to a center with the facilities available for PCI as opposed to an ischemia-guided approach. Moreover, our heightened awareness of the benefits of rescue PCI and the need to perform this before the development of hemodynamic complications is another critical aspect of the pharmacoinvasive strategy.[3]

This is a pilot study, and a larger randomized trial is certainly warranted. In such a trial, it would be advisable for patients receiving fibrinolytic therapy to receive pretreatment with clopidogrel given the results of other recent trials. Nonetheless, these data suggest that an approach focusing on prehospital care and other methods that ensure the prompt and early administration of fibrinolytic therapy followed by timely and effective postfibrinolytic rescue strategies seems to be a very promising therapeutic option.

**B. J. Gersh, MB, ChB, DPhil, FRCP**

*References*

1. ASSENT-4 Investigators: Primary verses tenecteplase facilitated percutaneous coronary intervention in patients with ST-elevation acute myocardial infarction: The ASSSENT 4 PCI Randomized Trial. *Lancet* 367:569-578, 2006.
2. Tgonnefoy E, Chabaud S, et al: Impact of time to treat the mortality of after prehospital fibrinolysis or primary angioplasty: Data from the CAPTIM randomized clinical trial. *Circulation* 108:2851-2856, 2003.
3. Holmes DR Jr, Gersh BJ, Ellis SG: Rescue percutaneous coronary intervention after failed fibrinolytic therapy: Have expectations been met? *Am Heart J* 151:779-785, 2006.

---

### Effect of Door-to-Balloon Time on Mortality in Patients With ST-Segment Elevation Myocardial Infarction

McNamara RL, for the NRMI Investigators (Yale Univ, New Haven, Conn; et al)
*J Am Coll Cardiol* 47:2180-2186, 2006                                    4–14

---

*Objectives.*—We sought to determine the effect of door-to-balloon time on mortality for patients with ST-segment elevation myocardial infarction (STEMI) undergoing primary percutaneous coronary intervention (PCI).

*Background.*—Studies have found conflicting results regarding this relationship.

*Methods.*—We conducted a cohort study of 29,222 STEMI patients treated with PCI within 6 h of presentation at 395 hospitals that participated in the National Registry of Myocardial Infarction (NRMI)-3 and -4 from 1999 to 2002. We used hierarchical models to evaluate the effect of door-to-balloon time on in-hospital mortality adjusted for patient characteristics in the entire cohort and in different subgroups of patients based on symptom onset-to-door time and baseline risk status.

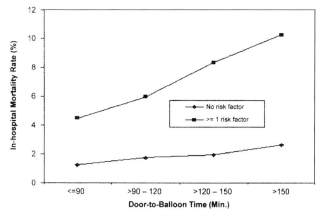

FIGURE 3.—In-hospital mortality and door-to-balloon time in patients stratified by risk factor status; p for trend < 0.001 for each line. Risk factors include anterior/septal location, diabetes mellitus, heart rate >100 beats/min, systolic blood pressure <100 mm Hg. (Courtesy of McNamara RL, for the NRMI Investigators: Effect of door-to-balloon time on mortality in patients with ST-segment elevation myocardial infarction. *J Am Coll Cardiol* 47:2180-2186. Copyright 2006 Elsevier.)

*Results.*—Longer door-to-balloon time was associated with increased in-hospital mortality (mortality rate of 3.0%, 4.2%, 5.7%, and 7.4% for door-to-balloon times of ≤90 min, 91 to 120 min, 121 to 150 min, and >150 min, respectively; p for trend <0.01) (Fig 3). Adjusted for patient characteristics, patients with door-to-balloon time >90 min had increased mortality (odds ratio 1.42; 95% confidence interval [CI] 1.24 to 1.62) compared with those who had door-to-balloon time ≤90 min. In subgroup analyses, increasing mortality with increasing door-to-balloon time was seen regardless of symptom onset-to-door time (≤1 h, >1 to 2 h, >2 h) and regardless of the presence or absence of high-risk factors.

*Conclusions.*—Time to primary PCI is strongly associated with mortality risk and is important regardless of time from symptom onset to presentation and regardless of baseline risk of mortality. Efforts to shorten door-to-balloon time should apply to all patients.

▶ The concept that "time is muscle" in regard to reperfusion therapy has been convincingly demonstrated by the correlations between mortality and time to drug administration in trials of fibrinolytic therapy.[1] In patients receiving primary PCI, the association, however, between door-to-balloon time (D-B) and mortality has been more controversial, with some studies suggesting no relationship at all and others implying that shorter D-B times may be beneficial, but only in patients at higher risk.[2,3]

This very large study from a United States database appears to settle the issue. Although there are a number of factors that are associated with D-B times, it would appear that this parameter is significantly and independently associated with mortality. One advantage of a study of this size is a wide distribution of an adequate number of patients in the various time periods under study. Smaller studies may have included relatively few patients with prolonged D-B times in excess of 90 minutes.

Shortening D-B times is an obvious target for quality assurance. Shortening the total duration of ischemia by getting patients to present earlier after the onset of symptoms is another attractive target, but efforts to reduce this have to date been disappointing. Nonetheless, there is good evidence that over time when the patient is on the "flat" part of the curve representing duration of ischemia, mortality, and salvage, time is less of a critical factor.[4] Yet the relationship between D-B time persists, irrespective of the duration of ischemia (at least in this study). Could it be that shorter D-B times are also a surrogate for overall quality of care and the relationship to mortality might reflect other unrecorded quality measures?

**B J. Gersh, MB, ChB, DPhil, FRCP**

*References*

1. Newby LK, Rutsch WR, Califf RM, et al: Time from symptom onset to treatment in outcomes after thrombolytic therapy. GUSTO-1 Investigators. *J Am Coll Cardiol* 27:1646-1655, 1996.
2. DeLuca G, Suryapranata H, Zijlstra F, et al: ZWOLLE Myocardial Infarction Study Group. Symptom onset-to-balloon time and mortality in patients with acute myocardial infarction treated by primary angioplasty. *J Am Coll Cardiol* 42:991-997, 2003.
3. Antoniucci D, Valenti R, Migliorini A, et al: Relation of time to treatment and mortality in patients with acute myocardial infarction undergoing primary coronary angioplasty. *Am J Cardiol* 89:1248-1252, 2002.
4. Gersh BJ, Stone GW, White HD, et al: Pharmacological facilitation of primary percutaneous coronary intervention for acute myocardial infarction. Is the slope of the curve the shape of the future? *JAMA* 293:979-986, 2005.

---

**Effects of Primary Angioplasty for Acute Myocardial Infarction on Early and Late Infarct Size and Left Ventricular Wall Characteristics**

Baks T, van Geuns R-J, Biagini E, et al (Erasmus Med Ctr, Rotterdam, The Netherlands)

*J Am Coll Cardiol* 47:40-44, 2006                                                    4–15

---

The effects of reperfusion on early and late infarct size and left ventricular wall characteristics were studied by performing cine–magnetic resonance imaging, first-pass perfusion, and delayed enhancement imaging in 22 patients at five days and five months after successful primary angioplasty for first acute myocardial infarction. Infarct size, end-diastolic wall thickness, and segmental wall thickening were quantified, and the extent of microvascular obstruction (MO) was evaluated qualitatively. Infarct size decreased by 31%. Segments without MO had early increased wall thickness and late partially normalized wall thickening. Segments with MO showed late wall thinning and no functional recovery at five months.

*Objectives.*—We aimed to study the effects of early successful primary angioplasty for ST-segment elevation acute myocardial infarction (AMI) on early and late infarct size and left ventricular (LV) wall characteristics.

*Background.*—Early reperfusion treatment for AMI preserves LV function, but the effects on early and late infarct size, end-diastolic wall thickness (EDWT), and segmental wall thickening (SWT) are not well known.

*Methods.*—In 22 patients with successful primary angioplasty for first AMI, cine–magnetic resonance imaging (MRI), first-pass perfusion, and delayed-enhancement imaging was performed at five days and five months. The extent of microvascular obstruction (MO) was evaluated on perfusion images. Infarct shrinkage was defined as the difference between the volume of delayed-enhancement at five days and five months. The EDWT and SWT were quantified on cine-MRI.

*Results.*—Infarct shrinkage occurred to the same extent in small and large infarctions [r = 0.92; p < 0.001], with a mean decrease of 31% (35 ± 21 g to 24 ± 17 g). Dysfunctional segments without MO had an increased EDWT at five days compared with remote myocardium (9.2 ± 1.7 mm vs. 8.4 ± 1.7 mm; p < 0.001). At five months, EDWT in these segments became comparable to the thickness of remote myocardium (7.8 ± 1.6 mm vs. 7.6 ± 1.4 mm; p = 0.60), and SWT improved (21 ± 15% to 40 ± 24%; p < 0.001) but remained impaired (40 ± 24% vs. 71 ± 29%; p < 0.001). Segments with MO demonstrated wall thinning at five months (6.4 ± 1.3 mm vs. 7.6 ± 1.4 mm; p = 0.006) and no significant recovery in SWT (12 ± 14% to 17 ± 20%; p = 0.15).

*Conclusions.*—Infarct size decreased by 31%. Segments without MO had early increased wall thickness and late partial functional recovery. Segments with MO showed late wall thinning and no functional recovery at five months.

▶ The contrast between the very impressive achievement in regard to TIMI (thrombolysis in myocardial infarction) grade 3 flow rates after primary percutaneous coronary intervention and the disappointingly low rates of normal myocardial perfusion and the high incidence of microvascular dysfunction remains an area of considerable interest but also concern.[1] It has recently been shown that contrast-enhanced MRI may be helpful in clarifying the interactions between the achievement of reperfusion and myocardial healing, by providing reproducible measurements of infarction size, myocardial perfusion and left ventricular wall thickness and function.[2]

This small study identifies a correlation between the presence of microvascular dysfunction at 5 days with wall thinning and no improvement in wall thickening at follow up. Another important aspect of this study is the approximate 25% reduction in infarct size and the spontaneous improvement in ejection fraction over a 5-month period. Similar figures are being used to support the benefits of the administration of bone marrow or adult progenitor cells in unblinded studies in post-myocardial infarction patients undergoing cell repair therapy.[3] Clearly we need additional blinded randomized trials in this area.

Microvascular dysfunction is an attractive topic for further enhancing the benefit of reperfusion therapy. Nonetheless, given the rather depressing outcomes of clinical trials to date, it would appear that the achievement of this goal is much more difficult than is the case in the experimental model. Perhaps an element of microvascular dysfunction, precedes the onset of myocardial infarction as part of a diffuse inflammatory state? This is speculative but certainly worth looking into.

**B. J. Gersh, MD, ChB, DPhil, FRCP**

*References*

1. Sorajja P, Gersh BJ, Costantini C, et al: Combined prognostic utility of ST-segment recovery and myocardial blush after primary percutaneous coronary intervention in acute myocardial infarction. *Eur Heart J* 26(7):667-674, 2005.
2. Kim RJ, Fieno DS, Parrish TB, et al: Relationship of MRI delayed contract enhancement to irreversible injury, infarct age, and contractile function. *Circulation* 100:1992-2002, 1999.
3. Wollert KC, Meyer GP, Lotz J, et al: Intracoronary autologous bone-marrow cell transfer after myocardial infarction: the BOOST randomised controlled clinical trial. *Lancet* 364:141-148, 2004.

# Non-ST-Elevation Acute Coronary Syndromes

**Excess Dosing of Antiplatelet and Antithrombin Agents in the Treatment of Non–ST-Segment Elevation Acute Coronary Syndromes**
Alexander KP, for the CRUSADE Investigators (Duke Univ Med Ctr, Durham, NC; et al)
*JAMA* 294:3108-3116, 2005                                                    4–16

---

*Context.*—Effective medical care assumes delivery of evidence-based medicines to appropriate patients with doses comparable to those studied.

*Objective.*—To investigate dosing of unfractionated heparin (UFH), low-molecular-weight heparin (LMWH), and glycoprotein IIb/IIIa inhibitors, and the association between dosing and major outcomes.

*Design, Setting, and Participants.*—A prospective observational analysis in 387 US academic and nonacademic hospitals of 30,136 patients from the CRUSADE (Can Rapid Risk Stratification of Unstable Angina Patients Suppress Adverse Outcomes With Early Implementation of the American College of Cardiology/American Heart Association Guidelines) National Quality Improvement Initiative Registry who had non–ST-segment elevation acute coronary syndromes (NSTE ACS) with chest pain and either positive electrocardiograms or cardiac biomarkers between January 1 and September 30, 2004.

*Main Outcome Measures.*—Excessive dosing of UFH, LMWH, and glycoprotein IIb/IIIa inhibitors and major clinical outcomes, including bleeding, in-hospital mortality, and length of stay.

*Results.*—A total of 3354 patients (42%) with NSTE ACS who were administered antithrombotic agents received at least 1 initial dose outside the recommended range. An excess dose was administered to 2934 patients (32.8%) treated with UFH, 1378 (13.8%) treated with LMWH, and 2784 (26.8%) treated with glycoprotein IIb/IIIa inhibitors. Factors associated with excess dosing included older age, as well as female sex, renal insufficiency, low body weight, diabetes mellitus, and congestive heart failure. Relative to those patients not administered excess dosages, patients with excess dosages of UFH, LMWH, and glycoprotein IIb/IIIa inhibitors either tended toward or had higher risks for major bleeding (adjusted odds ratio [OR], 1.08; 95% confidence interval [CI], 0.94-1.26; OR, 1.39; 95% CI, 1.11-1.74; and OR, 1.36; 95% CI, 1.10-1.68; respectively). Bleeding increased relative to the degree of excess dose and to the number of agents administered in excess (6.6% [237/3590] if neither heparin nor glycoprotein IIb/IIIa excess vs 22.2% [93/419] if both excess). Mortality and length of stay were also higher among those patients administered excess dosing. We estimated that 15% (400/2766) of major bleeding in this population may be attributable to excess dosing.

*Conclusions.*—Patients with NSTE ACS treated in the community often receive excess doses of antithrombotic therapy. Dosing errors occur more often in vulnerable populations and predict an increased risk of major bleeding.

▶ The trust of many quality improvement initiatives is to appropriately ensure that eligible patients receive evidence-based therapy. This is an important step in closing the quite large gap between guideline development and their widespread adoption and implementation in clinical practice. What also has to be kept in the forefront, however, is that these therapies not only be widely used but that this is done safely, expeditiously, and correctly. Multiple studies have demonstrated the efficacy of antiplatelet and antithrombin therapy in improving outcomes in patients with acute coronary syndromes.[1] Nonetheless, the therapeutic window is narrowing and bleeding complications remain a serious concern and are particularly frequent in patients who are elderly and with comorbidity.[2]

This analysis from a multicenter registry protects practice patents across a wide range of hospitals in the United States (28% for academic institutions). What is quite disturbing is that the correct dose of unfractionated heparin was administered only 30.3% of the time; this was 53.8% of time in the case of low molecular weight heparin and 72.3% were glycoprotein IIb/IIIa inhibitors. Of the patients receiving excess doses, the majority were categorized as "mild excess," but a major excess occurred in 2.1% to 25% of patients, depending on the drug, the lowest being the platelet inhibitors. Factors associated with excess dosing include older age, reduced body mass index, female sex, renal insufficiency, diabetes, and congestive heart failure—these are vulnerable populations with a greater risk of bleeding to begin with. The consequences of excess drug dosage were severe with a higher rate of bleeding and a longer hospital length of stay with the relationship to mortality was less clear.

The authors suggest that excess dosing accounts for approximately 15% of all bleeding. Given the greater than 1 million patients admitted to US hospitals annually with non-ST elevation acute coronary syndromes and the aging of our population, this is a very significant issue.

**B. J. Gersh, MD, ChB, DPhil, FRCP**

References

1. Boersma E, Harrington RA, Molitemo DJ, et al: Platelet glycoprotein IIb/IIIa inhibitors in acute coronary syndromes: A meta-analysis of all major randomised clinical trials. *Lancet* 359:189-198, 2002.
2. Moscucci M, Fox K, Cannon C, et al: Predictors of major bleeding in acute coronary syndromes: The Global Registry of Acute Coronary Events (GRACE). *Eur Heart J* 24:1815-1823, 2003.

**Acute Clopidogrel Use and Outcomes in Patients With Non-ST-Segment Elevation Acute Coronary Syndromes Undergoing Coronary Artery Bypass Surgery**

Mehta RH, Roe MT, Mulgund J, et al (Duke Clinical Research Inst, Durham, NC; Univ of North Carolina, Chapel Hill; Brigham and Women's Hosp, Boston; et al)
*J Am Coll Cardiol* 48:281-286, 2006                                      4–17

*Objectives.*—We sought to characterize patterns of clopidogrel use before coronary artery bypass grafting (CABG) and examine the drug's impact on risks for postoperative transfusions among patients with non–ST-segment elevation acute coronary syndromes (NSTE ACS).

*Background.*—Adherence in community practice to American College of Cardiology/American Heart Association guidelines for clopidogrel use among NSTE ACS patients has not been previously characterized.

*Methods.*—We evaluated 2,858 NSTE ACS patients undergoing CABG at 264 hospitals participating in the CRUSADE (Can Rapid Risk Stratification of Unstable Angina Patients Suppress Adverse Outcomes With Early Implementation of the ACC/AHA Guidelines) Initiative. We examined the patterns of acute clopidogrel therapy and its association with bleeding risks among those having "early" CABG ≤5 days and again among those having "late" surgery >5 days after catheterization.

*Results.*—Within 24 h of admission, 852 patients (30%) received clopidogrel. In contrast to national guidelines, 87% of clopidogrel-treated patients underwent CABG ≤5 days after treatment. Among those receiving CABG within ≤5 days of last treatment, the use of clopidogrel was associated with a significant increase in blood transfusions (65.0% vs. 56.9%, adjusted odds ratio [OR] 1.36, 95% confidence interval [CI] 1.10 to 1.68) as well as the need for transfusion of ≥4 U of blood (27.7% vs. 18.4%, OR 1.70, 95% CI 1.32 to 2.19). In contrast, acute clopidogrel therapy was not associated with higher bleeding risks if CABG was delayed >5 days (adjusted OR 1.18, 95% CI 0.54 to 2.58).

*Conclusions.*—Despite guideline recommendations, the overwhelming majority of NSTE ACS patients treated with acute clopidogrel needing CABG have their surgery within ≤5 days of treatment. A failure to delay surgery is associated with increased blood transfusion requirements that must be weighed against the potential clinical and economic impacts of such delays.

▶ One of the most surprising aspects of this article is the poor community adherence to the guidelines regarding the use of clopidogrel in patients undergoing CABG. Eighty-seven percent of patients undergoing CABG in this large registry had received clopidogrel within the preceding 5 days. One might have expected that patients undergoing surgery within the 5-day window were "sicker," but this did not appear to be the case—in fact, patients undergoing "delayed" CABG had a higher prevalence of high-risk features.

As has been shown in prior studies,[1] clopidogrel within 5 days is associated with a high rate of perioperative bleeding and an increased need for transfusions of red blood cells and platelets. If a cut-point of greater than or equal to 4 U of red blood cell transfusions is used as a marker of severe bleeding, this occurred in 28% of patients receiving clopidogrel versus 18% not treated with clopidogrel.

The increased bleeding with clopidogrel must be weighed against the documented potential benefits of the drug in patients awaiting surgery. This may be a particular dilemma in countries and centers where there is a considerable delay between angiography and surgery or between admission and angiography. In other centers such as my own and many in the United States, angiography is performed relatively early after admission, and if surgery is advised, this is performed without much delay. In this situation, among patients who are considered at a higher risk of undergoing CABG (eg, patients with prior angina, known multivessel disease, left ventricular dysfunction, prior myocardial infarction, marked ST-segment depression, or transient heart failure), it is reasonable to withhold clopidogrel until the angiographic anatomy has been documented and a decision for or against surgery has been made. Among patients in whom the preangiographic clinical picture suggests a very low likelihood of bipolar surgery, it would certainly be reasonable to administer clopidogrel before angiography, particularly if the patient is unstable.

**B. J. Gersh, MB, ChB, DPhil, FRCP**

*Reference*

1. Fox KAA, Mehta SR, Peters R, et al: Benefits and risks of the combination of clopidogrel and aspirin in patients undergoing surgical revascularization for non–ST elevation acute coronary syndrome: The Clopidogrel in Unstable Angina to Prevent Recurrent Ischemic Events (CURE) trial. *Circulation* 110:1202-1208, 2004.

## Chronic Coronary Artery Disease

### B-Type Natriuretic Peptide and the Risk of Cardiovascular Events and Death in Patients With Stable Angina: Results From the Athero*Gene* Study

Schnabel R, Lubos E, Rupprecht HJ, et al (Johannes Gutenberg Univ, Mainz, Germany; INSERM U525, Pitié-Salpétrière, Paris; Bundeswehrzentral-krankenhaus, Koblenz, Germany)

*J Am Coll Cardiol* 47:552-558, 2006                                          4–18

*Objectives.*—The aim of this study was to assess the predictive value of the cardiac hormone B-type natriuretic peptide (BNP) for long-term outcome in a large cohort of stable angina patients.

*Background.*—Recent data suggest a role of BNP in stable ischemic heart disease beyond its known value in heart failure and acute coronary syndromes.

*Methods.*—In 1,085 patients with coronary artery disease (CAD) baseline levels of BNP were prospectively associated with cardiovascular (CV) events during a mean follow-up of 2.5 years.

*Results.*—BNP concentrations were significantly elevated in patients with future CV events (median [25th/75th interquartile range] 119.2 [43.6/300.4] pg/ml vs. 36.2 [11.3/94.6] pg/ml; p < 0.001). Kaplan-Meier survival analysis showed a stepwise decrease in event-free survival across quartiles of BNP baseline concentration ($p_{log\ rank}$ < 0.001). Patients in the highest quartile revealed a 6.1-fold increased risk (p = 0.001) compared to patients in the

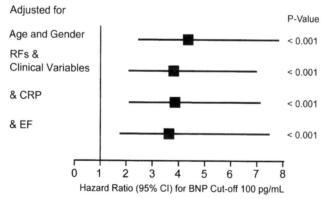

FIGURE 2.—Hazard ratio and 95 percent confidence interval (CI) of cardiovascular events associated with BNP concentrations above a chosen cut-off value of 100 pg/ml, the border of the upper quartile in this cohort being 100.35 pg/ml. Adjustment was performed in four consecutive models as outlined. The traditional risk factors (RFs) (models 2 to 4) comprised age, gender, a history of hypertension, diabetes, smoking status, body mass index, and high-density lipoprotein (the last two parameters entered the model as continuous variables). Presence of multivessel disease and therapy with angiotensin-converting enzyme inhibitors and statins entered the Cox regression analysis as clinical variables (models 2 to 4). BNP = B-type natriuretic peptide; CRP = C-reactive protein; EF = angiographically determined left ventricular ejection fraction. (Courtesy of Schnabel R, Lubos E, Rupprecht HJ, et al: B-type natriuretic peptide and the risk of cardiovascular events and death in patients with stable angina: Results from the Athero*Gene* study. *J Am Coll Cardiol* 47:552-558. Copyright 2006 Elsevier.)

lowest quartile after adjustment for potential confounders. For a cut-off value of 100 pg/ml, an independently increased risk of adverse outcome (hazard ratio [HR] 4.4; p < 0.001) could be demonstrated. One standard deviation (SD) decrease in ejection fraction implied the most prominent increase in risk of future CV events (HR 1.69; p < 0.001) followed by one SD increase in BNP (HR 1.53; p < 0.001). The highest prognostic accuracy could be demonstrated for BNP (area under the curve 0.671).

*Conclusions.*—The data of this large group of CAD patients provide independent evidence that BNP is a strong predictor of cardiovascular risk in patients with stable angina independent of left ventricular systolic performance and known risk factors (Fig 2).

▶ Much of the emphasis on the value of the cardiac hormone BNP has been on the diagnosis and perhaps prognosis of congestive heart failure, since BNP is a sensitive hormonal marker of cardiac stretch.[1] There is, however, increasing evidence that BNP may be a marker of ischemia and hypoxia, which could in turn influence myocardial stretch. BNP has been shown to be a predictor of outcome in patients with acute coronary syndromes, probably as an index of left ventricular dysfunction either chronic or ischemia induced, and in the case of the latter, increased BNP levels could be a surrogate for the severity of ischemia and extent of myocardial jeopardy.[2]

This large prospective study takes things a step further by demonstrating a high prognostic value for long-term outcome in a cohort of patients with chronic stable angina. After adjustment of demographic variables, risk factors, other inflammatory markers, left ventricular function, and angiographic variables, the predictive value persisted. It appears that BNP release is involved in a variety of cardiac abnormalities, but at this stage, its pathophysiologic role is not clearly understood. Further elucidation of this will likely lead to novel indications for its use as a multifaceted cardiac biomarker in the future. To what extent the measurement of BNP currently plays a role in the risk stratification of patients with chronic stable angina is unclear, but the results of the current study are promising and point in a direction for further investigation.

**B. J. Gersh, MB, ChB, DPhil, FRCP**

*References*

1. de Lemos JA, McGuire DK, Drazner MH: B-type natriuretic peptide and cardiovascular disease. *Lancet* 362:316-322, 2003.
2. de Lemos JA, Morrow DA, Bentley JH, et al: The prognostic value of B-type natriuretic peptide in patients with acute coronary syndromes. *N Engl J Med* 345:1014-1021, 2001.

## Clinical Judgment and Treatment Options in Stable Multivessel Coronary Artery Disease: Results From the One-Year Follow-Up of the MASS II (Medicine, Angioplasty, or Surgery Study II)

Pereira AC, Lopes NHM, Soares PR, et al (Univ of São Paulo, Brazil)
*J Am Coll Cardiol* 48:948-953, 2006          4–19

*Objectives.*—This study examined the predictive power of clinical judgment in the incidence of cardiovascular end points in a group of individuals with multivessel coronary artery disease (CAD) followed up in the MASS II (Medicine, Angioplasty, or Surgery Study II).

*Background.*—There is still no consensus on the best treatment for patients with stable multivessel CAD and preserved left ventricular function.

*Methods.*—Preferred treatment allocation was recorded for each of the 611 randomized patients in the MASS II trial before randomization. We have divided our sample according to physician-guided decision and randomization result into two categories: concordant or discordant. The incidence of the points of cardiac death, myocardial infarction, and refractory angina was compared between concordant and discordant patients.

*Results.*—The number of concordant individuals was 292 (48.2%), and this number was not different between the three studied treatments (p = 0.11). A significant difference (p = 0.02) was disclosed because of an increased incidence of combined end point events in discordant patients. In the multivariate Cox hazard model, clinical judgment was a powerful predictor of outcome (p = 0.01) even after adjustment for other covariates. The main subgroup explaining this difference was a significant shift toward a worse outcome in the subgroup of discordant patients who underwent percutaneous coronary intervention (PCI) (p = 0.003).

*Conclusions.*—Angiographic variables were more often used in making clinical decisions regarding PCI than clinical variables, and the only independent predictor of concordance status in the PCI group was the number of

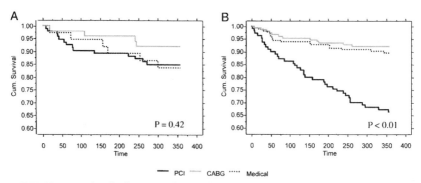

FIGURE 4.—Combined end points incident in individuals with a clinical decision in favor of PCI (A) and individuals with a clinical decision in favor of medical or CABG treatment (B). (Courtesy Pereira AC, Lopes NHM, Soares PR, et al: Clinical judgment and treatment options in stable multivessel coronary artery disease: Results from the one-year follow-up of the MASS II (Medicine, Angioplasty, or Surgery Study II). *J Am Coll Cardiol* 48:948-953. Copyright 2006 Elsevier.)

diseased vessels (p = 0.01). Our data are a reminder that physician judgment remains an important predictor of outcomes (Fig 4).

▶ This is an unusual and clever study in which, before randomization, 2 cardiologists independently made an assessment of which of 3 treatment strategies was preferred, from a clinical perspective: percutaneous coronary intervention (PCI), coronary artery bypass surgery (CABG), or medical therapy. Fundamental to the design of this trial was the requirement that patients would be suitable for all 3 treatment strategies; inclusion criteria were preserved left ventricular function and stable angina. Although the overall trial was negative, it is of interest that among patients who received PCI, but in whom the initial clinical impression was that this would not be the preferred strategy, there was a much higher rate of cardiac events, in particular revascularization for recurrence of ischemia. The single variable most strongly correlated with accordance regarding PCI as the preferred strategy was the presence of triple-vessel disease. The Bypass Angioplasty Revascularization Investigation (BARI), among diabetics, had a mortality difference in favor of CABG, but this fell away when treatment was based on physician and patient preference in the BARI registry.[1] In other words, in trials one might randomize to PCI patients who in clinical practice would be deemed more suitable for CABG.

This has been discussed in a recent editorial that compared the results of randomized control trials and registry studies.[2] Both kinds of studies are important but address different questions. Trials are confined to highly selected patients and introduce entry bias, whereas registry studies are subject to selection bias. Nonetheless, realization that evidence-based medicine must take its place alongside clinical judgment is refreshing. I believe that the best decision for an individual patient regarding the need for and preferred method of coronary revascularization requires widespread participation of physicians in the decision-making process, and this should include both interventional and noninterventional cardiologists and the cardiac surgeon.

**B. J Gersh, MB, ChB, DPhil, FRCP**

*References*

1. Detre KN, Guo P, Holubkov R, et al: Coronary revascularization in diabetic patients: A comparison of the randomized and observational components of the Bypass Angioplasty Revascularization Investigation (BARI). *Circulation* 99:633-640, 1999.
2. Gersh BJ, Frye RL: Methods of coronary revascularization—things may not be as they seem. *N Engl J Med* 352:2235-2237, 2005).

### Relationship Between C-Reactive Protein and Subclinical Atherosclerosis: The Dallas Heart Study

Khera A, de Lemos JA, Peshock RM, et al (Univ of Texas Southwestern Med Ctr, Dallas; Brigham and Women's Hosp, Boston)
*Circulation* 113:38-43, 2006 4-20

*Background.*—Elevated levels of C-reactive protein (CRP) are associated with increased risk for incident cardiovascular events on the basis of observations from several prospective epidemiological studies. However, less is known regarding the relationship between CRP levels and atherosclerotic burden.

*Method and Results.*—We measured CRP in 3373 subjects 30 to 65 years of age who were participating in the Dallas Heart Study, a multiethnic, population-based, probability sample. Electron-beam CT scans were used to measure coronary artery calcification (CAC) in 2726 of these subjects, and MRI was used to measure aortic plaque in 2393. CRP levels were associated with most traditional cardiovascular risk factors. Subjects with CAC had higher median CRP levels than those without CAC (men: median, 2.4 versus 1.8 mg/L, $P<0.001$; women: median, 5.2 versus 3.6 mg/L, $P<0.001$), and there was a modest trend toward increasing CRP levels with increased CAC levels in men ($P$ for trend=0.003) but not in women ($P$ for trend=0.08). Male subjects with aortic plaque also had higher CRP levels than those without (median, 2.3 versus 1.8; $P<0.001$). In multivariate analysis adjusted for traditional cardiovascular risk factors, body mass index, and estrogen and statin medication use, the associations between CRP levels and CAC and CRP levels and aortic plaque were no longer statistically significant.

*Conclusions.*—In a large, population-based sample, subjects with higher CRP levels had a modest increase in the prevalence of subclinical atherosclerosis, but this association was not independent of traditional cardiovascular risk factors. CRP is a poor predictor of atherosclerotic burden.

▶ There is a strong body of evidence demonstrating a consistent relationship between elevation of C-reactive protein (CRP) and an increased risk of cardiovascular events including myocardial infarction, stroke, and cardiovascular death.[1] Nonetheless, despite these persuasive epidemiologic data, the mechanisms underlying this relationship are unclear. On the one hand, increased CRP levels could be a reflection of the extent of atherosclerosis with a magnitude of the "atherosclerotic burden," but an alternative explanation is that the inflammatory marker identifies patients with high-risk, vulnerable plaques that are prone to rupture. There is accumulating evidence that measurements of the extent of coronary artery calcification by computed tomography and aortic plaque by magnetic resonance imaging are promising techniques for the quantification of the extent of atherosclerosis.[2]

This analysis for the multiethnic Dallas Heart Study provides important new data from a population-based perspective. Not unexpectedly, CRP levels are associated with most of the traditional risk factors. However, after multivariable adjustment for traditional risk factors, body mass index, and estrogen and statin use, the association between CRP levels and coronary arterial calcification and aortic plaque were not statistically significant, although there was a modest trend in the univariate analyses.

In summary, in this population of patients without overt cardiovascular disease, CRP levels are not a strong predictor of the burden of subclinical atherosclerosis. These data suggest that the association between CRP levels and cardiovascular events may primary reflect the composition from a morphology and "stability" of plaque rather than the overall cardiovascular, atherosclerotic burden.

**B. J. Gersh, MB, ChB, DPhil, FRCP**

*References*

1. Koenig W, Sund M, Frohilich M, et al: C-reactive protein, a sensitive marker of inflammation, predicts future risk of coronary heart disease in initially healthy middle-aged men: Results from the MONICA (Monitoring Trends and Determinants in Cardiovascular Disease) Augsburg Cohort Study, 1984 to 1992. *Circulation* 99:237-242, 1999.
2. Jaffer FA, O'Donnell CJ, Larson MG, et al: Age and sex distribution of subclinical aortic atherosclerosis: A magnetic resonance imaging examination of the Framingham Heart Study. *Arterioscler Thromb Vasc Biol* 22:849-854, 2002.

---

## Homocysteine Lowering with Folic Acid and B Vitamins in Vascular Disease

Lonn E, for The Heart Outcomes Prevention Evaluation (HOPE) 2 Investigators
(Population Health Research Inst, Hamilton, Ont, Canada; et al)
*N Engl J Med* 354:1567-1577, 2006                                     4–21

---

*Background.*—In observational studies, lower homocysteine levels are associated with lower rates of coronary heart disease and stroke. Folic acid and vitamins $B_6$ and $B_{12}$ lower homocysteine levels. We assessed whether supplementation reduced the risk of major cardiovascular events in patients with vascular disease.

*Methods.*—We randomly assigned 5522 patients 55 years of age or older who had vascular disease or diabetes to daily treatment either with the combination of 2.5 mg of folic acid, 50 mg of vitamin $B_6$, and 1 mg of vitamin $B_{12}$ or with placebo for an average of five years. The primary outcome was a composite of death from cardiovascular causes, myocardial infarction, and stroke.

*Results.*—Mean plasma homocysteine levels decreased by 2.4 μmol per liter (0.3 mg per liter) in the active-treatment group and increased by 0.8 μmol per liter (0.1 mg per liter) in the placebo group. Primary outcome events occurred in 519 patients (18.8 percent) assigned to active therapy and 547 (19.8 percent) assigned to placebo (relative risk, 0.95; 95 percent confidence interval, 0.84 to 1.07; P=0.41). As compared with placebo, active treatment did not significantly decrease the risk of death from cardiovascular causes (relative risk, 0.96; 95 percent confidence interval, 0.81 to 1.13), myocardial infarction (relative risk, 0.98; 95 percent confidence interval, 0.85 to 1.14), or any of the secondary outcomes. Fewer patients assigned to active treatment than to placebo had a stroke (relative risk, 0.75; 95 percent confidence interval, 0.59 to 0.97). More patients in the active-treatment group were hospitalized for unstable angina (relative risk, 1.24; 95 percent confidence interval, 1.04 to 1.49).

*Conclusions.*—Supplements combining folic acid and vitamins $B_6$ and $B_{12}$ did not reduce the risk of major cardiovascular events in patients with vascular disease.

▶ This large trial of folic acid and B vitamins on the secondary prevention of events in patients with established vascular disease or diabetes in addition to another secondary prevention trial on myocardial infarction survivors in the same issue of the journal is emphatically neutral.[1] It would appear that there is no role for supplements containing folic acid and vitamins $B_6$ and $B_{12}$ in the prevention of recurrent events in patients with cardiovascular disease. In fact, in the NORVIT Trial, a trend in the reverse direction was noted.

This was yet another example of a nice hypothesis destroyed by ugly facts. Similar lessons were learned from the trials of hormone replacement therapy, vitamin E, and betacarotene and reinforce the importance of the rigorous scrutiny of randomized, controlled trials. We also need to remember that an epidemiologic association does not necessarily imply a cause and effect relationship. In the case of homocysteine, prior epidemiologic studies did demonstrate an independent and graded association between homocysteine levels and cardiovascular risk.[2] In experimental studies, homocysteine causes oxidative stress, endothelial damage, and increased thrombogenicity, and all these are plausible mechanisms for the development of coronary events.

So the stage was set for trials that would identify a clinical role for folic acid supplementation, but as stated in the accompanying editorial, the answers are unambiguous, but for complex reasons.[3] In the HOPE 2 Trial, the apparent benefit on stroke and unstable angina is correctly discounted by the authors as a probable statistical artifact because there is no trend toward benefit with regard to transient ischemic attacks and other manifestations of coronary artery disease. Does this mean that there is no benefit to lowering homocysteine levels? This is not necessarily the case, as Loscalzo points out in the editorial, but what should be explored are alternative methods such as enhancing the conversion of homocysteine to cysteine in the liver or by increasing urinary secretion of the amino acids.

**B. J. Gersh, MB, ChB, DPhil, FRCP**

*References*

1. Bonaa KH, Ngølestad I, Ueland PM, et al: Homocysteine lowering and cardiovascular events after acute myocardial infarction. *N Engl J Med* 354:1-11, 2006.
2. Homocysteine Studies Collaboration: Homocysteine and risk of ischemic heart disease and stroke: A meta-analysis. *JAMA* 288:2015-2022, 2002.
3. Loscalzo J: Homocysteine trials: Clear outcomes for complex reasons [editorial]. *N Engl J Med* 354:1-3, 2006.

### Angiotensin-Converting Enzyme Inhibitors in Coronary Artery Disease and Preserved Left Ventricular Systolic Function: A Systematic Review and Meta-Analysis of Randomized Controlled Trials

Al-Mallah MH, Tleyjeh IM, Abdel-Latif AA, et al (Henry Ford Heart and Vascular Inst, Detroit; Mayo Clinic College of Medicine, Rochester, Minn; Univ of Louisville, Ky)
*J Am Coll Cardiol* 47:1576-1583, 2006                     4–22

*Objectives.*—This study sought to assess the efficacy of angiotensin-converting enzyme inhibitors (ACEIs) in patients with coronary heart disease and preserved left ventricular (LV) function.

*Background.*—The ACEIs have been shown to improve outcomes in patients with heart failure and myocardial infarction (MI). However, there is conflicting evidence concerning the benefits of ACEIs in patients with coronary artery disease (CAD) and preserved LV systolic function.

*Methods.*—An extensive search was performed to identify randomized, placebo-controlled trials of ACEI use in patients with CAD and preserved LV systolic function. Of 61 potentially relevant articles screened, 6 trials met the inclusion criteria. They were reviewed to determine cardiovascular mortality, nonfatal MI, all-cause mortality, and revascularization rates. We performed random-effect model meta-analyses and quantified between-studies heterogeneity with $I^2$.

*Results.*—There were 16,772 patients randomized to ACEI and 16,728 patients randomized to placebo. Use of ACEIs was associated with a decrease in cardiovascular mortality (relative risk [RR] 0.83, 95% confidence interval [CI] 0.72 to 0.96, p = 0.01), nonfatal MI (RR 0.84, 95% CI 0.75 to 0.94, p = 0.003), all-cause mortality (RR 0.87, 95% CI 0.81 to 0.94, p = 0.0003), and revascularization rates (RR 0.93, 95% CI 0.87 to 1.00, p = 0.04). There was no significant between-studies heterogeneity. Treatment of 100 patients for an average duration of 4.4 years prevents either of the adverse outcomes (one death, or one nonfatal myocardial infarction, or one cardiovascular death or one coronary revascularization procedure).

*Conclusions.*—The cumulative evidence provided by this meta-analysis shows a modest favorable effect of ACEIs on the outcome of patients with CAD and preserved LV systolic function.

▶ The angiotensin-converting enzyme inhibitor (ACE-I) story continues to be fascinating. This class of agents has run the full gamut from their use in patients with hypertension, severe congestive heart failure, asymptomatic left ventricular dysfunction, and diabetes to their role in the primary and secondary prevention of cardiac events in patients with cardiovascular disease but with preserved left ventricular function and no congestive heart failure. The latter category has, however, generated considerable controversy. The 2 largest trials (HOPE and EUROPA) demonstrated a significant benefit that was not noted in the other large trial, namely, PEACE.[1-3] There have been many explanations for the lack of benefit in the PEACE Trial, including suggestions that the wrong drug was used and in too low of a dose. This is, however, an unlikely explanation given the demonstrable biologic effect of the drug on blood pressure lowering, the development of heart failure, and diabetes in that trial.

I believe that the major cause of the differences in outcomes relates to the level of baseline risk. Patients in the PEACE Trial were at the lowest risk, having undergone a high rate of prior revascularization and among whom statin, aspirin, and β-blocker use was extremely high. Far fewer had peripheral vascular disease in comparison with the HOPE Trial. Nonetheless, it should be mentioned that even low-risk patients appear to have benefited in the EUROPA Trial.[4]

This meta-analysis shows a modest favorable effect in ACE-I on the outcome of patients with coronary artery disease and preserved left ventricular function. This is not surprising given the known beneficial effects of ACE-I on vascular inflammation, endothelial dysfunction, plaque stability, thrombogenicity, and fibrinolysis. Nonetheless, I agree with the conclusions of the PEACE Study, of which I was a member of the Writing Committee, and that is, although ACE-I should be considered in all patients with coronary artery disease, their use is not mandatory. This becomes particularly important in an elderly population in whom there is limit to the amount of drugs that will be tolerated. In those patients at higher risk or in those patients who need an ACE-I because they have diabetes, hypertension, or left ventricular dysfunction, the decision is very simple. Nonetheless, I believe there are some patients who appear to be at low risk and in whom the use of ACE-I is not mandatory.

**B. J. Gersh, MB, ChB, DPhil, FRCP**

*References*

1. Heart Outcomes Evaluation Study Investigators (THOESI): Effects of an angiotensin-converting-enzyme, ramipril, on cardiovascular events in high-risk patients. *N Engl J Med* 342:145-153, 2000.
2. Fox KM, European Trial on Reduction of Cardiac Events with Perindopril in Stable Coronary Artery Disease Investigators: Efficacy of perindopril in reduction of cardiovascular events among patients with stable coronary artery disease: Randomized, double-blind, placebo-controlled, multicenter trial (the EUROPA Study). *Lancet* 362:782-788, 2003.
3. PEACE Trial Investigators: Angiotensin-converting-enzyme inhibition in stable coronary artery disease. *N Engl J Med* 351:2058-2068, 2004.
4. Deckers JW, Goedhart DM, Boersma E, et al: Treatment benefit by perindopril in patients with stable coronary artery disease at different levels of risk. *Eur Heart J* 27:796-801, 2006.

## Sequence Variations in *PCSK9*, Low LDL, and Protection against Coronary Heart Disease

Cohen JC, Boerwinkle E, Mosley TH Jr, et al (Univ of Texas Southwestern Med Ctr, Dallas; Univ of Texas Health Science Ctr, Houston; Univ of Mississippi Med Ctr, Jackson)
*N Engl J Med* 354:1264-1272, 2006                    4–23

*Background.*—A low plasma level of low-density lipoprotein (LDL) cholesterol is associated with reduced risk of coronary heart disease (CHD), but the effect of lifelong reductions in plasma LDL cholesterol is not known. We examined the effect of DNA-sequence variations that reduce plasma levels of LDL cholesterol on the incidence of coronary events in a large population.

*Methods.*—We compared the incidence of CHD (myocardial infarction, fatal CHD, or coronary revascularization) over a 15-year interval in the Atherosclerosis Risk in Communities study according to the presence or absence of sequence variants in the proprotein convertase subtilisin/kexin type 9 serine protease gene (*PCSK9*) that are associated with reduced plasma levels of LDL cholesterol.

*Results.*—Of the 3363 black subjects examined, 2.6 percent had nonsense mutations in *PCSK9*; these mutations were associated with a 28 percent reduction in mean LDL cholesterol and an 88 percent reduction in the risk of CHD (P=0.008 for the reduction; hazard ratio, 0.11; 95 percent confidence interval, 0.02 to 0.81; P=0.03). Of the 9524 white subjects examined, 3.2 percent had a sequence variation in *PCSK9* that was associated with a 15 percent reduction in LDL cholesterol and a 47 percent reduction in the risk of CHD (hazard ratio, 0.50; 95 percent confidence interval, 0.32 to 0.79; P=0.003).

*Conclusions.*—These data indicate that moderate lifelong reduction in the plasma level of LDL cholesterol is associated with a substantial reduction in the incidence of coronary events, even in populations with a high prevalence of non-lipid-related cardiovascular risk factors.

▶ Although low levels of low-density lipoprotein (LDL) cholesterol are indisputably linked to a reduced risk of cardiovascular disease and the results of lowering cholesterol levels are impressive in regard to short and intermediate term outcomes,[1,2] the effects of lifelong reductions in LDL cholesterol upon the incidence of coronary artery disease are less-well established. Prior data from cross sectional and cohort studies support the hypothesis that low levels of LDL cholesterol are protective but these observations may be potentially confounded by other factors related to low LDL cholesterol.[3]

This fascinating study utilizes the presence of mutations present in 2% of black subjects that had previously been associated with a 40% reduction in mean LDL cholesterol levels.[4] In this study, over a 15-year period a 28% reduction in LDL cholesterol was associated with an 88% reduction in the risk of coronary artery disease in black subjects. In white subjects, the reduction in LDL cholesterol levels was 15% and in coronary events 47%. Although there is a possibility that the nonsense mutations reduce coronary heart disease by mechanisms other than LDL cholesterol lowering, there is no evidence in this analysis of an effect on non-lipid-related risk factors.

This and other studies suggest that the PCISK 9 gene and in particular the inhibition of its activity, is an attractive target for future LDL cholesterol therapies.

**B. J. Gersh, MB, ChB, DPhil**

*References*

1. Third report of the National Cholesterol Education Program (NCEP) Expert Panel on Detection, Evaluation, and Treatment of High Blood Cholesterol in Adults (Adult Treatment Panel III): Final Report. *Circulation* 106:3143-3421, 2002.
2. Lohr MR, Wald NJ, Rudnick AAR: Quantifying effects of statins on low-density lipoprotein cholesterol, ischaemic heart disease, and stroke: Systematic review and meta-analysis. *BMJ* 2003;326:1423-1427.
3. Stamler J, Dabigous ML, Garside DB, et al: Relationship of baseline serum cholesterol levels in three large cohorts of younger men to long-term coronary, cardiovascular, and all-cause mortality into longevity. *JAMA* 84:311-318, 2002.
4. Cohen J, Pertscmlidis A, Kotowski IK, et al: Low LDL cholesterol in individuals of African descent resulting from frequent nonsense mutations in *PCSK 9. Nat Genet* 37:161-165, 2005.

---

**The Risk Associated with Aprotinin in Cardiac Surgery**
Mangano DT, for the Multicenter Study of Perioperative Ischemia Research Group and the Ischemia Research and Education Foundation (Ischemia Research and Education Found, San Bruno Calif; et al)
*N Engl J Med* 354:353-365, 2006                                    4–24

---

*Background.*—The majority of patients undergoing surgical treatment for ST-elevation myocardial infarction receive antifibrinolytic therapy to limit blood loss. This approach appears counterintuitive to the accepted medical treatment of the same condition—namely, fibrinolysis to limit thrombosis. Despite this concern, no independent, large-scale safety assessment has been undertaken.

*Methods.*—In this observational study involving 4374 patients undergoing revascularization, we prospectively assessed three agents (aprotinin [1295 patients], aminocaproic acid [883], and tranexamic acid [822]) as compared with no agent (1374 patients) with regard to serious outcomes by propensity and multivariable methods. (Although aprotinin is a serine protease inhibitor, here we use the term antifibrinolytic therapy to include all three agents.)

*Results.*—In propensity-adjusted, multivariable logistic regression (C-index, 0.72), use of aprotinin was associated with a doubling in the risk of renal failure requiring dialysis among patients undergoing complex coronary-artery surgery (odds ratio, 2.59; 95 percent confidence interval, 1.36 to 4.95) or primary surgery (odds ratio, 2.34; 95 percent confidence interval, 1.27 to 4.31). Similarly, use of aprotinin in the latter group was associated with a 55 percent increase in the risk of myocardial infarction or heart

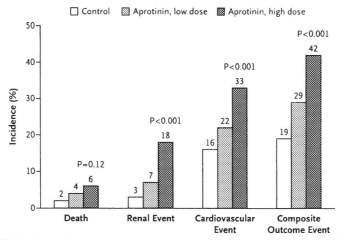

FIGURE 3.—**Aprotonin dose response.** P values shown are for the comparison between a high dose of aprotonin and either a low dose of aprotonin or no antifibrinolytic therapy (control). Pairwise comparison between a high dose of aprotonin and control was significant with respect to renal events, cardiovascular events, and composit outcome events (P<0.001 for all three comparisons by Bonferroni-adjusted analyses) but not for death (P = 0.12). Pairwise comparison between a low dose of aprotonin and no antifibrinolytic therapy was significant (in Bonferroni-adjusted analyses) with respect to renal events (P<0.001) and composite outcome events (P = 0.003) but not cardiovascular events (P = 0.08) or death (P = 0.14). Pairwise comparison between a high dose of aprotonin and a low dose of aprotonin was significant (in Bonferroni-adjust analyses) with respect to renal events (P<0.001) but not cardiovascular events (P = 0.04), composite outcome events (P = 0.3), or death (P = 0.38). (Reprinted by permission of *The New England Journal of Medicine* from Mangano DT, for the Multicenter Study of Perioperative Inschemia Research Group and the Ischemia Research and Education Foundation: The risk associated with aprotonin in cardiac surgery. *N Engl J Med* 354, 353-365, 2006. Copyright © 2006, Massachusetts Medical Society. All rights reserved.)

failure (P<0.001) and a 181 percent increase in the risk of stroke or encephalopathy (P=0.001). Neither aminocaproic acid nor tranexamic acid was associated with an increased risk of renal, cardiac, or cerebral events. Adjustment according to propensity score for the use of any one of the three agents as compared with no agent yielded nearly identical findings. All the agents reduced blood loss.

*Conclusions.*—The association between aprotinin and serious end-organ damage indicates that continued use is not prudent. In contrast, the less expensive generic medications aminocaproic acid and tranexamic acid are safe alternatives (Fig 3).

▶ In patients with coronary artery disease undergoing coronary bypass surgery with cardiopulmonary bypass, concerns regarding the dangers of excessive bleeding have led to the use of 2 classes of antifibrinolytic drugs that mitigate bleeding, namely, the lysine analogs (aminocaproic acid and transexamic acid) and the serine protease inhibitors (aprotinin). This approach is somewhat paradoxical in that the mainstay of medical therapy for the acute coronary syndromes is antithrombotic and fibrinolytic measures. Although antifibrinolytic drug use is fairly standard in patients undergoing cardiac surgery and prior studies have suggested safety,[1] the authors of this large, international, non–sponsor-supported study highlight the many limitations of prior studies.

This is an observational study and not a randomized controlled trial, although differences in baseline variables were adjusted by using propensity-adjusted multivariable logistic regression. Among patients undergoing elective coronary bypass surgery, aprotinin was associated with a disturbing increase in cardiovascular, cerebrovascular, and renal events, including a higher mortality rate. This was not the case with aminocaproic or transexamic acid. The differences persisted after multivariate adjustment. Among patients undergoing more complex cardiac surgery, the adverse affect of aprotinin on renal events was quite striking. All 3 drugs were similarly effective in reducing blood loss.

Although the aprotinin group was somewhat sicker to begin with, the results of this study are nonetheless quite impressive. First, it is well documented that aprotinin has a high affinity for the kidneys, unlike the lysine analog. Furthermore, prior studies have hinted at neprotoxicity and increased intravascular thrombosis.[2] Second, the relationship between the dose and adverse events involving kidneys, brain, and heart is extremely strong and consistent with a generalized pattern of ischemic injury.

The advantages of preventing excessive blood loss after cardiac surgery are not in dispute. Nonetheless, it would appear that this may be achieved with less expensive generic medications such as a minor caproic acid and tranexamic acid and with increased safety.

**B. J. Gersh, MB, ChB, DPhil, FRCP**

*References*

1. Sedrakyan A, Treasure T, Elefteriades JA: Effect of aprotinin on clinical outcomes in coronary artery bypass graft surgery: A systematic review and meta-analysis of randomized clinical trials. *J Thorac Cardiovasc Surg* 128:442-448, 2004.
2. Samama CM, Mazoyer E, Drunebal P, et al: Aprotinin could promote arterial thrombosis in pigs: A prospective, randomized, blind study. *Thromb Haemost* 71:663-669, 1994.

▶ One of the most controversial publications of the year was this analysis of risks associated with aprotinin use in cardiac surgery. This remarkable drug came on the scene over a decade ago with great fanfare and widespread celebration of its multiple beneficial effects. Initially introduced in the hopes that it would improve pulmonary function after cardiac surgery, this protease inhibitor was incidentally noted to have a remarkable effect on postoperative bleeding. Any surgeon who has used it will attest to its remarkable effect in this regard in most instances. Unfortunately, the drug was promoted with almost religious fervor, and early reports raising concerns about potential adverse effects were dismissed.[1] In the end, for aprotinin, as is the case for any other intervention pharmacologic or surgical, there are risks as well as a benefits. It is simply a matter of thermodynamics. The risks are well outlined in this study. What is unfortunate, however, is the benefits are not so clearly stated.

There is no question that aprotinin can have a life-saving impact in high risk patients. Its utility in the setting of active endocarditis, for example, or complex reoperative aortic surgery is beyond doubt. Its indiscriminate use, however, cannot be supported. The results of this study emphasize the importance of judgment in the application of any of these interventions.

**T. M. Sundt III, MD**

*Reference*

1. Sundt TM III, Kouchoukos NT, Saffitz JE, et al: Renal dysfunction and intravascular coagulation with aprotinin and hypothermic circulatory arrest. *Ann Thorac Surg* 55:1418-1424, 1993.

## Coronary Bypass Surgery and Percutaneous Coronary Intervention

### Prevalence, Predictors, and Outcomes of Premature Discontinuation of Thienopyridine Therapy After Drug-Eluting Stent Placement: Results From the PREMIER Registry

Spertus JA, Kettelkamp R, Vance C, et al (Univ of Missouri at Kansas City; Univ of Colorado Hosp/Denver VA Med Ctr; Univ of Colorado Health Sciences Ctr, Denver; et al)
*Circulation* 113:2803-2809, 2006                                    4–25

*Background.*—Although drug-eluting stents (DES) significantly reduce restenosis, they require 3 to 6 months of thienopyridine therapy to prevent stent thrombosis. The rate and consequences of prematurely discontinuing thienopyridine therapy after DES placement for acute myocardial infarction (MI) are unknown.

*Method and Results.*—We used prospectively collected data from a 19-center study of MI patients to examine the prevalence and predictors of thienopyridine discontinuation 30 days after DES treatment. We then compared the mortality and cardiac hospitalization rates for the next 11 months between those who stopped and those who continued thienopyridine therapy. Among 500 DES-treated MI patients who were discharged on thienopyridine therapy, 68 (13.6%) stopped therapy within 30 days. Those who stopped were older, less likely to have completed high school or be married, more likely to avoid health care because of cost, and more likely to have had preexisting cardiovascular disease or anemia at presentation. They were also less likely to have received discharge instructions about their medications or a cardiac rehabilitation referral. Patients who stopped thienopyridine therapy by 30 days were more likely to die during the next 11 months (7.5% versus 0.7%, $P<0.0001$; adjusted hazard ratio=9.0; 95% confidence interval=1.3 to 60.6) and to be rehospitalized (23% versus 14%, $P=0.08$; adjusted hazard ratio=1.5; 95% confidence interval=0.78 to 3.0).

*Conclusions.*—Almost 1 in 7 MI patients who received a DES were no longer taking thienopyridine by 30 days. Prematurely stopping thienopyridine therapy was strongly associated with subsequent mortality. Strategies to improve the use of thienopyridine are needed to optimize the outcomes of MI patients treated with DES.

▶ This is an interesting and unusual study that addresses several issues, among which patient compliance is probably the most important.

Patients who discontinue thienopyridine therapy within 30 days after DED for ST-elevation MI (STEMI) had higher mortality and hospitalization rates for cardiac reasons over the next 11 months. Some of these events may have been attributable to a direct effect on subacute stent thrombosis, but other adverse risk factors that were increased in the discontinuation group may have played a confounding role, such as older age, anemia, and preexisting cardiac disease. To my mind, the major message of the study is to reinforce the impact of social economic status on cardiac outcomes.[1] Patients who discontinued thienopyridine (14% of the total population) were less educated and less likely to be married, more likely to be affected by health care costs, and less likely to enter cardiac rehabilitation programs or to receive discharge instructions regarding medication usage. The mechanisms by which these factors affect outcomes are uncertain and obviously multifactorial, but to some extent may be related to stress, anger, depression, and lack of risk factor modification among other explanations.

Approaches to increasing drug compliance are a logical target for interventions aimed at improving long-term outcomes.[2] Nonetheless, one has the impression that drug adherence is, at least in part, a surrogate for other powerful modifying influences, namely socioeconomic status and the entire milieu surrounding this. Either way, these could have an adverse effect on cardiovascular outcome.

**B. J. Gersh, MB, ChB, DPhil, FRCP**

*References*

1. McDermott MM, Schmitt V, Wallner A: Impact of medication nonadherence on coronary heart disease outcomes: A critical review. *Arch Intern Med* 157:1921-1929, 1997.
2. Byrne M, Walsh J, Murphy AW: Secondary prevention of coronary heart disease; patient beliefs and health-related behavior. *J Psychosomat Res* 58:403-415, 2005.

---

**Late Thrombosis of Drug-Eluting Stents: A Meta-Analysis of Randomized Clinical Trials**
Bavry AA, Kumbhani DJ, Helton TJ, et al (Cleveland Clinic Found, Ohio; Univ of Pennsylvania, Philadelphia)
*Am J Med* 119:1056-1061, 2006                                              4–26

---

*Purpose.*—Drug-eluting stents are commonly used for percutaneous coronary intervention. Despite excellent clinical efficacy, the association between drug-eluting stents and the risk for late thrombosis remains imprecisely defined.

**Months**

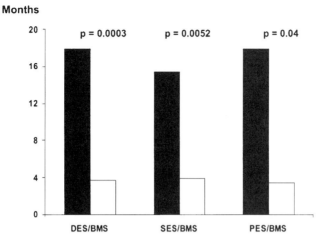

FIGURE 2.—Median time of late stent thrombosis. BMS = bare metal stent; DES = drug-eluting stent; PES = paclitaxel-eluting stent; SES = sirolimus-eluting stent. (Reprinted from Bavry AA, Kumbhani DJ, Helton TJ, et al: Late thrombosis of drug-eluting stents: A meta-analysis of randomized clinical trials. *Am J Med* 119:1056-1061. Copyright Elsevier 2006.)

*Methods.*—We performed a meta-analysis on 14 contemporary clinical trials that randomized 6675 patients to drug-eluting stents (paclitaxel or sirolimus) compared with bare metal stents. Eight of these trials have reported more than a year of clinical follow-up.

*Results.*—The incidence of very late thrombosis (>1 year after the index procedure) was 5.0 events per 1000 drug-eluting stent patients, with no events in bare metal stent patients (risk ratio [RR] = 5.02, 95% confidence interval [CI], 1.29 to 19.52, $P$ = .02). Among sirolimus trials, the incidence of very late thrombosis was 3.6 events per 1000 sirolimus stent patients, with no events in bare metal stent patients (RR = 3.99, 95% CI, .45 to 35.62, $P$ = .22). The median time of late sirolimus stent thrombosis was 15.5 months, whereas with bare metal stents it was 4 months (Fig 2). Among paclitaxel trials, the incidence of very late thrombosis was 5.9 events per 1000 paclitaxel stent patients, with no events in bare metal stent patients (RR = 5.72, 95% CI, 1.08 to 32.45, $P$ = .049). The median time of late paclitaxel stent thrombosis was 18 months, whereas it was 3.5 months in bare metal stent patients.

*Conclusions.*—Although the incidence of very late stent thrombosis more than 1 year after coronary revascularization is low, drug-eluting stents appear to increase the risk for late thrombosis. Although more of this risk was seen with paclitaxel stents, it remains possible that sirolimus stents similarly increase the risk for late thrombosis compared with bare metal stents.

▶ This meta-analysis addresses one of the most controversial and topical issues in interventional cardiology. It appears that although the risk of very late (greater than 1 year) stent thrombosis is low, drug-eluting stents (DES) clearly appeared to increase the risk approximately 5-fold. Whether this differs among sirolimus versus paclitaxel stents is undetermined. The importance of this analysis is that follow-up is beyond 1 year, since prior reports from the randomized controlled trials suggested a similar rate of stent thrombosis of 1 year between DES and bare-metal stents.[1]

There are several unresolved issues that led to a recent Food and Drug Administration panel. First, we do not have hard information on late stent thrombosis rates in patients receiving DES for off-label indications. It is likely that major adverse coronary events, including late stent thrombosis, will be substantially higher in these subgroups. Second, we really do not know whether Plavix should be continued for 1 year or indefinitely. There may be no safe period for DES after which Plavix can be discontinued, as suggested by this meta-analysis. The clinical implications in patients with DES undergoing noncardiac surgery are also substantial.

The limitations of DES are now increasingly recognized by patients and physicians, but these do not negate their substantial advantages in reducing restenosis in many subsets of patients. Moreover, restenosis should not necessarily be considered a benign event. Perhaps the next generation of bioabsorbable DES will eliminate the problem of delayed internal healing and a persistent thrombotic miler? New clinical trials will have to address not only the duration of Plavix but a long period of follow-up; 9 months of follow-up is acceptable if restenosis is the end point, but the issue of very late stent thrombosis will require many years of follow-up.

**B. J. Gersh, MB, ChB, DPhil, FRCP**

*Reference*

1. Moreno R, Fernandaz C, Ernandez R, et al: Drug-eluting stent thrombosis: Results from a pooled analysis including 10 randomized studies. *J Am Coll Cardiol* 45:954-959, 2005.

---

**Cognitive Outcomes in Elderly High-Risk Patients After Off-Pump Versus Conventional Coronary Artery Bypass Grafting: A Randomized Trial**
Jensen BO, Hughes P, Rasmussen LS, et al (Copenhagen Univ Hosp)
*Circulation* 113:2790-2795, 2006                                      4-27

---

*Background.*—It has been suggested that the risk of cerebral dysfunction is less with off-pump coronary artery bypass grafting (OPCAB) than with conventional coronary artery bypass grafting (CCAB). However, evidence for this statement is preliminary, and additional insight is needed.

*Method and Results.*—The study was a substudy of the randomized Best Bypass Surgery trial that compared OPCAB with CCAB treatment with respect to intraoperative and postoperative mortality and morbidity in patients with a moderate to high level of predicted preoperative risk. The outcome was cognitive function. A total of 120 elderly patients (mean age 76 years, SD 4.5 years) underwent psychometric testing before surgery and at a mean of 103 (SD 15) days postoperatively with a neuropsychological test battery that included 7 parameters from 4 tests. Cognitive dysfunction was defined as the occurrence of at least 2 of the 7 possible deficits. Secondary analysis was performed on the basis of the definition of a 20% decline in cognitive scores compared with baseline, and with z score analysis. Cognitive dysfunction was identified in 4 of the 54 patients (7.4%, 95% confidence interval [CI] 2.1% to 17.9%) in the OPCAB group and 5 of the 51 patients (9.8%, 95% CI 3.3% to 21.4%) in the CCAB group. We found no difference in incidence of cognitive dysfunction between the groups regardless of the definition applied.

*Conclusions.*—In elderly high-risk patients, no significant difference was found in the incidence of cognitive dysfunction 3 months after either OPCAB or CCAB.

▶ The results of this study come somewhat as a disappointment in that what one might have expected that OPCAB might have resulted in less cognitive dysfunction than CCAB. Although the number of patients is quite small, this study was adequately powered to detect a difference. Fortunately, however, the incidence of cognitive dysfunction is quite low, although by no means negligible, in both groups (7.4% to 9.8%) given the mean age of the study population of 76 ± 4.5 years. This is substantially less than has been quoted in some other prior studies.[1]

With modern techniques such as diffusion-weighted MRI, it appears that cerebral emboli are the major cause of brain injury during cardiac surgery, even in patients without overt evidence of stroke.[2] Watershed or border zone lesions caused by cerebral hypoperfusion secondary to hypotension are uncommon. This study shows that the majority of emboli cannot be caused by cardiopulmonary bypass, and it is likely that manipulation of the aorta and great vessels is the major culprit, resulting in the release of microemboli. As was pointed out in the editorial by Samuels, cardiac surgery can be likened to a stress test for cerebral reserve, and patients with preexisting cerebrovascular disease are the most vulnerable to cognitive dysfunction postoperatively.

Whether approaches such as sutureless anastomoses and others that may reduce aortic manipulation will lead to a deduction in the incidence of cognitive dysfunction remains to be seen. It is also possible that patient selection can be improved by the use of preoperative cognitive function testing and brain imaging methods. Fortunately, OPCAB surgery is not the solution.

**B. J. Gersh, MB, ChB, DPhil, FRCP**

*References*

1. Kirchner JL, Phillips-Bute B, et al: Longitudinal assessment of neurocognitive function after coronary-artery bypass surgery. *N Engl J Med* 344:395-402, 2001.
2. Samuels MA: Can cognition survive heart surgery [editorial]? *Circulation* 113:2784-1786, 2006.

## Comparison of Cardiovascular Risk of Noncardiac Surgery Following Coronary Angioplasty With Versus Without Stenting

Leibowitz D, Cohen M, Planer D, et al (Hadassah Univ Hosps of Mount Scopus and Ein Kerem, Jerusalem; Kaplan Med Ctr, Rehovot, Israel)
Am J Cardiol 97:1188-1191, 2006                                                    4–28

Previous studies have shown a high incidence of cardiovascular complications when noncardiac surgery (NCS) is performed after coronary stenting. No study has compared the outcomes of NCS after stenting compared with percutaneous transluminal coronary angioplasty (PTCA) alone. The records of all patients who underwent NCS within 3 months of percutaneous coronary intervention at our institution were reviewed for adverse clinical events with the end points of acute myocardial infarction, major bleeding, and death ≤6 months after NCS. A total of 216 consecutive patients were included in the study. Of these, 122 (56%) underwent PTCA and 94 (44%) underwent stenting. A total of 26 patients (12%) died, 13 in the stent group (14%) and 13 in the PTCA group (11%), a nonsignificant difference. The incidence of acute myocardial infarction and major bleeding was 7% and 16% in the stent group and 6% and 13% in the PTCA group (p = NS), respectively. Significantly more events occurred in the 2 groups when NCS was performed within 2 weeks of percutaneous coronary intervention. In conclusion, our study has demonstrated high rates of perioperative morbidity and mortality after NCS in patients undergoing PTCA alone, as well as stenting. These findings support the current guidelines regarding the risk of NCS after stenting but suggest they be extended to PTCA as well (Fig 2).

▶ The issue of the appropriate timing of NCS after prior revascularization is characterized by a paucity of data, and most of what we have emanates from small studies.[1,2] One large randomized trial designed to assess the impact of preoperative coronary revascularization in patients undergoing vascular surgery demonstrated no differences in death or perioperative events.[3] The conclusions of this trial were, however, limited in their generalizability, in that randomization was only performed after coronary angiography, with the results of

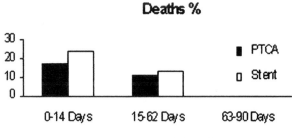

FIGURE 2.—Timing of perioperative death. (Courtesy of Leibowitz D, Cohen M, Planer D, et al: Comparison of cardiovascular risk of noncardiac surgery following coronary angioplasty with versus without stenting. Am J Cardiol 97:1188-1191. Copyright Elsevier 2006.)

this study confined to patients in whom the coronary anatomy and symptoms status were such that it was considered ethical to randomize to a strategy of revascularization versus no revascularization.

Recent reports have documented a high incidence of complications after NCS within 6 weeks of coronary stenting. After PTCA alone, several studies have demonstrated the relatively low rate of complications, particularly if the procedure was performed at least 2 weeks after percutaneous coronary intervention.[4,5]

This Israeli study makes several points. The mortality is relatively high, particularly in patients undergoing surgery within 2 weeks of percutaneous coronary intervention and in patients with left ventricular dysfunction. A limitation of this nonrandomized study, however, is the low rate of β-blocker use and, in the stent group, a rather low rate of thienopyridine use, presumably because of concerns regarding bleeding. Moreover, the study by and large antedates the use of drug-eluting stents.

Nonetheless, one comes away with the conclusion that the performance of NCS in a patient with coronary artery disease is *not* in itself an indication for coronary revascularization. A decision to perform the latter is based upon the standard indications—for example, the severity of symptoms or ischemia, and left ventricular dysfunction in the coronary anatomy. A noncardiac surgical procedure may affect the timing of coronary revascularization but is *not* the indication. We need a large randomized, controlled trial in which patients are randomized before the performance of angiography. A clinically relevant issue in patients with stable coronary disease is whether all should undergo preoperative stress testing, taking into account the cascade of events that often follows a positive test as opposed to a strategy of intensive perioperative monitoring including the use of β-blockers and statin therapy.

**B. J. Gersh, MB, ChB, DPhil, FRCP**

*References*

1. Kaluza GL, Joseph J, Lee JR, et al: Catastrophic outcomes of noncardiac surgery soon after coronary stenting. *J Am Coll Cardiol* 35:1288-1294, 2002.
2. Wilson SH, Fasseas P, Orford JL, et al: Clinical outcome of patients undergoing non-cardiac surgery in the two months following coronary stenting. *J Am Coll Cardiol* 42:234-240, 2003.
3. McFalls EO, Ward HB, Moritz TE, et al: Coronary-artery revascularization before elective major vascular surgery. *N Engl J Med* 351:2795-2804, 2004.
4. Brilakis ES, Orford JL, Faaseas P, et al: Outcome of patients undergoing balloon angioplasty in the two months prior to noncardiac surgery. *Am J Cardiol* 96:512-514, 2005.
5. Hassan SA, Hlatky MA, Boothroyd DB, et al: Outcomes of noncardiac surgery after coronary bypass surgery or coronary angioplasty in the Bypass Angioplasty Revascularization Investigation (BARI). *Am J Med* 110:260-266, 2001.

### Post-Reperfusion Myocardial Infarction: Long-Term Survival Improvement Using Adenosine Regulation With Acadesine

Mangano DT, for the Investigators of the Multicenter Study of Perioperative Ischemia (McSPI) Research Group and the Ischemia Research and Education Found (IREF) (Ischemia Research and Education Found (IREF), San Bruno, Calif)

*J Am Coll Cardiol* 48:206-214, 2006                                    4–29

*Objectives.*—The purpose of this study was to assess the safety and efficacy of the adenosine regulating agent (ARA) acadesine for reducing long-term mortality among patients with post-reperfusion myocardial infarction (MI).

*Background.*—No prospectively applied therapy exists that improves long-term survival after MI associated with coronary artery bypass graft (CABG) surgery—a robust model of ischemia/reperfusion injury. Pretreatment with the purine nucleoside autocoid adenosine mitigates the extent of post-ischemic reperfusion injury in animal models. Therefore, we questioned whether use of the ARA acadesine—by increasing interstitial adenosine concentrations in ischemic tissue—would improve long-term survival after post-reperfusion MI.

*Methods.*—At 54 institutions, 2,698 patients undergoing CABG surgery were randomized to receive placebo (n = 1,346) or acadesine (n = 1,352) by intravenous infusion (0.1 mg/kg/min; 7 h) and in cardioplegia solution (placebo or acadesine; 5 μg/ml). Myocardial infarction was prospectively defined as: 1) new Q-wave and MB isoform of creatine kinase (CK-MB) elevation (daily electrocardiography; 16 serial CK-MB measurements); or 2)

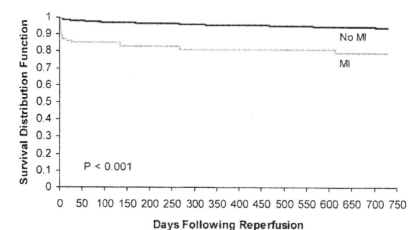

FIGURE 2.—Kaplan-Meier analysis of 2-year survival according to with or without postoperative myocardial infarction (MI) among the 2,698 study patients. (Reprinted with permission from the American College of Cardiology from Mangano DT, for the Investigators of the Multicenter Study of Perioperative Ischemia (McSPI) Research Group and the Ischemia Research and Education Foundation (IREF): Post-reperfusion myocardial infarction: Long-term survival improvement using adenosine regulation with acadesine. *J Am Coll Cardiol* 48:206-214. Copyright Elsevier, 2006.)

**B**

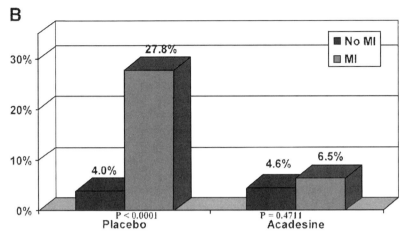

FIGURE 3.—Two-year mortality by-MI and by-treatment. (Reprinted with permission from the American College of Cardiology from Mangano DT, for the Investigators of the Multicenter Study of Perioperative Ischemia (McSPI) Research Group and the Ischemia Research and Education Foundation (IREF): Post-reperfusion myocardial infarction: Long-term survival improvement using adenosine regulation with acadesine. *J Am Coll Cardiol* 48:206-214. Copyright Elsevier, 2006.)

autopsy evidence. Vital status was assessed over 2 years, and outcomes were adjudicated centrally.

*Results.*—Perioperative MI occurred in 100 patients (3.7%), conferring a 4.2-fold increase in 2-year mortality (p < 0.001) compared with those not suffering MI. Acadesine treatment, however, reduced that mortality by 4.3-fold, from 27.8% (15 of 54; placebo) to 6.5% (3 of 46; acadesine) (p = 0.006), with the principal benefit occurring over the first 30 days after MI. The acadesine benefit was similar among diverse subsets, and multivariable analysis confirmed these findings.

*Conclusions.*—Acadesine is the first therapy proven to be effective for reducing the severity of acute post-reperfusion MI, substantially reducing the risk of dying over the 2 years after infarction (Figs 2 and 3).

▶ The entity of microvascular dysfunction after apparently successful reperfusion of the infarct-related artery is well delineated and common. Reperfusion injury, which implies additional injury to myocytes as a consequence of the reperfusion process per se is more controversial and its clinical relevance is the subject of considerable debate.[1] Irrespective, despite a large agenda of agents that have been shown to be successful in the experimental model, clinical trial results have been extremely disappointing. One explanation may be in the timing of therapy, which is often administered preocclusion in the experimental model of ischemia and reperfusion, whereas this is not possible in the clinical scenario of evolving myocardial infarction. It may well be that even potentially effective agents lose their beneficial impact if given 2 to 3 hours post occlusion, at a time when the majority of patients present for therapy.

This is a particularly interesting study in that adenosine, which targets a broad spectrum of the pathophysiology of ischemia-reperfusion injury, was administered 15 minutes before anesthesia and well before the processes of ischemia and reperfusion occurring during cardiopulmonary bypass. The results are impressive and certainly consistent with an effect on ischemic precondition leading to a reduction in infarct size and improvement in mortality.[2] This would also explain the relative lack of benefit when adenosine was given as an adjunct to reperfusion therapy but well after the onset of ischemia in the setting of acute myocardial infarction.[3]

This large trial is encouraging in that it appears to be one of the very few, if not the first, that demonstrates a clear and apparently clear clinical benefit for an agent aimed at modifying ischemia-reperfusion injury. The problem is, how can we translate this into the clinical setting of acute myocardial infarction given that the majority of patients present 2 to 3 hours after symptom onset because it is almost impossible to visualize a scenario in which the drug is given at the time of the onset of ischemia or myocardial infarction? In any event, reperfusion occurring that early in the infarct process is associated with such a low mortality rate and levels of necrosis that it would be almost impossible to demonstrate a benefit even if the agents were effective. This remains a field of great interest, but it certainly has its share of frustration.

**B. J. Gersh, MB, ChB, DPhil, FRCP**

*References*

1. Kloner RA, Jennings RV: Consequences of brief ischemia: Stunning, preconditioning, and their clinical implications: Part I. *Circulation* 104:2981-2989, 2001.
2. Gottlieb RA, Gruol DL, Zhu JY, et al: Preconditioning in rabbit cardiomyocytes role of pH, vacuolar proton ATPase, and apoptosis. *J Clin Invest* 97:2391-2398, 1996.
3. Ross AM, Gibbons RJ, Stone GW, et al: A randomized, double-blinded, placebo-controlled multicenter trial of adenosine as an adjunct to reperfusion in the treatment of acute myocardial infarction (AMISTAD-II). *J Am Coll Cardiol* 45:1775-1780, 2005.

## A Total of 1,007 Percutaneous Coronary Interventions Without Onsite Cardiac Surgery: Acute and Long-Term Outcomes

Ting HH, Raveendran G, Lennon RJ, et al (Mayo Clinic, Rochester, Minn)
*J Am Coll Cardiol* 47:1713-1721, 2006                                     4–30

*Objectives.*—We sought to compare clinical outcomes of elective percutaneous coronary intervention (PCI) and primary PCI for ST-segment elevation myocardial infarction (STEMI) at a community hospital without onsite cardiac surgery to those at a tertiary center with onsite cardiac surgery.

*Background.*—Disagreement exists about whether hospitals with cardiac catheterization laboratories, but without onsite cardiac surgery, should develop PCI programs. Primary PCI for STEMI at hospitals without onsite cardiac surgery have achieved satisfactory outcomes; however, elective PCI outcomes are not well defined.

*Methods.*—A total of 1,007 elective PCI and primary PCI procedures performed from March 1999 to August 2005 at the Immanuel St. Joseph's

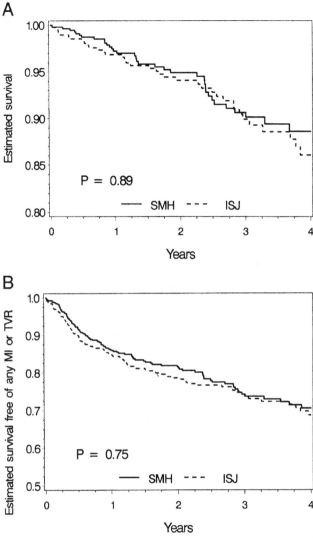

**FIGURE 1.**—Kaplan-Meier curves relating treatment location to (**A**) survival and to (**B**) freedom from recurrent myocardial infarction (MI) or target vessel revascularization (TVR) for matched patients undergoing elective percutaneous coronary intervention. ISJ = Immanuel St. Joseph's Hospital–Mayo Health System; SMH = St. Mary's Hospital. (Courtesy of Ting HH, Raveendran G, Lennon RJ, et al: A total of 1,007 percutaneous coronary interventions without onsite cardiac surgery: Acute and long-term outcomes. *J Am Coll Cardiol* 47:1713-1721. Copyright 2006 Elsevier.)

Hospital-Mayo Health System (ISJ) in Mankato, Minnesota, were matched one-to-one with those performed at St. Mary's Hospital (SMH) in Rochester, Minnesota. Strict protocols were followed for case selection and PCI program requirements. Clinical outcomes (in-hospital procedural success, death, any myocardial infarction, Q-wave myocardial infarction, and emergency coronary artery bypass surgery) and follow-up survival were compared between groups.

*Results.*—Among 722 elective PCIs, procedural success was 97% at ISJ compared with 95% at SMH (p = 0.046). Among 285 primary PCIs for STEMI, procedural success was 93% at ISJ and 96% at SMH (p = 0.085). No patients at ISJ undergoing PCI required emergent transfer for cardiac surgery. Survival at two years' follow-up by treatment location was similar for patients with elective PCI and primary PCI.

*Conclusions.*—Similar clinical outcomes for elective PCI and primary PCI were achieved at a community hospital without onsite cardiac surgery compared with those at a tertiary center with onsite cardiac surgery using a prospective, rigorous protocol for case selection and PCI program requirements (Fig 1).

▶ More than 1 million PCIs are performed annually in the United States. Irrespective of whether this number is considered to be the consequence of overutilization, the fact remains that procedural success rates have increased, complications have been reduced, and emergency coronary bypass surgery is a rare event. The expansion of PCI to community hospitals without onsite surgical backup is a controversial issue to say the least.[1] Current American College of Cardiology/American Heart Association guidelines grade elective PCI in the absence of cardiac surgical onsite backup as a class III indication (ie, not indicated), and a IIb indication when performed in patients with acute STEMI.[2]

This large study of 2 hospitals within a single health care system compared outcomes for elective and primary PCI in a community hospital without onsite surgical backup, with those obtained at a large referral center. The results are gratifying and support the hypothesis that PCI procedures can be performed safely in the absence of onsite surgical backup. No patient required emergency transfer for coronary bypass surgery. The key to these results, however, lies in the details. The community hospital program was developed systematically and involved cross-training and cross-credentialing of all operators, a telemedicine link for consultation, and strict protocols for case selection and PCI case requirements.

The expansion of PCI procedures to their performance in smaller community hospitals is not without its dangers and raises questions about overutilization. Nonetheless, this does have the potential to improve access to care for patients living in medically underserved regions or among those with geographic or other socioeconomic impediments to care at a large referral center. Patient preference may also be a factor, particularly in some rural areas.

It is imperative, however, that any institutions embarking upon this approach ensure that this is protocol-based and subject to regular and meticulous audit of their own results. Relying on a published series from other institutions could be a serious mistake.

**B. J. Gersh, MB, ChB, DPhil, FRCP**

*References*

1. Singh M, Ting HH, Berger PB, et al: Rationale for onsite cardiac surgery for primary angioplasty: A time for reappraisal. *J Am Coll Cardiol* 39:1881-1889, 2002.
2. Smith SC, Feldman TE, Hirshfeld JW, et al: ACC/AHA/SCAI 2005 guideline update for percutaneous coronary intervention. *J Am Coll Cardiol* 47:216-235, 2006.

## Percutaneous Treatment With Drug-Eluting Stent Implantation Versus Bypass Surgery for Unprotected Left Main Stenosis: A Single-Center Experience

Chieffo A, Morici N, Maisano F, et al (San Raffaele Scientific Inst, Milan, Italy; Univ of Milan, Italy)
*Circulation* 113:2542-2547, 2006                   4–31

*Background.*—Improvements in results with percutaneous coronary intervention (PCI) with drug-eluting stents (DES) may extend their use in patients with left main coronary artery (LMCA) stenosis.

*Method and Results.*—Two hundred forty-nine patients with LMCA stenosis were treated with PCI and DES implantation (n=107) or coronary artery bypass grafting (CABG) (n=142), in a single center, between March 2002 and July 2004. A propensity analysis was performed to adjust for baseline differences between the two cohorts. At 1 year, there was no statistical difference in the occurrence of death in PCI versus CABG both for the unadjusted (OR=0.291; 95% CI=0.054 to 1.085; $P$=0.0710) and adjusted analyses (OR=0.331; 95% CI=0.055 to 1.404; $P$=0.1673). PCI was correlated to a lower occurrence of the composite end points of death and myocardial infarction (unadjusted OR=0.235; 95% CI=0.048 to 0.580; $P$=0.0002; adjusted OR=0.260; 95% CI=0.078 to 0.597; $P$=0.0005) and death, myocardial infarction, and cerebrovascular events (unadjusted OR=0.300; 95% CI=0.102 to 0.617; $P$=0.0004; adjusted OR=0.385; 95% CI=0.180 to 0.819; $P$=0.01). No difference was detected in the occurrence of major adverse cardiac and cerebrovascular event at the unadjusted (OR=0.675; 95% CI=0.371 to 1.189; $P$=0.1891) and adjusted analyses (OR=0.568; 95% CI=0.229 to 1.344; $P$=0.2266).

*Conclusions.*—At 1 year, in this single-center, retrospective experience, there was no difference in the degree of protection against death, stroke, myocardial infarction, and revascularization between PCI with DES and CABG for LMCA disease.

▶ The role of coronary revascularization for LMCA disease was established approximately 30 years ago by the Veterans' Administration trial of coronary bypass surgery versus medical therapy.[1] Current guidelines recommend surgical revascularization for this disorder,[2] since technical limitations, stent thrombosis, and restenosis pose formidable challenges for the strategy of PCI. Nonetheless, preliminary results in selected cases have been somewhat promising.[3]

The availability of drug-eluting stenting has altered the playing field and certainly has renewed interest in a percutaneous approach to LMCA disease. This single-center, 1-year follow-up study demonstrates no difference in rates of death, stroke, and myocardial infarction, although there is a high rate of repeat revascularization of the drug-eluting stenting versus coronary bypass surgery.

The major limitation is the short follow-up and the fact that this is a nonrandomized study, which is subject to all the imperfections of selection bias. No amount of statistical adjustment can fully compensate for the impact of confounding variables. The ongoing Synergy between Percutaneous Intervention with TAXUS and Cardiac Surgery (SYNTAX) trial will include 1800 patients with either LMCA or triple-vessel disease, and has extended follow-up for at least 5 years. This trial should provide conclusive information about the optimal treatment of LMCA disease. Nonetheless, an accompanying editorial discusses many of the technical limitations of LMCA stenting, including the problem of bifurcation as stenoses.[4] If ongoing technical developments result in the availability of DES, which are designed specifically for branch vessel application, this could increase the reliability of percutaneous revascularization strategies in the setting of LMCA and other vessel disease and, to some extent, may reduce the clinical impact of ongoing trials including SYNTAX. Another issue that will have to be resolved is the optimal antiplatelet therapeutic strategy in patients with DES. As stated in the editorial, at this point in time revascularization for LMCA disease is perhaps really at the crossroads.

**B. J. Gersh, MB, ChB, DPhil, FRCP**

*References*

1. Takaro T, Hultgren HN, Lipton MJ, et al: VA-Cooperative randomized study of surgery for coronary arterial occlusive disease: II. Subgroup with significant main lesions. *Circulation* 54:III107S-III117S, 1976.
2. Eagle KA, Guyton RA, Davidoff R, et al: ACC/AHA 2004 Guidelines updates for coronary artery bypass graft surgery. *Circulation* 110:1168-1176, 2004.
3. Ellis SG, Tamai H, Nobuyoshi M, et al: Contemporary percutaneous treatment of unprotected left main coronary stenosis: Initial results from a multicenter registry analysis 1994-1996. *Circulation* 96:3867-3872, 1997.
4. Kereiakes DJ, Faxon DP: Left main coronary revascularization at the crossroads (editorial). *Circulation* 113:2480-2484, 2006.

---

**Effect of Clopidogrel Premedication in Off-Pump Cardiac Surgery: Are We Forfeiting the Benefits of Reduced Hemorrhagic Sequelae?**
Kapetanakis EI, Medlam DA, Petro KR, et al (Washington Hosp Ctr, DC; MedStar Research Inst, Washington, DC)
*Circulation* 113:1667-1674, 2006                                                    4–32

---

*Background.*—Premedication with clopidogrel has reduced thrombotic complications after percutaneous coronary revascularization procedures. However, because of the enhanced and irreversible platelet inhibition by clopidogrel, patients requiring surgical revascularization have a higher risk of bleeding complications and transfusion requirements. A principal benefit of surgical coronary revascularization without cardiopulmonary bypass is its lower hemorrhagic sequelae. The purpose of this study was to evaluate the effect of preoperative clopidogrel administration in the incidence of hemostatic reexploration, blood product transfusion rates, morbidity, and mortality in patients undergoing off-pump coronary artery bypass graft surgery using a large patient sample and a risk-adjusted approach.

*Method and Results.*—Two hundred eighty-one patients (17.9%) did and 1291 (82.1%) did not receive clopidogrel before their surgery, for a total of 1572 patients undergoing isolated off-pump coronary artery bypass graft surgery between January 2000 and June 2002. Risk-adjusted logistic regression analyses and a matched pair analyses by propensity scores were used to assess the association between clopidogrel administration and reoperation as a result of bleeding, intraoperative and postoperative blood transfusions received, and the need for multiple transfusions. Hemorrhage-related preoperative risk factors identified in the literature and those found significant in a univariate model were used. The clopidogrel group had a higher likelihood of hemostatic reoperations (odds ratio [OR], 5.1; 95% confidence interval [CI], 2.47 to 10.47; $P<0.01$) and an increased need in overall packed red blood cell (OR, 2.6; 95% CI, 1.94 to 3.60; $P<0.01$), multiple unit (OR, 1.6; 95% CI, 1.07 to 2.48; $P=0.02$), and platelet (OR, 2.5; 95% CI, 1.77 to 3.66; $P<0.01$) transfusions. Surgical outcomes and operative mortality (1.4% versus 1.4%; $P=1.00$) were not statistically different.

*Conclusions.*—Clopidogrel administration in the cardiology suite increases the risk for hemostatic reoperation and the requirements for blood product transfusions during and after off-pump coronary artery bypass graft surgery.

▶ This large single-center study has the advantage of comparing patients undergoing coronary bypass surgery with and without cardiopulmonary bypass. This confirms prior reports of significant increased bleeding after cardiac surgery within 15 days of taking clopidogrel.[1,2]

Although perioperative mortality was not increased in this study, clopidogrel had a substantial unfavorable impact upon reoperation rates for bleeding (approximately 5-fold increase) and the transfusion of blood products. This was noted in patients undergoing conventional cardiopulmonary bypass as well as off-pump cardiac surgery.

This places us squarely on a whole new clinical dilemma. Prior large trials of patients with acute coronary syndromes have unequivocally documented the efficacy of clopidogrel. There appears to be an incremental benefit of the drug if given before the procedure.[3,4] However, in the event that the patient requires bypass surgery, the price to be paid is either a substantially increased rate of bleeding or postponement of surgery for at least 5 days. One approach, therefore, is to use 2B/3A inhibitors pre-procedure and hold off clopidogrel until the coronary anatomy is known.

The other is to recognize that in the current era, emergency or urgent coronary artery bypass grafting (CABG) is a relatively uncommon event. Perhaps there is a role for clinical judgment based upon an estimate of the likelihood of CABG (eg, in patients who are elderly, diabetics, prior myocardial infarction, a

history of prior chronic angina, impaired ejection fraction or transient congestive heart failure, and marked ST-segment depression on ECGs). All of these
are strong predictors of multivessel disease, and in such patients, it would be
prudent to accept the increased risk of events by not administering clopidogrel
and to proceed with angiography as soon as possible. For the remainder and
given the likelihood of a percutaneous coronary intervention is high, it would
be reasonable to administer clopidogrel before the procedure; and in this situation, preprocedural 2B/3A inhibitors or bivalirudin might be beneficial.

**B. J. Gersh, MB, ChB, DPhil, FRCP**

*References*

1. Fox KA, Mehta SR, Peters R, et al: Benefits and risks of the combination of
   clopidogrel and aspirin in patients undergoing surgical revascularization for
   non-ST elevation acute coronary syndrome: The Clopidogrel in Unstable Angina to
   Prevent Recurrent Ischemic Events (CURE) trial. *Circulation* 110:1202-1208,
   2004.
2. Sabbatine MS, Cannon CP, Gibson CM, et al: Addition of clopidogrel to aspirin
   and fibrolytic therapy for myocardial infarction with ST segment elevation. *N Engl
   J Med* 352:1179-1189, 2005.
3. Yusuf S, Zhao F, Mehta SR, et al: Effects of clopidogrel in addition to aspirin in
   patients with acute coronary syndromes without ST segment elevation. *N Engl J
   Med* 345:494-502, 2001.
4. Steinhubl SR, Berger PB, Mann JT III, et al: Early and sustained dual oral antiplatelet therapy following percutaneous coronary intervention: A randomized controlled trial. *JAMA* 288:2411-2420, 2002.

## Impact of Completeness of Percutaneous Coronary Intervention Revascularization on Long-Term Outcomes in the Stent Era

Hannan EL, Racz M, Holmes DR, et al (State Univ of New York, Univ at Albany;
New York State Dept of Health, Albany; Mayo Clinic, Rochester, Minn; et al)
*Circulation* 113:2406-2412, 2006                                    4–33

*Background.*—The importance of completeness of revascularization by
percutaneous coronary intervention in patients with multivessel disease is
unclear in that there is little information on the impact of incomplete revascularization outside of randomized trials. The objective of this study is to
compare long-term mortality and subsequent revascularization for percutaneous coronary intervention patients receiving stents who were completely
revascularized (CR) with those who were incompletely revascularized (IR).

*Method and Results.*—Patients from New York State's Percutaneous Coronary Interventions Reporting System were subdivided into patients who
were CR and IR. Then subsets of IR patients were contrasted with CR patients. Differences in long-term survival and subsequent revascularization
for CR and IR patients were compared after adjustment for differences in
preprocedural risk. A total of 68.9% of all stent patients with multivessel
disease who were studied were IR, and 30.1% of all patients had total occlusions and/or ≥2 IR vessels. At baseline, the following patients were at higher
risk: those who were older and those with more comorbid conditions, worse

ejection fraction, and more renal disease and stroke. After adjustment for these baseline differences, IR patients were significantly more likely to die at any time (adjusted hazard ratio=1.15; 95% confidence interval, 1.01 to 1.30) than CR patients. IR patients with total occlusions and a total of ≥2 IR vessels were at the highest risk compared with CR patients (hazard ratio=1.36; 95% confidence interval, 1.12 to 1.66).

*Conclusions.*—IR with stenting is associated with an adverse impact on long-term mortality, and consideration should be given to either achieving CR, opting for surgery, or monitoring percutaneous coronary intervention patients with IR more closely after discharge.

▶ This study using the large New York State registry database between 1997 and 2000 addresses the perennial question of the completeness of revascularization upon outcome. Prior surgical series from an earlier era identified better long-term outcomes for patients who were CR versus IR. In one large registry study on patients with triple-vessel disease, there was a statistically significant difference in survival and event-free survival from CR, but the magnitude of the absolute difference and its clinical impact appeared to be small.[1]

The current study, which is confined to patients undergoing percutaneous coronary intervention with stenting, demonstrates an adverse effect of IR on mortality and makes a case for the more frequent use of coronary bypass surgery, more committed attempts to achieve CR with percutaneous coronary intervention, and more careful monitoring of patients who were IR. The problem with all the studies that aimed to address this issue are the multiple reasons underlying IR. In many situations, IR may be a surrogate for a "sicker" patient—for example, a patient with chronic total occlusion supplying an area of akinesis/scar; a patient with diffuse disease with poor distal vessels secondary to diabetes and older age; or a frail patient with renal dysfunction, limiting the length and scope of the procedure. In this analysis, the authors have attempted to adjust for these factors by performing risk-adjusted and propensity analyses and by excluding patients with a prior myocardial infarction. Nonetheless, no amount of statistical adjustment can get around the basic problem of whether IR is a direct cause of adverse outcomes or a consequence of other factors that drive prognosis.

From a clinical standpoint, CR is always a desirable goal, and judgment is needed. I would not use these data, however, to advocate for the more frequent use of coronary bypass surgery, although there are subsets of patients (eg, younger patients with diabetes) among whom CR with arterial grafts is an attractive option. An accompanying editorial appropriately draws attention to the problem of chronic total occlusions and calls for action for interventionists to improve their skills at opening chronically occluded arteries.[2]

**B. J. Gersh, MB, ChB, DPhil, FRCP**

*References*

1. Bell MR, Gersh BJ, Schaff HV: Effect of completeness of revascularization on long-term outcome in patients with three-vessel disease undergoing coronary artery bypass surgery: A report from the Coronary Artery Surgery Study (CASS) Registry. *Circulation* 86:446-457, 1992.
2. Teirstein PS: The dueling hazards of incomplete revascularization and incomplete data. *Circulation* 113:2380-2382, 2006.

---

### Geographical Differences in the Rates of Angiographic Restenosis and Ischemia-Driven Target Vessel Revascularization After Percutaneous Coronary Interventions: Results From the Prevention of Restenosis With Tranilast and its Outcomes (PRESTO) Trial

Singh M, Williams BA, Gersh BJ, et al (Mayo Clinic and Mayo Found, Rochester, Minn; Harvard Clinical Research Inst, Boston; Texas Heart Inst, Houston; et al)

*J Am Coll Cardiol* 47:34-39, 2006

4–34

---

*Objectives.*—This study assessed the geographical differences in target vessel revascularization (TVR) after percutaneous coronary intervention (PCI) in the Prevention of Restenosis With Tranilast and its Outcomes (PRESTO) trial.

*Background.*—An aggressive approach to PCI is more common in the U.S. than in other countries. The impact of this approach on restenosis outcomes has not been studied.

*Methods.*—Using the PRESTO trial, we compared nine-month ischemic TVR after PCI in U.S.-treated patients (n = 5,026) with rates in other countries (n = 6,458). We defined TVR as repeat intervention for chest pain/positive stress test. Additionally, angiographic restenosis (>50% narrowing or >50% loss of gain at nine-month follow-up) was compared between U.S. and non-U.S. patients within the prespecified angiographic subset (n = 2,823). Regression models were developed to adjust for clinical and lesion-related characteristics.

*Results.*—Higher rates of TVR (18% vs. 11%), and angiographic restenosis (65% vs. 48%) were observed in patients treated in the U.S. as compared with the other patients (p < 0.01 for both comparisons). Patients treated in the U.S. were more likely to be female, diabetic, not currently smoking, to have unstable angina, and to have a prior PCI. In U.S. patients, lesions tended to be longer, but less likely to be American College of Cardiology/American Heart Association class C. After adjusting for clinical and angiographic variables, PCI in the U.S. was still associated with increased angiographic restenosis and ischemic TVR.

*Conclusions.*—Angiographic restenosis and ischemia-driven TVR rates were higher in patients treated in the U.S. The difference could only partially be explained by the higher prevalence of measured adverse clinical and angiographic features.

▶ The Prevention of Restenosis with Tranilast and its Outcomes (PRESTO) Trial is the largest published trial of restenosis and an important resource for information on clinical and angiographic outcomes in patients undergoing a PCI (percutaneous coronary intervention) in the current area (although this does antedate the use of drug eluting stents). Of the 11,484 patients, 44% were treated in the United States and the remainder in Western Europe, Canada, Eastern Europe, Australia, and South Africa. This provides an ideal international perspective for comparison of angiographic rates of restenosis and ischemia-driven target vessel revascularization (TVR) in patients treated in the United States and in other countries.

Rates of TVR vary considerably from a low of 4% in Estonia and the Czech Republic to a high of 16% in Germany and 18% in the United States. Nonetheless, rates of angiographic restenosis were also highest in the United States, suggesting that the increased rates of TVR are driven by factors other than economics and practice tactics.

To some extent, the increased rates of restenosis and TVR in patients treated in the United States may be related to the increased frequency of baseline angiographic variables, which have been shown to indicate higher risk in prior studies.[1] That the international differences continue to exist after multivariable adjustment may simply be a function of the limited discriminatory power of statistical models in identifying restenotic events.[2]

Another explanation may lie in the greater proportion of patients in the United States with unstable angina plus the earlier performance of PCI in the United States in comparison with the non-US sites. A prior study has shown a relationship between earlier revascularization after the onset of symptoms and repeat revascularization in patients with acute coronary syndromes.[3]

In summary, these interesting differences are not fully explained by the data from this trial. This is certainly an area that warrants further studies.

**B. J. Gersh, MB, ChB, DPhil, FRCP**

*References*

1. Mercado N, Boersma E, Wijns W, et al: Clinical and quantitative coronary angiographic predictors of coronary restenosis: A comparative analysis from the balloon-to-stent era. *J Am Coll Cardiol* 38:645-652, 2001.
2. Singh M, Gersh BJ, McClelland RL, et al: Clinical and angiographic predictors of restenosis after percutaneous coronary intervention: Insights from the Prevention of Restenosis With Tranilast and Its Outcomes (PRESTO) trial. *Circulation* 109:2727-2731, 2004.
3. Ronner E, Boersma E, Laarman GJ, et al: Early angioplasty in acute coronary syndromes without persistent ST-segment elevation improves outcome but increases in the need for six-month repeat revascularization: An analysis of the PURSUIT trial: Platelet glycoprotein IIB/IIIA in Unstable angina: Receptor Suppression Using Integrilin Therapy. *J Am Coll Cardiol* 39:1924-1929, 2002.

## Clinical Pharmacology

**NSAID use and the risk of hospitalization for first myocardial infarction in the general population: a nationwide case–control study from Finland**
Helin-Salmivaara A, Virtanen A, Vesalainen R, et al (Univ of Turku, Helsinki; Social Insurance Inst, Turku, Finland; Turku Univ Hosp, Finland; et al)
*Eur Heart J* 27:1657-1663, 2006                                                    4–35

*Aims.*—To evaluate the risk of first myocardial infarction (MI) associated with the use of various non-steroidal anti-inflammatory drugs (NSAIDs) in the general population.

*Method and Results.*—We conducted a population-based matched case-control study over the years 2000–3 in outpatient residents of Finland. In the nationwide Hospital Discharge Register 33 309 persons with first time MI were identified. A total of 138 949 controls individually matched for age, gender, hospital catchment area, and index day were selected from the Population Register. For combined NSAIDs, the adjusted odds ratio for the risk of first MI with current use was 1.40 (95% CI, 1.33–1.48). The risk was similar for conventional (1.34; 1.26–1.43), semi-selective (etodolac, nabumetone, nimesulide, and meloxicam) (1.50; 1.32–1.71), and cyclo-oxygenase-2 (COX-2) selective NSAIDs (rofecoxib, celecoxib, valdecoxib, and etoricoxib) (1.31; 1.13–1.50). Age of current user did not consistently modify the risk. No NSAID was associated with an MI-protective effect. All durations from 1 to 180 days of conventional NSAIDs and from 31 to 90 days duration of COX-2 selective NSAIDs were associated with an elevated risk of MI.

*Conclusion.*—Current use of all NSAIDs is associated with a modest risk of first time MI.

▶ This population-based study from Finland of 3309 patients is the largest case-controlled study of NSAIDs to date. Aspirin has been shown unequivocally to reduce MI in patients with established coronary artery disease. Literature on the cardiovascular effects of NSAIDs, excluding the Coxibs, has been conflicting, and in regard to the COX-2 inhibitors, this is an area that has been controversial to say the least.[1]

This study strongly suggests an approximately 40% increase in risk of a first MI, with a similar increase in risk noted for conventional NSAIDs as well as for COX-2 inhibitors. Moreover, the increasing likelihood of adverse effects in association with a shorter duration of NSAID discontinuation and heavy NSAID use in the prior year is supportive of a causal relationship. This is a very complex area that could be made even more complex if the pharmacologic interactions between aspirin and ibuprofen or naproxen are indeed clinically relevant.[2]

Studies such as this have many limitations but are nonetheless a useful adjunct to the literature. These data certainly suggest that all NSAIDs have the potential to help in many ways but also to cause harm. An extensive body of evidence suggests that NSAIDs and COX-2 inhibitors may be beneficial, harmful, or neutral, and to explore these reasons a clinical trial is both needed and ethical. Recently, the Prospective Randomized Evaluation of Celecoxib Integrated Safety versus Ibuprofen or Naproxen (PRECISION) trial has been launched.[3] This trial will enroll approximately 20,000 patients with osteoarthritis or rheumatoid arthritis who either have cardiovascular disease or are at high risk of it, and the end points will be rates of cardiovascular death, MI, or stroke. Both aspirin users and nonusers will be included, and additional end points will be gastrointestinal and renal safety as well as arthritis effects. Potentially and hopefully, this pilot trial will settle the question of the optimal therapy for pain relief in patients with degenerative or rheumatoid arthritis. The results will be of interest to patients and physicians encompassing many disciplines.

**B. J. Gersh, MB, ChB, DPhil, FRCP**

*References*

1. Mukherjee D, Nissen SE, Topol EJ: Risk of cardiovascular events associated with the selective COX-II inhibitors. *JAMA* 2:954-959, 2001.
2. Capone ML, Sciull MG, Tacconelli S, et al: Pharmacodynamic interaction of naproxen with low-dose aspirin in healthy subjects. *J Am Coll Cardiol* 45:1295-1300, 2005.
3. Bhatt DL: NSAIDs and the risk of myocardial infarction: Do they help or harm? *Eur Heart J* 27:1635-1636, 2006.

---

**Clopidogrel and Aspirin versus Aspirin Alone for the Prevention of Atherothrombotic Events**
Bhatt DL, for the CHARISMA Investigators (Cleveland Clinic, Ohio; Univ and Royal Infirmary of Edinburgh, Scotland; Univ of Heidelberg, Germany; et al)
*N Engl J Med* 354:1706-1717, 2006                                      4–36

---

*Background.*—Dual antiplatelet therapy with clopidogrel plus low-dose aspirin has not been studied in a broad population of patients at high risk for atherothrombotic events.

*Methods.*—We randomly assigned 15,603 patients with either clinically evident cardiovascular disease or multiple risk factors to receive clopidogrel (75 mg per day) plus low-dose aspirin (75 to 162 mg per day) or placebo plus low-dose aspirin and followed them for a median of 28 months. The primary efficacy end point was a composite of myocardial infarction, stroke, or death from cardiovascular causes.

*Results.*—The rate of the primary efficacy end point was 6.8 percent with clopidogrel plus aspirin and 7.3 percent with placebo plus aspirin (relative risk, 0.93; 95 percent confidence interval, 0.83 to 1.05; P=0.22). The respective rate of the principal secondary efficacy end point, which included hospitalizations for ischemic events, was 16.7 percent and 17.9 percent (relative risk, 0.92; 95 percent confidence interval, 0.86 to 0.995; P=0.04), and the rate of severe bleeding was 1.7 percent and 1.3 percent (relative risk, 1.25; 95 percent confidence interval, 0.97 to 1.61 percent; P=0.09). The rate of the primary end point among patients with multiple risk factors was 6.6

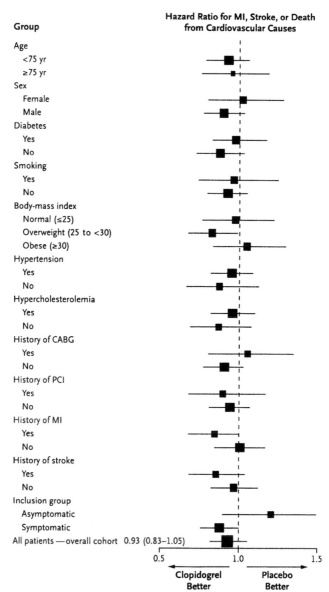

FIGURE 2.—Hazard Ratios for Myocardial Infarction (MI), Stroke, or Death from Cardiovascular Causes in Each of the Subgroups Examined. Hazard ratios are shown with their 95 percent confidence intervals. The sizes of the symbols are roughly proportional to the number of patients in the analysis. Body-mass index is the weight in kilograms divided by the square of the height in meters. CABG denotes coronary-artery bypass grafting, and PCI percutaneous coronary intervention. (Reprinted by permission of *The New England Journal of Medicine* from Bhatt DL, for the CHARISMA Investigators: Clopidogrel and aspirin versus aspirin alone for the prevention of atherothrombotic events. *N Engl J Med* 354:1706-1717, 2006. Copyright © 2006, Massachusetts Medical Society. All rights reserved.)

percent with clopidogrel and 5.5 percent with placebo (relative risk, 1.2; 95 percent confidence interval, 0.91 to 1.59; P=0.20) and the rate of death from cardiovascular causes also was higher with clopidogrel (3.9 percent vs. 2.2 percent, P=0.01). In the subgroup with clinically evident atherothrombosis, the rate was 6.9 percent with clopidogrel and 7.9 percent with placebo (relative risk, 0.88; 95 percent confidence interval, 0.77 to 0.998; P=0.046).

*Conclusions.*—In this trial, there was a suggestion of benefit with clopidogrel treatment in patients with symptomatic atherothrombosis and a suggestion of harm in patients with multiple risk factors. Overall, clopidogrel plus aspirin was not significantly more effective than aspirin alone in reducing the rate of myocardial infarction, stroke, or death from cardiovascular causes (Fig 2).

▶ This is a large, well-conducted but neutral trial comparing the combination of aspirin and clopidogrel versus aspirin alone in the secondary prevention of cardiovascular events in patients with either stable cardiovascular disease or multiple risk factors for cardiovascular disease. A prior trial has emphasized the benefits of clopidogrel as monotherapy in patients with chronic stable vascular disease.[1] Moreover, multiple trials have documented the benefits of clopidogrel or ticlopidine in patients with "acute vascular injury" such as ST-elevation myocardial infarction, coronary stenting, and non-ST-elevation acute coronary syndromes, and the benefits were not accompanied by increased rates of bleeding.[2]

The CHARISMA Trial was a logical extension to groups at lower risk with presumed "chronic vascular injury." Although there is a marginal benefit in patients with overt heart disease and a trend in favor of placebo in the "asymptomatic group," the significance of this is unclear and should be regarded as nothing more than hypothesis generating at this time. I agree with the editorial and the author's comment that such subgroup analysis can lead to inappropriate conclusions.

In summary, the addition of clopidogrel to aspirin in patients with stable vascular disease or in those with multiple risk factors should be avoided. Of course, there will be clinically driven exceptions, for example, multiple prior myocardial infarctions in patients with premature disease. Nonetheless, the avoidance of this treatment regimen on a routine basis will generate substantial cost savings.

**B. J. Gersh, MB, ChB, DPhil, FRCP**

*References*

1. CAPRIE Steering Committee: A randomized, blinded trial of Clopidogrel versus Aspirin in Patients at Risk of Ischaemic Events (CAPRIE). *Lancet* 348:1329-1339, 1996.
2. Pfeffer MA, Jarcho JA: The charisma of subgroups and the subgroups of CHARISMA. *N Engl J Med* DOI:10.1056/NEJMe068057. Available at http://www.nejm.org.

# Epidemiology

## Seasonality and Daily Weather Conditions in Relation to Myocardial Infarction and Sudden Cardiac Death in Olmsted County, Minnesota, 1979 to 2002

Gerber Y, Jacobsen SJ, Killian JM, et al (Mayo Clinic, Rochester, Minn)
*J Am Coll Cardiol* 48:287-292, 2006                                                4–37

*Objectives.*—We assessed the relationship of season and weather types with myocardial infarction (MI) and sudden cardiac death (SCD) in a geographically defined population, and tested the hypothesis that the increased risk in winter was related to weather.

*Background.*—Winter peaks in coronary heart disease (CHD) have been documented. Yet, it is uncertain if seasonality exists for both incident events and deaths, and the role of weather conditions is not clear.

*Methods.*—The daily occurrence of incident MI and SCD in Olmsted County was examined with data from the National Weather Service. Poisson regression models were used to assess the relative risks (RRs) associated with season and climatic variables. Subsequent analysis stratified SCD into those with and without antecedent CHD (unexpected SCD).

TABLE 2.—Standardized Rates and RRs (95% CI) of MI and SCD for Seasonal and Climatic Variables

| | | Incident MI | | SCD | |
|---|---|---|---|---|---|
| | Days | Rate* | RR (95% CI)† | Rate* | RR (95% CI)† |
| Season | | | | | |
| Fall | 2,184 | 5.18 | 1.02 (0.92-1.14) | 4.10 | 1.12 (0.99-1.27) |
| Winter | 2,190 | 5.32 | 1.04 (0.94-1.16) | 4.26 | 1.17 (1.03-1.32) |
| Spring | 2,208 | 5.36 | 1.06 (0.95-1.17) | 3.99 | 1.09 (0.97-1.24) |
| Summer | 2,184 | 5.06 | 1 (reference) | 3.66 | 1 (reference) |
| Temperature | | | | | |
| >30°C | 362 | 4.98 | 0.93 (0.76-1.14) | 3.67 | 1.02 (0.81-1.29) |
| 18°C-30°C | 3,220 | 5.21 | 1 (reference) | 3.83 | 1 (reference) |
| 0°C-17°C | 3,422 | 5.18 | 0.97 (0.89-1.06) | 3.92 | 1.05 (0.95-1.16) |
| <0°C | 1,762 | 5.43 | 1.03 (0.92-1.14) | 4.54 | 1.20 (1.07-1.35) |
| Rain‡ | | | | | |
| Heavy rain | 1,421 | 5.00 | 0.94 (0.85-1.05) | 3.92 | 0.97 (0.86-1.09) |
| Mild rain | 1,100 | 5.25 | 0.99 (0.88-1.11) | 3.87 | 0.95 (0.83-1.09) |
| No rain | 6,245 | 5.28 | 1 (reference) | 4.04 | 1 (reference) |
| Snow‡ | | | | | |
| Heavy snow | 384 | 5.37 | 1.02 (0.85-1.23) | 4.07 | 1.00 (0.81-1.24) |
| Mild snow | 633 | 5.47 | 1.04 (0.90-1.20) | 4.28 | 1.06 (0.90-1.25) |
| No snow | 7,749 | 5.20 | 1 (reference) | 3.98 | 1 (reference) |

*Rates per $10^6$ person-days are directly standardized to the age and gender distribution of the 2000 US population.

†The relative risks (95% confidence intervals [CI]) are derived from Poisson regression models adjusting for age, gender, year, and all other variables within each season or weather group.

‡Rain and snow categories are defined as follows (values represent daily amount in cm): heavy rain ≥0.25; mild rain 0.025 to <0.25; heavy snow ≥2.5; mild snow 0.25 to <2.5.

MI = myocardial infarction; RR = relative risk; SCD = sudden cardiac death.

(Courtesy of Gerber Y, Jacobsen SJ, Killian JM, et al: Seasonality and daily weather conditions in relation to myocardial infarction and sudden cardiac death in Olmsted County, Minnesota, 1979 to 2002. *J Am Coll Cardiol* 48:287-292. Copyright Elsevier 2006.)

*Results.*—Between 1979 and 2002, 2,676 MI and 2,066 SCD occurred. The age-, gender-, and year-adjusted RR of SCD, but not of MI, was increased in winter versus summer (1.17, 95% confidence interval [CI] 1.03 to 1.32) and in low temperatures (1.20, 95% CI 1.07 to 1.35, for temperatures below 0°C vs. 18°C to 30°C) (Table 2). These associations were stronger for unexpected SCD than for SCD with prior CHD (p < 0.05). After adjustment for all climatic variables, low temperature was associated with a large increase in the risk of unexpected SCD (RR = 1.38, 95% CI 1.10 to 1.73), while the association with winter declined (RR = 1.06, 95% CI 0.83 to 1.35).

*Conclusions.*—These data suggest that the winter peak in SCD can be accounted for by daily weather.

▶ This is a rather extraordinary article that utilizes the daily records from the National Weather Service to analyze the impact of seasonality and weather conditions on the incidence of SCD and MI in Olmsted County, Minnesota, from 1979 to 2002. A winter peak and summer nadir for CHD events is well documented and is being demonstrated among diverse populations in many countries.[1]

What this study adds is to distinguish between seasons and actual weather conditions, namely, rain, snow, and temperature. This community surveillance approach demonstrates a seasonal variation in SCD but not incident MI. Moreover, the SCD relationship is greatest among patients without a history of prior CHD, perhaps reflecting a greater degree of exposure among apparently healthy individuals, since coronary patients may have been advised against exposure to outdoor cold stress. After adjustment, it appears that the seasonal variation is primarily temperature dependent, and there are multiple plausible biological mechanisms that could be involved in the association between cold weather and SCD.[2]

The gender and SCD interactions are of interest in that heavy snow appears to increase the risk for SCD in men but not for women. Increased CHD mortality after snowfall has been demonstrated in other studies.[3] A possible explanation for the gender difference in this study could involve the acute exertion of snow shoveling shortly after a snowfall, in that one would expect that the majority of snow shoveling is carried out by men.

Although there are limitations to this study in that actual outdoor exposure to these conditions cannot be measured and the possibility that the associations may be due to other unmeasured cofounders, this study does suggest that the winter peak in SCD can be accounted for by lower temperatures and, perhaps in some situations, snow shoveling.

**B. J. Gersh, MB, ChB, DPhil, FRCP**

*References*

1. Kloner RA, Poole WK, Perritt RL: When throughout the year is coronary death most likely to occur? A 12-year population-based analysis of more than 220,000 cases. *Circulation* 100:1630-1634, 1999.

2. Kawahra J, Sano H, Fukuzaki H: Acute effects of the exposure to cold and blood pressure, platelet function and sympathetic nervous activity in humans. *Am J Hypertens* 2:724-726, 1989.

3. Baker-Blocker A: Winter weather and cardiovascular mortality in Minneapolis-Saint Paul. *Am J Public Health* 72:261-265, 1982.

### Coffee, CYP1A2 Genotype, and Risk of Myocardial Infarction

Cornelis MC, El-Sohemy A, Kabagambe EK, et al (Univ of Toronto; Harvard School of Public Health, Boston; Universidad de Costa Rica, San Pedro de Montes de Oca)

*JAMA* 295:1135-1141, 2006

*Context.*—The association between coffee intake and risk of myocardial infarction (MI) remains controversial. Coffee is a major source of caffeine, which is metabolized by the polymorphic cytochrome P450 1A2 (CYP1A2) enzyme. Individuals who are homozygous for the *CYP1A2\*1A* allele are "rapid" caffeine metabolizers, whereas carriers of the variant *CYP1A2\*1F* are "slow" caffeine metabolizers.

*Objective.*—To determine whether CYP1A2 genotype modifies the association between coffee consumption and risk of acute nonfatal MI.

*Design, Setting, and Participants.*—Cases (n = 2014) with a first acute nonfatal MI and population-based controls (n = 2014) living in Costa Rica between 1994 and 2004, matched for age, sex, and area of residence, were genotyped by restriction fragment-length polymorphism polymerase chain reaction. A food frequency questionnaire was used to assess the intake of caffeinated coffee.

*Main Outcome Measure.*—Relative risk of nonfatal MI associated with coffee intake, calculated using unconditional logistic regression.

*Results.*—Fifty-five percent of cases (n = 1114) and 54% of controls (n = 1082) were carriers of the slow *\*1F* allele. For carriers of the slow *\*1F* allele, the multivariate-adjusted odds ratios (ORs) and 95% confidence intervals (CIs) of nonfatal MI associated with consuming less than 1, 1, 2 to 3, and 4 or more cups of coffee per day were 1.00 (reference), 0.99 (0.69-1.44), 1.36 (1.01-1.83), and 1.64 (1.14-2.34), respectively. Corresponding ORs (95% CIs) for individuals with the rapid *\*1A/\*1A* genotype were 1.00, 0.75 (0.51-1.12), 0.78 (0.56-1.09), and 0.99 (0.66-1.48) (*P* = .04 for gene × coffee interaction). For individuals younger than the median age of 59 years, the ORs (95% CIs) associated with consuming less than 1, 1, 2 to 3, or 4 or more cups of coffee per day were 1.00, 1.24 (0.71-2.18), 1.67 (1.08-2.60), and 2.33 (1.39-3.89), respectively, among carriers of the *\*1F* allele. The corresponding ORs (95% CIs) for those with the *\*1A/\*1A* genotype were 1.00, 0.48 (0.26-0.87), 0.57 (0.35-0.95), and 0.83 (0.46-1.51).

*Conclusion.*—Intake of coffee was associated with an increased risk of nonfatal MI only among individuals with slow caffeine metabolism, suggesting that caffeine plays a role in this association.

▶ Prior epidemiologic studies documenting an association between coffee consumption and the development of cardiovascular disease have been somewhat inconclusive.[1,2] Confounding factors include an unhealthy lifestyle that may be associated with increased coffee intake plus other risk factors. Moreover, it is unclear even if coffee is a putative risk factor, whether this is due to caffeine or other compounds present in coffee.

This case-controlled study in a patient population from Costa Rica (an appropriate choice of country for a study on coffee consumption) aimed to determine whether nonfatal MI was associated with the CYP1A2 genotype, which is strongly related to the rate of metabolism of caffeine. The data suggest that increased coffee consumption is associated with a higher rate of nonfatal MI (slow metabolizers), and by implication, caffeine is the culprit. This is an interesting study and an example of an epidemiologic application of pharmacogenetics. Nonetheless, adjustments for major risk factors do not incriminate other potentially confounding variables. The message is that caffeine, for the present, should be ingested "in moderation, as in most things."

Another recent and more convincing study in 120,000 participants in 2 US studies in which individuals were followed up for as long as 2 decades, identified no link whatsoever between heart disease and coffee consumption ranging from less than 1 cup per month to as many as 6 or more cups per day.[3] Among men after adjustment for age, smoking, and other coronary heart disease risk factors, the trend for relative risks across categories of cumulative coffee consumption was 0.41, and among women the relative risks were 0.01. Stratification by smoking status, alcohol consumption, and a history of type 2 diabetes mellitus and body mass index gave similar results. Moreover, when most recent coffee consumption was examined, the results were the same.

This does not exclude an association between coffee consumption and cardiovascular risk in some subsets of people, as in those particular genotypes. Moreover, this may not apply to the heavy consumption of unfiltered coffee, and one should also emphasize what one puts into the coffee cup—for example, sugar, cream, and other dairy products.

The message in regard to caffeine is "moderation as in most things." Certainly in individuals who develop symptoms such as difficulty in falling asleep and palpitations, this may be a sign that caffeine intake is excessive, and women who are pregnant or nursing should limit their caffeine intake.

**B. J. Gersh, MB, ChB, DPhil, FRCP**

*References*

1. Ranheim T, Halborsen B: Coffee consumption and human health—beneficial or detrimental? Mechanisms for effects of coffee consumption on different risk factors for cardiovascular disease and type 2 diabetes mellitus. *Mol Nutr Food Res* 49:274-284, 2005.
2. Kleemola P, Jousilahti P, Pietinen P, et al: Coffee consumption and the risk of coronary heart disease and death. *Arch Intern Med* 160:3393-3400, 2000.
3. Garcia E, VanDam RM, Willett WC: Coffee consumption and coronary heart disease in men and women: A prospective cohort study. *Circulation* 113:2045-2053, 2006.

### Relation between age and cardiovascular disease in men and women with diabetes compared with non-diabetic people: a population-based retrospective cohort study

Booth GL, Kapral MK, Fung K, et al (Univ of Toronto; Inst for Clinical Evaluative Sciences, Toronto)

*Lancet* 368:29-36, 2006

4–39

*Background.*—Adults with diabetes are thought to have a high risk of cardiovascular disease (CVD), irrespective of their age. The main aim of this study was to find out the age at which people with diabetes develop a high risk of CVD, as defined by: an event rate equivalent to a 10-year risk of 20%

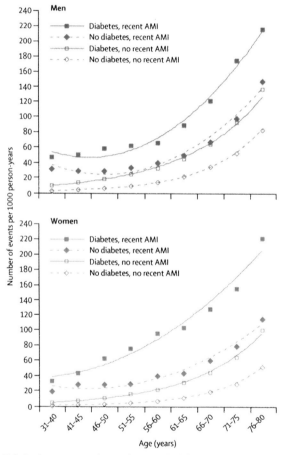

FIGURE 2.—Relation between age and rates of AMI or death from any cause in men and women according to presence of diabetes and previous AMI. Recent AMI: polynomial distribution. No recent AMI: exponential distribution. $R^2 > 0.97$ for each fitted line. Recent AMI = within 3 years of baseline. (Courtesy of Booth GL, Kapral MK, Fung K, et al: Relation between age and cardiovascular disease in men and women with diabetes compared with non-diabetic people: A population-based retrospective cohort study. *Lancet* 368:29-36. Copyright Elsevier 2006.)

or more; or an event rate equivalent to that associated with previous myocardial infarction.

*Methods.*—We did a population-based retrospective cohort study using provincial health claims to identify all adults with (n=379 003) and (n=9 018 082) without diabetes mellitus living in Ontario, Canada, on April 1, 1994. Individuals were followed up to record CVD events until March 31, 2000.

*Findings.*—The transition to a high-risk category occurred at a younger age for men and women with diabetes than for those without diabetes (mean difference 14.6 years). For the outcome of acute myocardial infarction (AMI), stroke, or death from any cause, diabetic men and women entered the high-risk category at ages 47.9 and 54.3 years respectively. When we used a broader definition of CVD that also included coronary or carotid revascularisation, the ages were 41.3 and 47.7 years for men and women with diabetes respectively.

*Interpretation.*—Diabetes confers an equivalent risk to ageing 15 years. However, in general, younger people with diabetes (age 40 or younger) do not seem to be at high risk of CVD. Age should be taken into account in targeting of risk reduction in people with diabetes (Fig 2).

▶ This massive population-based study from Ontario, Canada, emphasizes the cardiovascular risks of diabetes but adds new information. Diabetes confers an equivalent risk of coronary heart disease as 15 years of aging in both men and women. In older men over the age of 50 years, rates of MI and death in diabetics without prior MI were almost identical to those for nondiabetics with prior MI—a finding previously described.[1] However, in younger men and women of all ages, those with diabetes had lower coronary heart disease event rates than in those with recent MI but who were not diabetic. The transition to a high-risk category for coronary heart disease events occurred at a much younger age in diabetics, and using a broad definition of events, this occurred at ages 41.1 and 47.7 years, respectively, in men and women. Diabetics younger than 40 years are at relatively low risk of coronary events at least in the short to intermediate term.

Obviously these data could be used in the decision to use drugs for primary prevention of CVD in younger patients, given their low risk of developing the disease in the short to intermediate term. On the other hand, is it really prudent to wait for an age when such patients fall into a high-risk subgroup? It may make sense from a cost-effective standpoint, but we do not know the potential benefits of aggressive primary prevention at an earlier age. After all, once atherosclerosis is overtly detected, the disease is well advanced. There is, however, certainly a need for appropriate algorithms for primary and secondary prevention in young adults with type 1 and 2 diabetes.

**B. J. Gersh, MB, ChB, DPhil, FRCP**

*Reference*

1. Haffner SM, Lehto S, Ronnemaa T, et al: Mortality from coronary heart disease in subjects with type 2 diabetes and in non-diabetic subjects with and without prior myocardial infarction. *N Engl J Med* 339:229-234, 1998.

---

**Effects of Selenium Supplementation on Cardiovascular Disease Incidence and Mortality: Secondary Analyses in a Randomized Clinical Trial**
Stranges S, Marshall JR, Trevisan M, et al (State Univ of New York at Buffalo; Roswell Park Cancer Inst, Buffalo, NY; US Dept of Agriculture Human Nutrition Research Ctr, Grand Forks, ND; et al)
*Am J Epidemiol* 163:694-699, 2006                                    4–40

---

Despite the documented antioxidant and chemopreventive properties of selenium, studies of selenium intake and supplementation and cardiovascular disease have yielded inconsistent findings. The authors examined the effect of selenium supplementation (200 µg daily) on cardiovascular disease incidence and mortality through the entire blinded phase of the Nutritional Prevention of Cancer Trial (1983–1996) among participants who were free of cardiovascular disease at baseline (randomized to selenium: $n = 504$; randomized to placebo: $n = 500$). Selenium supplementation was not significantly associated with any of the cardiovascular disease endpoints during 7.6 years of follow-up (all cardiovascular disease: hazard ratio (HR) = 1.03, 95% confidence interval (CI): 0.78, 1.37; myocardial infarction: HR = 0.94, 95% CI: 0.61, 1.44; stroke: HR = 1.02, 95% CI: 0.63, 1.65; all cardiovascular disease mortality: HR = 1.22, 95% CI: 0.76, 1.95). The lack of significant association with cardiovascular disease endpoints was also confirmed when analyses were further stratified by tertiles of baseline plasma selenium concentrations. These findings indicate no overall effect of selenium supplementation on the primary prevention of cardiovascular disease in this population.

▶ Selenium, which is an essential component of a number of enzymes with antioxidant functions, has long generated interest in its potential "chemopreventive" and, in particular, in regard to its cardioprotective functions. Several earlier studies have demonstrated associations between low selenium levels and an increased risk of coronary artery disease[1] and of dilated cardiomyopathy of Keshan's disease, as it is named in China.[2] Nonetheless, in regard to the latter, the extent to which this is a consequence of a viral infection is still unknown.[3]

In this large randomized trial with a dermatologic primary end point, this subset analysis of secondary end points, however, demonstrates no evidence whatsoever of selenium supplementation in the development of cardiovascular disease, cardiovascular disease mortality, stroke, and myocardial infarction. Moreover, this is the largest randomized controlled trial to date of selenium supplementation. Other prospective trials have also had negative results, including a large nutritional interventional study in China.[4]

**B. J Gersh, MB, ChB, DPhil, FRCP**

*References*

1. Suadicani P, Hein HO, Gyntelberg F: Serum selenium concentration and risk of ischemic heart disease in a prospective cohort study of 3000 males. *Atherosclerosis* 96:33-42, 1992.
2. Xu GL, Wang SC, Gu BQ, et al: Further investigation on the role of selenium deficiency in the aetiology and pathogenesis of Keshan disease. *Biomed Environ Sci* 10:316-326, 1997.
3. Li Y, Ping T, Wang W, et al: High prevalence of enteroviral genomics sequences in myocardium from cases of endemic cardiomyopathy (Keshan disease) in China. *Heart* 83:696-701, 2000.
4. Blot WJ, Li JY, Taylor PR, et al: Nutrition interventional trials in Linxian, China: Supplementation with specific vitamin/mineral combinations, cancer incidences, and disease-specific mortality in the general population. *J Natl Cancer Inst* 85:1483-1492, 1993.

**Risk of Myocardial Infarction in Patients With Psoriasis**
Gelfand JM, Neimann AL, Shin DB, et al (Univ of Pennsylvania, Philadelphia)
*JAMA* 296:1735-1741, 2006                                                4–41

*Context.*—Psoriasis is the most common T-helper cell type 1 ($T_H1$) immunological disease. Evidence has linked $T_H1$ diseases to myocardial infarction (MI). Psoriasis has been associated with cardiovascular diseases, but has only been investigated in hospital-based studies that did not control for major cardiovascular risk factors.

*Objective.*—To determine if within a population-based cohort psoriasis is an independent risk factor for MI when controlling for major cardiovascular risk factors.

*Design, Setting, and Patients.*—A prospective, population-based cohort study in the United Kingdom of patients with psoriasis aged 20 to 90 years, comparing outcomes among patients with and without a diagnosis of psoriasis. Data were collected by general practitioners as part of the patient's medical record and stored in the General Practice Research Database between 1987 and 2002, with a mean follow-up of 5.4 years. Adjustments were made for hypertension, diabetes, history of myocardial infarction, hyperlipidemia, age, sex, smoking, and body mass index. Patients with psoriasis were classified as severe if they ever received a systemic therapy. Up to 5 controls without psoriasis were randomly selected from the same practices and start dates as the patients with psoriasis. A total of 556,995 control patients and patients with mild (n = 127,139) and severe psoriasis (n = 3837) were identified.

*Main Outcome Measure.*—Incident MI.

*Results.*—There were 11,194 MIs (2.0%) within the control population and 2319 (1.8%) and 112 (2.9%) MIs within the mild and severe psoriasis groups, respectively. The incidences per 1000 person-years for control patients and patients with mild and severe psoriasis were 3.58 (95% confidence interval [CI], 3.52-3.65), 4.04 (95% CI, 3.88-4.21), and 5.13 (95% CI, 4.22-6.17), respectively. Patients with psoriasis had an increased adjusted relative risk (RR) for MI that varied by age. For example, for a 30-year-old patient with mild or severe psoriasis, the adjusted RR of having an MI is 1.29 (95% CI, 1.14-1.46) and 3.10 (95% CI, 1.98-4.86), respectively. For a 60-year-old patient with mild or severe psoriasis, the adjusted RR of having an MI is 1.08 (95% CI, 1.03-1.13) and 1.36 (95% CI, 1.13-1.64), respectively.

*Conclusions.*—Psoriasis may confer an independent risk of MI. The RR was greatest in young patients with severe psoriasis.

▶ Psoriasis, which affects 2% to 3% of the population, is a $T_H1$ immunological disturbance associated with a systemic inflammatory state, including elevated levels of C-reactive protein. These immunological abnormalities suggest that patients may be at increased risk of other diseases associated with inflammation, including atherosclerosis and myocardial infarction.[1] Several prior hospital-based studies that did not control for confounding variables have suggested that psoriasis is associated with a higher prevalence of cardiovascular diseases, including myocardial infarction.[2]

This very large population-based study from the United Kingdom, with a mean follow-up of 5.4 years, adjusted for the presence of hypertension, diabetes, prior history of myocardial infarction, hyperlipidemia, age, sex, smoking, and body mass index. Patients were also categorized according to the severity of psoriasis. The findings are novel and make a strong case that psoriasis confers an independent risk of myocardial infarction, particularly in younger patients and in those with severe disease. To what extent the link is attributable to inflammation as opposed to other factors such as psychologic stress, sedentary lifestyle, or poor compliance with management of cardiovascular risk factors is uncertain. Irrespective, the clinical message is unambiguous, and that is one should aggressively look for and treat cardiovascular risk factors in all patients with psoriasis.

**B. J. Gersh, MB, ChB, DPhil, FRCP**

*References*

1. Hansson GK: Inflammation, atherosclerosis, and coronary artery disease. *N Engl J Med* 352:1685-95, 2005.
2. McDonald CJ, Calabresi P: Complication of psoriasis. *JAMA* 224:629, 1973.

---

**Midlife Body Mass Index and Hospitalization and Mortality in Older Age**
Yan LL, Daviglus ML, Liu K, et al (Northwestern Univ, Chicago; Peking Univ, Beijing, China; Centers for Disease Control and Prevention, Atlanta, Ga; et al)
*JAMA* 295:190-198, 2006                                              4–42

*Context.*—Abundant evidence links overweight and obesity with impaired health. However, controversies persist as to whether overweight and obesity have additional impact on cardiovascular outcomes independent of their strong associations with established coronary risk factors, eg, high blood pressure and high cholesterol level.

*Objective.*—To assess the relation of midlife body mass index with morbidity and mortality outcomes in older age among individuals without and with other major risk factors at baseline.

*Design.*—Chicago Heart Association Detection Project in Industry study, a prospective study with baseline (1967-1973) cardiovascular risk classified as low risk (blood pressure ≤120/≤80 mm Hg, serum total cholesterol level <200 mg/dL [5.2 mmol/L], and not currently smoking); moderate risk (nonsmoking and systolic blood pressure 121-139 mm Hg, diastolic blood pressure 81-89 mm Hg, and/or total cholesterol level 200-239 mg/dL [5.2-6.2 mmol/L]); or having any 1, any 2, or all 3 of the following risk factors: blood pressure ≥140/90 mm Hg, total cholesterol level ≥240 mg/dL (6.2 mmol/L), and current cigarette smoking. Body mass index was classified as normal weight (18.5-24.9), overweight (25.0-29.9), or obese (≥30). Mean follow-up was 32 years.

*Setting and Participants.*—Participants were 17,643 men and women aged 31 through 64 years, recruited from Chicago-area companies or organizations and free of coronary heart disease (CHD), diabetes, or major electrocardiographic abnormalities at baseline.

*Main Outcome Measures.*—Hospitalization and mortality from CHD, cardiovascular disease, or diabetes, beginning at age 65 years.

*Results.*—In multivariable analyses that included adjustment for systolic blood pressure and total cholesterol level, the odds ratio (95% confidence interval) for CHD death for obese participants compared with those of normal weight in the same risk category was 1.43 (0.33-6.25) for low risk and 2.07 (1.29-3.31) for moderate risk; for CHD hospitalization, the corresponding results were 4.25 (1.57-11.5) for low risk and 2.04 (1.29-3.24) for moderate risk. Results were similar for other risk groups and for cardiovascular disease, but stronger for diabetes (eg, low risk: 11.0 [2.21-54.5] for mortality and 7.84 [3.95-15.6] for hospitalization).

*Conclusion.*—For individuals with no cardiovascular risk factors as well as for those with 1 or more risk factors, those who are obese in middle age have a higher risk of hospitalization and mortality from CHD, cardiovascular disease, and diabetes in older age than those who are normal weight.

▶ Although there is abundant evidence linking obesity to coronary heart disease and other cardiovascular diseases, in addition to a strong association with other cardiovascular risk factors, the issue whether obesity is an adverse predictor independent of other risk factors remain controversial.[1] It is an important clinical question that needs to be addressed in the obese patient in whom blood pressure and cholesterol levels are not elevated.

This important large population study with lengthy follow up (mean 32 years) emphatically answers the questions. For individuals who are obese at middle age, irrespective of whether they have 1 or more cardiovascular risk factors, obesity in middle age is associated with a higher risk of hospitalization and mortality from coronary heart disease, cardiovascular disease and diabetes in older age (age ≥65) in comparison to individuals who are at normal weight. In those with 1 or more risk factors, the presence of obesity appeared to be additive. In general, the results were consistent from both sexes. Clarification of this issue is needed because indices such as the Framingham Risk Score does not include obesity on the basis of the argument that the effects of obesity are mediated primarily through other major cardiovascular risk factors.[2]

The endemic of obesity poses an amebicidal public health challenge and it is possible that obesity may soon over take smoking as the major cause of death.[3] It is even being postulated that obesity could potential result in a decline in life expectancy in the United States in the 21st century.[4] The way forward is clear and this study provides overwhelming support for population-wide, multifaceted, primary prevention strategies that need to start at a young age.

**B. J. Gersh, MB, ChB, DPhil, FRCP**

*References*

1. Willet WC, Manson JE, Stampfer MJ, et al: Weight, weight change, and coronary heart disease in women: Risk within the "normal" weight range. *JAMA* 273:461-465, 1995.
2. Wilson PW, D'Agostino RB, Levy D, et al: Prediction of coronary heart disease using risk factor categories. *Circulation* 97:1837-1847, 1998.
3. Mokdad AH, Marks JS, Stroup DF, et al: Actual causes of death in the United States, 2000 [published correction appears in *JAMA* 293:298, 2005]. *JAMA* 291:1238-1245, 2004.
4. Olshansky SK, Passaro DJ, Hershow RC, et al: A potential decline in life expectancy in the United States in the 21st century. *N Engl J Med* 352:1138-1145, 2005.

---

**Low-Fat Dietary Pattern and Risk of Cardiovascular Disease: The Women's Health Initiative Randomized Controlled Dietary Modification Trial**

Howard BV, Van Horn L, Hsia J, et al (Howard Inst, Washington, DC; Northwestern Univ, Chicago; George Washington Univ, Washington, DC; et al)
*JAMA* 295:655-666, 2006 4–43

---

*Context.*—Multiple epidemiologic studies and some trials have linked diet with cardiovascular disease (CVD) prevention, but long-term intervention data are needed.

*Objective.*—To test the hypothesis that a dietary intervention, intended to be low in fat and high in vegetables, fruits, and grains to reduce cancer, would reduce CVD risk.

*Design, Setting, and Participants.*—Randomized controlled trial of 48 835 postmenopausal women aged 50 to 79 years, of diverse backgrounds and ethnicities, who participated in the Women's Health Initiative Dietary Modification Trial. Women were randomly assigned to an intervention (19 541 [40%]) or comparison group (29 294 [60%]) in a free-living setting. Study enrollment occurred between 1993 and 1998 in 40 US clinical centers; mean follow-up in this analysis was 8.1 years.

*Intervention.*—Intensive behavior modification in group and individual sessions designed to reduce total fat intake to 20% of calories and increase intakes of vegetables/fruits to 5 servings/d and grains to at least 6 servings/d. The comparison group received diet-related education materials.

*Main Outcome Measures.*—Fatal and nonfatal coronary heart disease (CHD), fatal and nonfatal stroke, and CVD (composite of CHD and stroke).

*Results.*—By year 6, mean fat intake decreased by 8.2% of energy intake in the intervention vs the comparison group, with small decreases in saturated (2.9%), monounsaturated (3.3%), and polyunsaturated (1.5%) fat; increases occurred in intakes of vegetables/fruits (1.1 servings/d) and grains (0.5 serving/d). Low-density lipoprotein cholesterol levels, diastolic blood pressure, and factor VIIc levels were significantly reduced by 3.55 mg/dL, 0.31 mm Hg, and 4.29%, respectively; levels of high-density lipoprotein cholesterol, triglycerides, glucose, and insulin did not significantly differ in the intervention vs comparison groups. The numbers who developed CHD, stroke, and CVD (annualized incidence rates) were 1000 (0.63%), 434 (0.28%), and 1357 (0.86%) in the intervention and 1549 (0.65%), 642 (0.27%), and 2088 (0.88%) in the comparison group. The diet had no significant effects on incidence of CHD (hazard ratio [HR], 0.97; 95% confidence interval [CI], 0.90-1.06), stroke (HR, 1.02; 95% CI, 0.90-1.15), or CVD (HR, 0.98; 95% CI, 0.92-1.05). Excluding participants with baseline CVD (3.4%), the HRs (95% CIs) for CHD and stroke were 0.94 (0.86-1.02) and 1.02 (0.90-1.17), respectively. Trends toward greater reductions in CHD risk were observed in those with lower intakes of saturated fat or trans fat or higher intakes of vegetables/fruits.

*Conclusions.*—Over a mean of 8.1 years, a dietary intervention that reduced total fat intake and increased intakes of vegetables, fruits, and grains did not significantly reduce the risk of CHD, stroke, or CVD in postmenopausal women and achieved only modest effects on CVD risk factors, suggesting that more focused diet and lifestyle interventions may be needed to improve risk factors and reduce CVD risk.

▶ This is the longest long-term dietary interventional trial ever conducted, and the results come as a disappointment, and certainly at first glance, as a surprise. A diet that lowered the daily intake of fat and increased the intake of fruits, vegetables, and grains had no effect on the primary end point of the risk of breast and colon cancer and there was no reduction in cardiovascular events.[1] Indeed, among patients with preexisting cardiovascular disease, the trend was in the reverse direction, but this could have been a statistical aberration or artifact. As pointed out in the discussion and in a accompanying editorial, the intervention had only a very small effect on cardiovascular risk factors, including LDL cholesterol, blood pressure, and obesity.[2] This is a problem for all trials that are concluded over a prolonged period of time and against the backdrop of changing therapies and lifestyle considerations.

In summary, dietary guidelines need to be adapted in conjunction with modifications of other risk factors, for example, hypertension, sedentary lifestyle and obesity, and smoking cessation. In this respect, the Women's Health Initiative should not dissuade anyone from following the 2005 dietary guidelines for Americans.[3]

**B. J. Gersh, MB, ChB, DPhil, FRCP**

*References*

1. Prentice RL, Cwan B, Chlebowski R, et al: Low-fat dietary pattern in risk of invasive breast cancer: The Women's Health Initiative Randomized, Controlled Dietary Modification Trial. *JAMA* 295:629-642, 2006.
2. Anderson CAM, Appell J: Dietary modification in CDD prevention: A matter of fat. *JAMA* 295:693-695, 2006.
3. U.S. Department of Health and Human Services: *U.S. Department of Agriculture: Dietary guidelines for Americans 2005*, ed 6. Washington, DC, 2005, U.S. Government Printing Office.

---

### Reduction in the Incidence of Acute Myocardial Infarction Associated With a Citywide Smoking Ordinance

Bartecchi C, Alsever RN, Nevin-Woods C, et al (Univ of Colorado Health Sciences Ctr, Pueblo; Parkview Med Ctr, Pueblo, Colo; Pueblo City-County Health Dept, Colo; et al)
*Circulation* 114:1490-1496, 2006                                                    4–44

---

*Background.*—Secondhand smoke exposure increases the risk of acute myocardial infarction (AMI). One study (Helena, Mont) examined the issue and found a decrease in AMI associated with a smoke-free ordinance. We sought to determine the impact of a smoke-free ordinance on AMI admission rates in another geographically isolated community (Pueblo, Colo).

*Method and Results.*—We assessed AMI hospitalizations in Pueblo during a 3-year period, 1.5 years before and 1.5 years after implementation of a smoke-free ordinance. We compared the AMI hospitalization rates among individuals residing within city limits, the area where the ordinance applied, versus those outside city limits. We also compared AMI rates during this time period with another geographically isolated but proximal community, El Paso County, Colo, that did not have an ordinance. A total of 855 patients were hospitalized with a diagnosis of primary AMI in Pueblo between January 1, 2002, and December 31, 2004. A reduction in AMI hospitalizations was observed in the period after the ordinance among Pueblo city limit residents (relative risk [RR]=0.73, 95% confidence interval [CI] 0.63 to 0.85). No significant changes in AMI rates were observed among residents outside city limits (RR=0.85, 95% CI 0.63 to 1.16) or in El Paso County during the same period (RR=0.97, 95% CI 0.89 to 1.06). The reduction in AMI rate within Pueblo differed significantly from changes in the external control group (El Paso County) even after adjustment for seasonal trends ($P<0.001$).

*Conclusions.*—A public ordinance reducing exposure to secondhand smoke was associated with a decrease in AMI hospitalizations in Pueblo, Colo, which supports previous data from a smaller study.

▶ Although it is well established that chronic exposure to secondhand cigarette smoke is associated with an increased risk of acute myocardial infarction,[1] only one prior study has demonstrated the beneficial impact of a smoke-free ordinance on rates of AMI.[2] That study, in Helena, Mont, demonstrated a 40% decline in hospital admissions during a 6-month smoking ordinance within the city limits. The study was limited by a small sample size and lifting of the ban after 6 months after a legal challenge.

This study from Colorado on a larger population demonstrates a very impressive reduction in AMI hospitalization rates within months after imposition of the ordinance. Moreover, this is significantly different from changes noted in a regional control population, even after adjustment for seasonal trends. What is quite remarkable is the extent and rapidity of the impact of secondhand smoke on atherothrombotic events.[3] It is perhaps not surprising, therefore, that limiting secondhand smoke reduces the incidence of AMI, but the magnitude of the effect is gratifying. In addition, it is possible that imposition of the ordinance may help current smokers either quit or reduce the number of cigarettes smoked. To what extent the changes noted will persist with time is unknown.

Nonetheless, the data do suggest that an antismoking ordinance may really benefit community health. It is hard to believe that it was not that long ago when smoking was permitted on aircraft.

**B. J. Gersh, MB, ChB, DPhil, FRCP**

*References*

1. Barnoya J, Goantz SA: Cardiovascular effects of secondhand smoke nearly as large as smoking. *Circulation* 111:2684-2698, 2005.
2. Sargent RP, Shepard RM, Glantz SA: Reduced incidence of admissions from myocardial infarction associated with public smoking ban: Before and after study. *BMJ* 328:977-980, 2004.
3. Pechacek TF, Babb S: How acute and reversible are the cardiovascular risks of secondhand smoke? *BMJ* 328:980-983, 2004.

## Psychosocial and Economic Issues

### Reduced Cardiocirculatory Complications With Unrestrictive Visiting Policy in an Intensive Care Unit: Results From a Pilot, Randomized Trial

Fumagalli S, Boncinelli L, Lo Nostro A, et al (Univ of Florence, Italy)
*Circulation* 113:946-952, 2006                                          4–45

*Background.*—Observational studies suggest that open visiting policies are preferred by most patients and visitors in intensive care units (ICUs), but no randomized trial has compared the safety and health outcomes of unrestrictive (UVP) and restrictive (RVP) visiting policies. The aim of this pilot, randomized trial was to compare the complications associated with UVP (single visitor with frequency and duration chosen by patient) and RVP (single visitor for 30 minutes twice a day).

*Method and Results.*—Two-month sequences of the 2 visiting policies were randomly alternated for 2 years in a 6-bed ICU, with 226 patients enrolled (RVP/UVP, n=115/111). Environmental microbial contamination, septic and cardiovascular complications, emotional profile, and stress hormones response were systematically assessed. Patients admitted during the randomly scheduled periods of UVP received more frequent (3.2±0.2 versus 2.0±0.0 visits per day, mean±SEM) and longer (2.6±0.2 versus 1.0±0.0 h/d) visits (P<0.001 for both comparisons). Despite significantly higher environmental microbial contamination during the UVP periods, septic complications were similar in the 2 periods. The risk of cardiocirculatory complications was 2-fold (odds ratio 2.0; 95% CI, 1.1 to 3.5; P=0.03) in the RVP periods, which were also associated with a nonsignificantly higher mortality rate (5.2% versus 1.8%; P=0.28). The UVP was associated with a greater reduction in anxiety score and a significantly lower increase in thyroid stimulating hormone from admission to discharge.

*Conclusions.*—Despite greater environmental microbial contamination, liberalizing visiting hours in ICUs does not increase septic complications, whereas it might reduce cardiovascular complications, possibly through reduced anxiety and more favorable hormonal profile.

▶ This is a rather unique study that could serve as a pilot for a larger trial. A number of emotional factors may contribute to what is being termed, "the ICU psychosis and delirium," and these include fear, sleep deprivation, pain, restricted mobility, and limited family contact.[1] Moreover, delirium is a powerful independent predictor of an adverse prognosis.

The results of this trial are perhaps surprising but, nonetheless, quite promising. Despite greater environmental microbial contamination, liberalizing visiting hours in a cardiac intensive care unit (single visitor with frequency in duration chosen by patient) did not increase septic complications, which was associated with a marked reduction in hemodynamic complications in comparison with a more restricted policy (single visitor for 30 minutes twice a day).

The mechanisms of benefit remain speculative, but reduction in anxiety could certainly lead to a more favorable autonomic milieu with a beneficial impact on vasomotor tone, platelet activity, and left ventricular wall stress. The extent to which a reduction in anxiety results in a more favorable hormonal profile is uncertain, although there were higher TSh levels in the restricted visit group.

**B. J Gersh, MB, ChB, DPhil, FRCP**

*Reference*

1. Simini B: Patients' perceptions of intensive care. *Lancet* 354:571-572, 1999.

## Socioeconomic status and ischaemic heart disease mortality in 10 western European populations during the 1990s

Avendano M, Kunst AE, Huisman M, et al (Erasmus Med Centre, Rotterdam, The Netherlands; Univ of Zurich, Switzerland; Univ of Madrid; et al)

*Heart* 92:461-467, 2006                                            4–46

*Objective.*—To assess the association between socioeconomic status and ischaemic heart disease (IHD) mortality in 10 western European populations during the 1990s.

*Design.*—Longitudinal study.

*Setting.*—10 European populations (95 009 822 person years).

*Methods.*—Longitudinal data on IHD mortality by educational level were obtained from registries in Finland, Norway, Denmark, England/Wales, Belgium, Switzerland, Austria, Turin (Italy), Barcelona (Spain), and Madrid (Spain). Age standardised rates and rate ratios (RRs) of IHD mortality by educational level were calculated by using Poisson regression.

*Results.*—IHD mortality was higher in those with a lower socioeconomic status than in those with a higher socioeconomic status among men aged 30–59 (RR 1.55, 95% confidence interval (CI) 1.51 to 1.60) and 60 years and over (RR 1.22, 95% CI 1.21 to 1.24), and among women aged 30–59 (RR 2.13, 95% CI 1.98 to 2.29) and 60 years and over (RR 1.36, 95% CI 1.33 to 1.38). Socioeconomic disparities in IHD mortality were larger in the Scandinavian countries and England/Wales, of moderate size in Belgium, Switzerland, and Austria, and smaller in southern European populations among men and younger women (p < 0.0001). For elderly women the north-south gradient was smaller and there was less variation between populations. No socioeconomic disparities in IHD mortality existed among elderly men in southern Europe.

*Conclusions.*—Socioeconomic disparities in IHD mortality were larger in northern than in southern European populations during the 1990s. This partly reflects the pattern of socioeconomic disparities in cardiovascular risk factors in Europe. Population wide strategies to reduce risk factor prevalence combined with interventions targeted at the lower socioeconomic groups can contribute to reduce IHD mortality in Europe.

▶ It is well accepted that socioeconomic status has a major impact upon the mortality of coronary heart disease.[1] Individuals comprising a lower socioeconomic class have a greater risk of dying of coronary artery disease, and this relationship has been noted in the United States, Canada, and Europe.

What is particularly interesting in this study of 10 western European populations is the "North-South gradient," and that disparities in mortality according to educational levels (as a surrogate of socioeconomic status) were larger in the Scandinavian countries and the United Kingdom; of moderate size in Switzerland, Belgium, and Austria; and smaller in the southern European countries, particularly among men and younger women. The potential explanations in the light of current knowledge of risk factors are interesting. Smoking patterns differ among countries, and in the more northern countries, smoking has declined among the higher classes but is still rampant in those of lower socio-economic groups.[2] This progression in the pattern of the smoking epidemic is less evident in southern European countries, with higher rates of smoking.

Another potential factor is the widespread availability of the Mediterranean diet in the South, whereas this may be more prevalent only among the higher classes in the North. These socioeconomic differences were less evident among elderly women who have a low prevalence of smoking. Obesity, however, which is higher in lower socioeconomic classes, may account for some of the differences still present among the elderly. Lastly, disproportions in access to care probably play a role, although widespread access to specialists' care is high in the Scandinavian countries where the disparities in mortality according to class were also the largest.

This study provides food for thought and raises concerns in regard to the smoldering epidemic of coronary artery disease in the developing world with its very large population that falls into the lowest socioeconomic group.

**B. J. Gersh, MB, ChB, DPhil, FRCP**

*References*

1. 1. Huisman N, Kunst AE, Bopp MO: Educational inequalities in cause-specific mortality in middle-aged men and women in 8 western European populations. *Lancet* 365:493-500, 2005.
2. Opaters AD, Collishaaw NE, Piha T: A descriptive model of the cigarette epidemic in developed countries. *Tab Control* 3:242-247, 1994.

---

**Socioeconomic Status and Mortality After Acute Myocardial Infarction**
Alter DA, for the SESAMI Study Group (Inst for Clinical Evaluative Sciences, Toronto; et al)
*Ann Intern Med* 144:82-93, 2006                                                4–47

---

*Background.*—Gradients that link socioeconomic status and cardiovascular mortality have been observed in many populations, including those of countries that provide publicly funded comprehensive medical coverage. The intermediary causes of such gradients remain poorly elucidated.

*Objective.*—To examine the relationships among socioeconomic status, other health factors, and 2-year mortality rates after acute myocardial infarction (MI).

*Design.*—Prospective cohort study.

*Setting.*—Ontario, Canada.

*Patients.*—3407 patients who were hospitalized for acute MI in 53 large-volume hospitals in Canada from December 1999 to February 2003.

*Measurements.*—The authors obtained self-reported measures of income and education and developed profiles of the patients' prehospitalization cardiac risks and comorbid conditions. To create these profiles, the authors used the patients' self-reports and retrospectively linked no less than 12 years' worth of previous hospitalization data. Mortality rates 2 years after acute MI were examined with and without sequential risk adjustment for age, sex, ethnicity, social support, cardiovascular history and risk, comorbid conditions, and selected in-hospital process factors.

*Results.*—Income was strongly and inversely correlated with 2-year mortality rate (crude hazard ratio for high-income vs. low-income tertile, 0.45 [95% CI, 0.35 to 0.57]; *P* < 0.001). However, after adjustment for age and preexisting cardiovascular events or conventional vascular risk factors, the effect of income was greatly attenuated (adjusted hazard ratio for high-income vs. low-income tertile, 0.77 [CI, 0.54 to 1.10]; *P* = 0.150). Noncardiovascular comorbid conditions and in-hospital process factors had negligible explanatory effect.

*Limitations.*—Previous cardiovascular risks were ascertained through self-report or retrospectively through the longitudinal tracking of the hospitals' administrative databases. The study began with a cohort of patients who had an index cardiac event rather than with asymptomatic individuals.

*Conclusions.*—Age, past cardiovascular events, and current vascular risk factors accounted for most of the income-mortality gradient after acute MI. This observation suggests that the "wealth-health gradient" in cardiovascular mortality may be partially ameliorated by more rigorous management of known risk factors among less affluent persons.

▶ In some ways, the results of this study from a single payor system in Canada are at variance with prior reports. The literature is replete with studies which demonstrate a strong association between "wealth health" gradient and the prevalence of cardiovascular disease and cardiac mortality.[1] The beneficial impact of higher socioeconomic status has been demonstrated using multiple definitions and among both private and publicly funded health systems.[2]

This study from two large-volume hospitals in Ontario, Canada, is in some ways encouraging. It suggests that most of the impact of income on post-infarction mortality is accounted for by age, prior cardiovascular events, and current cardiovascular risk factors. The latter provides a target for modification, irrespective of wealth and social status. To what extent other factors, such as stress, anger, lack of job control, etc., play a role cannot be ascertained from this study, but there are other studies which suggest that these factors which are associated with cardiovascular disease and mortality are more prevalent among patients of lower socioeconomic status.

**B. J. Gersh, MB, ChB, DPhil, FRCP**

*References*

1. Wolfson M, Captain G, Lynch J, et al: Relation between income inequality and mortality: Empirical demonstration. *BJM* 319:953-955, 1999.
2. Alter DA, Naylor CD, Austin P, et al: Effects of socioeconomic status on access to invasive cardiac procedures and on mortality after acute myocardial infarction. *N Engl J Med* 341:1359-1367, 1999.

## Pathophysiology

### Postconditioning Protects Against Endothelial Ischemia-Reperfusion Injury in the Human Forearm

Loukogeorgakis SP, Panagiotidou AT, Yellon DM, et al (Univ College London)
*Circulation* 113:1015-1019, 2006
4–48

*Background.*—Hypoxic cell death follows interruption of blood supply to tissues. Although successful restoration of blood flow is mandatory for salvage of ischemic tissues, reperfusion can paradoxically place tissues at risk of further injury. Brief periods of ischemia applied at the onset of reperfusion have been shown to reduce ischemia-reperfusion (IR) injury, a phenomenon called postconditioning. The aim of this study was to determine whether postconditioning protects against endothelial IR injury in humans, in vivo.

*Method and Results.*—Brachial artery endothelial function was assessed by vascular ultrasound to measure flow-mediated dilation (FMD) in response to forearm reactive hyperemia. FMD was measured before and after IR (20 minutes of arm ischemia followed by 20 minutes of reperfusion) in healthy volunteers. To test the protective effects of postconditioning, 3 cycles of reperfusion followed by ischemia (each lasting 10 or 30 seconds) were applied immediately after 20 minutes of arm ischemia. To determine whether postconditioning needs to be applied at the onset of reperfusion, a 1-minute period of arm reperfusion was allowed before the application of the 10-second postconditioning stimulus. IR caused endothelial dysfunction (FMD $9.1 \pm 1.2\%$ pre-IR, $3.6 \pm 0.7\%$ post-IR, $P<0.001$; n=11), which was prevented by postconditioning applied as 10-second cycles of reperfusion/ischemia (FMD $9.9 \pm 1.7\%$ pre-IR, $8.3 \pm 1.4\%$ post-IR, $P=NS$; n=11) and 30-second cycles of reperfusion/ischemia (FMD $10.8 \pm 1.7\%$ pre-IR, $9.5 \pm 1.5\%$ post-IR, $P=NS$; n=10) immediately at the onset of reperfusion. No protection was observed when the application of the 10-second postconditioning stimulus was delayed for 1 minute after the onset of reperfusion (FMD $9.8 \pm 1.2\%$ pre-IR, $4.0 \pm 0.9\%$ post-IR, $P<0.001$; n=8).

*Conclusions.*—This study demonstrates for the first time that postconditioning can protect against endothelial IR injury in humans. Postconditioning might reduce tissue injury when applied at the onset of reperfusion by modifying the reperfusion phase of IR.

▶ Although restoration of blood flow in the infarct-related artery is the cornerstone of reperfusion therapy, the presence of microvascular dysfunction and perhaps reperfusion injury has been a limiting factor in the achievement of optimal myocardial perfusion. The protective effect of the phenomenon of ischemic preconditioning is well recognized, but from a practical therapeutic standpoint, this approach is seriously limited by the need to apply these measures before the onset of infarction and reperfusion.

This has stimulated great interest in the strategy of postconditioning, which is restricted to the reperfusion phase of myocardial injury[1] and as such can be incorporated into a strategy of primary percutaneous coronary intervention (PPCI) in acute evolving ST-segment elevation myocardial infarction. One recent clinical study has shown that a postconditioning protocol of intermittent reperfusion does indeed reduce infarct size in patients undergoing PPCI.[2]

The current study in humans demonstrates rather convincingly that postconditioning can protect against endothelial IR injury in the brachial artery vascular beds. The mechanisms underlying the striking benefits are speculative, but it is likely that preconditioning and postconditioning share common signaling pathways.[3] The identification and isolation of the molecular mechanism could herald a new approach to the treatment of acute ischemic injury.

**B. J. Gersh, MB, ChB, DPhil, FRCP**

*References*

1. Zhao ZQ, Corvera JS, Halkof ME, et al: Inhibition of myocardial injury by ischemic postconditioning during reperfusion: Comparison with ischemic preconditioning. *Am J Physiol Heart Circ Physiol* 285:H579-H588, 2003.
2. Staat B, Rioufol G, Poit C, et al: Post deconditioning of the human heart. *Circulation* 112:2143-2148, 2005.
3. Tsang A, Hausenloy DJ, Yellon DM: Myocardial post-conditioning: Reperfusion injury revisited. *Am J Physiol Heart Circ Physiol* 289:H2-H7, 2005.

## Miscellaneous

### Should Major Vascular Surgery Be Delayed Because of Preoperative Cardiac Testing in Intermediate-Risk Patients Receiving Beta-Blocker Therapy With Tight Heart Rate Control?

Poldermans D, for the Dutch Echocardiographic Cardiac Risk Evaluation Applying Stress Echo Study Group (Erasmus Med Ctr, Rotterdam, The Netherlands; et al)

*J Am Coll Cardiol* 48:964-969, 2006                                          4–49

*Objectives.*—The purpose of this study was to assess the value of preoperative cardiac testing in intermediate-risk patients receiving beta-blocker therapy with tight heart rate (HR) control scheduled for major vascular surgery.

*Background.*—Treatment guidelines of the American College of Cardiology/American Heart Association recommend cardiac testing in these patients to identify subjects at increased risk. This policy delays surgery, even though test results might be redundant and beta-blockers with tight HR control provide sufficient myocardial protection. Furthermore, the benefit of revascularization in high-risk patients is ill-defined.

*Methods.*—All 1,476 screened patients were stratified into low-risk (0 risk factors), intermediate-risk (1 to 2 risk factors), and high-risk ($\geq$3 risk factors). All patients received beta-blockers. The 770 intermediate-risk patients were randomly assigned to cardiac stress-testing (n = 386) or no testing. Test results influenced management. In patients with ischemia, physicians aimed to control HR below the ischemic threshold. Those with extensive stress-induced ischemia were considered for revascularization.

The primary end point was cardiac death or myocardial infarction at 30-days after surgery.

*Results.*—Testing showed no ischemia in 287 patients (74%); limited ischemia in 65 patients (17%), and extensive ischemia in 34 patients (8.8%). Of 34 patients with extensive ischemia, revascularization before surgery was feasible in 12 patients (35%). Patients assigned to no testing had similar incidence of the primary end point as those assigned to testing (1.8% vs. 2.3%; odds ratio [OR] 0.78; 95% confidence interval [CI] 0.28 to 2.1; p = 0.62). The strategy of no testing brought surgery almost 3 weeks forward. Regardless of allocated strategy, patients with a HR <65 beats/min had lower risk than the remaining patients (1.3% vs. 5.2%; OR 0.24; 95% CI 0.09 to 0.66; p = 0.003).

*Conclusions.*—Cardiac testing can safely be omitted in intermediate-risk patients, provided that beta-blockers aiming at tight HR control are prescribed.

▶ The American College of Cardiology/American Heart Association guidelines state that patients scheduled for major vascular surgery who have clinical features associated with increased cardiac risk should undergo noninvasive stress testing. Although this is a reasonable approach, it has the potential to create a "cascade" effect in which a positive stress test leads to angiography, which in turn may result in coronary revascularization, despite the fact that the patient was initially referred for a noncardiac surgical procedure.[1] Furthermore, the cardiac procedures may lead to a delay in surgery with a theoretical risk of aneurysm rupture or exacerbation of critical limb ischemia.

A prior multicenter, randomized, controlled trial demonstrated that coronary revascularization before elective vascular surgery was not associated with any improvement in perioperative or long-term outcomes.[2] In this trial, patients were enrolled after angiography, and high-risk subsets were excluded. The current study from Holland addresses a more important clinical issue, mainly whether patients at intermediate risk based on 1 or 2 risk factors for coronary artery disease should undergo stress testing with all the potential consequences after a positive stress test versus the approach of β-blocker therapy and proceeding directly to vascular surgery. From a clinical standpoint, this is a very important question that could lead to a reduction in the performance of an unnecessary angiography.

The results are quite emphatic. Patients assigned to no testing have a similar but low evidence of the primary end point, and surgery was performed 3 weeks earlier. Although β-blockers have become a mainstay of therapy in this setting, randomized control trials have provided discordant findings.[3] This study does, however, suggest that tight heart rate control (65 beats/min or less) could be beneficial.

To my mind, the performance of noncardiac surgery has never been an indication for coronary revascularization. Coronary revascularization should be performed for all the standard indications, namely the severity of ischemia and symptoms, left ventricular dysfunction, and severity of anatomic obstructive coronary disease. Once a decision has been made to proceed with angiography with a view to revascularization for underlying cardiac reasons, the vascular procedure can then be brought back into the picture in that it may influence the timing of coronary revascularization and the vascular procedure.

**B. J. Gersh, MB, ChB, DPhil, FRCP**

*References*

1. Mold JW, Stein HF: The cascade effect in the clinical care of patients. *N Engl J. Med* 314:512-514, 1986.
2. McFalls EO, Ward HB, Moritz TE, et al: Coronary-artery revascularization before elective major vascular surgery. *N Engl J Med* 351:2795-2804, 2004.
3. Juul AB, Wetterslev J, Kofoed-Enevoldsen, A, et al: Randomized blinded trauma in perioperative metoprolol versus placebo for diabetic patients undergoing non-cardiac surgery. *Circulation* 111:1725-1728, 2005.

---

**Redefinition of Myocardial Infarction: Prospective Evaluation in the Community**

Roger VL, Killian JM, Weston SA, et al (Mayo Clinic College of Medicine, Rochester, Minn; Erasmus Univ Med Ctr, Rotterdam, The Netherlands; Univ of Dundee, Scotland; et al)
*Circulation* 114:790-797, 2006                                                4–50

---

*Background.*—The 2000 European Society of Cardiology/American College of Cardiology definition for myocardial infarction (MI) combines ischemic symptoms, electrocardiographic changes, and troponin rather than creatine kinase levels. The use of troponins will increase the detection of MI by a magnitude to be quantified, and the clinical acceptance of the new definition is unknown.

*Method and Results.*—Subjects presenting to an Olmsted County facility with a troponin T value ≥0.03 ng/mL between November 2002 and March 2005 were prospectively classified through the use of standardized MI criteria, relying on cardiac pain, Minnesota coding of the ECG, and troponin, creatine kinase, and its MB fraction measured simultaneously. Through the use of dynamic changes in troponin, 538 MIs were identified versus 327 with creatine kinase and 427 with only the MB fraction of creatine kinase. This represents a 74% (95% confidence interval [CI], 69% to 79%) increase above the number of MIs identified with creatine kinase and a 41% (95% CI, 37% to 46%) increase above the number identified with criteria including only its MB fraction. When relying on single values of troponin, increases in the number of MIs were always large but varied widely according to the threshold used for troponin. Cases meeting only troponin-based criteria were less likely to have electrocardiographic ST-segment elevation and had better survival than those identified with previous criteria. Clinician diagnoses mentioned MI in 42% (95% CI, 34% to 49%) of cases meeting only troponin-based criteria versus 74% (95% CI, 69% to 78%) for MIs meeting the previous criteria ($P<0.001$).

*Conclusions.*—The prospective application of the new criteria in the community results in a large increase in the number of MIs and a change in case mix. The clinical acceptance of the new criteria is incomplete, and studies that rely exclusively on dismissal diagnoses to assess MI rates may underestimate the burden of disease as presently defined.

▶ In the year 2000 the European Society of Cardiology and the American College of Cardiology recommended a new definition of myocardial infarction that used the troponins as biomarkers of cardiac necrosis. This change in definition acknowledges the increased sensitivity and specificity of the troponins compared with measurements of creatinine kinase and its NB fraction. The implications of this new definition on the increase in the number of cases classified as myocardial infarction and their more benign prognosis are substantial and have widespread public health implications. This study from Olmsted County, Minn, demonstrates that when dynamic changes in troponin, as opposed to single measurements, are taken into account, this results in a 74% increase in the number of myocardial infarctions identified with creatinine kinase and a 41% over the number identified by the MB fraction of creatinine kinase.

The adoption of troponins in clinical practice has been rapid and widespread.[1] Nonetheless, coding practices (code 410) have not changed at the same rate, which means that some patients will be classified as myocardial infarction on the basis of elevated troponin values, whereas the diagnosis in others may be based on more traditional criteria. The economic, social, and research implications of this lack of consistency are a great concern. During 2007, a new and revised definition of myocardial infarction will be published, and this is the subject of current deliberations of a second task force. One has to agree with the sentiments in the editorial accompanying this study and that hopefully the redefinition of myocardial infarction will be universally adopted and used in clinical practice.[2]

**B. J. Gersh, MB, ChB, DPhil, FRCP**

*References*

1. Rosamond WD, Chambless LE, Sorlie PD, et al: Trends in the sensitivity, positive predictive value, false-positive rate, and comparability ratio of hospital discharge diagnosis codes for acute myocardial infarction in four US communities, 1987-2000. *Am J Epidemiol* 160:1137-1146, 2004.
2. Alpert JS, Thygesen K: A call for universal definitions in cardiovascular disease [editorial]. *Circulation* 114:757-758, 2006.

---

**The simplest statistical test: how to check for a difference between treatments**
Pocock SJ (London School of Hygiene and Tropical Medicine)
*BMJ* 332:1256-1258, 2006                                                  4–51

---

*Background.*—Interpretation for clinical trial reports can be a challenge for many readers, given the complexity of the statistical methods used to analyze clinical data. However, the key result of many trials could be presented and interpreted by using simple, readily accessible statistical methods. The primary outcome in many trials is a disease event. In the standard statistical methods, such as Cox proportional hazards modeling and log-rank tests, variation in patient follow-up times is accounted for, but the consequent hazard ratios, confidence intervals, and $P$ values may seem mysterious to some readers. A method for testing statistical significance is described that is much easier to use than Cox proportional hazard modeling and log-rank tests.

*Overview.*—The example given is that of a randomized clinical trial with 2 treatment groups of roughly equal size. The outcome of interest is a clinical event. The key data are the numbers of patients experiencing the clinical event by treatment group. A statistical test of significance can be performed based solely on these 2 numbers. The difference in the 2 numbers of events is calculated and divided by the square root of the their sum. The resulting number is referred to as $z$. Under the null hypothesis that the 2 treatments have identical influence on the risk of an event, $z$ is approximately a standardized normal deviate; in other words, it has a normal distribution with mean 0 and variance 1. Using commonly available normal distribution tables, $z$ can be converted into a $P$ value. This test can be performed in approximately 15 seconds on a calculator and gives an instant feel for the strength of evidence in a treatment difference. However, there are 2 limitations to the test. First, if the denominators differ by a nonnegligible amount, then the test will be biased in the obvious direction. Second, if event rates are high, the test becomes conservative, and the $P$ values are larger than they should be. In most published trials, however, these potential limitations appear negligible.

*Conclusions.*—Many sophisticated, complex statistical methods are appropriately used in the analysis of medical data, but it is important to identify the key information used to derive a study's conclusion. For clinical trials with equal randomization and event outcomes, this simple test can facilitate a better understanding of the key findings.

▶ This report by Dr Stuart Pocock, an internationally recognized biostatus physician, is a "must" for anyone interested in clinical trials. This simple test allows one to eyeball the data and come to a pretty accurate conclusion as to the likelihood and magnitude of statistical significance in approximately 15 seconds. This does not, however, take the place of the more complex biostatistical analysis required in the actual publication of trial data.

The test has 2 major limitations in that one assumption is that the numbers of patients enrolled in each of the 2 groups is roughly equal. In addition, if the event rates are high the test becomes more conservative—that is, the $P$ values are higher than they really are.

So learn to use these "statistics" and impress your friends and colleagues. Since Dr Pocock demonstrated the use of this simple test to me several years ago, I have found it invaluable in a variety of situations in which data are being presented.

**B. J. Gersh, MB, ChB, DPhil, FRCP**

# 5 Non-Coronary Heart Disease in Adults

## Introduction

This year there continue to be studies reported concerning the pathogenesis and prognosis of patients with congestive heart failure (CHF). Levy et al (Abstract 5–7) have reported yet another prognostic index, the Seattle Heart Failure model, derived from 1,100 patients over 17,000 patient-years follow-up. It also has the advantage of estimating the effect on survival by adding or subtracting medications or devices. Since it includes 24 variables in its calculations for survival, calculating the score by hand is impractical and there is a Web-based calculator available. Casolo et al (Abstract 5–8) have reported the use of MRI and late gadolinium enhancement in identifying ischemia as the etiology in patients with CHF. There is an intriguing paper by Blanc et al (Abstract 5–10) on the possibility of primary left bundle branch block eventually leading to CHF, termed left ventricular-induced dyssynchrony cardiomyopathy. With cardiac resynchronization therapy, the cardiomyopathy appears to be reversible. The abnormal response of heart rate reduction after exercise was examined by Nanas et al (Abstract 5–12), who report that a reduction ≤12 beats/min at 1 minute after exercise in a follow-up of almost 2 years predicted a mortality of 65% compared to 11% in those with >12 beats/minute reduction. Lima et al (Abstract 5–13) associated this abnormal heart rate response to exercise to greater myocardial scarring and decreased left ventricular ejection fraction. Anemia and its association with poor prognosis in patients with CHF was addressed in papers by Go et al (Abstract 5–14) and Ralli et al (Abstract 5–6). Whether therapy with erythropoietin is justified remains to be seen, especially with the recent reports of increased mortality with high doses of erythropoietin.

The medical treatment of patients with CHF continues to be a subject of great interest. Statins and their possible effect on prognosis in CHF was addressed by Sola et al (Abstract 5–18) and Mozaffarian et al (Abstract 5–21), in another paper, described the effect of atorvasatin on ventricular function and inflammatory markers in patients with CHF. Vrtovec et al (Abstract 5–20) showed that statins increase heart rate variability and improve repolarization as manifested by QT interval in such a way to decrease arrhythmogenesis and possibly sudden death in patients with CHF. Yancey et al (Abstract 5–17) reported a database of >100,000 CHF patients allowing comparison of therapies and mortality in those with preserved LV function to those with LV dysfunction. The mortality of those with preserved LV function was almost twice that of patients with LV systolic dysfunction, emphasizing the need for more effective therapy in patients with CHF and preserved systolic function. Therapy for diabetic cardiomyopathy continues to be a problem. Grandi et al (Abstract 5–19) presented evidence that good glycemic control improves left ventricular diastolic function in patients with Type 1 diabetes mellitus who were poorly controlled and had normal systolic function. The effect of good glycemic control needs to be studied in diabetic patients with cardiomyopathy to see if the favorable observed effect on diastolic function improves the patient with heart failure. Costello-Boerrigter et al (Abstract 5–22) described the effect of a vasopressin-2-receptor antagonist, tolvaptan, which augments free-water clearance in patients with CHF without changes in renal hemodynamics or sodium, potassium excretion. The effect of perhexilene, a metabolic modulator, was described by Lee et al (Abstract 5–23), and Adamopoulos et al (Abstract 5–24) described the advantages of levosimendan over dobutamine on the inflammatory and apoptotic pathways.

Papers reporting the use of technology in the therapy of CHF continue to be important. By using cardiac resynchronization therapy, Fantoni et al (Abstract 5–26) (CRT) reported improved heart rate variability in patients with moderate to severe CHF consistent with decreased sympathetic activation that may decrease the incidence of malignant arrhythmias and possibly sudden death. Waggoner et al (Abstract 5–3) showed that in patients with CHF, improved diastolic function by CRT is coupled to improved systolic function. If the LV ejection fraction did not increase by 5% or more, there was no improvement in the parameters of diastolic function. In patients with end-stage CHF, Vanderheyden et al (Abstract 5–29) showed that CRT could delay the time that cardiac transplantation was necessary, and Xydas et al (Abstract 5–30) reported that patients supported with left ventricular assist devices (LVAD) had LV unloading that led to a degree of functional, neurohormonal and histologic myocardial recovery. Enhanced external counterpulsation (EECP) has been shown to be useful in patients with refractory angina pectoris. Soran et al (Abstract 5–31) reported the clinical outcome of a 2-year trial of EECP in patients with angina pectoris and LV dysfunction refractory to medical management. Surgical ventricular remodeling in patients with severe CHF continues to be explored. Patel et al (Abstract 5–33) reported 32 patients with CHF, Functional Class III-IV who had surgical exclusion of all LV asynergic areas and restoration of an elliptical geometry to the LV, with marked improvement in LV function and functional status.

Studies concerning valvular disease and infective endocarditis include papers on the effectiveness of repeat mitral valvotomy in patients with recurrent mitral stenosis, the results of aortic valve replacement in patients with poor LV function, the prognosis of patients with prosthesis-patient mismatch, and the value of brain natriuretic peptides in following patients with mitral regurgitation (MR). The significance of MR after an acute myocardial infarction is still questionable. Studies have been inconsistent in finding that new MR after an acute myocardial infarction is an independent predictor of higher late mortality. Hillis et al (Abstract 5–39) reported a large prospective study that finds on multivariate analysis that MR is not an independent predictor of late mortality, and that late mortality depends on the extent of myocardial damage and the residual LV function.

There is still great interest in percutaneous valve replacement. The best results have occurred with percutaneous pulmonic valve replacement. Webb et al (Abstracts 5–40 and 5–41) reported small numbers of patients with percutaneous aortic valve replacement together with results and complications. Feldman et al described a percutaneous technique for doing mitral annuloplasty in patients with MR. The long-term fate of mechanical mitral valve prostheses depends on mechanical valves replacement in large numbers of relatively young patients. DeSanto et al reported (Abstract 5–43) up to a 27-year follow-up of a large number of women who had mechanical mitral valve replacement at average age 30 years. The follow-up gives a very good idea of the frequency of valve-related complications such as thromboembolism and maternal and fetal complications in pregnant women with mechanical prostheses.

With patients who have severe MR and the possibility of mitral valve repair, there is a strong tendency to send such people to surgery, even if asymptomatic with good LV function. Rosenhek et al (Abstract 5–46) managed 132 consecutive asymptomatic patients with severe MR with LV ejection fraction $\geq 60\%$ with watchful waiting, sending patients to surgery only when symptoms occurred of beginning signs of LV dysfunction. The follow-up was almost 7 years and the survival was similar to that of the general population of the same age. This study is an important validation of the ACC/AHA Guidelines for the Management of Patients With Valvular Heart Disease.

Papers by Jassal et al (Abstract 5–48) and Anguera et al evaluated variables that predict the need for surgery in patients with infective endocarditis in large series of patients. Anguera et al focused on the prognosis of patients with periannular abscesses and in a large series of patients found on multivariable analysis that the perivalvular abscess was not an independent predictor of mortality.

The problem of diagnosing and treating patients with myocarditis is addressed in several papers. Magnani et al (Abstract 5–50) examined the role of myocardial biopsy in managing patients with suspected myocarditis that the histopathology was more important than the clinical presentation, the early LV function, or the presence of malignant arrhythmias. A paper by Kůhl et al in a large series of myocarditis patients with myocardial biopsies, all with viral genomes in their cells, reported the follow-up outcomes of those where viral genomes had cleared on rebiopsy compared to those where the viral genomes persisted.

The diagnosis of myocarditis in the absence of myocardial biopsy presents a problem. De Cobelli et al (Abstract 5–52) reported a study showing the value of delayed gadolinium enhanced MRI in identifying myocardial inflammation. Since similar delayed gadolinium enhancement occurs with myocardial infarction, ischemic heart disease must first be ruled out.

In many trials of implantable cardioverter defibrillators (ICD) the number of appropriate shocks is accepted as a surrogate for sudden death. Ellenbogen et al (Abstract 5–51) reported a study of the effectiveness of ICD in patients with non-ischemic cardiomyopathy and showed that compared to a group of medically treated patients that the ICD group had twice as many shocks as the number of fatal events in the medically treated group. The difference in the medically treated group is the number of syncopal episodes. Therefore it is inappropriate to equate appropriate shocks with the number of sudden death episodes avoided.

Izawa et al (Abstract 5–55) explored the mechanism by which mineralocorticoid receptor antagonists (spironolactone and eplerenone) improve LV diastolic function in patients with idiopathic dilated cardiomyopathy. Statins with their pleiotropic activities have been found to be useful in patients with cardiomyopathy. Goldberger et al (Abstract 5–56) reported a 78% reduction in mortality in patients with dilated cardiomyopathy on statins compared to those not on statins, in part because of a decrease in arrhythmic deaths, supporting a role for statins in the therapy of dilated cardiomyopathy.

There are papers on the pregnancy and outcomes of patients with postpartum cardiomyopathy by Mielniczuk et al (Abstract 5–54) and Amos et al (Abstract 5–53). Finally, there are papers on cryptogenic stroke and the possible role of a patent foramen ovale with paradoxical embolism, the role of the endothelin antagonist bosentan in the therapy of pulmonary hypertension related to congenital heart disease, the effectiveness of colchicines in the therapy of acute pericarditis, and the long-term outcomes in difficult-to-treat recurrent pericarditis. As is the case every year, there were at least twice as many interesting and important articles published that could not be included because of space limitations.

M. D. Cheitlin, MD

## Pathogenesis and Prognosis

### Mechanical Dyssynchrony Assessed by Tissue Doppler Imaging Is a Powerful Predictor of Mortality in Congestive Heart Failure With Normal QRS Duration

Cho G-Y, Song J-K, Park W-J, et al (Univ of Hallym, Seoul, Korea; Univ of Ulsan, Seoul, Korea)
*J Am Coll Cardiol* 46:2237-2243, 2005                                              5–1

*Objectives.*—We sought to test whether the mechanical dyssynchrony assessed by tissue Doppler imaging (TDI) is a predictor of cardiac events in patients with congestive heart failure (CHF) and QRS duration ≤120 ms.

*Background.*—The prevalence and prognostic value of mechanical dyssynchrony in patients with CHF and normal QRS duration have not been well clarified.

*Methods.*—A total of 106 patients (age 63 ± 11 years) with CHF and ejection fraction (EF) <35% were followed serially; TDI was performed using

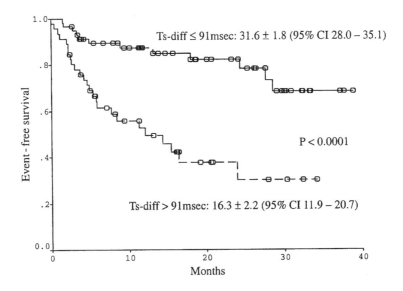

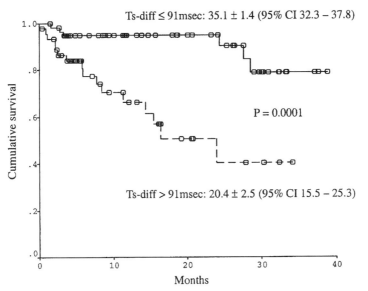

**FIGURE 4.**—Clinical event-free survival (**top**) and mortality-free survival (**bottom**) by Kaplan-Meier analysis. Patients with maximal temporal difference of time to peak systolic point from R-wave on electrocardiogram (Ts-diff) >91 ms were expressed in a **dashed line** and those with Ts-diff ≤91 ms in a **solid line**. CI = confidence interval. (Reprinted with permission from the American College of Cardiology from Cho G-Y, Song J-K, Park W-J, et al: Mechanical dyssynchrony assessed by tissue Doppler imaging is a powerful predictor of mortality in congestive heart failure with normal QRS duration. *J Am Coll Cardiol* 46:2237-2243. Copyright Elsevier 2005.)

four basal and four mid-left ventricular segments to assess the time to peak systolic point from R-wave on electrocardiogram (Ts). The standard deviation of Ts (Ts-SD) and the maximal temporal difference of Ts (Ts-diff) of eight segments were used as an indicator of mechanical dyssynchrony. Clinical events included readmission due to worsening of CHF, cardiac transplantation, and death.

*Results.*—After 17 ± 11 months of follow-up, the clinical event rate was 33% including all-cause mortality of 19%. Prolonged Ts-SD (>37 ms) and Ts-diff (>91 ms) were associated with a significant increase in all clinical events. By multivariate analysis, Ts-diff (>91 ms) was an independent risk factor of clinical events and mortality regardless of age, EF, QRS duration, and use of beta-blocking agents. Mean event-free survival was 16.3 months (95% confidence interval [CI] 11.9 to 20.7) in patients with Ts-diff >91 ms and 31.6 months (95% CI 28.0 to 35.1) in those with Ts-diff ≤91 ms, respectively (p < 0.001).

*Conclusions.*—Myocardial dyssynchrony assessed by TDI is a powerful predictor of clinical events in CHF with normal QRS (Fig 4).

---

### Diastolic Asynchrony Is More Frequent Than Systolic Asynchrony in Dilated Cardiomyopathy and Is Less Improved by Cardiac Resynchronization Therapy

Schuster I, Habib G, Jego C, et al (La Timone Hosp, Marseille, France; Hôpital Louis Pradel, Lyon, France)
*J Am Coll Cardiol* 46:2250-2257, 2005                                   5–2

---

*Objectives.*—To compare the incidence of diastolic and systolic asynchrony, assessed by tissue Doppler imaging (TDI), in patients with congestive heart failure (CHF) and severe left ventricular (LV) dysfunction, and to assess TDI changes induced by cardiac resynchronization therapy (CRT).

*Background.*—Thirty percent of CRT candidates are nonresponders. Besides QRS width, the presence of echographic systolic asynchrony has been used to identify future responders. Little is known about diastolic asynchrony and its change after CRT.

*Methods.*—Tissue Doppler imaging was performed in 116 CHF patients (LV ejection fraction 26 ± 8%). Systolic and diastolic asynchrony was calculated using TDI recordings of right ventricular and LV walls.

*Results.*—The CHF group consisted of 116 patients. Diastolic asynchrony was more frequent than systolic, concerning both intraventricular (58% vs. 47%; p = 0.0004) and interventricular (72 vs. 45%; p < 0.0001) asynchrony. Systolic and diastolic asynchrony were both present in 41% patients, but one-third had isolated diastolic asynchrony. Although diastolic delays increased with QRS duration, 42% patients with narrow QRS presented with diastolic asynchrony. Conversely, 27% patients with large QRS had no diastolic asynchrony. Forty-two patients underwent CRT. Incidence of systolic intraventricular asynchrony decreased from 71% to 33% after CRT (p < 0.0001), but diastolic asynchrony decreased only from 81% to

55% (p < 0.0002). Cardiac resynchronization therapy induced new diastolic asynchrony in eight patients.

*Conclusions.*—Diastolic asynchrony is weakly correlated with QRS duration, is more frequent than systolic asynchrony, and may be observed alone. Diastolic asynchrony is less improved by CRT than systolic. Persistent diastolic asynchrony may explain some cases of lack of improvement after CRT despite good systolic resynchronization.

---

**Improvements in Left Ventricular Diastolic Function After Cardiac Resynchronization Therapy Are Coupled to Response in Systolic Performance**
Waggoner AD, Faddis MN, Gleva MJ, et al (Washington Univ School of Medicine, St Louis)
*J Am Coll Cardiol* 46:2244-2249, 2005                                    5–3

---

*Objectives.*—To determine the short-term effects of cardiac resynchronization therapy (CRT) on measurements of left ventricular (LV) diastolic function in patients with severe heart failure.

*Background.*—Cardiac resynchronization therapy improves systolic performance; however, the effects on diastolic function by load-dependent pulsed-wave Doppler transmitral indices has been variable.

*Methods.*—Fifty patients with severe heart failure were evaluated by two-dimensional Doppler echocardiography immediately prior to and 4 ± 1 month after CRT. Measurements included LV volumes and ejection fraction (EF), pulsed-wave Doppler (PWD)-derived transmitral filling indices (E- and A-wave velocities, E/A ratio, deceleration time [DT], diastolic filling time [DFT], and isovolumic relaxation time). Tissue Doppler imaging was used for measurements of systolic and diastolic (Em) velocities at four mitral annular sites; mitral E-wave/Em ratio was calculated to estimate LV filling pressure. Color M-mode flow propagation velocities were also obtained.

*Results.*—After CRT, LV volumes decreased significantly (p < 0.001) and LVEF increased >5% in 28 of 50 patients (56%) and were accompanied by reduction in PWD mitral E-wave velocity and E/A ratio (both p < 0.01), increased DT and DFT (both p < 0.01), and lower filling pressures (i.e., E-wave/Em septal; p < 0.01). Patients with LVEF response ≤5% after CRT had no significant changes in measurements of diastolic function; LV relaxation (i.e., Em velocities) worsened in this group.

*Conclusions.*—In heart failure patients receiving CRT, improvement in LV diastolic function is coupled to the improvement in LV systolic function.

▶ Cardiac resynchronization (CR) in patients with congestive heart failure (CHF) and prolonged QRS complexes has been a major advance in therapy. Cho et al (Abstract 5–1) using tissue Doppler imaging in patients with CHF and a QRS ≤120 ms, not all with a "normal duration QRS" as advertised in the title of the article, have shown that mechanical dyssynchrony by multivariate analysis is a powerful independent predictor for adverse clinical events, including hospitalization for worsening CHF, serious ventricular arrhythmias, heart transplantation, and all-cause mortality. The mean QRS duration was longer in those with clinical events (103 ± 12 ms) compared with those without (45 ± 12 msec). Whether CR in patients with QRS duration ≤120 msec and mechanical dyssynchrony will have the same improvement in exercise capacity and decrease in clinical events mentioned remains to be seen.

Other papers of interest in this field are those by Schuster et al (Abstract 5–2) and Waggoner et al (Abstract 5–3). Schuster et al, by using tissue Doppler imaging in patients with dilated cardiomyopathy with an ejection fraction of 26% ± 8%, showed that diastolic asynchrony is more frequent than systolic asynchrony, both between the 2 ventricles (72% vs 45%) and between any 2 parts of the left ventricle (58% vs 47%). Although diastolic delays increased with QRS duration, 42% of patients with narrow QRS had diastolic asynchrony. With CR therapy in 42 patients, the incidence of systolic intraventricular asynchrony decreased from 71% to 33% (*P* < .0001), but diastolic asynchrony only decreased from 81% to 55% (*P* < .0002). Therefore, diastolic asynchrony is less improved by CR than systolic dysynchrony is. Also, CR produced diastolic asynchrony in 7% of patients. These findings may explain to some extent the 30% of CR candidates who are nonresponders.

Waggoner et al showed that improvement in left ventricular diastolic function after CR is coupled to a response in systolic performance. With CR patients, an ejection fraction increase >5% was accompanied by reduction in pulsed-wave Doppler mitral E-wave velocity and E/A ratio, increased deceleration time and diastolic filling time, and lower filling pressures, as measured by E wave/Em septal tissue Doppler velocities. Patients with an ejection fraction response <5% after CR had no significant changes in measurements of diastolic function.

**M. D. Cheitlin, MD**

---

**QT dispersion is determined by the relative extent of normal, hibernating, and scarred myocardium in patients with chronic ischemic cardiomyopathy. A dobutamine stress echocardiography study before and after surgical revascularization**

Papadopoulos CE, Zaglavara T, Karvounis HI, et al (Freeman Hosp, Newcastle upon Tyne, England; Aristotle Univ of Thessaloniki, Greece)
*J Electrocardiol* 39:103-109, 2006                         5–4

---

*Introduction.*—The aim of the present study was to evaluate a possible association between QT dispersion (QTd) and the amount of viable and scarred myocardial tissue after revascularization in patients with coronary artery disease and impaired left ventricular (LV) function.

*Methods.*—Twenty-two patients with ischemic LV dysfunction underwent dobutamine stress echocardiography (DSE) before and 6 months after surgical revascularization. Mean corrected QT-interval value and QTd were calculated at baseline and follow-up. Segments consisting of transmural scar were determined as the segments that remained akinetic in all stages of DSE despite reperfusion. Patients were divided into 2 groups according to the number of definitive segments consisting of transmural scar (minor scar group, ≤2 scarred segments; major scar group, >2 scarred segments).

*Results.*—QTd was significantly lower in the minor compared with the major scar group at baseline and follow-up (mean [SD], 61 [22] vs 98 [33] milliseconds, $P = .008$, and 45 [18] vs 68 [21] milliseconds, $P = .01$, respectively). Segments consisting of transmural scar positively correlated to QTd at baseline ($r = 0.53, P = .01$) and follow-up ($r = 0.62, P = .002$).

*Conclusions.*—QTd is positively correlated with the extent of scarred myocardial tissue assessed by DSE. Surgical revascularization results in reduction of QTd in all patients with hibernating myocardium and LV dysfunction.

▶ QT dispersion (QTd) as a predictor of cardiac mortality or arrhythmic mortality in patients with severe left ventricular (LV) dysfunction resulting from coronary artery disease is still controversial.[1-3] Most of these studies did not consider the extent of hibernating or ischemic myocardium or the effect of revascularization. The unique feature of this study that shows that the duration of QTd is determined by the relative extent of scarred hibernating myocardium in the patient with chronic LV dysfunction is that the myocardial scar was determined by resting akinesis and the absence of contractile reserve at 6 months after successful revascularization. Revascularization showed the greatest decrease in QTd in the group with major scar, a group also with a significant amount of hibernating myocardium. The QTd reduction occurred even with a lack of improvement in resting LV ejection fraction. Previous studies have shown a marked improvement in long-term prognosis in patients with hibernating myocardium.[4,5] Decreasing the QTd and arrhythmogenisity could partly account for this prognostic benefit.[6]

**M. D. Cheitlin, MD**

*References*

1. Brendorp B, Elming H, Jun L, et al: Qt dispersion has no prognostic information for patients with advanced congestive heart failure and reduced left ventricular systolic function. *Circulation* 103:831-835, 2001.
2. Spargias KS, Lindsay SJ, Kawar GI, et al: QT dispersion as a predictor of long-term mortality in patients with acute myocardial infarction and clinical evidence of heart failure. *Eur Heart J* 20:1158-1165, 1999.
3. Padmanabhan S, Silvet H, Amin J, et al: Prognostic value of QT interval and QT dispersion in patients with left ventricular systolic dysfunction: Results from a cohort of 2265 patients with an ejection fraction of ≤40%. *Am Heart J* 145:132-138, 2003.
4. Pasquet A, Robert A, D'Hondt AM, et al: Prognostic value of myocardial ischemia and viability in patients with chronic left ventricular. *Circulation* 100:141-148, 1999.
5. Senior R, Kaul S, Lahiri A: Myocardial viability on echocardiography predicts long-term survival after revascularization in patients with ischemic congestive heart failure. *J Am Coll Cardiol* 33:1848-1854, 1999.
6. Bonow RO: Identification of viable myocardium. *Circulation* 94:2674-2680, 1996.

## Depression predicts mortality and hospitalization in patients with myocardial infarction complicated by heart failure

Rumsfeld JS, Jones PG, Whooley MA, et al (Denver VA Med Ctr; Univ of Colorado Health Sciences Ctr, Denver; Mid-America Heart Inst, Kansas City, Mo; et al)

*Am Heart J* 150:961-967, 2005                                                    5–5

*Background.*—To evaluate whether depressive symptoms are independently predictive of mortality and hospitalization among patients with acute myocardial infarction (AMI) complicated by heart failure.

*Methods.*—The EPHESUS trial enrolled patients with AMI complicated by heart failure. Patients from Canada, the UK, and the United States completed a Medical Outcomes Study-Depression questionnaire at baseline in addition to a comprehensive clinical examination. Cox proportional hazards regression was used to determine the relationship between depressive symptoms and outcomes, including 2-year all-cause mortality and cardiovascular death or hospitalization, adjusting for baseline clinical variables.

*Results.*—Overall, 143 of 634 patients (22.6%) had significant depressive symptoms at baseline (Medical Outcomes Study-Depression score ≥0.06). Depressed patients had higher 2-year mortality (29% vs 18%; $P$ = .004) and cardiovascular death or hospitalization (42% vs 33%; $P$ = .016). After risk adjustment, depressive symptoms remained significantly associated with mortality (hazard ratio 1.75, 95% CI 1.15-2.68, $P$ = .01) and cardiovascular death or hospitalization (hazard ratio 1.41, 95% CI 1.03-1.93, $P$ = .03). Results were consistent across demographic and clinical subgroups.

*Conclusions.*—Depression is an independent predictor of all-cause mortality and cardiovascular death or hospitalization after AMI complicated by

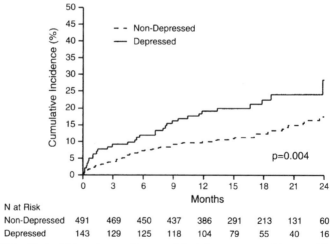

FIGURE 1.—Kaplan-Meier estimates of the rate of death from any cause. (Courtesy of Rumsfeld JS, Jones PG, Whooley MA, et al: Depression indicates mortality and hospitalization in patients with myocardial infarction complicated by heart failure. *Am Heart J* 150:961-967. Copyright Elsevier 2005.)

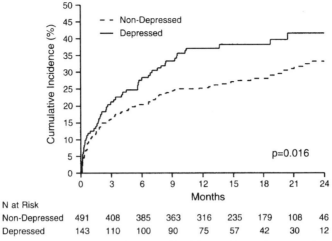

FIGURE 2.—Kaplan-Meier estimates of the rate of death from cardiovascular causes or hospitalization for cardiac events. (Courtesy of Rumsfeld JS, Jones PG, Whooley MA, et al: Depression indicates mortality and hospitalization in patients with myocardial infarction complicated by heart failure. *Am Heart J* 150:961-967. Copyright Elsevier 2005.)

heart failure. Although many factors may mediate outcomes in patients with AMI, studies are warranted to evaluate whether a depression intervention can improve survival and/or reduce hospitalizations (Figs 1 and 2).

▶ Heart failure commonly complicates acute myocardial infarction (AMI) and results in an elevated risk of adverse outcomes including mortality and rehospitalization. Depression also commonly complicates AMI and is associated with increased mortality and morbidity,[1,2] but most studies did not adequately adjust for left ventricular (LV) function, so it is uncertain whether the adverse outcomes are due to LV dysfunction or to depression. The current study from the Eplerenone Post-Acute Myocardial Infarction Heart Failure Efficacy and Survival Study (EPHESUS) surveyed patients with acute myocardial infarction with LV dysfunction and heart failure before discharge for depression, using the MOS-D questionnaire. They found that the presence of depression was an independent predictor of all-cause mortality, cardiovascular death, or rehospitalization. The association between depression and all-cause mortality was consistent among subgroups of age, gender, prior myocardial infarction or heart failure, and diabetes. Depression remained predictive of adverse outcome after adjustment for cardiac and noncardiac history, presentation, cardiac function, revascularization, and discharge medications. It remains to be seen whether treatment of depression in patients with AMI and heart failure will improve outcome.

**M. D. Cheitlin, MD**

*References*

1. Ziegelstein RC: Depression after myocardial infarction. *Cardiol Rev* 9:45-51, 2001.

2. Lesperance F, Frasure-Smith N, Talajic M, et al: Five-year risk of cardiac mortality in relation to initial severity and one-year changes in depression symptoms after myocardial infarction. *Circulation* 105:1049-1053, 2002.

---

**Relationship between anemia, cardiac troponin I, and B-type natriuretic peptide levels and mortality in patients with advanced heart failure**
Ralli S, Horwich TB, Fonarow GC (Ahmanson-UCLA Cardiomyopathy Ctr, Los Angeles)
*Am Heart J* 150:1220-1227, 2005                                         5–6

---

*Background.*—Anemia has been associated with worse symptoms and increased mortality in patients with advanced HF. The association between anemia and biomarkers of increased HF risk is unknown. This study aimed to evaluate the relationship between hemoglobin (Hb), cardiac troponin I (cTnI), B-type natriuretic peptide (BNP), and mortality in patients with advanced heart failure (HF).

*Methods.*—A cohort of 264 patients with advanced HF referred to a single university HF center was analyzed. Hb, cTnI, and BNP levels were drawn at time of initial evaluation. Patients were divided into groups based on the presence or absence of anemia, detectable cTnI ($\geq$0.04 ng/mL), and elevated BNP ($\geq$485 pg/mL).

*Results.*—Mean Hb was 13.0 and the values ranged from 7.7 to 17.9 g/dL. Anemic patients were more likely to have elevated BNP (65.7% vs 47.4%, $P = .002$). Cardiac troponin I levels were detectable in 50.9% and 46.8% of anemic and non-anemic patients, respectively ($P = .3$). Anemic patients were at 2.3-fold increased risk of mortality ($P = .04$). Low Hb, detectable cTnI, and elevated BNP remained independent predictors of mortality on multivariate analysis. Anemia in the setting of detectable cTnI, elevated BNP, or both, was associated with markedly increased mortality.

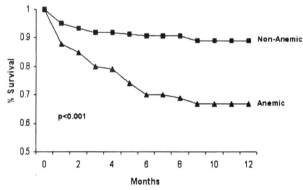

FIGURE 2.—Kaplan-Meier survival analysis by anemia classification. (−)Anemia, Hb $\geq$13 mg/dL (male) and $\geq$12 mg/dL (female); (+anemia, Hb <13 mg/dL (male) and <12 mg/dL (female). (Courtesy of Ralli S, Horwich TB, Fonarow GC: Relationship between anemia, cardiac troponin I, and B-type natriuretic peptide levels and mortality in patients with advanced heart failure. *Am Heart J* 150:1220-1227. Copyright Elsevier 2005.)

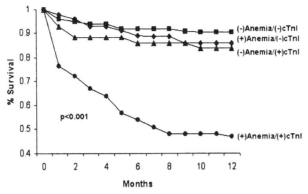

FIGURE 3.—Kaplan-Meier survival analysis by stratification of anemia and detectable cTnI. (−)Anemia, Hb ≥13 mg/dL (male) and ≥12 mg/dL (female); (+)anemia, Hb <13 mg/dL (male) and <12 mg/dL (female); (−)cTnI, cTnI <0.04 ng/mL.; (+)cTnI, cTnI ≥0.04 ng/mL. (Courtesy of Ralli S, Horwich TB, Fonarow GC: Relationship between anemia, cardiac troponin I, and B-type natriuretic peptide levels and mortality in patients with advanced heart failure. *Am Heart J* 150:1220-1227. Copyright Elsevier 2005.)

*Conclusions.*—Anemia is associated with elevated BNP and increased mortality in HF. Furthermore, elevation of the cardiac biomarkers, BNP and cTnI, in patients with HF and anemia identifies patients at particularly high risk of future events (Figs 2, 3, 4, and 5).

▶ Anemia in congestive heart failure is common, occurring in 25% to 50% of patients, and a linear, inverse relationship has been identified between hemoglobin levels and heart failure mortality rates.[1] Elevation of troponin I and B-type natriuretic peptide (BNP) levels are also predictive of death in patients with heart failure. This article is about 246 patients with "advanced" heart failure, which is never definitely defined, 28% with NYHA class IV symptoms. The heart failure was due to ischemic heart disease in 50%, idiopathic cardiomy-

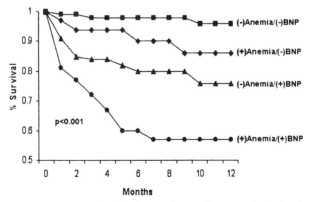

FIGURE 4.—Kaplan-Meier survival analysis by stratification of anemia and BNP elevation. (−)Anemia, Hb ≥13 mg/dL (male) and ≥12 mg/dL (female); (+)anemia, Hb <13 mg/dL (male) and <12 mg/dL (female); (−)BNP, BNP <485 pg/mL; (+)BNP, BNP ≥485 pg/mL. (Courtesy of Ralli S, Horwich TB, Fonarow GC: Relationship between anemia, cardiac troponin I, and B-type natriuretic peptide levels and mortality in patients with advanced heart failure. *Am Heart J* 150:1220-1227. Copyright Elsevier 2005.)

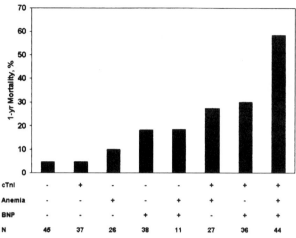

FIGURE 5.—One-year mortality rates by stratification of anemia, detectable cTnI, and BNP elevation. (−)Anemia, Hb ≥13 mg/dL (male) and ≥12 mg/dL (female); (+)anemia, Hb <13 mg/dL (male) and <12 mg/ dL (female); (−)cTnI, cTnI <0.04 ng/mL; (+)cTnI, cTnI ≥0.04 ng/mL; (−)BNP, BNP <485 pg/mL; (+)BNP, BNP ≥485 pg/mL. N indicates number of patients in each group. (Courtesy of Ralli S, Horwich TB, Fonarow GC: Relationship between anemia, cardiac troponin I, and B-type natriuretic peptide levels and mortality in patients with advanced heart failure. *Am Heart J* 150:1220-1227. Copyright Elsevier 2005.)

opathy in 17%, and other etiologies in 33%. Anemia was defined as < 13 g/dL in men and <12 g/dL in women. Elevated BNP was defined as >485 pg/ml$^2$ and detectable tropnin I as ≤0.04 ng/mL. The authors found that patients with anemia had a relative risk (RR) of a 2.3 increase in the 1-year mortality rate. Each 1 g/dL decrease in hemoglobin was associated with an age- and sex-adjusted 43% increase in the mortality rate. If the BNP was also increased, there was a 10.4-fold increase in the risk of death, a 1-year mortality rate of 35.3%. In anemic patients with a detectable troponin I, there was a 5.3-fold increase in death, and with all 3 abnormalities, the 1-year mortality rate was the highest (58.4%). With the absence of all 3 abnormalities, the 1-year mortality rate was an exceptionally low 3.7%. Whether treating the anemia would lower the incidence of BP and troponin I levels and thus, the mortality rate, is a question that should be investigated.

**M. D. Cheitlin, MD**

*References*

1. Horwich TB, Fonarow GC, Hamilton MA, et al. Anemia is associated with worse symptoms, greater impairment in functional capacity and a significant increase in mortality in patients with advanced heart failure. *J Am Coll Cardiol* 39:1780-1786, 2002.
2. Horwich TB, Patel J, MacLellan WR, et al: Cardiac troponin I is associated with impaired hemodynamics, progressive left ventricular dysfunction, and increased mortality rates in advanced heart failure. *Circulation* 108:833-838, 2003.

### The Seattle Heart Failure Model: Prediction of Survival in Heart Failure

Levy WC, Mozaffarian D, Linker DT, et al (Univ of Washington, Seattle; Harvard Med School; Merck Research Labs, Blue Bell, Pa; et al)
*Circulation* 113:1424-1433, 2006                                            5–7

*Background.*—Heart failure has an annual mortality rate ranging from 5% to 75%. The purpose of the study was to develop and validate a multivariate risk model to predict 1-, 2-, and 3-year survival in heart failure patients with the use of easily obtainable characteristics relating to clinical status, therapy (pharmacological as well as devices), and laboratory parameters.

*Method and Results.*—The Seattle Heart Failure Model was derived in a cohort of 1125 heart failure patients with the use of a multivariate Cox model. For medications and devices not available in the derivation database, hazard ratios were estimated from published literature. The model was prospectively validated in 5 additional cohorts totaling 9942 heart failure patients and 17,307 person-years of follow-up. The accuracy of the model was excellent, with predicted versus actual 1-year survival rates of 73.4% versus 74.3% in the derivation cohort and 90.5% versus 88.5%, 86.5% versus 86.5%, 83.8% versus 83.3%, 90.9% versus 91.0%, and 89.6% versus 86.7% in the 5 validation cohorts. For the lowest score, the 2-year survival was 92.8% compared with 88.7%, 77.8%, 58.1%, 29.5%, and 10.8% for scores of 0, 1, 2, 3, and 4, respectively. The overall receiver operating characteristic area under the curve was 0.729 (95% CI, 0.714 to 0.744). The model also allowed estimation of the benefit of adding medications or devices to an individual patient's therapeutic regimen.

*Conclusions.*—The Seattle Heart Failure Model provides an accurate estimate of 1-, 2-, and 3-year survival with the use of easily obtained clinical, pharmacological, device, and laboratory characteristics.

▶ Heart failure from a variety of heart diseases affects more than 5 million people in the United States. Each year more than one half million new cases are diagnosed and ~1 million are hospitalized.[1] There are a numerous prognostic scores available in the literature, many of which have problems in that they have been derived from hospitalized patients, patients with a single etiology of their heart failure, and, especially, failure to validate in a general population of patients with different etiologies and severities of heart failure. This article reports the Seattle Heart Failure Model (SHFM), which was derived from the Prospective Randomized Amlodopine Survival Evaluation (PRAISE 1) study and validated in 5 other heart failure studies. The aggregate patient population is therefore more than 11,000 patients with more than 17,000 patient-years of follow-up.The SHFM score performs very well in all the validation cohorts. Although many heart failure scores include variables such as peak oxygen consumption or even invasive measures of cardiac performance,[2] the SHFM uses commonly assessed clinical and laboratory variables as well as heart failure medications and devices (defibrillators and biventricular pacemakers). An additional benefit is that the effect on survival by adding or subtracting medications or devices can be estimated. Because the calculation of survival includes 14 continuous variables and 10 categorical values, it is impractical to calculate the score by hand. A Web-based calculator (*http://www.SeattleHeartFailureModel.org*) is available, allowing an interactive calculation of estimated survival as well as the effects of adding or subtracting medication or devices. This is the most comprehensive validated congestive heart failure survival score to date addressing the general population of patients with congestive heart failure.

**M. D. Cheitlin, MD**

*References*

1. Heart disease and stroke statistics: 2004 update. Available at: http://www.american heart.org. Accessed April 28, 2007.
2. Aaronson KD, Schwartz JS, Chen TM, et al: Development and prospective validation of a clinical index to predict survival in ambulatory patients referred for cardiac transplant evaluation. *Circulation* 1795:2660-2667, 1997.

---

**Identification of the ischemic etiology of heart failure by cardiovascular magnetic resonance imaging: Diagnostic accuracy of late gadolinium enhancement**
Casolo G, Minneci S, Manta R, et al (Azienda Universitaria Ospedaliera Careggi, Florence, Italy; Nuovo Ospedale San Giovanni di Dio, Florence, Italy)
*Am Heart J* 151:101-108, 2006                                                   5–8

---

*Background.*—A large proportion of patients with heart failure (HF) have a large and poorly contracting left ventricle. The noninvasive recognition of the ischemic etiology of such patients is difficult, and for this purpose, usually patients undergo coronary angiography. It has been shown that cardiovascular magnetic resonance (CMR) imaging can detect myocardial scarring by evaluating late gadolinium enhancement (LGE). The diagnostic accuracy of such a method in differentiating the etiology of HF has not been previously tested in an unselected HF ambulatory population.

*Methods.*—We studied 60 ambulatory patients consecutively enrolled from a specialized HF clinic. We included HF patients who were found to have increased left ventricular (LV) dimensions and reduced function. CMR was performed in these patients by operators who were unaware of patients' history and clinical conditions. LV dimensions and global and regional function, as well as the pattern of LGE, were obtained in each subject. Coronary angiography was subsequently performed in all the patients. The diagnostic accuracy of clinical history and electrocardiographic patterns, as well as regional wall motion abnormalities, wall thinning, and LGE, in differentiating coronary artery disease (CAD) from non-CAD patients were evaluated.

*Results.*—The majority of CAD patients (98%) showed LV contrast hyperenhancement with respect to non-CAD HF subjects (16%). The detection of LGE by CMR had a sensitivity of 98% and a specificity of 84% and an overall accuracy of 93% in detecting CAD etiology among HF patients.

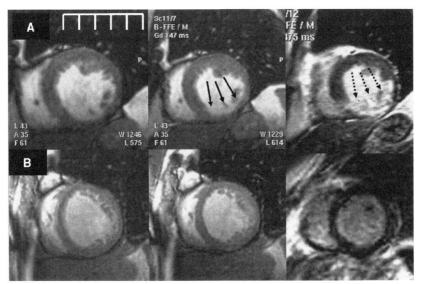

FIGURE 1.—The upper part of the image (**A**) refers to the diastolic (left) and systolic (center) frame of the cine series in the short-axis plane of the left ventricle of a CAD patient. The dark arrows indicate the thinned inferior wall also showing absence of systolic thickening. On the right is shown the LGE image corresponding to the same level of the other images. The arrows with dotted lines indicate the transmural delayed hyperenhancement at this level consistent with an irreversibly damaged myocardium. The lower part of the image (**B**) refers to a non-CAD HF patient. Note the absence of WT and homogeneous wall thickening in the absence of myocardial contrast uptake. Each segment of the distance marker corresponds to 1 cm. (Courtesy of Casolo G, Minneci S, Manta R, et al: Identification of the ischemic etiology of heart failure by cardiovascular magnetic resonance imaging: Diagnostic accuracy of late gadolinium enhancement. *Am Heart J* 151:101-108. Copyright Elsevier 2006.)

*Conclusions.*—LGE is able to accurately differentiate CAD from non-CAD etiology of HF and may represent a clinically useful noninvasive tool for this purpose. As it provides relevant functional information as well as insight into the etiology, CMR may be included among the most important diagnostic tools in the workup of patients with HF (Fig 1).

▶ Congestive heart failure and a dilated hypocontractile left ventricle (LV) can be due to coronary artery disease (CAD) or nonischemic cardiomyopathy. Differentiating the two can be difficult clinically. The usual approach is to do a myocardial perfusion stress test to detect the presence of myocardial ischemia or localized fibrosis or to do a coronary arteriogram. This study of 600 patients with congestive heart failure and a hypocontractile LV studied with magnetic resonance imaging (MRI) with gadolinium injection showed that late gadolinium enhancement (LGE) of the myocardium was present in 98% of patients with CAD and only 16% of patients with non-CAD etiology. LGE correlates with the presence of fibrosis and therefore is nonspecific for CAD, although that is the most frequent reason for regional scarring of the LV. Gadolinium enhancement is seen in patients with hypertrophic obstructive cardiomyopathy[1] and myocarditis, where the enhancement is in the area of active inflammatory infiltrate,[2] but the pattern of enhancement differs from that found in fibrosis resulting from CAD. MRI with LGE has been described as a diagnostic tool for CAD in congestive heart failure before.[3,4] The major feature of this study is the blind examination of the MRI gadolinium scan and the confirmation of the presence or absence of CAD by coronary arterioraphy. More important than the identification of CAD as the cause of the dilated heart and heart failure is the fact that the presence of CAD in such patients and the absence of LGE predicts viability and reversibility of the LV dysfunction after revascularization. This is another method to evaluate myocardial viability. Such a study was reported by Kim et al[5] who showed that reversible myocardial dysfunction can be identified by contrast-enhanced MRI and that the percentage of the LV that was both dysfunctional and not hyperenhanced before revascularization was strongly related to the degree of improvement in the global mean wall motion score and LV ejection fraction after revascularization.

**M. D. Cheitlin, MD**

*References*

1. Moon JC, McKenna WJ, McCrohon JA, et al: Toward clinical risk assessment in hypertrophic cardiomyopathy with gadolinium cardiovascular magnetic resonance. *J Am Coll Cardiol* 41:1561-1567, 2003.
2. Mahrholdt H, Goedecke C, Wagner A, et al: Cardiovascular magnetic resonance assessment of human myocarditis: A comparison to histology and molecular pathology. *Circulation* 109:1250-1258, 2004.
3. Wu E, Judd RM, Vargas JD, et al: Visualisation of presence, location, and transmural extent of healed Q-wave and non-Q-wave myocardial infarction. *Lancet* 357:21-28, 2001.
4. McCrohon JA, Moon JC, Prasad SK, et al: Differentiation of heart failure enhanced cardiovascular magnetic resonance. *Circulation* 108:54-59, 2003.
5. Kim RJ, Wu E, Rafael A, et al: The use of contrast-enhanced magnetic resonance imaging to identify reversible myocardial dysfunction. *N Engl J Med* 343:1445-1453, 2000.

---

**Electrocardiographic Strain Pattern and Prediction of New-Onset Congestive Heart Failure in Hypertensive Patients: The Losartan Intervention for Endpoint Reduction in Hypertension (LIFE) Study**
Okin PM, for the LIFE Study Investigators (Weill Med College of Cornell Univ, New York; et al)
*Circulation* 113:67-73, 2006                                                                      5–9

---

*Background.*—The ECG strain pattern of ST depression and T-wave inversion is strongly associated with left ventricular hypertrophy (LVH) independently of coronary heart disease and with an increased risk of cardiovascular morbidity and mortality in hypertensive patients. However, whether ECG strain is an independent predictor of new-onset congestive heart failure (CHF) in the setting of aggressive antihypertensive therapy in unclear.

*Method and Results.*—The relationship of ECG strain at study baseline to the development of CHF was examined in 8696 patients with no history of CHF who were enrolled in the Losartan Intervention for Endpoint Reduction in Hypertension (LIFE) study. All patients had ECG LVH by Cornell product and/or Sokolow-Lyon voltage criteria on a screening ECG, were treated in a blinded manner with atenolol- or losartan-based regimens, and were followed up for a mean of 4.7±1.1 years. Strain was defined as a downsloping convex ST segment with inverted asymmetrical T-wave opposite the QRS axis in lead $V_5$ or $V_6$. ECG strain was present in 923 patients (10.6%), and new-onset CHF occurred in 265 patients (3.0%), 26 of whom had a CHF-related death. Compared with patients who did not develop CHF, hypertensive patients who developed CHF were older; were more likely to be black, current smokers, and diabetic; were more like to have a history of myocardial infarction, ischemic heart disease, stroke, or peripheral vascular disease; and had greater baseline severity of LVH by Cornell product and Sokolow-Lyon voltage, higher baseline body mass indexes, higher serum glucose levels and albuminuria, similar baseline systolic and diastolic pressures, and reductions in diastolic pressure with treatment but greater reductions in systolic pressure. In univariate Cox analyses, ECG strain was a significant predictor of new-onset CHF (hazard ratio [HR], 3.27; 95% CI, 2.49 to 4.29) and CHF mortality (HR, 4.74; 95% CI, 2.11 to 10.64). In Cox multivariable analyses adjusting for baseline differences between patients with and without new-onset CHF, in-treatment differences in systolic and diastolic pressures, Sokolow-Lyon voltage, and Cornell product, and the impact of treatment with losartan versus atenolol on outcomes, ECG strain remained a significant predictor of incident CHF (HR, 1.80; 95% CI, 1.30 to 2.48) and CHF-related death (HR, 2.78; 95% CI, 1.02 to 7.63).

*Conclusions.*—ECG strain identifies hypertensive patients at increased risk of developing CHF and dying as a result of CHF, even in the setting of aggressive blood pressure.

▶ With the geometric increase in the number and complexity of technologies capable of imaging the heart and aiding in cardiovascular diagnosis together with the escalating number of serum markers to predict prognosis in patients with heart disease, it is refreshing to see that there is still value and new potential uses in one of the oldest technologies for the diagnosis for heart disease, the ECG. In a substudy from the Losartan Intervention for Endpoint reduction in Hypertension (LIFE) study, which included 8696 hypertensive patients without a history of congestive heart failure, the predictors of those patients who would develop heart failure were examined. On multivariate Cox analysis adjusting for the other significant prognostic factors for new-onset congestive heart failure such as in-treatment differences in systolic and diastolic blood pressure, QRS voltage, and impact of treatment with losartan versus atenolol, ECG strain (downward ST depression and T wave inversion in $V_5$ and $V_6$) remained a significant predictor of new-onset heart failure (hazard ratio [HR] 1.80, 95% CI 1.30-2.48) and congestive heart failure related death (HR 2.78, 95% CI 1.02-7.63).

Aside from its invaluable primary use in diagnosing arrhythmias, the elderly ECG is still one of the most useful tools we have in cardiology.

**M. D. Cheitlin, MD**

### Evaluation of left bundle branch block as a reversible cause of non-ischaemic dilated cardiomyopathy with severe heart failure. A new concept of left ventricular dyssynchrony-induced cardiomyopathy

Blanc J-J, Fatemi M, Bertault V, et al (Brest Univ Hosp, France)
*Europace* 7:604-610, 2005                                          5–10

*Objectives.*—We sought to determine if amelioration of left bundle branch block (LBBB)-induced contraction disturbances achieved by left ventricular (LV)-based pacing could result in sustained reversal of severe LV dysfunction in certain patients with chronic heart failure due to non-ischaemic cardiomyopathy.

*Background.*—It has been shown that LBBB induces asynchronous contraction of LV. However, whether such a functional contraction disturbance, if present for an extended period of time, could account for a dilated cardiomyopathy remains unknown.

*Methods.*—The study population comprised 29 patients with dilated cardiomyopathy, sinus rhythm, LBBB and severe heart failure (14 patients in New York Heart Association (NYHA) class III and 15 in class IV). Patients were followed prospectively after resynchronization therapy. LV function was considered to be normalized when ejection fraction (EF) was 50% at 1 year.

*Results.*—Five among the 29 patients (17%: group 1) demonstrated both complete normalization of LV function following resynchronization therapy (EF: from $19 \pm 6$ to $55 \pm 3\%$, $P = 0.001$) and clinical improvement (mean NYHA class: $3.4 \pm 0.5$ to $1.8 \pm 0.4$, $P = 0.02$; 6-min walk distance: $300 \pm 136$ to $444 \pm 75$ m, $P = 0.12$; peak $VO_2$: $11.9 \pm 4$ to $15.8 \pm$ ml/min/kg, $p = 0.03$). Among the remaining 24 patients (83%: group 2) EF improved but did not normalize (from $21 \pm 8$ to $23 \pm 11\%$, ns). Baseline clinical features could not predict which patients would exhibit the reversal of LV dysfunction.

*Conclusions.*—Normalization of LV function 1 year after resynchronization therapy in a small but important number of patients suggests that long-standing LBBB may be a newly identified reversible cause of cardiomyopathy.

▶ Resynchronization with biventricular pacing in patients with left bundle branch block (LBBB), a wide QRS, and congestive heart failure has been shown to markedly improve symptoms and cardiac function and even prolong survival in patients with cardiomyopathy. The assumption has been that LBBB is a consequence of the underlying cardiomyopathy. However, it is possible that the conduction defect and abnormal depolarization sequence of the left ventricle over a prolonged period of time is the inducing cause of the cardiomyopathy. The only way to show this is to reverse the abnormal LBBB ventricular depolarization sequence and demonstrate that left ventricle function returns to normal and the congestive heart failure abates. The current observational study in 29 patients with persistent LBBB and severe heart failure, functional class III and IV, lasting >6 months in spite of optimal medical management with a QRS >140 ms recorded multiple times for a minimum of 1 year, who had a pacemaker lead in the lateral coronary vein pacing the LV and an atrial lead in the right atrial appendage. The A-V delay was individually programmed for optimal LV contraction. Five patients (17%) had completely normalized LV function after resynchronization, with the ejection fraction going from 19% ± 6% to 55% ± 3%, accompanied by marked clinical improvement. The other 24 patients (83%) did not have a significant change in their ejection fractions. Such an experience, although still small in numbers, is consistent with the explanation that in some patients long-standing LBBB may be a newly recognized reversible cause of cardiomyopathy.

**M. D. Cheitlin, MD**

---

**Mode of Death in Advanced Heart Failure: The Comparison of Medical, Pacing, and Defibrillation Therapies in Heart Failure (COMPANION) Trial**
Carson P, Anand I, O'Connor C, et al (Veterans Affairs Med Ctr, Washington, DC; Veterans Affairs Med Ctr, Minneapolis, Minn; Duke Univ, Durham, NC; et al)
*J Am Coll Cardiol* 46:2329-2334, 2005                                                     5–11

---

*Objectives.*—The aim of this study was to evaluate the mode of death in patients with advanced chronic heart failure (HF) and intraventricular conduction delay treated with optimal pharmacologic therapy (OPT) alone or OPT with biventricular pacing to provide cardiac resynchronization therapy (CRT) or CRT + an implantable defibrillator (CRT-D).

*Background.*—Limited data are available on mode of death in advanced HF. No data have existed on mode of death in these patients who also have an intraventricular conduction delay and are treated with CRT or CRT-D.

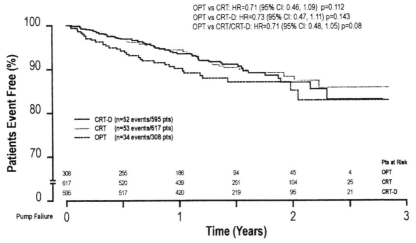

FIGURE 2.—Kaplan-Meier estimate of the time to first pump failure death. CI = confidence interval; HR = hazard ratio; other abbreviations as in Figure 1. (Reprinted with permission from the American College of Cardiology from Carson P, Anand I, O'Connor C, et al: Mode of death in advanced heart failure: The Comparison of Medical, Pacing, and Defibrillaion Therapies in Heart Failure (COMPANION) Trial. *J Am Coll Cardiol* 46:2329-2334. Copyright Elsevier 2005.)

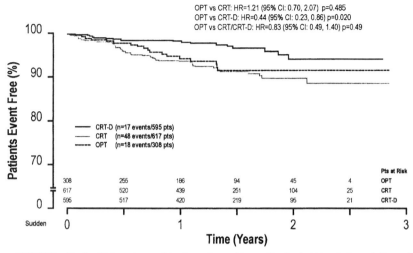

OPT vs CRT: HR=1.21 (95% CI: 0.70, 2.07) p=0.485
OPT vs CRT-D: HR=0.44 (95% CI: 0.23, 0.86) p=0.020
OPT vs CRT/CRT-D: HR=0.83 (95% CI: 0.49, 1.40) p=0.49

CRT-D (n=17 events/595 pts)
CRT (n=48 events/617 pts)
OPT (n=18 events/308 pts)

| | | | | | | |
|---|---|---|---|---|---|---|
| 308 | 255 | 186 | 94 | 45 | 4 | OPT |
| 617 | 520 | 439 | 251 | 104 | 25 | CRT |
| 595 | 517 | 420 | 219 | 95 | 21 | CRT-D |

FIGURE 3.—Kaplan-Meier estimate of the time to first sudden cardiac death. Abbreviation as in Figure 1. (Reprinted with permission from the American College of Cardiology from Carson P, Anand I, O'Connor C, et al: Mode of death in advanced heart failure: The Comparison of Medical, Pacing, and Defibrillaion Therapies in Heart Failure (COMPANION) Trial. *J Am Coll Cardiol* 46:2329-2334. Copyright Elsevier 2005.)

*Methods.*—Using prespecified definitions and source materials, seven cardiologists assessed mode of death among the 313 deaths that occurred in the Comparison of Medical, Pacing, and Defibrillation Therapies in Heart Failure (COMPANION) trial.

*Results.*—A primary cardiac cause was present in 78% of deaths. Pump failure (44.4%) was the most common mode of death followed by sudden cardiac death (SCD) (26.5%). Compared with OPT, CRT-D significantly reduced the number of cardiac deaths (38%, p = 0.006), whereas CRT alone was associated with a non-significant 14.5% reduction (p = 0.33). Both CRT and CRT-D tended to reduce pump failure deaths (29%, p = 0.11 and 27%, p = 0.14, respectively). The CRT-D significantly reduced SCD (56%, p = 0.02), but CRT alone did not.

*Conclusions.*—Pump failure deaths are the predominant mode of death in patients with advanced HF and are modestly reduced by both CRT and CRT-D. Only CRT-D reduced SCD and thus produced a favorable effect on cardiac mortality (Figs 2 and 3).

▶ With understanding of the pathophysiology of congestive heart failure (CHF), there has been the development of medical therapy aimed at neurohormonal blockade, which has been successful in reducing the annual mortality rate in patients with mild to moderate CHF from 16% to 6% to 8%.[1] To further reduce mortality rates, both implantable cardioverter-defibrillators (ICD) and, for those with a wide QRS, biventricular pacing for cardiac resynchronization (CRT) have been developed. This study, a substudy of the COMPANION trial, looked at patients with advanced cardiac failure (functional therapeutic class III-IV) and QRS >120 ms who were randomly assigned to optimal medical therapy, CRT alone, or CRT with Defibrillator (CRT-D). In 1510 patients there were 313 deaths (20.6%) during the period of follow-up and the mode of death was determined. Pump failure was the mode in almost half the patients and sudden death in just over one fourth of the patients. It appears in this study that pump failure is little reduced by these interventional tools, whereas only CRT-D but not CRT reduced sudden death by 56%. A much larger study may be needed to show a significant reduction in pump failure.

**M. D. Cheitlin, MD**

*Reference*

1. Cohn JN, Tognoni G, Valsartan Heart Failure Trial Investigators: A randomized trial of the angiotensin-receptor blocker valsartan in chronic heart failure. *N Engl Med* 345:1667-1675, 2001.

---

**Early heart rate recovery after exercise predicts mortality in patients with chronic heart failure**
Nanas S, Anastasiou-Nana M, Dimopoulos S, et al (Univ of Athens, Greece)
*Int J Cardiol* 110:393-400, 2006                                                    5–12

*Background.*—Patients with chronic heart failure (CHF) have multiple abnormalities of autonomic regulation that have been associated to their high mortality rate. Heart rate recovery immediately after exercise is an index of parasympathetic activity, but its prognostic role in CHF patients has not been determined yet.

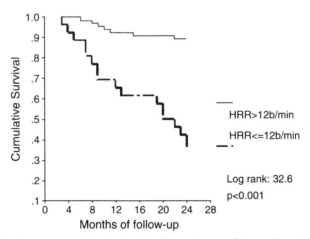

FIGURE 1.—Two-year actuarial survival analysis of 92 patients stratified according to HRR$_1$≤12 bpm versus>12 bpm. HRR$_1$=HR recovery for the 1st minute of recovery. (Reprinted by permission of the publisher from Nanas S, Anastasiou-Nana M, Dimopoulos S, et al: Early heart rate recovery after exercise predicts mortality in patients with chronic heart failure. *Int J Cardiol* 110:393-400, 2006. Copyright Elsevier 2006.)

*Methods.*—Ninety-two stable CHF patients (83M/9F, mean age: 51±12 years) performed an incremental symptom-limited cardiopulmonary exercise testing. Measurements included peak $O_2$ uptake ($VO_2p$), ventilatory response to exercise ($V_E/VCO_2$ slope), the first-degree slope of $VO_2$ for the 1st minute of recovery ($VO_2$/t-slope), heart rate recovery [($HRR_1$, bpm): HR difference from peak to 1 min after exercise] and chronotropic response to exercise [%chronotropic reserve (CR, %)=(peak HR–resting HR/220–age–resting HR)× 100]. Left ventricular ejection fraction (LVEF, %) was also measured by radionuclide ventriculography.

*Results.*—Fatal events occurred in 24 patients (26%) during 21±6 months of follow-up. $HRR_1$ was lower in non-survivors (11.4±6.4 vs. 20.4±8.1; $p<0.001$). All cause-mortality rate was 65% in patients with $HRR_1 \le 12$ bpm versus 11% in patients with $HRR_1 > 12$ bpm (log-rank: 32.6; $p<0.001$). By multivariate survival analysis, $HRR_1$ resulted as an independent predictor of mortality ($X^2=19.2$; odds ratio: 0.87; $p<0.001$) after adjustment for LVEF, $VO_2p$, $V_E/VCO_2$ slope, CR and $VO_2$/t-slope. In a subgroup of patients with intermediate exercise capacity ($VO_2p$: 10–18, ml/kg/min), $HRR_1$ was a strong predictor of mortality ($X^2$: 14.3; odds ratio: 0.8; $p<0.001$).

*Conclusions.*—Early heart rate recovery is an independent prognostic risk indicator in CHF patients and could be used in CHF risk stratification (Fig 1).

---

### Relation Between Postexercise Abnormal Heart Rate Recovery and Myocardial Damage Evidenced by Gated Single-Photon Emission Computed Tomography

Lima RSL, De Lorenzo A, Soares AJ (Universidade Estácio de Sá and Cintilab, Rio de Janeiro, Brazil)
*Am J Cardiol* 97:1452-1454, 2006                                    5–13

---

Abnormal heart rate recovery (HRR) after exercise has been associated with increased cardiac mortality. The ability of gated myocardial perfusion single-photon emission computed tomography (SPECT) to evaluate myocardial perfusion and function simultaneously might make it helpful in determining possible mechanisms that are involved in this finding. This study investigated the association between abnormal HRR and other indicators of risk for cardiovascular events. Patients (n = 1,296, 784 men; 57 ± 11 years of age) who underwent exercise/technetium-99m sestamibi gated myocardial perfusion SPECT at rest were prospectively enrolled. Exercise treadmill testing was performed according to a symptom-limited Bruce's protocol. HRR was obtained from the subtraction of heart rate in the first minute of recovery after exercise treadmill testing from maximal heart rate during exercise. Myocardial perfusion SPECT was semi-quantitatively analyzed using a 17-segment left ventricular model. Left ventricular ejection fraction was automatically calculated using quantitative gated SPECT software. In our study, patients with abnormal HRR were older, more frequently diabetic, and hypertensive and had previous myocardial infarction and myocardial revascularization, higher heart rate at rest and perfusion defect quantification scores, lower left ventricular ejection fraction, and larger left ventricular volumes than did patients with normal HRR. In multivariable analysis, age (p <0.0001), heart rate at rest (p <0.0001), left ventricular ejection fraction (p <0.0001), and perfusion defect extent and severity at rest (p = 0.038) were independent predictors of abnormal HRR. In conclusion, abnormal HRR was significantly associated with lower left ventricular ejection fraction and with perfusion defect extent and severity at rest, but not with gated SPECT markers of myocardial ischemia. Therefore, abnormal HRR may reflect myocardial damage.

▶ One of the most important pathophysiologic associations of mortality in congestive heart failure is neuroendocrine dysregulation[1] manifested by an imbalance in control of the autonomic nervous system,[2] characterized by increasing sympathetic activation,[3] cardiac β adrenoreceptor down-regulation,[4] parasympathetic withdrawal,[5] and decreased heart rate variability.[6] Attenuation of heart rate recovery after exercise is a marker of decreased parasympathetic activity[7] and is blunted in patients with heart failure.[8] The article by Nanas et al (Abstract 5–12) examines the HRR after exercise as a marker for increased mortality in patients with heart failure. The authors used a symptom-limited treadmill stress test with the Bruce protocol or the modified Naughton protocol depending on the patient's New York Heart Association (NYHA) functional class. On follow-up of 21 ± 6 months, the patients whose heart rate at 1 minute postexercise (HRR$_1$ had decreased 12 beats or less per minute had a mortality rate of 65% compared to 11% in those with HRR$_1$ of more than 12 beats/min after adjustment for left ventricular ejection fraction and measurements of peak O$_2$ uptake and ventilatory response to exercise. Therefore, the simple measurement of HRR$_1$ is an independent prognostic indicator for mortality rate and can be used for risk stratification.

In an article by Lima and colleagues (Abstract 5–13) in which SPECT was used to evaluate myocardial perfusion and ventricular function simultaneously in heart failure patients with abnormal HRR$_1$ after exercise, a response of 12 beats or less per minute was associated with a lower left ventricular ejection fraction and greater perfusion defect extent and severity at rest, a measure of myocardial scar, than patients with HRR$_1$ response greater than 12 beats/min.

**M. D. Cheitlin, MD**

*References*

1. Packer M: The neurohormonal hypothesis: A theory to explain the mechanism of disease progression in heart failure. *J Am Coll Cardiol* 20:248-254, 1992.
2. Ishise H, Asanoi H, Ishizaka S, et al: Time course of sympathovagal imbalance and left ventricular dysfunction in conscious dogs with heart failure. *J Appl Physiol* 84:1234-1241, 1998.
3. Cohn JN, Levine TB, Olivari MT, et al: Plasma norepinephrine as a guide to prognosis in patients with chronic congestive heart failure. *N Engl J Med* 311:819-823, 1984.
4. Bristow MR, Ginsburg R, Minobe W, et al: Decreased catecholamine sensitivity and beta-adrenergic-receptor density in failing human hearts. *N Engl J Med* 307:205-211, 1982.

5. Binkley PF, Nunziata E, Haas GJ, et al: Parasympathetic withdrawal is an integral component of autonomic imbalance in congestive heart failure: Demonstration in human subjects and verification in a paced canine model of ventricular failure. *J Am Coll Cardiol* 18:464-472, 1991.

6. Brouwer J, van Veldhuisen DJ, Man in 't Veld AJ, et al: Prognostic value of heart rate variability during long-term follow-up in patients with mild to moderate heart failure. The Dutch Ibopamine Multicenter Trial Study Group. *J Am Coll Cardiol* 28:1183-1189, 1996.

7. Arai Y, Saul JP, Albrecht P, et al: Modulation of cardiac autonomic activity during and immediately after exercise. *Am J Physiol* 256: 132S-141S, 1989.

8. Imai K, Sato H, Hori M, et al: Vagally mediated heart rate recovery after exercise is accelerated in athletes but blunted in patients with chronic heart failure. *J Am Coll Cardiol* 24:1529-1535, 1994.

---

## Hemoglobin Level, Chronic Kidney Disease, and the Risks of Death and Hospitalization in Adults With Chronic Heart Failure. The Anemia in Chronic Heart Failure: Outcomes and Resource Utilization (ANCHOR) Study

Go AS, Yang J, Ackerson LM, et al (Kaiser Permanente of Northern California, Oakland; Univ of California at San Francisco; Amgen, Thousand Oaks, Calif; et al)
*Circulation* 113:2713-2723, 2006                                     5–14

---

*Background.*—Previous studies have associated reduced hemoglobin levels with increased adverse events in heart failure. It is unclear, however, whether this relation is explained by underlying kidney disease, treatment differences, or associated comorbidity.

*Method and Results.*—We examined the associations between hemoglobin level, kidney function, and risks of death and hospitalization in persons with chronic heart failure between 1996 and 2002 within a large, integrated, healthcare delivery system in northern California. Longitudinal outpatient hemoglobin and creatinine levels and clinical and treatment characteristics were obtained from health plan records. Glomerular filtration rate (GFR; mL·min$^{-1}$·1.73 m$^{-2}$) was estimated from the Modification of Diet in Renal Disease equation. Mortality data were obtained from state death files; heart failure admissions were identified by primary discharge diagnoses. Among 59,772 adults with heart failure, the mean age was 72 years and 46% were women. Compared with that for hemoglobin levels of 13.0 to 13.9 g/dL, the multivariable-adjusted risk of death increased with lower hemoglobin levels: an adjusted hazard ratio (HR) of 1.16 and 95% confidence interval (CI) of 1.11 to 1.21 for hemoglobin levels of 12.0 to 12.9 g/dL; HR, 1.50 and 95% CI, 1.44 to 1.57 for 11.0 to 11.9 g/dL; HR, 1.89 and 95% CI, 1.80 to 1.98 for 10.0 to 10.9; HR, 2.31 and 95% CI, 2.18 to 2.45 for 9.0 to 9.9; and HR, 3.48 and 95% CI, 3.25 to 3.73 for <9.0 g/dL. Hemoglobin levels ≥ 17.0 g/dL were associated with an increased risk of death (adjusted HR, 1.42; 95% CI, 1.24 to 1.63). Compared with those with a GFR ≥ 60 mL· min$^{-1}$·1.73 m$^{-2}$, persons with a GFR <45 mL·min$^{-1}$·1.73 m$^{-2}$ had an increased mortality risk: adjusted HR, 1.39 and 95% CI, 1.34 to 1.44 for 30 to

44; HR, 2.28 and 95% CI, 2.19 to 2.39 for 15 to 29; HR, 3.26 and 95% CI, 3.05 to 3.49 for <15; and HR, 2.44 and 95% CI, 2.28 to 2.61 for those on dialysis. Relations were similar for the risk of hospitalization. The findings did not differ among patients with preserved or reduced systolic function, and hemoglobin level was an independent predictor of outcomes at all levels of kidney function.

*Conclusions.*—Very high ($\geq$17 g/dL) or reduced (<13 g/dL) hemoglobin levels and chronic kidney disease independently predict substantially increased risks of death and hospitalization in heart failure, regardless of the level of systolic function. Randomized trials are needed to evaluate whether raising hemoglobin levels can improve outcomes in chronic heart failure.

---

**Clinical Correlates and Consequences of Anemia in a Broad Spectrum of Patients With Heart Failure: Results of the Candesartan in Heart Failure: Assessment of Reduction in Mortality and Morbidity (CHARM) Program**

O'Meara E, for the CHARM Committees and Investigators (Western Infirmary, Glasgow, England; et al)

*Circulation* 113:986-994, 2006                                             5–15

---

*Background.*—We wished to determine the prevalence of, potential mechanistic associations of, and clinical outcomes related to anemia in patients with heart failure and a broad spectrum of left ventricular ejection fraction (LVEF).

*Method and Results.*—In multivariable analyses, we examined the associations between hemoglobin and baseline characteristics, laboratory variables, and outcomes in 2653 patients randomized in the CHARM Program in the United States and Canada. Anemia was equally common in patients with preserved (27%) and reduced (25%) LVEF but was more common in black and older patients. Anemia was associated with ethnicity, diabetes, low body mass index, higher systolic and lower diastolic blood pressure, and recent heart failure hospitalization. More than 50% of anemic patients had a glomerular filtration rate <60 mL·min$^{-1}$·1.73 m$^{-2}$ compared with <30% of nonanemic patients. Despite an inverse relationship between hemoglobin and LVEF, anemia was associated with an increased risk of death and hospitalization, a relationship observed in patients with both reduced and preserved LVEF. There were 133 versus 69 deaths and 527 versus 352 hospitalizations per 1000 patient-years of follow-up in anemic versus nonanemic patients (both $P<0.001$). The effect of candesartan in reducing outcomes was independent of hemoglobin.

*Conclusions.*—Anemia was common in heart failure, regardless of LVEF. Lower hemoglobin was associated with higher LVEF yet was an independent predictor of adverse mortality and morbidity outcomes. In heart failure, the causes of anemia and the associations between anemia and outcomes are probably multiple and complex.

▶ Anemia in patients with congestive heart failure (CHF) has been well documented to contribute to adverse outcomes, including in several studies,[1,2] mortality, probably through increased myocardial and peripheral $O_2$ demand, accelerated progression of left ventricular hypertrophy, increased edema and promotion of inflammation.[3] Renal dysfunction in patients with CHF also increases morbidity and mortality rates,and the possible interaction of these 2 negative prognostic factors is evaluated in the present study of over 59,000 ambulatory and hospitalized patients' records from an integrated health care delivery system in Northern California (Abstract 5–14). The authors found that both the levels of hemoglobin (Hgb) and underlying kidney function independently predicted risks for death and hospitalization for CHF even after accounting for differences in other patient characteristics and types of treatment. Both high ($\geq$17 g/dL) and low (<13.0 g/dL) Hgb levels and an estimated glomerular filtration rate less than 45 mL/min/m$^2$) were independent, graduated risk factors for hospitalization for CHF and mortality in patients with chronic CHF. The findings were similar for patients with preserved or reduced LVEF, and Hgb levels were independent negative predictors at all levels of renal function.

The article by O'Meara and colleagues (Abstract 5–15) used data from the Candesartan in Heart Failure: Assessment of Reduction in Mortality and Morbidity (CHARM) program and also showed that anemia was common in CHF regardless of LVEF and the level of Hgb was negatively associated with LVEF and an independent predictor of adverse events including mortality. They concluded that although anemia was associated with renal dysfunction, the causes of anemia in patients with CHF were probably multiple and complex.

The treatment of anemia in patients with CHF with a combination of erythropoietin and IV or oral iron has been shown to improve symptoms, cardiac function and peak $O_2$ consumption.[2,3] A study of a small number of patients with CHF and anemia reported by Bolger and colleagues[4] were treated as outpatients with 200-mg boluses given IV during 10 minutes of undiluted iron sucrose to a maximum of 1 g over a 12-day treatment phase. Following up for 3 months, they found an increase in Hgb from 11.2±0.7 to 12.6±1.2 g/dL ($P$=0.0007), improvement in the Minnesota Living with Heart Failure score and the 6-minute walk distance. A larger, placebo-controlled trial will have to be done to further assess the efficacy of this approach.

**M. D. Cheitlin, MD**

*References*

1. Anand I, McMurray JJV, Whitmore J, et al: Anemia and its relationship to clinical outcome in heart failure. *Circulation* 110:149-154, 2004.
2. Silverberg DS, Wexler D, Sheps D, et al: The effect of correction of mild anemia in severe, resistant congestive heart failure using subcutaneous erythropoietin and intravenous iron: A randomized controlled study. *J Am Coll Cardiol* 37:1775-1780, 2001.

3. Mancini DM, Katz SD, Lang CC, et al: Effect of erythropoietin on exercise capacity in patients with moderate to severe chronic heart failure. *Circulation* 107:294-299, 2003.
4. Bolger AP, Bartlett FR, Chapman CM, et al: Intravenous iron alone for the treatment of anemia in patients with chronic heart failure. *J Am Coll Cardiol* 48:1225-1227, 2006.

---

### Renal Function as a Predictor of Outcome in a Broad Spectrum of Patients With Heart Failure

Hillege HL, for the Candesartan in Heart Failure: Assessment of Reduction in Mortality and Morbidity (CHARM) Investigators (Univ of Groningen, the Netherlands; et al)

*Circulation* 113:671-678, 2006

5–16

---

*Background.*—Decreased renal function has been found to be an independent risk factor for cardiovascular outcomes in patients with chronic heart failure (CHF) with markedly reduced left ventricular ejection fraction (LVEF). The aim of this analysis was to evaluate the prognostic importance of renal function in a broader spectrum of patients with CHF.

*Method and Results.*—The Candesartan in Heart Failure:Assessment of Reduction in Mortality and Morbidity (CHARM) program consisted of three component trials that enrolled patients with symptomatic CHF, based on use of ACE inhibitors and reduced ($\leq$40%) or preserved LVEF (>40%). Entry baseline creatinine was required to be below 3.0 mg/dL (265 $\mu$mol/L). Routine baseline serum creatinine assessments were done in 2680 North American patients. An analysis of the estimated glomerular filtration rate (eGFR), using the Modification of Diet in Renal Disease equation and LVEF on risk of cardiovascular death or hospitalization for heart failure, as well as on all-cause mortality, was conducted on these 2680 patients. The proportion of patients with eGFR <60 mL/min per 1.73 m$^2$ was 36.0%; 42.6% for CHARM-Alternative, 33.0% for CHARM-Added, and 34.7% for CHARM-Preserved. During the median follow-up of 34.4 months (total 6493 person-years), the primary outcome of cardiovascular death or hospital admission for worsening CHF occurred in 950 of 2680 subjects. Both reduced eGFR and lower LVEF were found to be significant independent predictors of worse outcome after adjustment for major confounding baseline clinical characteristics. The risk for cardiovascular death or hospitalization for worsening CHF as well as the risk for all-cause mortality increased significantly below an eGFR of 60 mL/min per 1.73 m$^2$ (adjusted hazard ratio, 1.54 for 45 to 60 mL/min per 1.73 m$^2$ and 1.86 for <45 mL/min per 1.73 m$^2$ for the primary outcome, both $P<0.001$, and hazard ratio of 1.50, $P=0.006$, and 1.91, $P=0.001$, respectively, for all-cause mortality). The prognostic value of eGFR was not significantly different among the three component trials. There was no significant interaction between renal function, the effect of candesartan, and clinical outcome.

*Conclusions.*—Impaired renal function is independently associated with heightened risk for death, cardiovascular death, and hospitalization for heart failure in patients with CHF with both preserved as well as reduced LVEF. There was no evidence that the beneficial effect of candesartan was modified by baseline eGFR.

▶ Renal dysfunction has been demonstrated to be an independent risk factor for cardiovascular disease outcomes and all-cause mortality in patients with left ventricular systolic dysfunction (LVSD) as well as with CHF.[1-3] Most of these studies were done in patients with severe LVSD and markedly reduced LVEF. The CHARM study included 3 distinct types of CHF populations: CHARM preserved with LVEF more than 40%; CHARM added with LVEF 40% or less and treated with angiotensin converting enzyme inhibitors (ACEI); and CHARM alternative with LVEF 40% or less and not treated with ACEI because of previous intolerance. Entry into the study required a serum creatinine to be less than 3 mg/dL. An eGFR was calculated on entry. The proportion of patients with eGFR less than 60 ml/dL/1.73 m² was relatively common in all 3 groups. In addition, there was a wide range of LVEFs from 15% to 45% or more. They found that eGFR was inversely related to the risk of death, cardiovascular death, and recurrent hospitalization for CHF, and this was independent of LVEF. They also found that the beneficial effect of candesartan was not affected by the baseline eGFR. The independent effect of eGFR on outcomes with relation to LVEF may indicate that eGFR may be a marker for generalized vascular disease and reflects severity of atherosclerosis in both kidney and heart, rather than a dependence on cardiac function.

**M. D. Cheitlin, MD**

*References*

1. Mahon NG, Blackstone EH, Francis GS, et al: The prognostic value of estimated creatinine clearance alongside functional capacity in ambulatory patients with chronic congestive heart failure. *J Am Coll Cardiol* 40:1106-1113, 2002.
2. Smilde TD, Hillege HL, Voors AA, et al: Prognostic importance of renal function in patients with early heart failure and mild left ventricular dysfunction. *Am J Cardiol* 94:240-243, 2004.
3. McAlister FA, Ezekowitz J, Tonelli M, et al: Renal insufficiency and heart failure: Prognostic and therapeutic implications from a prospective cohort study. *Circulation* 109:1004-1009, 2004.

## Medical Treatment of Congestive Heart Failure

**Clinical Presentation, Management, and In-Hospital Outcomes of Patients Admitted With Acute Decompensated Heart Failure With Preserved Systolic Function: A Report From the Acute Decompensated Heart Failure National Registry (ADHERE) Database**

Yancy CW, for the ADHERE Scientific Advisory Committee and Investigators (Univ of Texas Southwest Med Ctr, Dallas; et al)

*J Am Coll Cardiol* 47:76-84, 2006                                       5–17

*Objectives.*—The aims of this analysis were to describe the clinical characteristics, management, and outcomes of patients hospitalized for acute decompensated heart failure (HF) with preserved systolic function (PSF).

*Background.*—Clinically meaningful characteristics of these patients have not been fully studied in a large database.

*Methods.*—Data from >100,000 hospitalizations from the Acute Decompensated Heart Failure National Registry (ADHERE) database were analyzed.

*Results.*—Heart failure with PSF was present in 50.4% of patients with in-hospital assessment of left ventricular function. When compared with patients with systolic dysfunction, patients with PSF were more likely to be older, women, and hypertensive and less likely to have had a prior myocardial infarction or be receiving an angiotensin-converting enzyme inhibitor or angiotensin II receptor blocker. In-hospital mortality was lower in patients with PSF compared with patients with systolic dysfunction (2.8% vs. 3.9%; adjusted odds ratio [OR]: 0.86; $p = 0.005$), but duration of intensive care unit stay and total hospital length of stay were similar. Serum creatinine >2 mg/dl was associated with increased in-hospital mortality in both systolic function groups (PSF: 4.8%; systolic dysfunction: 8.4%; $p < 0.0001$), and the most powerful predictors of in-hospital mortality in both groups were blood urea nitrogen >37 mg/dl (OR: 2.53; 95% confidence interval [CI]: 2.22 to 2.87) and systolic blood pressure $\leq$125 mm Hg (OR: 2.58; 95% CI: 2.33 to 2.86).

*Conclusions.*—Heart failure with PSF is common and is characterized by a unique patient profile. Event rates are worrisome and reflect a need for more effective management strategies.

▶ The management and outcome of patients with acute decompensated heart failure and preserved systolic function (PSF) compared with those with systolic dysfunction is of great interest. From this data bank of >100,000 patients hospitalized for decompensated heart failure, half the patients had PSF. The clinical picture of the patients with PSF differed from that of those with systolic dysfunction in that the patients were older, most often women with hypertension, and less likely to be taking angiotensin-converting enzyme inhibitors. Their duration of stay in the intensive care unit and total hospitalization time were similar to those with systolic dysfunction. As is true with many patients with heart disease, the presence of renal dysfunction is a powerful predictor of the in-hospital mortality rate. Because the in-hospital mortality rate in those with PSF was almost twice that of those with systolic dysfunction, it is clear that more effort must be made to find the best medical management in patients with acute decompensated heart failure.

**M. D. Cheitlin, MD**

## Atorvastatin Improves Left Ventricular Systolic Function and Serum Markers of Inflammation in Nonischemic Heart Failure

Sola S, Mir MQS, Lerakis S, et al (Emory Univ School of Medicine, Atlanta, Ga; Louisiana State Univ Health Sciences Ctr, Shreveport)
*J Am Coll Cardiol* 47:332-337, 2006          5–18

*Objectives.*—This study examined the effect of statin therapy on vascular markers of inflammation and echocardiographic findings in patients with nonischemic forms of cardiomyopathy.

*Background.*—Despite advances in therapy, morbidity and mortality from heart failure (HF) remain high. We wished to determine whether treatment with atorvastatin affects left ventricular (LV) systolic function and markers of inflammation in patients with nonischemic HF.

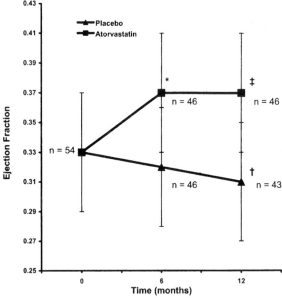

FIGURE 1.—Change in ejection fraction in the placebo and atorvastatin groups during the 12-month study follow up. *p = 0.01 for the difference in ejection fraction between baseline and 6 or 12 months within the atorvastatin group; †p = 0.04 for the difference in ejection fraction between baseline as 12 months within the placebo group; ‡p = 0.004 for the difference in ejection fraction at 12 months between the placebo and the atorvastatin groups. (Reprinted with permission from the American College of Cardiology from Sola S, Mir MQS, Lerakis S, et al: Atorvastatin improves left ventricular systolic function and serum markers of inflammation in nonischemic heart failure. *J Am Coll Cardiol* 47:332-337. Copyright Elsevier 2006.)

*Methods.*—A total of 108 patients with nonischemic HF and a left ventricular ejection fraction (LVEF) ≤35% were randomized to either atorvastatin 20 mg/day or placebo in a double-blinded fashion for a 12-month period. The LVEF and LV end-diastolic diameter (LVEDD) and left ventricular end-systolic diameter (LVESD) were determined by echocardiography. Serum markers of inflammation and oxidation were also measured.

*Results.*—The LVEF increased from 0.33 ± 0.05 to 0.37 ± 0.04 (p = 0.01) in the atorvastatin group over the 12-month follow-up period, whereas those patients in the placebo group experienced a decline in ejection fraction during the same time period. In addition, LVEDD was reduced from 57.1 ± 5.9 mm to 53.4 ± 5.1 mm (p = 0.007) and LVESD was reduced from 42.4 ± 3.8 mm to 39.1 ± 3.8 mm (p = 0.02) in the cohort of patients treated with atorvastatin; these dimensions increased in the placebo group. There was an increase in erythrocyte superoxide dismutase (E-SOD) activity, and there were significant reductions in serum levels of high sensitivity C-reactive protein, interleukin-6 (IL-6), and tumor necrosis factor-alpha receptor II (TNF-alpha RII) in the atorvastatin group.

*Conclusions.*—The use of atorvastatin in patients with nonischemic HF improves LVEF and attenuates adverse LV remodeling. The effects on soluble levels of several inflammatory markers with atorvastatin suggest, in part, mechanisms by which statins might exert their beneficial effects in nonischemic HF (Fig 1).

▶ Hydromethylglutaryl CoA reductase inhibitors (statins) have been shown to reduce morbidity and mortality in patients with coronary artery disease, even in patients without coronary disease but with multiple risk factors for coronary disease.[1,2] This study explores the effects of statin drugs on patients with nonischemic congestive heart failure, functional class II-III, and shows that statins improve left ventricular (LV) ejection fraction, decrease LV end-diastolic and end-systolic volumes, decrease levels of a number of inflammatory serum markers, and increase erythrocyte superoxide dismutase, a powerful antioxidant. This pilot study is underpowered, too small (108 patients) with too short a follow-up period (1 year), to show an effect on functional class or morbidity or mortality rates. However, the pleiotropic effects of statins produce a favorable reduction in LV remodeling, evidence of decreased inflammatory markers, improvement in endothelial function and increased production of antioxidants. All these actions are consistent with the possibility that there will be a reduction in adverse events in functional class II-III patients with congestive heart failure, possibly including a reduction in mortality rate. Statins are turning out to be useful in a wide variety of pathologic conditions. A larger randomized, controlled study of statins in patients with congestive heart failure is warranted.

There is an accompanying Editorial by Rammasubbu and Mann[3] that is worth reading.

**M. D. Cheitlin, MD**

*References*

1. Sacks FM, Pfeffer MA, Moye LA, et al: The effect of pravastatin on coronary events after myocardial infarction in patients with average cholesterol levels: Cholesterol and Recurrent Events Trial investigators. *N Engl J Med* 335:1001-1009, 1996.
2. Heart Protection Study Collaborative Group: The MRC/BHF Heart Protection Study of cholesterol lowering with simvstatinin 20,536 high-risk individuals: A randomized placebo controlled trial. *Lancet* 360:7-22, 2002.
3. Ramasubbu K, Mann DL: The emerging role of statins in the treatment of heart failure. *J Am Coll Cardiol* 47:342-344, 2006.

**Effect of Glycemic Control on Left Ventricular Diastolic Function in Type 1 Diabetes Mellitus**
Grandi AM, Piantanida E, Franzetti I, et al (Univ of Insubria, Italy; Ospedale di Circolo, Varese, Italy)
*Am J Cardiol* 97:71-76, 2006                                    5–19

Left ventricular (LV) diastolic dysfunction is a main feature of diabetic heart disease. The aim of this prospective study was to evaluate the influence of glycemic control on diastolic function in type 1 diabetes mellitus. Thirty-six normotensive (24-hour blood pressure <130/80 mm Hg) subjects with inadequately controlled (glycated hemoglobin >7%) type 1 diabetes, without clinically detectable heart disease, were enrolled. After the basal evaluation, insulin therapy was modified to improve glycemic control. Glycated hemoglobin, LV echocardiography, 24-hour blood pressure monitoring, and laboratory tests were repeated after 6 months in all patients and after 12 months in 27 patients. At the basal evaluation, LV anatomy and systolic

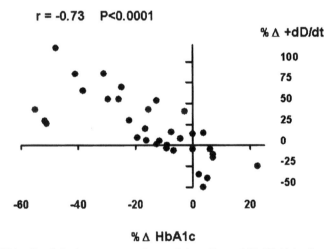

FIGURE 1.—Correlation between percent changes of glycated hemoglobin (HbA1c) and percent changes of the peak lengthening rate of LV diameter (+dD/dt) from the basal to the 6-month evaluation. (Reprinted from *American Journal of Cardiology* courtesy of Grandi AM, Piantanida E, Franzetti I, et al: Effect of glycemic control on left ventricular diastolic function in type 1 diabetes mellitus. *Am J Cardiol* 97:71-76. Copyright Elsevier 2006.)

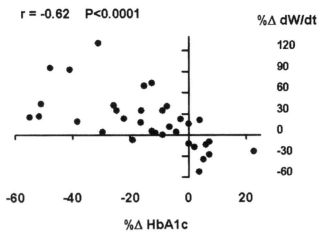

FIGURE 2.—Correlation between percent changes of glycated hemoglobin (HbA1c) and percent changes of the peak thinning rate of the LV posterior wall (dW/dt) from the basal to the 6-month evaluation. (Reprinted from *American Journal of Cardiology* courtesy of Grandi AM, Piantanida E, Franzetti I, et al: Effect of glycemic control on left ventricular diastolic function in type 1 diabetes mellitus. *Am J Cardiol* 97:71-76. Copyright Elsevier 2006.)

function were normal in all, and diastolic function was impaired in 14 patients. After 6 months, the mean values of body mass index, 24-hour blood pressure, and LV anatomy and systolic function were unchanged; mean glycated hemoglobin was decreased (p <0.001), and mean values of diastolic parameters were significantly improved. After 12 months, the mean values of all blood pressure, metabolic, and LV parameters were unchanged. Percent changes of diastolic parameters were inversely correlated with percent

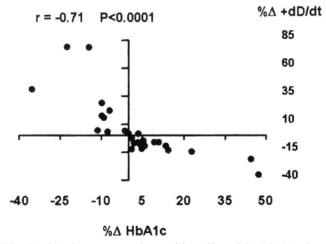

FIGURE 3.—Correlation between percent changes of glycated hemoglobin (HbA1c) and percent changes of the peak lengthening rate of LV diameter (+dD/dt) from the 6- to the 12-month evaluation. (Reprinted from *American Journal of Cardiology* courtesy of Grandi AM, Piantanida E, Franzetti I, et al: Effect of glycemic control on left ventricular diastolic function in type 1 diabetes mellitus. *Am J Cardiol* 97:71-76. Copyright Elsevier 2006.)

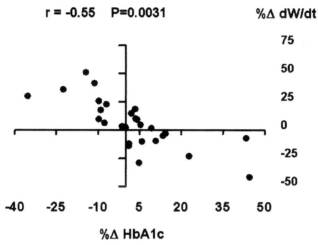

r = -0.55   P=0.0031

%Δ dW/dt

%Δ HbA1c

**FIGURE 4.**—Correlation between percent changes of glycated hemoglobin (HbA1c) and percent changes of the peak thinning rate of the LV posterior wall (dW/dt) from the 6- to the 12-month evaluation. (Reprinted from *American Journal of Cardiology* courtesy of Grandi AM, Piantanida E, Franzetti I, et al: Effect of glycemic control on left ventricular diastolic function in type 1 diabetes mellitus. *Am J Cardiol* 97:71-76. Copyright Elsevier 2006.)

changes of glycated hemoglobin, considering changes from the basal to the 6-month evaluation, as well as changes from the 6- to the 12-month evaluation. In conclusion, in normotensive patients with type 1 diabetes, a close relation was found between glycemic control and LV diastolic function, which improves when glycemic control improves. Therefore, diastolic dysfunction can be prevented or reversed, at least partly, by tight glycemic control (Figs 1, 2, 3, and 4).

▶ In diabetic patients, left ventricular function, including diastolic function, may be impaired. The exact cause in any individual patient may be due to a number of reasons, including ventricular hypertrophy, glycolated proteins, or coronary artery disease. Whether good glycemic control can improve diastolic function has been examined in type 2 diabetics with negative results.[1,2] However, many of these patients had hypertension or myocardial hypertrophy or were obese, all of which could influence diastolic function. This is the first longitudinal study in type 1 diabetic patients who were poorly controlled diabetics with elevated $HgbA_{1c}$ levels, who proved normotensive, without clinical evidence of coronary artery disease, normal LV systolic function, and without myocardial hypertrophy. In the basal study, 39% had diastolic dysfunction and after 6 and 12 months of good glycemic control with multiple doses of regular insulin, there was marked improvement in diastolic function and a significant inverse correlation was found between the percent changes in $HgbA_{1c}$ levels and percent changes of diastolic parameters. The fact that diastolic impairment in these patients, even with a long history of diabetes, was reversible with good glycemic control may indicate that the impairment is to a great extent functional rather than the result of irreversible anatomic changes.

**M. D. Cheitlin, MD**

*References*

1. Beljic T, Miric M: Improved metabolic control does not reverse left ventricular filling abnormalities in newly diagnosed non-insulin-dependent diabetes patients. *Acta Diabetol* 31:147-150, 1994.
2. Gough SC, Smyllie J, Barker M, et al: Diastolic dysfunction is not related to changes in glycaemic control over 6 months in type 2 (non-insulin-dependent) diabetes mellitus: A cross-sectional study. *Acta Diabetol* 32:110-115, 1995.

**Atorvastatin Therapy Increases Heart Rate Variability, Decreases QT Variability, and Shortens QTc Interval Duration in Patients With Advanced Chronic Heart Failure**

Vrtovec B, Okrajsek R, Golicnik A, et al (Ljubljana Univ Med Ctr, Slovenia; Texas Heart Inst at St Luke's Episcopal Hosp, Houston)

*J Card Fail* 11:684-690, 2005                                                5–20

*Background.*—Although statins decrease the incidence of ventricular arrhythmias in patients with atherosclerotic heart disease, their potential antiarrhythmic effects in heart failure remain undefined.

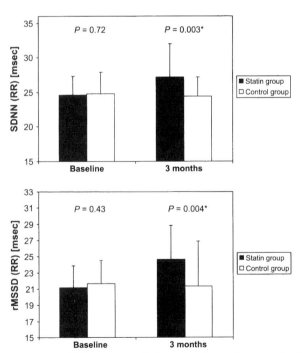

FIGURE 1.—Heart rate variability parameters in the statin and control groups at baseline and after 3 months of the study (the results are presented as mean + SD). Abbreviations: *SD,* Standard deviation; *SDNN (RR),* standard deviation of normal-to-normal RR intervals; *rMSSD (RR),* square root of the mean of squared differences between successive RR intervals. (Courtesy of Vrtovec B, Okrajsek R, Golicnik A, et al: Atorvastatin therapy increases heart rate variability, decreases QT variability, and shortens QTc interval duration in patients with advanced chronic heart failure. *J Card Fail* 11:684-690. Copyright Elsevier 2005.)

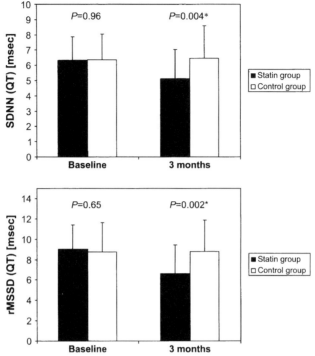

FIGURE 2.—QT variability parameters in the statin and control groups at baseline and after 3 months of the study (the results are presented as mean + SD). Abbreviations: *SD*, Standard deviation; *SDNN (RR)*, standard deviation of normal-to-normal RR intervals; *rMSSD (RR)*, square root of the mean of squared differences between successive RR intervals. (Courtesy of Vrtovec B, Okrajsek R, Golicnik A, et al: Atorvastatin therapy increases heart rate variability, decreases QT variability, and shortens QTc interval duration in patients with advanced chronic heart failure. *J Card Fail* 11:684-690. Copyright Elsevier 2005.)

*Method and Results.*—Of 80 heart failure patients enrolled, 40 were randomized to receive atorvastatin (statin group); the remaining 40 served as controls. At baseline and after 3 months, we measured heart rate variability (HRV), QT variability (QTV), and QTc interval using interactive high-resolution electrocardiogram analysis. The 2 groups did not differ in baseline HRV standard deviation of normal-to-normal intervals (SDNN) (RR): 24.6 ± 2.8 ms in statin group versus 24.8 ± 3.1 ms in controls, $P = .72$; square root of the mean of squared differences between successive intervals (rMSSD) (RR): 21.2 ± 2.7 ms versus 21.7 ± 2.9 ms, $P = .43$), QTV SDNN (QT): 6.4 ± 1.5 ms versus 6.4 ± 1.7, $P = .96$; rMSSD QT): 9.0 ± 2.4 ms versus 8.7 ± 2.9 ms, $P = .65$, and QTc interval 450 ± 30 ms versus 446 ± 27 ms, $P = .59$. At 3 months, the statin group displayed higher HRV SDNN RR): 27.2 ± 4.9 ms versus 24.4 ± 2.8 ms in controls, $P = .003$; rMSSD RR: 24.7 ± 4.2 ms versus 21.3 ± 5.6 ms, $P = .004$, lower QTV SDNN (QT): 5.1 ± 1.9 ms versus 6.5 ± 2.1, $P = .004$; rMSSD (QT): 6.6 ± 2.8 ms versus 8.8 ± 3.1 ms, $P = .002$, and shorter QTc interval 437 ± 29 ms versus 450 ± 25 ms, $P = .03$ than the control group.

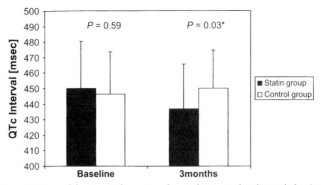

FIGURE 3.—QTc interval duration in the statin and control groups at baseline and after 3 months of the study (the results are presented as means). (Courtesy of Vrtovec B, Okrajsek R, Golicnik A, et al: Atorvastatin therapy increases heart rate variability, decreases QT variability, and shortens QTc interval duration in patients with advanced chronic heart failure. *J Card Fail* 11:684-690. Copyright Elsevier 2005.)

*Conclusions.*—Atorvastatin increases HRV, decreases QTV, and shortens QTc interval, and may thereby reduce the risk of arrhythmias in patients with advanced heart failure (Figs 1, 2, and 3).

## The Effects of *Atorvastatin* (10 mg) on Systemic Inflammation in Heart Failure

Mozaffarian D, Minami E, Letterer RA, et al (Harvard Med School, Boston; Univ of Washington, Seattle; Fred Hutchinson Cancer Research Ctr, Seattle)
*Am J Cardiol* 96:1699-1704, 2005                                                    5–21

In observational studies, statins are associated with lower mortality in patients with heart failure (HF), including those with nonischemic HF. Such benefits could be related to anti-inflammatory effects; however, the effects of statins on systemic inflammation in HF are not well-established. We conducted a 16-week, single-center, randomized, double-blind, placebo-controlled, crossover clinical trial of the effects of atorvastatin 10 mg/day on concentrations of systemic inflammatory markers in 22 patients with HF (including 20 with nonischemic HF) with New York Heart Association class II or III symptoms and left ventricular ejection fraction of <40%. The absolute and percentage of changes in inflammatory marker levels were evaluated using analysis of variance. Statin treatment reduced the concentrations of soluble tumor necrosis factor receptor-1 by 132 pg/ml (p = 0.04) and 8% (p = 0.056), C-reactive protein by 1.6 mg/L (p = 0.006) and 37% (p = 0.0002), and, after adjustment for treatment order, endothelin-1 by 0.21 pg/ml (p = 0.007) and 17% (p = 0.01). In post hoc analyses, the reduction in tumor necrosis factor receptor-1 levels was highest among patients with elevated levels at baseline (at or higher than the median of 1,055 pg/ml, p interaction = 0.001), among whom statin therapy reduced the levels by 306 pg/ml (p <0.001) and 22% (p <0.001). Statin treatment did not significantly affect the levels of other inflammatory markers, including interleukin-6 and brain natriuretic peptide. In conclusion, short-term atorvastatin therapy reduced the levels of several important inflammatory markers in patients with HF.

▶ Up to half the deaths that occur in patients with heart failure are sudden deaths, presumably resulting from malignant ventricular arrhythmias.[1] Ventricular arrhythmogenesis appears to be related to increased sympathetic tone and disturbances in ventricular repolarization.[2] In patients with heart failure, brain natriuretic peptide (BNP) levels >400 pg/mL and QTc interval prolongation of 440 ms predicted death from both pump failure and sudden death.[3] Statin drugs have recently been shown to improve exercise tolerance and increase left ventricular ejection fraction in heart failure.[4] Also, statins have been associated with lower mortality rates in patients with congestive heart failure[5] and also with a decrease in systemic inflammation. In the article by Mozaffarian et al (Abstract 5–21) a randomized, double-blind, placebo-controlled, cross-over clinical trial in 22 patients with cardiomyopathy (20 non-ischemic, 2 ischemic) showed that 10 mg of atorvastatin reduced soluble tumor necrosis factor (TNF) receptor-1 by 8% , C-reactive protein by 37%, and endothelin-1 by 17%. The current study in 80 patients with heart failure showed that atorvastatin increased heart rate variability (decreased sympathetic tone) and QT variability and shortened QTc interval, all consistent with reduction in the risk of ventricular arrhythmias in patients wit advanced chronic heart failure.

The statins, developed to decrease low-density lipoproteins, have remarkable pleiotropic effects on inflammatory markers and now on the substrate of ventricular arrhythmias, which may account, in part, for reduction in mortality rates in patients with advanced heart failure.

**M. D. Cheitlin, MD**

*References*

1. Tomaselli GF, Beuckelmann DJ, Calkins HG, et al: Sudden cardiac death in heart failure: The role of abnormal repolarization. *Circulation* 90:2534-2539, 1994.
2. Verrier RL, Antzelevitch C: Autonomic aspects of arrhythmogenesis: The enduring and the new. *Curr Opin Cardiol* 19:2-11, 2004.
3. Vrtovec B, Delgado R, Zewail A, et al: Prolonged QTc interval and high B-type natriuretic peptide levels together predict mortality in patients with advanced heart failure. *Circulation* 107:1764-1769, 2003.
4. Ridker PM, Rifai N, Lowenthal SP: Rapid reduction in C-reactive protein with cerivastatin among 785 patients with primary hypercholesterolemia. *Circulation* 103:1191-1193, 2001.
5. Miyauchi T, Masaki T: Pathophysiology of endothelin in the cardiovascular system. *Annu Rev Physiol* 61:391-415, 1999.

## Vasopressin-2-receptor antagonism augments water excretion without changes in renal hemodynamics or sodium and potassium excretion in human heart failure

Costello-Boerrigter LC, Smith WB, Boerrigter G, et al (Mayo Clinic, Rochester, Minn; New Orleans Ctr for Clin Research, La; Otsuka Maryland Research Inst, Rockville)

*Am J Physiol Renal Physiol* 290:273-278, 2006                    5–22

Diuretics are frequently required to treat fluid retention in patients with congestive heart failure (CHF). Unfortunately, they can lead to a decline in renal function, electrolyte depletion, and neurohumoral activation. Arginine vasopressin (AVP) promotes renal water reabsorption via the $V_2$ receptor, and its levels are increased in CHF. This study was designed to assess the effects of a single oral dose of tolvaptan, a selective $V_2$-receptor blocker, in the absence of other medications, on renal function in human CHF and to compare this to the effects of a single oral dose of furosemide. We hypothesized that $V_2$-receptor antagonism would yield a diuresis comparable to furosemide but would not adversely affect renal hemodynamics, plasma electrolyte concentration, or neurohumoral activation in stable human CHF. Renal and neurohumoral effects of tolvaptan and furosemide were assessed in an open-label, randomized, placebo-controlled crossover study in 14 patients with NYHA II-III CHF. Patients received placebo or 30 mg of tolvaptan on *day 1* and were crossed over to the other medication on *day 3*. On *day 5*, all subjects received 80 mg of furosemide. Tolvaptan and furosemide induced similar diuretic responses. Unlike tolvaptan, furosemide increased urinary sodium and potassium excretion and decreased renal blood flow. Tolvaptan, furosemide, and placebo did not differ with respect to mean arterial pressure, glomerular filtration rate, or serum sodium and potassium. We conclude that tolvaptan is an effective aquaretic with no adverse effects on renal hemodynamics or serum electrolytes in patients with mild to moderate heart failure (Figs 2, 3, and 4).

▶ Diuretics are a mainstay of therapy in congestive heart failure. Loop diuretics such as furosemide are very effective but can result in some undesirable and even serious side effects, such as potassium depletion and hypokalemia, which can predispose to malignant arrhythmias, hyponatremia, and renal insufficiency, which is a powerful predictive factor for congestive heart failure.[1] Because loop diuretics are saluretics, by increasing distal tubular delivery of sodium, loop diuretics activate the tubuloglomerular feedback mechanism that causes vasoconstriction of the afferent arterioles and a reduction in renal blood flow, leading to renal dysfunction and decreased effectiveness of the diuretic.[2-4] Arginine vasopressin promotes water reabsorbtion by the $V_2$ receptor located in the renal collecting duct.[5] This study evaluates the comparative

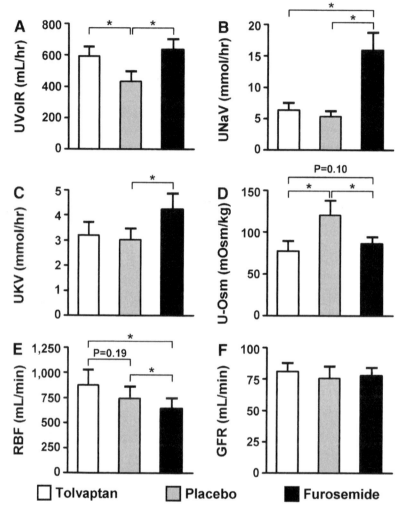

FIGURE 2.—Effect of tolvaptan, placebo, and furosemide on urine flow ($U_{Vol}R$; $A$), urinary sodium excretion ($U_{Na}V$; $B$), urinary potassium excretion ($U_KV$; $C$), urine osmolality (U-Osm; $D$), renal blood flow (RBF; $E$), and glomerular filtration rate (GFR; $F$). Bars represent weighted averages ± SE over an observation period of 9 h. *$P < 0.05$. (Courtesy of Costello-Boerrigter LC, Smith WB, Boerrigter G, et al: Vasopressin-2-receptor antagonism augments water excretion without changes in renal hemodynamics or sodium and potassium excretion in human heart failure. *Am J Physiol Renal Physiol* 290: F273-F278, 2006. Used with permission.

effect of tolvaptan, a selective $V_2$ blocker, and furosemide on the volume of diuresis, urinary sodium and potassium excretion, glomerular filtration rate, and renal blood flow in patients with heart failure. The 2 diuretics show equal effectiveness on urinary volume but no difference with tolvaptan from placebo on sodium and potassium serum levels or urinary excretion and no decrease in

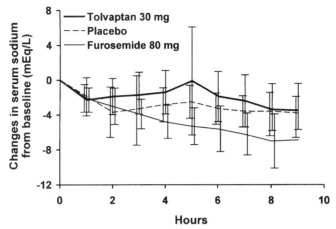

FIGURE 3.—Changes in serum sodium concentration from baseline. Thick line, tolvaptan; dashed line, placebo; thin line, furosemide. (Courtesy of Costello-Boerrigter LC, Smith WB, Boerrigter G, et al: Vasopressin-2-receptor antagonism augments water excretion without changes in renal hemodynamics or sodium and potassium excretion in human heart failure. *Am J Physiol Renal Physiol* 290: F273-F278, 2006. Used with permission.

renal blood flow. Gheorghiade et al[5] performed the first studies of tolvaptan in patients with heart failure, but this is the first study in humans to examine its renal effects compared with furosemide. Tolvaptan could be a valuable addition to the therapy of patients with congestive heart failure.

**M. D. Cheitlin, MD**

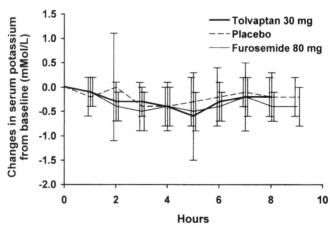

FIGURE 4.—Changes in serum potassium concentration from baseline. Thick line, tolvaptan; dashed line, placebo; thin line, furosemide. (Courtesy of Costello-Boerrigter LC, Smith WB, Boerrigter G, et al: Vasopressin-2-receptor antagonism augments water excretion without changes in renal hemodynamics or sodium and potassium excretion in human heart failure. *Am J Physiol Renal Physiol* 290: F273-F278, 2006. Used with permission.

*References*

1. Dries DL, Exner DV, Domanski MJ, et al: The prognostic implications of renal insufficiency in asymptomatic and symptomatic patients with left ventricular systolic dysfunction. *J Am Coll Cardiol* 35:681-689, 2000.
2. Chen HH, Redfield MM, Nordstrom LJ, et al: Angiotensin II AT1 receptor antagonism prevents detrimental renal actions of acute diuretic therapy in human heart failure. *Am J Physiol Renal Physiol* 284:F1115-F1119, 2003.
3. Gottlieb SS, Brater DC, Thomas I, et al: BG9719 (CVT-124), an A1 adenosine receptor antagonist, protects against the decline in renal function observed with diuretic therapy. *Circulation* 105:1348-1353, 2002.
4. Vallon V: Tubuloglomerular feedback and the control of glomerular filtration rate. *News Physiol Sci* 18:169-174, 2003.
5. Gheorghiade M, Niazi I, Ouyang J, et al: Vasopressin V2-receptor blockade with tolvaptan in patients with chronic heart failure: Results from a double-blind, randomized trial. *Circulation* 107:2690-2696, 2003.

---

**Metabolic Modulation With Perhexiline in Chronic Heart Failure: A Randomized, Controlled Trial of Short-Term Use of a Novel Treatment**
Lee L, Campbell R, Scheuermann-Freestone M, et al (Univ of Nottingham, England; Univ of Birmingham, England; Univ of Oxford, England; et al)
*Circulation* 112:3280-3288, 2005                                   5–23

---

*Background.*—Chronic heart failure (CHF) is a major cause of morbidity and mortality that requires a novel approach to therapy. Perhexiline is an antianginal drug that augments glucose metabolism by blocking muscle mitochondrial free fatty acid uptake, thereby increasing metabolic efficiency. We assessed the effects of perhexiline treatment in CHF patients.

*Method and Results.*—In a double-blind fashion, we randomly assigned patients with optimally medicated CHF to either perhexiline (n=28) or placebo (n=28). The primary end point was peak exercise oxygen consumption ($\dot{V}O_2$max), an important prognostic marker. In addition, the effect of perhexiline on myocardial function and quality of life was assessed. Quantitative stress echocardiography with tissue Doppler measurements was used to assess regional myocardial function in patients with ischemic CHF. $^{31}$P magnetic resonance spectroscopy was used to assess the effect of perhexiline on skeletal muscle energetics in patients with nonischemic CHF. Treatment with perhexiline led to significant improvements in $\dot{V}O_2$max ($16.1\pm0.6$ to $18.8\pm1.1$ mL $\cdot$ kg$^{-1}$ $\cdot$ min$^{-1}$; $P<0.001$), quality of life (Minnesota score reduction from $45\pm5$ to $34\pm5$; $P=0.04$), and left ventricular ejection fraction ($24\pm1\%$ to $34\pm2\%$; $P<0.001$). Perhexiline treatment also increased resting and peak dobutamine stress regional myocardial function (by $15\%$ and $24\%$, respectively) and normalized skeletal muscle phosphocreatine recovery after exercise. There were no adverse effects during the treatment period.

*Conclusions.*—In patients with CHF, metabolic modulation with perhexiline improved $\dot{V}O_2$max, left ventricular ejection fraction, symptoms, resting and peak stress myocardial function, and skeletal muscle energetics. Perhexiline may therefore represent a novel treatment for CHF with a good safety profile, provided that the dosage is adjusted according to plasma levels.

▶ Perhexiline maleate is a new class of antianginal drugs that inhibits the mitochondrial free fatty acid (FFA) uptake enzymes carnitine palmitoyl transferase (CPT)-1 and -2, thereby shifting muscle substrate utilization from FFA to glucose.[1] In congestive heart failure exercise capacity and oxygen consumption during peak exercise ($\dot{V}O_2$max) are reduced because of abnormal myocardial and skeletal muscle function.[2,3] In this study in patients with both ischemic and nonischemic heart failure on maximal medical therapy, perhexiline treatment caused a remarkable improvement in symptoms, cardiac function exercise tolerance, peak $\dot{V}O_2$ with exercise and normalized skeletal muscle energetics. Although perhexiline is an effective antianginal drug,[4,5] its use has been associated with hepatotoxicity and peripheral neuropathy, probably related to "slow hydroxylators" causing a progressive drug accumulation in patients with a variant of cytochrome P-450-2D6. With levels monitored between 0.15 and 0.16 mg/L the risk of hepatotoxicity is markedly reduced. The study was small (56 patients) and lasted only 8 weeks. This novel treatment of patients with congestive heart failure deserves a longer, larger study.

**M. D. Cheitlin, MD**

*References*

1. Jeffrey FM, Alvarez L, Diczku V, et al: Direct evidence that perhexiline modifies myocardial substrate utilization from fatty acids to lactate. *J Cardiovasc Pharmacol* 25:469-472, 1995.
2. Harrington D, Coats AJ: Skeletal muscle abnormalities and evidence for their role in symptom generation in chronic heart failure. *Eur Heart J* 18:1865-1872, 1997.
3. Clark AL, Poole-Wilson PA, Coats AJ: Exercise limitation in chronic heart failure: Central role of the periphery. *J Am Coll Cardiol* 28:1092-1102, 1996.
4. Horowitz JD, Mashford ML: Perhexiline maleate in the treatment of severe angina pectoris. *Med J Aust* 1:485-488, 1979.
5. Cole PL, Beamer AD, McGowan N, et al: Efficacy and safety of perhexiline maleate in refractory angina: A double-blind placebo-controlled clinical trial of a novel antianginal agent. *Circulation* 81:1260-1270, 1990.

**Effects of *Levosimendan* Versus *Dobutamine* on Inflammatory and Apoptotic Pathways in Acutely Decompensated Chronic Heart Failure**
Adamopoulos S, Parissis JT, Iliodromitis EK, et al (Attikon Univ, Athens, Greece; Northwestern Univ, Chicago)
*Am J Cardiol* 98:102-106, 2006                                                5–24

A single levosimendan administration has recently been shown to result in clinical and hemodynamic improvement in patients with decompensated heart failure (HF), but without survival benefits. In this study, the effects of levosimendan and dobutamine on plasma levels of proinflammatory and proapoptotic mediators in decompensated HF were compared and correlated with the concomitant effects on cardiac function and prognosis. Sixty-nine patients were randomized to received 24-hour intravenous infusions of levosimendan (n − 23), dobutamine (n = 23), or placebo (n = 23). Echocardiographic, hemodynamic, and biochemical assessments were performed at

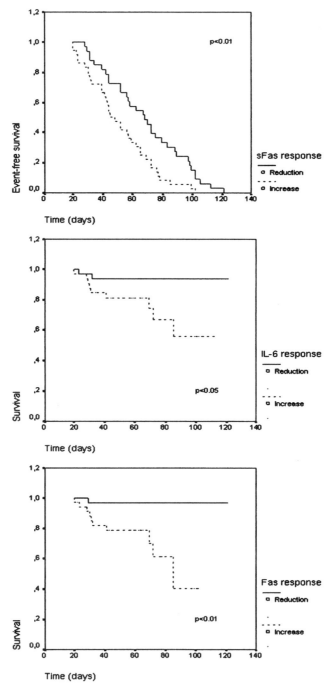

FIGURE 1.—Kaplan-Meier estimates for event-free survival (*top panel*) and overall survival (*middle and bottom panels*) according to the response of proinflammatory or proapoptotic markers to therapy. (Reprinted by permission of the publisher from Adamopoulos S, Parissis JT, Iliodromitis EK, et al: Effects of ***levosimendan*** versus ***dobutamine*** on inflammatory and apoptotic pathways in acutely decompensated chronic heart failure. *Am J Cardiol* 98:102-106. Copyright Elsevier 2006.)

baseline, immediately after treatment, and 48 hours later. Patients were subsequently followed for 4 months for disease progression. End-systolic wall stress, the left ventricular ejection fraction, pulmonary capillary wedge pressure, and cardiac index were significantly improved in the levosimendan group but remained practically unaffected in the other groups. Plasma N-terminal–pro-B-type natriuretic peptide, tumor necrosis factor-$\alpha$, and soluble Fas ligand levels were significantly decreased only in the levosimendan group (from $1,900 \pm 223$ to $1,378 \pm 170$ pg/ml, $13.4 \pm 1.0$ to $12.3 \pm 1.2$ pg/ml, and $68.2 \pm 3.7$ to $59.8 \pm 3.6$ pg/ml, respectively; p <0.05 for all); interleukin-6 was also borderline reduced (p = 0.051). Levosimendan-induced reduction in end-systolic wall stress was significantly correlated with respective decreases in N-terminal–pro-B-type natriuretic peptide (r = 0.671, p <0.01), tumor necrosis factor-$\alpha$ (r = 0.586, p <0.01), soluble Fas (r = 0.441, p <0.05), and soluble Fas ligand (r = 0.614, p <0.01). Event-free survival was significantly longer in the levosimendan group (p <0.05). In conclusion, the superiority of levosimendan over dobutamine in improving central hemodynamics and left ventricular performance in decompensated HF seems to be related to its anti-inflammatory and antiapoptotic effects (Fig 1).

► Since a basic mechanism for the development of congestive heart failure (CHF) is a decrease in myocardial contractility, it is intuitively reasonable that drugs increasing contractility should be beneficial in patients with CHF. β-Adrenergic agonists, catecholamines, such as dobutamine, and phosphodiesterase-3 (PDE-3) inhibitors, such as milrinone, increase contractility and improve symptoms and hemodynamics in patients with CHF. Unfortunately, these drugs also promote cellular and biochemical pathways for progression of HF resulting in maladaptive ventricular remodeling and decrease in survival in placebo-controlled trials. Levosimendan is a new class of calcium-sensitizing drugs that do not increase intracellular $Ca^{2+}$ overloading in cardiomyocytes. In the present study, patients with decompensated CHF were randomized to receive 24-hour IV infusions of dobutamine, levosimendan, or placebo. They were studied by echocardiography and biochemical assessment before, immediately after, and 48 hours after infusion and then followed up for 4 months. At 48 hours end-systolic wall stress (ESWS), left ventricular ejection fraction (LVEF), cardiac index, and pulmonary artery wedge pressure were improved in the levosimendan group but not in those with dobutamine. Also N-terminal–pro-B-type natriuretic peptide, tumor necrosis factor-$\alpha$ and soluble Fas ligand levels were decreased only in the levosimendan group, and the decrease was significantly correlated with a decrease in ESWS. Although follow-up was very short, event-free survival rate was also significantly greater in the levosimendan group. The advantage of levosimendan over dobutamine seems to be related to its anti-inflammatory and antiapoptotic effects, probably related to a decrease in ESWS and improvement of peripheral tissue hypoperfusion, leading to the downregulation of extracardiac cytokine production by transcriptional factors, such as nuclear factor κB.[1] Survival advantage needs to be investigated.

**M. D. Cheitlin, MD**

*Reference*

1. Goren N, Cuenca J, Martin-Sanz P, et al: Attenuation of NF-kappaB signalling in rat cardiomyocytes at birth restricts the induction of inflammatory genes *Cardiovasc Res* 64:289-297, 2004.

---

**Angiotensin-converting-enzyme inhibitors in stable vascular disease without left ventricular systolic dysfunction or heart failure: a combined analysis of three trials**
Dagenais GR, Pogue J, Fox K, et al (Laval Univ, Quebec, Canada; McMaster Univ, Hamilton, Canada; Royal Brompton Hosp, London; et al)
*Lancet* 368:581-588, 2006                                                              5–25

---

*Background.*—Angiotensin-converting-enzyme (ACE) inhibitors reduce cardiovascular mortality and morbidity in patients with heart failure or left ventricular systolic dysfunction (LVSD). Three large trials have assessed the effect of ACE inhibitors in stable patients without these conditions but with atherosclerosis. We undertook a systematic review of the Heart Outcomes Prevention Evaluation (HOPE), the European trial on Reduction Of cardiac events with Perindopril among patients with stable coronary Artery disease (EUROPA), and the Prevention of Events with ACE inhibition (PEACE) studies to determine the consistency with which ACE inhibitors reduce total mortality and fatal and non-fatal cardiovascular events.

*Methods.*—We computed cardiovascular outcomes and total mortality in the 29,805 patients of these three trials, randomly assigned an ACE inhibitor

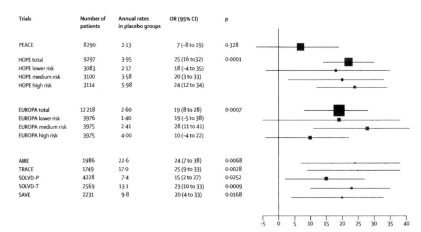

| Trials | Number of patients | Annual rates in placebo groups | OR (95% CI) | p |
|---|---|---|---|---|
| PEACE | 8290 | 2·13 | 7 (-8 to 19) | 0·328 |
| HOPE total | 9297 | 3·95 | 25 (16 to 32) | 0·0001 |
| HOPE lower risk | 3083 | 2·17 | 18 (-4 to 35) | |
| HOPE medium risk | 3100 | 3·58 | 20 (3 to 33) | |
| HOPE high risk | 3114 | 5·98 | 24 (12 to 34) | |
| EUROPA total | 12 218 | 2·60 | 19 (8 to 28) | 0·0007 |
| EUROPA lower risk | 3976 | 1·40 | 19 (-5 to 38) | |
| EUROPA medium risk | 3975 | 2·41 | 28 (11 to 41) | |
| EUROPA high risk | 3975 | 4·00 | 10 (-4 to 22) | |
| AIRE | 1986 | 22·6 | 24 (7 to 38) | 0·0068 |
| TRACE | 1749 | 17·0 | 25 (9 to 33) | 0·0028 |
| SOLVD-P | 4228 | 7·4 | 15 (2 to 27) | 0·0252 |
| SOLVD-T | 2569 | 13·1 | 23 (10 to 33) | 0·0009 |
| SAVE | 2231 | 9·8 | 20 (4 to 33) | 0·0168 |

FIGURE 1.—Percentage reduction in odds of cardiovascular death, non-fatal myocardial infarction, or stroke for PEACE, HOPE, and EUROPA, and for trials of patients with heart failure or left ventricular systolic dysfunction. Total mortality was used instead of cardiovascular death in patients with heart failure or left ventricular dysfunction. Heterogeneity p=0.083 for PEACE, HOPE, and EUROPA. Heterogeneity p=0.835 for the trials of patients with heart failure or left ventricular systolic dysfunction. (Courtesy of Dagenais GR, Pogue J, Fox K, et al: Angiotensin-converting-enzyme inhibitors in stable vascular disease without left ventricular systolic dysfunction or heart failure: a combined analysis of three trials. *Lancet* 368:581-588. Copyright Elsevier 2006.)

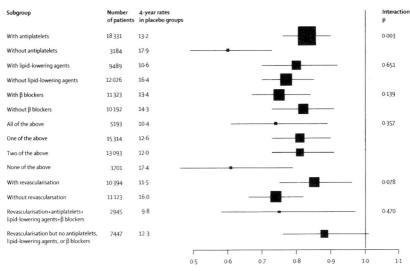

| Subgroup | Number of patients | 4-year rates in placebo groups | | Interaction p |
|---|---|---|---|---|
| With antiplatelets | 18 331 | 13·2 | | 0·003 |
| Without antiplatelets | 3184 | 17·9 | | |
| With lipid-lowering agents | 9489 | 10·6 | | 0·651 |
| Without lipid-lowering agents | 12 026 | 16·4 | | |
| With β blockers | 11 323 | 13·4 | | 0·139 |
| Without β blockers | 10 192 | 14·3 | | |
| All of the above | 5193 | 10·4 | | 0·357 |
| One of the above | 15 314 | 12·6 | | |
| Two of the above | 13 093 | 12·0 | | |
| None of the above | 1701 | 17·4 | | |
| With revascularisation | 10 394 | 11·5 | | 0·078 |
| Without revascularsation | 11 123 | 16·0 | | |
| Revascularisation+antiplatelets+ lipid-lowering agents+β blockers | 2945 | 9·8 | | 0·470 |
| Revascularisation but no antiplatelets, lipid-lowering agents, or β blockers | 7447 | 12·3 | | |

FIGURE 2.—Effects of ramipril or perindopril on cardiovascular mortality, non-fatal myocardial infarction, or stroke in patients taking antiplatelet agents, lipid-lowering agents, βblockers individually or together, in patients who underwent coronary revascularization or not, and in patients who underwent coronary revascularization and were taking all three drugs or fewer than three drugs at trial entry. Odds ratios are shown with 95% CI. (Courtesy of Dagenais GR, Pogue J, Fox K, et al: Angiotensin-converting-enzyme inhibitors in stable vascular disease without left ventricular systolic dysfunction or heart failure: a combined analysis of three trials. *Lancet* 368:581-588. Copyright Elsevier 2006.)

or placebo and followed up for a mean of about 4.5 years. The results were also analysed within the context of five large trials of ACE inhibitors in patients with heart failure or LVSD.

*Findings.*—When the findings of the HOPE, EUROPA, and PEACE trials were combined, ACE inhibitors significantly reduced all-cause mortality (7.8 *vs* 8.9%, p=0.0004), cardiovascular mortality (4.3 *vs* 5.2%, p=0.0002), non-fatal myocardial infarction (5.3 *vs* 6.4%, p=0.0001), all stroke (2.2 *vs* 2.8%, p=0.0004), heart failure (2.1 *vs* 2.7%, p=0.0007), coronary-artery bypass surgery (6.0 *vs* 6.9%, p=0.0036) but not percutaneous coronary intervention (7.4 *vs* 7.6%, p=0.481). The composite outcomes of cardiovascular mortality, non-fatal myocardial infarction, or stroke occurred in 1599 (10.7%) of the patients allocated ACE inhibitor and in 1910 (12.8%) of those allocated placebo (odds ratio, 0.82; 95% CIs 0.76–0.88; p<0.0001). Except for stroke and revascularisation, these results were similar to those of the five trials in patients with heart failure or LVSD.

*Interpretation.*—ACE inhibitors reduce serious vascular events in patients with atherosclerosis without known evidence of LVSD or heart failure. Results showing these benefits in intermediate-risk patients complement existing evidence of similar benefit in higher-risk patients with LVSD or heart failure. Therefore, use of ACE inhibitors should be considered in all patients with atherosclerosis (Figs 1 and 2).

▶ There is extensive evidence from randomized, placebo-controlled trials that ACE inhibitors reduce mortality, hospital readmissions for heart failure, and subsequent myocardial infarction in patients with heart failure or low left ventricular ejection fraction (LVEF).[1] This article combined the results of 3 large, randomized, placebo-controlled trials of patients with atherosclerosis but no evidence of heart failure of low LVEF, treated with ACE inhibitors. Overall, there was a highly significant 18% reduction in odds ratio for combined outcomes of cardiovascular mortality, non-fatal myocardial infarction, or strokes compared with that of placebo, with narrow confidence compared with that of placebo. The benefit was shown in addition to the other proved therapies of antiplatelet agents—β-blockers and lipid-lowering agents. The benefits were shown across a wide range of risk groups of patients for cardiovascular events from as high as 10% per year to as low as 1.7% per year, indicating a lack of threshold at least in patients with vascular disease. They performed a similar analysis of 5 randomized, placebo-controlled trials of ACE inhibitors in patients with heart failure or low LVEF. The reductions in the above endpoints were similar, except for stroke and revascularization.[1]

The implication of these studies is that for every 1000 patients treated over 4.5 years, 211 patients will avoid any of these serious vascular complications. These findings were consistent with the findings of previous trials in patients with heart failure or low LVEF, where ACE inhibitos significantly improved the outcomes with an odds ratio reduction of 21%. For every 100 patients treated for about 3 years, about 50 would be protected from a fatal event, nonfatal myocardial infarction or stroke. Since the trials in patients with systolic dysfunction were higher-risk patients, the benefit seen with ACE inhibitors was slightly greater in those patients than in patients with normal LV systolic function.

These data provide support for the use of ACE inhibitors in patients with vascular disease in spite of the absence of heart failure of low LVEF.

**M. D. Cheitlin, MD**

*Reference*

1. Flather MD, Yusuf S, Kober L, et al: Long-term ACE-inhibitor therapy in patients with heart failure or left-ventricular dysfunction: A systematic overview of data from individual patients. ACE-Inhibitor Myocardial Infarction Collaborative Group. Lancet. 355:1575-1581, 2000.

## Congestive Heart Failure Therapy and Technology

**Cardiac Resynchronization Therapy Improves Heart Rate Profile and Heart Rate Variability of Patients With Moderate to Severe Heart Failure**
Fantoni C, Raffia S, Regoli F, et al (Univ Hosp, Magdeburg, Germany; Univ of Insubria, Varese, Italy; Centro Cardiologico Monzino, Milan, Italy; et al)
*J Am Coll Cardiol* 46:1875-1882, 2005                                            5–26

*Objectives.*—This study sought to report long-term changes of cardiac autonomic control by continuous, device-based monitoring of the standard deviation of the averages of intrinsic intervals in the 288 five-min segments

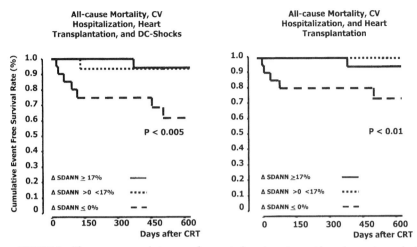

FIGURE 2.—The two-year cumulative event-free survival rate in patients with no changes in standard deviation of the average of intrinsic intervals in the 288 five-minute segments of a day (SDANN) four weeks after implantation (first tertile, Δ change ≤0%), in patients with some SDANN changes (seond tertile, Δ change from 1 to 17%), and in those with large SDANN changes (third tertile, Δ change ≥17%). CRT = cardiac resynchronization therapy; CV hospitalization = hospitalizations for cardiovascular reasons. (Reprinted with permission from the *American College of Cardiology* from Fantoni C, Raffia S, Regoli F, et al: Cardiac resynchronization therapy improves heart rate variability of patients with moderate to severe heart failure. *J Am Coll Cardiol* 46:1875-1882. Copyright Elsevier 2005.)

of a day (SDANN) and of heart rate (HR) profile in heart failure (HF) patients treated with cardiac resynchronization therapy (CRT).

*Background.*—Data on long-term changes of time-domain parameters of heart rate variability (HRV) and of HR in highly symptomatic HF patients treated with CRT are lacking.

*Methods.*—Stored data were retrieved for 113 HF patients (New York Heart Association functional class III to IV, left ventricular ejection fraction ≤35%, QRS >120 ms) receiving a CRT device capable of continuous assessment of HRV and HR profile.

*Results.*—The CRT induced a reduction of minimum HR (from 63 ± 9 beats/min to 58 ± 7 beats/min, p < 0.001) and mean HR (from 76 ± 10 beats/min to 72 ± 8 beats/min, p < 0.01) and an increase of SDANN (from 69 ± 23 ms to 93 ± 27 ms, p < 0.001) at three-month follow-up, which were consistent with improvement of functional capacity and structural changes. Different kinetics were observed among these parameters. The SDANN reached the plateau before minimum HR, and mean HR was the slowest parameter to change. Suboptimal left ventricular lead position was associated with no significant functional and structural improvement as well as no change or even worsening of HRV. The two-year event-free survival rate was significantly lower (62% vs. 94%, p < 0.005) in patients without any SDANN change (Δ change ≤0%) compared with patients who showed an increase in SDANN (Δ change >0%) four weeks after CRT initiation.

*Conclusions.*—Cardiac resynchronization therapy is able to significantly modify the sympathetic-parasympathetic interaction to the heart, as defined by HR profile and HRV. Lack of HRV improvement four weeks after CRT identifies patients at higher risk for major cardiovascular events (Fig 2).

---

**Cost Effectiveness of Cardiac Resynchronization Therapy in the Comparison of Medical Therapy, Pacing, and Defibrillation in Heart Failure (COMPANION) Trial**

Feldman AM, de Lissovoy G, Bristow MR, et al (Jefferson Med College, Philadelphia; MEDTAP Inst at UBC, Bethesda, Md; Johns Hopkins School of Public Health, Baltimore, Md; et al)

*J Am Coll Cardiol* 46:2311-2321, 2005                                    5–27

---

*Objectives.*—The analysis goal was to estimate incremental cost-effectiveness ratios (ICERs) for the Comparison of Medical Therapy, Pacing, and Defibrillation in Heart Failure (COMPANION) trial patients who received cardiac resynchronization therapy (CRT) via pacemaker (CRT-P) or pacemaker-defibrillator (CRT-D) in combination with optimal pharmacological therapy (OPT) relative to patients with OPT alone.

*Background.*—In the COMPANION trial, CRT-P and CRT-D reduced the combined risk of all-cause mortality or first hospitalization among patients with advanced heart failure and intraventricular conduction delays, but the cost effectiveness of the therapy remains unknown.

*Methods.*—In this analysis, intent-to-treat trial data were modeled to estimate the cost effectiveness of CRT-D and CRT-P relative to OPT over a base-case seven-year treatment episode. Exponential survival curves were derived from trial data and adjusted by quality-of-life trial results to yield quality-adjusted life-years (QALYs). For the first two years, follow-up hospitalizations were based on trial data. The model assumed equalized hospitalization rates beyond two years. Initial implantation and follow-up hospitalization costs were estimated using Medicare data.

*Results.*—Over two years, follow-up hospitalization costs were reduced by 29% for CRT-D and 37% for CRT-P. Extending the cost-effectiveness analysis to a seven-year base-case time period, the ICER for CRT-P was 19,600 dollars per QALY and the ICER for CRT-D was 43,000 dollars per QALY relative to OPT.

*Conclusions.*—For the COMPANION trial patients, the use of CRT-P and CRT-D was associated with a cost-effectiveness ratio below generally accepted benchmarks for therapeutic interventions of 50,000 dollars per QALY to 100,000 dollars per QALY. This suggests that the clinical benefits of CRT-P and CRT-D can be achieved at a reasonable cost.

▶ Sudden death is a common mode of exodus in patients with congestive heart failure (CHF). Cardiac resynchronization therapy (CRT) was shown in the COMPANION trial[1] (CRT in the Comparison of Medical Therapy, Pacing, and Defibrillation in Heart Failure) to decrease the all-cause mortality rate or the first hospitalization relative to patients with optimal medical therapy alone. Fantoni et al (Abstract 5–27) in patients with moderate to severe heart failure and a QRS >120 ms and EF ≤35% by using measures of sympathetic/parasympathetic cardiac interaction have shown that the heart rate profile (minimum and mean heart rate) is reduced and heart rate variability increased by CRT, consistent with improvement in functional capacity, decrease in left ventricular diastolic diameter, and increase in EF. With the increase in heart rate variability there was a decrease in the 2-year event-free survival rate (62% without change vs 94% with >0% change) 4 weeks after CRT initiation. This decrease in sympathetic drive would be consistent with a decrease in life-threatening ventricular arrhythmias.

Another article of interest is that of Feldman et al (Abstract 5–28) who, by using the patients in the COMPANION trial, estimated that use of CRT-P (with pacemaker) and CRT-D (with pacemaker-defibrillator) was associated with a cost-effectiveness rate below the generally accepted value for therapeutic interventions of $50,000 per QALY with incremental cost-effective ratios (ICERs of $19,000 per QALY for CRT-P and $43,000 per QALY for CRT-D relative to optimal medical therapy.

**M. D. Cheitlin, MD**

*Reference*

1. Bristow MR, Saxon LA, Boehmer J, et al: Comparison of Medical Therapy, Pacing, and Defibrillation in Heart Failure (COMPANION) Investigators: Cardiac-resynchronization therapy with or without an implantable defibrillator in advanced chronic heart failure. *N Engl J Med* 350:2140-2150, 2004.

---

**Myocardial Viability Testing and the Effect of Early Intervention in Patients With Advanced Left Ventricular Systolic Dysfunction**
Tarakji KG, Brunken R, McCarthy PM, et al (Cleveland Clinic Found, Ohio; Case Western Reserve Univ School of Medicine, Cleveland, Ohio)
*Circulation* 113:230-237, 2006                                                     5–28

---

*Background.*—The clinical value of revascularization and other procedures in patients with severe systolic heart failure is unclear. It has been suggested that assessing ischemia and viability by positron emission tomography (PET) with fluorodeoxyglucose (FDG) imaging may identify patients for whom revascularization may lead to improved survival. We performed a propensity analysis to determine whether there might be a survival advantage from revascularization.

*Method and Results.*—We analyzed the survival of 765 consecutive patients (age 64±11 years, 80% men) with advanced left ventricular systolic dysfunction (ejection fraction ≤35%) and without significant valvular heart disease who underwent PET/FDG study at the Cleveland Clinic between 1997 and 2002. Early intervention was defined as any cardiac intervention (surgical or percutaneous) within the first 6 months of the PET/FDG study. In the entire cohort, 230 patients (30%) underwent early intervention (188 [25%] had open heart surgery, most commonly coronary artery bypass grafting, and 42 [5%] had percutaneous revascularization); 535 (70%) were treated medically. Using 39 demographic, clinical and PET/FDG variables, we were able to propensity-match 153 of the 230 patients with 153 patients who did not undergo early intervention. Among the propensity-matched group, there were 84 deaths during a median of 3 years follow-up. Early intervention was associated with a markedly lower risk of death (3-year mortality rate of 15% versus 35%, propensity adjusted hazard ratio 0.52, 95% CI 0.33 to 0.81, $P=0.0004$).

*Conclusions.*—Among systolic heart failure patients referred for PET/FDG, early intervention may be associated with improved survival irrespective of the degree of viability

▶ This is an interesting study that sheds light on the "open artery" hypothesis. Intuitively it makes sense that survival after revascularization in patients with coronary artery disease and advanced left ventricular (LV) dysfunction would be dependent on the amount of ischemic viable myocardium revascularized. The CASS study[1] (Coronary Artery Surgery Study) reported that in patients with poor LV function symptomatic improvement with surgery occurred only in patients with angina, implying that viable myocardium had to be present for benefit to occur from revascularization. The current study of a large number of patients with ejection fraction ≤35% reports that the percentage of ischemic and hibernating myocardium was the best predictor of survival after revascularization. Most interesting, even with a small percentage of ischemic/hibernating myocardium, there was a distinct survival advantage over medical management. Because only 34 patients were revascularized with no ischemic/hibernating myocardium, this study cannot address the ultimate question of the value of opening an occluded coronary artery serving only scar, the basic question of the "open artery" hypothesis. This propensity-matched controlled study does not definitively answer the question of whether it was early intervention or early intervention in a patient with ischemic but viable myocardium that resulted in improved long-term survival because the degree of viability was the strongest predictor of early intervention. To answer such a question would require a very large prospective, randomized study. Such trials are in progress,[2,3] but the results from these studies are years away.

**M. D. Cheitlin, MD**

*References*

1. Alderman EL, Fisher L, Litwin L, et al: Results of coronary artery surgery in patients with poor left ventricular function (CASS). *Circulation* 4:785-795, 1983.
2. Cleland JG, Freemantle N, Ball SG, et al: The heart failure revascularisation trial (HEART): Rationale, design and methodology. *Eur J Heart Fail* 5:295-303, 2003.
3. Joyce D, Loebe M, Noon GP, et al: Revascularization and ventricular restoration in patients with ischemic heart failure: The STICH trial. *Curr Opin Cardiol* 18:454-457, 2003.

### Cardiac Rsynchronization Therapy Delays Heart Transplantation in Patients With End-stage Heart Failure and Mechanical Dyssynchrony

Vanderheyden M, Wellens F, Bartunek J, et al (Onze Lieve Vrouw Ziekenhuis, Aalst, Belgium)

*J Heart Lung Transplant* 25:447-453, 2006                                        5–29

*Background.*—Cardiac dyssynchrony is frequent in advanced heart failure, and cardiac resynchronization therapy (CRT) may offer an alternative to heart transplantation. We aimed to investigate the impact of CRT on freedom from Tx and death in transplant candidates with end-stage heart failure.

*Methods.*—Over a period of 2 years, 46 consecutive patients with refractory congestive heart failure due to dilated cardiomyopathy were referred for heart transplant evaluation. Patients with cardiac dyssynchrony >107 milliseconds according to tissue Doppler imaging (TDI) or QRS duration >150 milliseconds were treated with CRT (CRT group, $n = 24$), whereas patients without dyssynchrony were not treated (non-CRT group, $n = 22$).

*Results.*—At baseline, both groups showed similar hemodynamic and functional parameters, including ejection fraction ($19 \pm 10\%$ vs $21 \pm 12\%$, not statistically significant [NS]) and $VO_2$max ($11.9 \pm 2.0$ vs $12.0 \pm 1.8$ ml/kg/min, NS). After a follow-up of $488 \pm 346$ days, cumulative survival with freedom from transplantation and death was higher in CRT vs non-CRT patients (92% vs 39%; $p < 0.001$). CRT patients showed a decrease in New York Heart Association (NYHA) class from $3.2 \pm 1.1$ to $2.2 \pm 0.9$ ($p = 0.003$) and an increase in $VO_2$max from $11.9 \pm 2.0$ to $13.1 \pm 1.8$ ml/kg/min ($p = 0.02$), and 71% (17 of 24) of these patients were successfully removed from the waiting list.

*Conclusions.*—In heart transplant candidates with significant dyssynchrony, CRT delays heart transplantation and improves NYHA class and exercise capacity. For these patients, CRT should be considered before heart transplantation (Fig 4).

▶ This is an observational study of 46 consecutive patients with dilated cardiomyopathy and refractory heart failure referred for cardiac transplantation, 24 with dyssynchrony and 22 without. The patients with cardiac dyssynchrony were treated with cardiac resynchronization therapy (CRT). An internal cardioverter defibrillator was implanted in 24 patients with aborted sudden death or with inducible ventricular tachycardia or fibrillation by electrophysiologic study. Freedom from death or cardiac transplantation after $488 \pm 346$ days was 92% in those with CRT and 39% in those without ($P < .001$). The mortality rate was the same in both groups. This article provides evidence that, even in the patients with the most advanced heart failure, those with ventricular dyssynchrony, defined as total dyssynchrony of >107 ms by tissue Doppler imaging or QRS duration, >150 ms should be treated with CRT before considering cardiac transplantation.

**M. D. Cheitlin, MD**

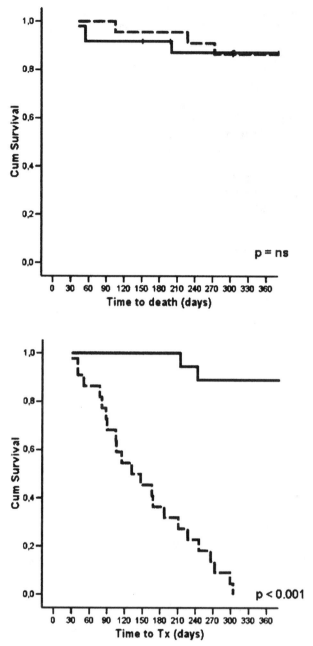

**FIGURE 4.**—Upper panel: Kaplan–Meier survival curves of patients with CRT (solid line) and without CRT (dotted line). Lower panel: Kaplan–Meier freedom-from-transplant curves for CRT and non-CRT patients. Dotted line: non-CRT; solid line: CRT patients. (Courtesy of Vanderheyden M, Wellens F, Bartunek J, et al: Cardiac resynchronization therapy delays heart transplantation in patients with end-stage heart failure and mechanical dyssyncrony. *J Heart Lung Transplant* 25:447-453. Copyright Elsevier 2006.)

SUGGESTED READING

Penicka M, Bartunek J, De Bruyne B, et al: Improvement of left ventricular function after cardiac resynchronization therapy is predicted by tissue Doppler imaging echocardiography. *Circulation* 109:978-983, 2004.

## Mechanical Unloading Leads to Echocardiographic, Electrocardiographic, Neurohormonal, and Histologic Recovery

Xydas S, Rosen RS, Ng C, et al (Columbia Univ College of Physicians and Surgeons, New York)
*J Heart Lung Transplant* 25:7-15, 2006                                    5–30

*Background.*—Mechanical unloading during left ventricular assist device (LVAD) support may lead to cardiac recovery. Predictors of recovery, however, have not been identified. We aimed to evaluate the time course and durability of echocardiographic, electrocardiographic (ECG), histologic, and neurohormonal changes that occur with LVAD support and to screen for non-invasive markers of cardiac recovery.

*Methods.*—LVAD patients underwent monthly testing, including echocardiographic, ECG, and serum B-type natriuretic peptide (BNP) measurement. Paired myocardial tissue samples from implant and explant were also analyzed.

*Results.*—Thirty-six LVAD patients were prospectively followed for an average of 101 ± 99 days. Left ventricular ejection fraction (LVEF) and end-diastolic diameter (LVEDD) significantly improved at 30 days compared with pre-LVAD (19% ± 6.6% vs 33% ± 8.1%, 7.1 ± 1.2 cm vs 4.9 ± 1.0 cm, respectively; both $p < 0.001$), with no improvement thereafter. At 30 days,

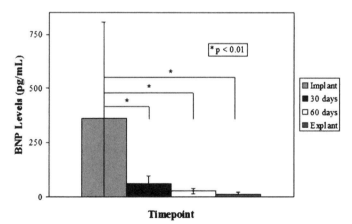

**FIGURE 1.**—Serial neurohormonal levels during left ventricular assist device (LVAD) support. There was a substantial decrease in B-type natriuretic peptide (BNP) levels at all time points compared with pre-LVAD. No differences were found, however, between 30-, 60-, or 90-day values. Data are shown as the mean value ± SD. *$p < 0.01$, as analyzed by repeated measures analysis of variance. (Courtesy of Xydas S, Rosen RS, Ng C: Mechanical unloading leads to echocardiographic, electrocardiographic, neurohormonal, and histologic recovery. *J Heart Lung Transplant* 25:7-15. Copyright Elsevier 2006.)

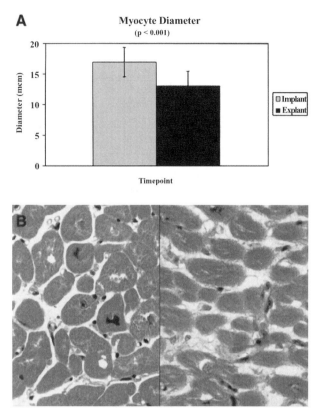

**A**

**Myocyte Diameter**
(p < 0.001)

Diameter (mcm)

□ Implant
■ Explant

Timepoint

**B**

FIGURE 2.—Myocyte diameter from time of left ventricular device (LVAD) implantation to time of explantation (*n* = 17). (A) There was a significant decrease in myocyte diameter between these time points. Data are shown as the mean value ± SD; the *p* value was determined from paired *t*-tests. (B) A representative photograph of the Masson's trichrome staining pattern is shown at high magnification (20× original magnification) depicting the decreas in the myocyte size before (left) and after (right) LVAD support. (Courtesy of Xydas S, Rosen RS, Ng C: Mechanical unloading leads to echocardiographic, electrocardiographic, neurohormonal, and histologic recovery. *J Heart Lung Transplant* 25:7-15. Copyright Elsevier 2006.)

QRS duration and QTc interval were significantly decreased from pre-LVAD (both *p* ± 0.05). There was a marked reduction in BNP, myocyte size, and collagen deposition with LVAD support (all *p* < 0.01). In screening for markers of recovery, the decrease in QTc was inversely related to LVEDD at 60 days. Changes in QRS and myocyte diameter also correlated with the improvement in LVEF at 30 days. No patients had sufficient recovery for device explantation.

*Conclusions.*—We demonstrate echocardiographic, ECG, histologic, and neurohormonal improvement during LVAD support. Cardiac recovery peaked by 60 days, and there was a trend toward progressive improvement in QRS duration with ongoing support. We report the association of ECG changes with echocardiographic and histologic improvements. Future prospective studies may yield important markers of recovery (Figs 1, 2, and 3 and Table 4).

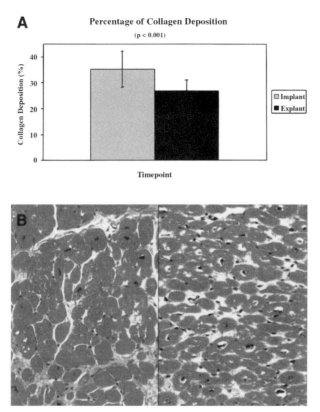

**FIGURE 3.**—The degree of collagen deposition from time of left ventricular assist device (LVAD) implantation to time of explantation ($n = 17$). (A) There was a significant decrease in collagen deposition between these time points, as determined from digital image analysis. Data are presented as the mean value ± SD; the *p* value was determined from paired *t*-tests. (B) A representative photograph of the Masson's trichrome staining pattern is shown at low magnification ($10\times$ original magnification). The amount of collagen, which stains blue with the trichrome stain, deposited at the time of LVAD implantation (left) decreases by the time of explantation (right) after a period of LVAD support. (Courtesy of Xydas S, Rosen RS, Ng C: Mechanical unloading leads to echocardiographic, electrocardiographic, neurohormonal, and histologic recovery. *J Heart Lung Transplant* 25:7-15. Copyright Elsevier 2006.)

▶ Left ventricular assist devices (LVAD) in patients with end-stage heart failure provide dramatic pressure and volume unloading of the left ventricle (LV) and restore adequate systemic blood flow. Currently it finds most use as a bridge to cardiac transplantation. Heerdt et al[1] have shown that with the use of LVAD in patients with severe heart failure there is normalization of genes regulating $Ca^{++}$ handling, with up-regulation of sarcoplasmic endoreticular $Ca^{++}$ ATPase-subtype 2A (SERCA-2A), the ryanodine receptor and the sarcolemmal $Na^+$-$Ca^{++}$ exchanger. Torre-Amione et al[2] have shown, in heart failure patients on LVAD, a decrease in myocardial tumor necrosis factor-α (TNF-α), an inflammatory cytokine that promotes hypertrophy, fibrosis, and progression of heart failure. Bruckner et al[3] have shown a decrease in myocardial hypertrophy and myocardial collagen in heart failure patients on LVAD. The current prospective study shows electrocardiographic and echocardiographic changes in patients

TABLE 4.—Correlations Between Electrocardiographic and
Echocardiographic Parameters

| | LVEDD at 60 Days | % $\triangle$ LVEF (pre-LVAD to 30 Days) |
|---|---|---|
| % $\triangle$ QTc (pre-LVAD to 60 days) | −0.6 (0.048*) | |
| % $\triangle$ QRS (48 hours post-LVAD to 30 days) | | 0.6 (0.036*) |

Data are presented for Spearman correlation coefficients and associated *p* values (in parentheses).
*$p < 0.05$.
LVAD, left ventricular assist device; LVEDD, left ventricular end-diastolic diameter; LVEF, left ventricular ejection fraction; QTc, corrected QT.
(Courtesy of Xydas S, Rosen RS, Ng C: Mechanical unloading leads to echocardiographic, electrocardiographic, neurohormonal, and histologic recovery. *J Heart Lung Transplant* 25:7-15. Copyright Elsevier 2006.)

with end-stage heart failure on LVAD, including a decrease in QRS duration and QTc and a decrease in LV end-diastolic diameter and an increase in LV ejection fraction. There was also a marked decrease in B-type natriuretic peptide (BNP) and a decrease in myocardial hypertrophy and myocardial collagen. They also showed that the QTc decrease between pre-LVAD and 60 days on LVAD correlated with the decrease in LV end-diastolic diameter at 60 days and that the decrease in QRS duration 48 hours of LVAD correlated at 30 days with an increase in LV ejection fraction.

No patient was felt to be recovered sufficiently to avoid transplantation, although this was not designed to be a weaning study. Mancini et al[4] have reported a low incidence of myocardial recovery on LVAD support to avoid transplantation. In 111 LVAD patients, only 5 were successfully weaned. However, there is evidence that in patients with end-stage heart failure LVAD support combined with maximal therapy with β-blockers and angiotensin-converting enzyme inhibitors may be more successful in producing myocardial recovery sufficient to avoid transplantation.

**M. D. Cheitlin, MD**

*References*

1. Heerdt PM, Holmes JW, Cai B, et al: Chronic unloading by left ventricular assist device reverses contractile dysfunction and alters gene expression in end-stage heart failure. *Circulation* 102:2713-2719, 2000.
2. Torre-Amione G, Stetson SJ, Youker KA, et al: Decreased expression of tumor necrosis factor-alpha in failing human myocardium after mechanical circulatory support: A potential mechanism for cardiac recovery. *Circulation* 100:1189-1193, 1999.
3. Bruckner BA, Stetson SJ, Perez-Verdia A, et al: Regression of fibrosis and hypertrophy in failing myocardium following mechanical circulatory support. *J Heart Lung Transplant* 20:457-464, 2001.
4. Mancini DM, Beniaminovitz A, Levin H, et al: Low incidence of myocardial recovery after left ventricular assist device implantation in patients with chronic heart failure. *Circulation* 98:2383-2389, 1998.

**Two-Year Clinical Outcomes After Enhanced External Counterpulsation (EECP) Therapy in Patients With Refractory Angina Pectoris and Left Ventricular Dysfunction (Report from the International EECP Patient Registry)**

Soran O, Kennard ED, Kfoury AG, et al (Univ of Pittsburgh Med Ctr, Pa; Utah Cardiac Transplant Program LDS Hosp, Salt Lake City)

*Am J Cardiol* 97:17-20, 2006                                          5–31

Enhanced external counterpulsation (EECP) is a noninvasive circulatory assist device that has recently emerged as a treatment option for refractory angina in left ventricular (LV) dysfunction. This 2-year cohort study describes the long-term follow-up of patients who had severe LV dysfunction that was treated with EECP for angina pectoris and reports clinical outcomes, event-free survival rates, and the incidence of repeat EECP. This study included 363 patients who had refractory angina and LV ejection fraction ≤35%. Most patients reported quality of life as poor. After completion of treatment, there was a significant decrease in severity of angina class (p <0.001), and 72% improved from severe angina to no angina or mild angina. Fifty-two percent of patients discontinued nitroglycerin use. Quality of life improved substantially. At 2 years this decrease in angina was maintained in 55% of patients. The 2-year survival rate was 83%, and the major adverse cardiovascular event-free survival rate was 70%. Forty-three per-

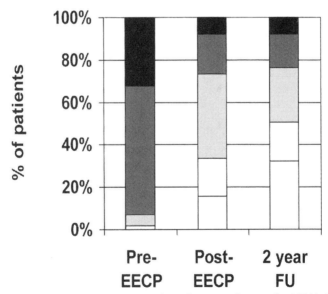

FIGURE 1.—Angina classes 0 (*white bars*), I (*pale gray bars*), II (*medium gray bars*), III (*dark gray bars*), and IV (*black bars*) before EECP (n = 363), after EECP (n = 358, and at 2-year follow-up (FU; n = 265). (Reprinted from *American Journal of Cardiology* from Soran O, Kennard ED, Kfoury AG, et al: Two-year clinical outcomes after enhanced external counterpulsation [EECP] therapy in patients with refractory angina pectoris and left ventricular dysfunction [report from the International EECP Patient Registry]. *Am J Cardiol* 97:17-20. Copyright Elsevier 2006.)

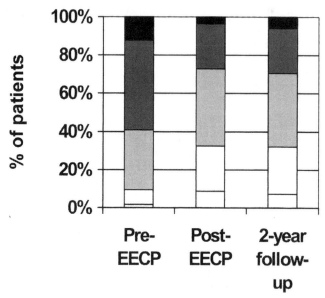

**FIGURE 2.**—Quality of life rated as poor (*black bars*), fair (*dark gray bars*), good (*medium gray bars*), very good (*pale gray bars*), and excellent (*white bars*) before and after EECP and at 2-year follow-up. (Reprinted from *American Journal of Cardiology* from Soran O, Kennard ED, Kfoury AG, et al: Two-year clinical outcomes after enhanced external counterpulsation [EECP] therapy in patients with refractory angina pectoris and left ventricular dysfunction [report from the International EECP Patient Registry]. *Am J Cardiol* 97:17-20. Copyright Elsevier 2006.)

cent had no reported cardiac hospitalization; 81% had no reported congestive heart failure events. Repeat EECP was performed in 20% of these patients. The only significant independent predictor of repeat EECP in a proportional hazard model was failure to complete the first EECP treatment course (hazard ratio 2.9, 95% confidence interval 1.7 to 4.9). Improvements in angina symptoms and quality of life were maintained at 2 years. In conclusion, for patients who have high-risk LV dysfunction, EECP offers an effective, durable therapeutic approach for refractory angina. Decreased angina and improvement in quality of life were maintained at 2 years, with modest repeat EECP and low major cardiovascular event rates (Figs 1 and 2).

▶ This study reports the 2-year follow-up of 363 patients with refractory angina and poor left ventricular (LV) function with an EF ≥35% treated with enhanced external counterpulsation (EECP). EECP has hemodynamic effects similar to those of intra-aortic counterpulsation: diastolic augmentation and decreased afterload.[1] In a 2-year follow-up almost three fourths of the patients improved from severe angina to mild or no angina and the major event-free survival rate was 70% with an improved quality of life. This is the largest report of long-term results of consecutive patients with refractory angina and LV dysfunction treated with EECP. The therapy is time-consuming, requiring 35 one-hour sessions offered once a day. The EECP was repeated in 20% of patients with the only significant independent predictor for repeat EECP being failure to complete the first EECP series of treatments. The 363 patients were selected from >5000 patients in the Interventional EECP Patient Registry (IEPR) on the basis of the presence of refractory angina and an EF ≥35%. Ninety-three percent of patients were not candidates for revascularization because of the extent of coronary disease. Therefore, this is an unusual type of patient. Yet, in such patients, EECP seems to be an effective mode of therapy.

**M. D. Cheitlin, MD**

*Reference*

1. Taguchi I, Ogawa K, Oida A, et al: Comparison of hemodynamic effects of enhanced external counterpulsation and intra-aortic balloon pumping in patients with acute myocardial infarction. *Am J Cardiol* 86:1139-1141, 2000.

## Surgical Ventricular Remodeling for Patients with Clinically Advanced Congestive Heart Failure and Severe Left Ventricular Dysfunction

Patel ND, Barreiro CJ, Williams JA, et al (Johns Hopkins Med Institutions, Baltimore, Md)
*J Heart Lung Transplant* 24:2202-2210, 2005                    5–32

*Background.*—Surgical ventricular remodeling (SVR) is an accepted therapy for post-infarction ventricular remodeling. Current literature on SVR outcomes has focused on heterogeneous populations with regard to left ventricular function and New York Heart Association (NYHA) class. We assessed outcomes after SVR in patients with advanced congestive heart fail-

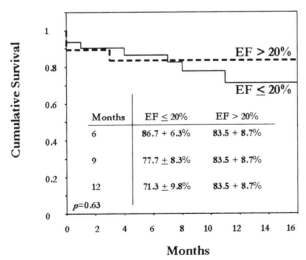

| Months | EF ≤ 20% | EF > 20% |
|--------|----------|----------|
| 6 | 86.7 + 6.3% | 83.5 + 8.7% |
| 9 | 77.7 ± 8.3% | 83.5 + 8.7% |
| 12 | 71.3 ± 9.8% | 83.5 + 8.7% |

$p$=0.63

**FIGURE 1.**—Actuarial survival of SVR patients with a pre-operative EF ≤ 20% vs >20%. (Courtesy of Patel ND, Barreiro CJ, Williams JA, et al: Surgical ventricular remodeling for patients with clinically advanced congestive heart failure and severe left ventricular dysfunction. *J Heart Lung Transplant* 24:2202-2210. Copyright Elsevier 2005.)

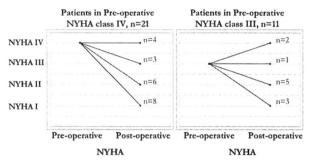

FIGURE 2.—Improvement in NYHA class for SVR patients with an EF ≤ 20%. (Courtesy of Patel ND, Barreiro CJ, Williams JA, et al: Surgical ventricular remodeling for patients with clinically advanced congestive heart failure and severe left ventricular dysfunction. *J Heart Lung Transplant* 24:2202-2210. Copyright Elsevier 2005.)

ure (CHF) (NYHA Class III/IV) and a pre-operative ejection fraction (EF) ≤20%.

*Methods.*—Data were analyzed for 51 consecutive SVR patients from January 2002 to June 2004. Cardiac catheterization, echocardiography and magnetic resonance imaging (MRI) identified 62.7% (32 of 51) of patients with an EF ≤20%, with the majority having an EF ≤15% (65.6%; 21 of 32). Cox regression analysis was performed to determine predictors of mortality in patients with an EF ≤20%. Follow-up was 100% (32 of 32) complete.

*Results.*—Mean age was 61.9 ± 10.3 (range 40 to 80) years with a male:female ratio of 27:5. Operative mortality was 6.3% (2 of 32). Twenty-two percent (7 of 32) had concomitant mitral valve procedures. Follow-up demonstrated a statistically significant improvement in left ventricular volumes and EF in survivors. Cox regression analysis identified the following to be significant predictors of mortality: pre-operative left ventricular end-systolic volume index >130 ml/m$^2$; pre-operative diabetes; and intra-aortic balloon pump usage. Pre-operatively, all patients (32 of 32) were categorized as NYHA Class III/IV, with 69% (22 of 32) improving to NYHA Class I/II at follow-up ($p < 0.01$). Survival did not differ statistically between patients with an EF ≤20% and an EF >20% ($n = 19$).

*Conclusions.*—Our results indicate that SVR improves left ventricular function and functional status for patients with advanced CHF and a pre-operative EF ≤20%. Therefore, SVR is a viable surgical alternative for patients with severe left ventricular dysfunction (Figs 1 and 2).

## Surgical ventricular remodeling for multiterritory myocardial infarction: Defining a new patient population

Patel ND, Williams JA, Barreiro CJ, et al (Johns Hopkins Med Institutions, Baltimore, Md)
*J Thorac Cardiovasc Surg* 130:1698-1706, 2005

5–33

*Objective.*—Because of limited medical and surgical options for patients with end-stage congestive heart failure, we expanded the criteria for surgical ventricular remodeling to include patients with multiterritory myocardial infarction, a group historically considered high-risk candidates. We present our series of patients with multiterritory myocardial infarction who underwent surgical ventricular remodeling and propose a new patient population who may benefit from this procedure.

*Methods.*—Data were analyzed for 51 consecutive patients undergoing surgical ventricular remodeling from January 2002 to June 2004, with 100% follow-up. Three left ventricular vascular territories were defined: anteroapicoseptal (left anterior descending), lateral (circumflex), and inferior (right coronary artery). Infarction was assessed with magnetic resonance imaging and intraoperative findings.

*Results.*—Multiterritory myocardial infarction was found in 64.7% of patients (33/51) undergoing surgical ventricular remodeling. Mean age was $61.6 \pm 11.1$ years (range 40-81 years). Sixty-one percent (20/33) demonstrated evidence of myocardial infarction in all three territories. Five patients underwent concomitant mitral valve repair or replacement. Operative mortality was 6.1% (2/33) and did not differ from that of patients with single-territory infarction (11.1%, $P = .61$). Surgical ventricular remodeling significantly improved left ventricular volumes and ejection fraction in patients with multiterritory myocardial infarction. Three patients required assist device implantation, and 2 patients required defibrillator placement. Sixty-nine percent of patients in preoperative New York Heart Association functional class III or IV (22/32) had improvement to class I or II at follow-up ($P < .01$). Cox regression analysis discriminated a preoperative left ventricular end-systolic volume index greater than $100 \text{ mL/m}^2$ as a significant risk factor for mortality (odds ratio 12.1, 95% confidence interval 1.27-114.51, $P = .03$). Thirty-month survival of patients with multiterritory myocardial infarction (73.5% ± 8.3%) did not differ statistically from that of patients with single-territory infarction (n = 18).

*Conclusion.*—Surgical ventricular remodeling improves cardiac function and New York Heart Association functional status in patients with multiterritory myocardial infarction. Our initial results are promising and should prompt further studies to confirm our results and potentially expand the surgical ventricular remodeling inclusion criteria to include patients with multiterritory myocardial infarction.

---

**Surgical ventricular reverse remodeling in severe ischemic dilated cardiomyopathy: The relevance of the left ventricular equator as a prognostic factor**
Ferrazzi P, Matteucci MLS, Merlo M, et al (Ospedali Riuniti Bergamo, Italy; Univ of South Carolina, Columbia)
*J Thorac Cardiovasc Surg* 131:357-363, 2006                                    5–34

---

*Objectives.*—Surgical ventricular reverse remodeling has been shown to possibly improve hemodynamics and symptoms, but effects on long-term mortality are not established. No consistent data are available on which patients will benefit most from this procedure. This study was designed to analyze the predictors of long-term survival after surgical ventricular reverse remodeling in patients with ischemic cardiomyopathy.

*Methods.*—Eighty-five patients who underwent surgical ventricular reverse remodeling between May 1991 and October 2003 were retrospectively analyzed. Left ventricular wall motion and left ventricular equatorial diameter were assessed by means of angioventriculography. Left ventricular ejection fraction and volumes were measured by means of echocardiography. Cox regression analysis was used in several combinations to create a final model for identifying predictors of death.

*Results.*—Actuarial survival after 1, 3, 5, and 10 years was 89%, 79%, 75%, and 75%, respectively. New York Heart Association class improved from 2.9 ± 1.0 to 1.3 ± 0.5 ($P < .0001$), left ventricular ejection fraction increased from 27.6% ± 6.3% to 43.0% ± 10.1% ($P < .0001$), and left ventricular end-systolic volume index decreased from 89.6 ± 27.6 mL/m$^2$ to 56.5 ± 34.5 mL/m$^2$ ($P < .0001$). Multivariate analysis identified left ventricular equatorial diameter of 70 mm or greater (hazard ratio, 5.28; 95% confidence interval, 1.79-11.71; $P = .020$) and segmental akinesia (hazard ratio, 4.46; 95% confidence interval, 1.23-17.12; $P = .024$) as the only independent predictors of death.

*Conclusions.*—In this analysis of a single cohort of patients, surgical ventricular reverse remodeling improves the symptoms of ischemic cardiomyopathy, as well as left ventricular function, shape, and volume, with encouraging long-term outcomes, particularly in patients with dyskinesia. A left ventricular equatorial diameter of 70 mm or greater appears to be an important independent prognostic factor, which suggests the relevance of the left ventricular equatorial region for effective surgical reverse remodeling.

▶ In postmyocardial infarction patients with areas of akinesis and dyskinesis, surgical ventricular remodeling (SVR) in addition to complete revascularization and, if necessary, correction of mitral regurgitation, has demonstrated beneficial in terms of improved left ventricular (LV) function, decreased symptoms, and prolonged survival.[1-5]

The first study (Abstract 5–33) focused on the subset of postmyocardial infarction patients with advanced congestive heart failure, functional class III-IV, and ejection fraction ≤20%. Such patients have an extremely poor prognosis and are candidates for cardiac transplantation. This small study of 32 such patients compared with 19 patients who either were functional class I-II or had an ejection fraction of >20% showed that surgery can be done with a relatively low operative mortality (6.3%) and that the surgery markedly improves LV function and functional status, even in these severely ill patients. It is not totally clear that SVR alone (that is, the exclusion of all asynergic areas and restoration of a more physiologic elliptical geometry and LV volume) is sufficient and that total revascularization and, if necessary, repair of mitral regurgitation is not also required.

Actuarial survival at 16 months was not significantly different in patients with EF ≤20% from those with EF >20%. It appears that SVR in such patients is a viable alternative to cardiac transplantation.

Another article by the same group (Abstract 5–34) reported SVR in patients with multiterritorial myocardial infarction and ventricular fibrous scar in multiple areas and that the results were similar to those with single territory infarction, with a 30-month survival rate of 73.5% compared to 82.5% for single-territory infarction (*P* = .64, not significant).

The final article by Ferrazzi et al (Abstract 5–35) where 85 postmyocardial infarction patients underwent SVR, complete revascularization, and, if necessary, repair of mitral regurgitation. They reported similar results as above, particularly good long-term results, in those with dyskinesia compared with akinesia. The most important preoperative independent prognostic factor was an LV equatorial diameter ≥70 mm. The association of an equatorial LV diameter ≥70 mm and segmental akinesia carried the worst prognosis at 10-year follow-up compared with those with an LV equatorial diameter of ≤70 mm and dyskinesia (survival 18% vs 88%).

**M. D. Cheitlin, MD**

*References*

1. Athanasuleas CL, Buckberg GD, Stanley AW, et al: RESTORE group: Surgical ventricular restoration in the treatment of congestive heart failure due to post-infarction ventricular dilation. *J Am Coll Cardiol* 44:1439-1445, 2004.
2. Kono T, Sabbah HN, Stein PD, et al: Left ventricular shape as a determinant of functional mitral regurgitation in patients with severe heart failure secondary to either coronary artery disease or idiopathic dilated cardiomyopathy. *Am J Cardiol* 68:355-359, 1991.
3. Dor V, Sabatier M, Di Donato M, et al: Efficacy of endoventricular patch plasty in large postinfarction akinetic scar and severe left ventricular dysfunction: Comparison with a series of large dyskinetic scars. *J Thorac Cardiovasc Surg* 116:50-59, 1998.
4. Di Donato M, Toso A, Maioli M, et al: RESTORE Group: Intermediate survival and predictors of death after surgical ventricular restoration. *Semin Thorac Cardiovasc Surg* 13:468-475, 2001.
5. Mickleborough LL, Merchant N, Ivanov J, et al: Left ventricular reconstruction: Early and late results. *J Thorac Cardiovasc Surg* 128:27-37, 2004.

---

**Benefit of Combined Resynchronization and Defibrillator Therapy in Heart Failure Patients With and Without Ventricular Arrhythmias**
Ypenburg C, van Erven L, Bleeker GB, et al (Leiden Univ, the Netherlands)
*J Am Coll Cardiol* 48:464-470, 2006                                    5–35

---

*Objectives.*—We attempted to assess the efficacy of combined cardiac resynchronization therapy-implantable cardioverter-defibrillator (CRT-ICD) in heart failure patients with and without ventricular arrhythmias.

*Background.*—Because CRT and ICDs both lower all-cause mortality in patients with advanced heart failure, combination of both therapies in a single device is challenging.

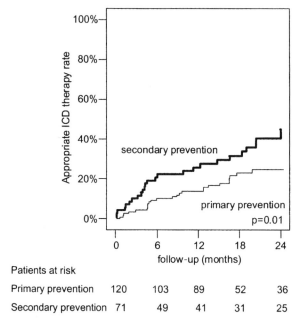

FIGURE 1.—Appropriate implantable cardioverter-defibrillator (ICD) therapy rate in primary and secondary prevention patients. (Courtesy of Ypenburg C, van Erven L, Bleeker GB, et al: Benefit of combined resynchronization and defibrillator therapy in heart failure patients with and without ventricular arrhythmias. *J Am Coll Card* 48:464-470. Copyright Elsevier 2006.)

*Methods.*—A total of 191 consecutive patients with advanced heart failure, left ventricular ejection fraction <35%, and a QRS duration >120 ms received CRT-ICD. Seventy-one patients had a history of ventricular arrhythmias (secondary prevention); 120 patients did not have prior ventricular arrhythmias (primary prevention). During follow-up, ICD therapy rate, clinical improvement after 6 months, and mortality rate were evaluated.

*Results.*—During follow-up (18 ± 4 months), primary prevention patients experienced less appropriate ICD therapies than secondary prevention patients (21% vs. 35%, p < 0.05). Multivariate analysis revealed, however, no predictors of ICD therapy. Furthermore, a similar, significant, improvement in clinical parameters was observed at 6 months in both groups. Also, the mortality rate in the primary prevention group was lower than in the secondary prevention group (3% vs. 18%, p < 0.05).

*Conclusions.*—As 21% of the primary prevention patients and 35% of the secondary prevention patients experienced appropriate ICD therapy within 2 years after implant, and no predictors of ICD therapy could be identified, implantation of a CRT-ICD device should be considered in all patients eligible for CRT (Figs 1, 2, and 3).

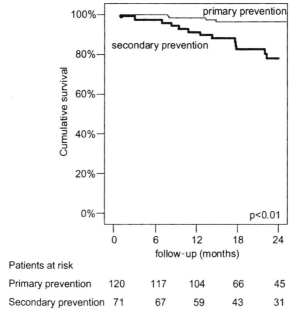

Patients at risk

| | 0 | 6 | 12 | 18 | 24 |
|---|---|---|---|---|---|
| Primary prevention | 120 | 117 | 104 | 66 | 45 |
| Secondary prevention | 71 | 67 | 59 | 43 | 31 |

FIGURE 2.—Survival curve for primary and secondary patients. (Courtesy of Ypenburg C, van Erven L, Bleeker GB, et al: Benefit of combined resynchronization and defibrillator therapy in heart failure patients with and without ventricular arrhythmias. *J Am Coll Card* 48:464-470. Copyright Elsevier 2006.)

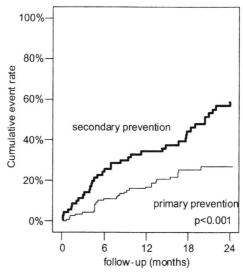

FIGURE 3.—Cardiac event curve for primary and secondary prevention patients. (Courtesy of Ypenburg C, van Erven L, Bleeker GB, et al: Benefit of combined resynchronization and defibrillator therapy in heart failure patients with and without ventricular arrhythmias. *J Am Coll Card* 48:464-470. Copyright Elsevier 2006.)

### A history of heart failure predicts arrhythmia treatment efficacy: Data from the Antiarrythmics versus Implantable Defibrillators (AVID) Study

Brodsky MA, for the AVID Investigators (Kaiser Permanente, Honolulu, Hawaii; et al)
*Am Heart J* 152:724-730, 2006                                                   5–36

*Background.*—In survivors of life-threatening ventricular tachycardia (VT), a history of CHF (H×CHF) before the VT episode may provide different prognostic information than their measured left ventricular ejection fraction (LVEF).

*Methods.*—We evaluated outcomes from patients in the AVID study. Patients were included in the study if they presented with ventricular fibrillation, VT with syncope or VT with hemodynamic compromise, and LVEF ≤ 40%. Treatment options included implantable cardioverter defibrillator (ICD) or antiarrhythmic drugs (AAD), usually amiodarone.

*Results.*—As expected, a H×CHF is associated with an increased and high risk of arrhythmic and nonarrhythmic death. However, an interaction was observed between arrhythmia treatment (ICD or AAD) and H×CHF status: the survival advantage with an ICD, as compared with AAD therapy, is largely restricted to H×CHF patients.

*Conclusions.*—The ICD is no better than AAD therapy in preventing arrhythmic death in patients with no H×CHF. In this data set, a H×CHF is somewhat more accurate in predicting prognosis and the response to therapy than a reduced LVEF.

▶ At present, the common indications for cardiac resynchronization therapy (CRT) are NYHA functional class III-IV, LVEF < 35% and a wide QRS complex >120 ms with a left bundle branch block pattern on ECG.[1] Classic indications for implantable ICD are those patients who have survived a cardiac arrest or with proved sustained hemodynamically significant VT. Furthermore, the Sudden Cardiac Death in Heart Failure (SCD-HeFT) trial showed that patients with low LVEF even without prior ventricular arrhythmias benefited from an ICD in addition to optimal medical management.[2] Patients who would benefit from a combination CRT-ICD might only be those with both indications. To examine this question, Ypenburg and colleagues (Abstract 5–36) implanted a CRT-ICD device in 191 consecutive patients with advanced congestive heart failure, an LVEF of less than 35% and a QRS duration more than 120 ms. Seventy-one (37%) had had a history of malignant ventricular arrhythmias (secondary prevention), and 120 (63%) did not (primary prevention). During 1½ years of follow-up, the primary prevention group received fewer appropriate shocks than the secondary prevention group (21% vs 35%), but multivariate analysis revealed no predictors of appropriate ICD therapy. Also, clinical improvement was seen equally in both groups at 6 months and the mortality rate was lower (3%) in the primary prevention group than in the secondary prevention group (18%). Since no predictors of appropriate ICD therapy were found, the authors recommend the implantation of combined CRT-ICD devices in all patients eligible for CRT. Should these findings be substantiated by other studies and, hopefully, a randomized trial, this recommendation will certainly be appropriate.

The article by Brodsky and colleagues (Abstract 5–37) used data from the AVID study, which randomized survivors of a malignant ventricular arrhythmic event and an LVEF less than 40% to either an ICD or AAD, usually amiodarone. Those patients with a history of heart failure had a high risk of arrhythmic and nonarrhythmic death. However, they found that there was an interaction between arrhythmic treatment (ICD or drugs) and a history of heart failure. The advantage with an ICD as compared with that of drugs is largely limited to those with a history of heart failure and that ICD treatment is no better than drugs in preventing arrhythmic death in patients without a history of heart failure. The history of heart failure in this study was more accurate in predicting prognosis and response to therapy than a reduced LVEF.

**M. D. Cheitlin, MD**

*References*

1. Abraham WT, Fisher WG, Smith AL, et al: Cardiac resynchronization in chronic heart failure. *N Engl J Med* 346:1845-1853, 2002.
2. Bardy GH, Lee KL, Mark DB, et al: Sudden Cardiac Death in Heart Failure Trial (SCD-HeFT) Investigators. Amiodarone or an implantable cardioverter-defibrillator for congestive heart failure. *N Engl J Med* 352:225-237, 2005.

---

**Cardiac Resynchronization Therapy in Patients With Systolic Left Ventricular Dysfunction and Symptoms of Mild Heart Failure Secondary to Ischemic or Nonischemic Cardiomyopathy**

Bleeker GB, Schalij MJ, Holman ER, et al (Leiden Univ, The Netherlands; Interuniv Cardiology Inst of The Netherlands, Utrecht)
*Am J Cardiol* 98:230-235, 2006                                         5–37

---

Cardiac resynchronization therapy (CRT) is beneficial in selected patients with moderate to severe heart failure (New York Heart Association [NYHA] classes III to IV). Patients with mildly symptomatic heart failure (NYHA class II) are currently not eligible for CRT and the potential beneficial effects in these patients have not been well studied. Fifty consecutive patients in NYHA class II heart failure and 50 consecutive patients in NYHA classes III to IV (control group) were prospectively included. All patients had left ventricular (LV) ejection fraction $\leq 35\%$ and QRS duration >120 ms. The effects of CRT in NYHA class II patients were compared with the results obtained in both groups. The severity of baseline LV dyssynchrony (assessed with color-coded tissue Doppler imaging) was comparable between patients in NYHA class II versus those in NYHA classes III to IV ($83 \pm 49$ vs $96 \pm 51$ ms, p = NS); resynchronization was achieved in all patients. NYHA class II patients showed a significant improvement in LV ejection fraction (from $25 \pm 7\%$ to $33 \pm 10\%$, p <0.001) and reduction in LV end-systolic volume (from $168 \pm 55$ to $132 \pm 51$ ml, p <0.001) after CRT, similar to patients in NYHA classes III to IV. In addition, only 8% of NYHA class II patients had progres-

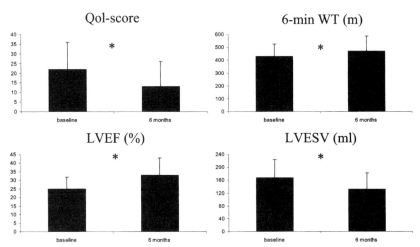

FIGURE 2.—Improvements in clinical and echocardiographic parameters at 6 months of follow-up in patients in NYHA Class II. *p <0.05. 6-minute WT = 6-minute walking test; LVESV = left ventricular end-systolic volume; Qol = quality-of-life. (Reprinted by permission of the publisher from Bleeker GB, Schalij MJ, Holman ER, et al: Cardiac resynchronization therapy in patients with systolic left ventricular dysfunction and symptoms of mild heart failure secondary to ischemic or nonischemic cardiomyopathy. *Am J Cardiol* 98:230-235. Copyright Elsevier 2006.)

sion of heart failure symptoms. In conclusion, CRT had comparable effects in patients in NYHA class II and in NYHA classes III to IV heart failure in terms of LV resynchronization, improvement in LV ejection fraction, and LV reverse remodeling (Fig 2).

▶ At present, the conventional indications for CRT are patients with moderate to severe CHF, New York Heart Association (NYHA) class III-IV, a QRS more than 120 ms, and an LV ejection fraction (LVEF equal to or less than 35%.[1] This study compared the results of CRT in patients with NYHA class II symptoms with those of patients with NYHA class III-IV symptoms. They found on 6 months' follow-up an improvement in LVEF and reduction in LV end-systolic volume that was similar in both groups. Symptomatic improvement was more evident in those with NYHA class III-IV symptoms. However, progression in patients with class II symptoms to class III symptoms only occurred in 8% of the patients. The degree of LV dyssynchrony (LVD), measured by tissue Doppler imaging (TDI) was similar in both groups at baseline, as was the immediate reduction in LVD post CRT. As in previous studies,[2] only patients with substantial LVD in both groups (LVD ≥65 ms) improved in LV function and showed reduction in LVD from baseline. Those without LVD ≥65 ms at baseline showed no improvement in LV function. It appears that in selecting patients with CHF for CRT, a wide QRS and decreased LVEF, especially with marked LVD, is more important than the severity of the symptoms.

**M. D. Cheitlin, MD**

*References*

1. Swedberg K, Cleland J, Dargie H, et al: Task Force for the Diagnosis and Treatment of Chronic Heart Failure of the European Society of Cardiology. Guidelines for the diagnosis and treatment of chronic heart failure: executive summary (update 2005): The Task Force for the Diagnosis and Treatment of Chronic Heart Failure of the European Society of Cardiology. *Eur Heart J* 26:1115-1140, 2005.
2. Bax JJ, Bleeker GB, Marwick TH, et al: Left ventricular dyssynchrony predicts response and prognosis after cardiac resynchronization therapy. *J Am Coll Cardiol* 44:1834-1840, 2004.

## Left Ventricular Assist Device and Drug Therapy for the Reversal of Heart Failure

Birks EJ, Tansley PD, Hardy J, et al (Royal Brompton and Harefield Natl Health Service Trust, Middlesex, England; Imperial College, London)
*N Engl J Med* 355:1873-1884, 2006                                     5–38

*Background.*—In patients with severe heart failure, prolonged unloading of the myocardium with the use of a left ventricular assist device has been reported to lead to myocardial recovery in small numbers of patients for varying periods of time. Increasing the frequency and durability of myocardial recovery could reduce or postpone the need for subsequent heart transplantation.

*Methods.*—We enrolled 15 patients with severe heart failure due to non-ischemic cardiomyopathy and with no histologic evidence of active myocarditis. All had markedly reduced cardiac output and were receiving inotropes. The patients underwent implantation of left ventricular assist devices and were treated with lisinopril, carvedilol, spironolactone, and losartan to enhance reverse remodeling. Once regression of left ventricular enlargement had been achieved, the $\beta_2$-adrenergic–receptor agonist clenbuterol was administered to prevent myocardial atrophy.

*Results.*—Eleven of the 15 patients had sufficient myocardial recovery to undergo explantation of the left ventricular assist device a mean (±SD) of 320±186 days after implantation of the device. One patient died of intractable arrhythmias 24 hours after explantation; another died of carcinoma of the lung 27 months after explantation. The cumulative rate of freedom from recurrent heart failure among the surviving patients was 100% and 88.9% 1 and 4 years after explantation, respectively. The quality of life as assessed by the Minnesota Living with Heart Failure Questionnaire score at 3 years was nearly normal. Fifty-nine months after explantation, the mean left ventricular ejection fraction was 64±12%, the mean left ventricular end-diastolic diameter was 59.4±12.1 mm, the mean left ventricular end-systolic diameter was 42.5±13.2 mm, and the mean maximal oxygen uptake with exercise was 26.3±6.0 ml per kilogram of body weight per minute.

*Conclusions.*—In this single-center study, we found that sustained reversal of severe heart failure secondary to nonischemic cardiomyopathy could be achieved in selected patients with the use of a left ventricular assist device and a specific pharmacologic regimen.

▶ Patients with advanced, end-stage congestive heart failure (CHF) have had their survival extended by the prolonged myocardial unloading provided by the implantation of left ventricular assist devices (LVAD). There is evidence that prolonged, nearly complete unloading of the LV by LVADs is associated with reverse remodeling of the LV[1] that is accompanied by clinical improvement,[2,3] at times sufficient to allow explantation of the LVAD in 5% to 24% of patients[4,5] and with a high incidence of recurrence of CHF.[5] Mechanical unloading of the LV leads to a reduction in neuroendocrine activation[6] and myocyte hypertrophy.[1] β-Blockers, angiotensin converting enzyme inhibitors (ACE-I), angiotensin II receptor blockers, and aldosterone antagonists can all reduce LV remodeling.[7-9]

In the present study, 15 patients with severe CHF caused by nonischemic cardiomyopathy and with no histologic evidence of active myocarditis were implanted with an LVAD and placed on the above pharmacologic regimen. Because there is evidence that prolonged LVAD unloading of the LV can result in myocyte atrophy1,[10] a $\beta_2$-adrenergic receptor agonist, clenbuterol, was used to cause minimal cardiac hypertrophy.[11] Clembuterol is a drug released in Europe but not in the United States for the treatment of asthma. The patients sufficiently recovered after 320±186 days that LVAD explantation was possible. Cumulative freedom from recurrent CHF at 4 years after explantation was 88.9%, and after almost 5 years, the mean LV ejection fraction was 64±12%. This is a remarkable result.

Possibly the role of the $\beta_2$-adrenergic receptor agonist has made the difference from other studies. Whether these excellent results will be obtained in studies with larger numbers, will be very long-lasting, or will be obtained in patients with other etiologies of CHF, such as ischemic cardiomyopathy, hypertension, and end-stage valve disease are all important questions for the future.

**M. D. Cheitlin, MD**

*References*

1. Zafeiridis A, Jeevanandam V, Houser SR, et al: Regression of cellular hypertrophy after left ventricular assist device support. *Circulation* 98:656-662, 1998.
2. Terracciano CM, Harding SE, Adamson D, et al: Changes in sarcolemmal Ca entry and sarcoplasmic reticulum Ca content in ventricular myocytes from patients with end-stage heart failure following myocardial recovery after combined pharmacological and ventricular assist device therapy. *Eur Heart J* 24:1329-1339, 2003.
3. Terracciano CM, Hardy J, Birks EJ, et al: Clinical recovery from end-stage heart failure using left-ventricular assist device and pharmacological therapy correlates with increased sarcoplasmic reticulum calcium content but not with regression of cellular hypertrophy. *Circulation* 109:2263-2265, 2004.
4. Mancini DM, Beniaminovitz A, Levin H, et al: Low incidence of myocardial recovery after left ventricular assist device implantation in patients. *Circulation* 98:2383-2389, 1998.
5. Dandel M, Weng Y, Siniawski H, et al: Long-term results in patients with idiopathic dilated cardiomyopathy after weaning from left ventricular assist devices. *Circulation* 112: 37S-45S, 2005.

6. James KB, McCarthy PM, Thomas JD, et al: Effect of the implantable left ventricular assist device on neuroendocrine activation in heart failure. *Circulation* 92: 191S-195S, 1995.
7. Groenning BA, Nilsson JC, Sondergaard L, et al: Antiremodeling effects on the left ventricle during beta-blockade with metoprolol in the treatment of chronic heart failure. *J Am Coll Cardiol* 36:2072-2080, 2000.
8. Wong M, Staszewsky L, Latini R, et al: Val-HeFT Heart Failure Trial Investigators. Valsartan benefits left ventricular structure and function in heart failure: Val-HeFT echocardiographic study. *J Am Coll Cardiol* 40:970-975, 2002.
9. Tsutamoto T, Wada A, Maeda K, et al: Effect of spironolactone on plasma brain natriuretic peptide and left ventricular remodeling in patients with congestive heart failure. *J Am Coll Cardiol* 37:1228-1233, 2001.
10. Soloff LA: Atrophy of myocardium and its myocytes by left ventricular assist device. *Circulation* 100:1012, 1999.
11. Wong K, Boheler KR, Bishop J, et al: Clenbuterol induces cardiac hypertrophy with normal functional, morphological and molecular features. *Cardiovasc Res* 37:115-122, 1998.

# Valvular Heart Disease and Infective Endocarditis

### Prognostic significance of echocardiographically defined mitral regurgitation early after acute myocardial infarction

Hillis GS, Møller JE, Pellikka PA, et al (Mayo Clinic, Rochester, Minn)
*Am Heart J* 150:1268-1275, 2005                    5–39

*Background.*—There are limited data regarding the clinical correlates and prognostic significance of echocardiographically defined mitral regurgitation (MR) early after acute myocardial infarction (MI). The current study addressed these issues.

*Methods.*—Seven hundred thirty-seven patients with acute MI who underwent transthoracic echocardiography with assessment of MR during

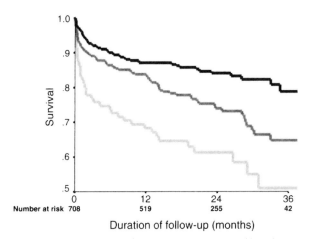

FIGURE 1.—The effect of MR on survival after acute MI. — No MR. – Mild (grade 1) MR - Moderate or severe (grade 2 or 3) MR. (Courtesy of Hills GS, Møller JE, Pellikka PA, et al: Prognostic significance of echocardiographically defined mitral regurgitation early after acute myocardial infarction. *Am Heart J* 150:1268-1275. Copyright Elsevier 2005.)

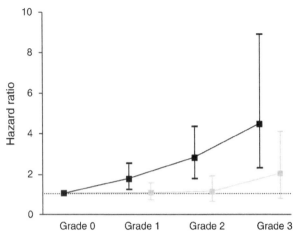

FIGURE 4.—The effect of MR on survival after acute MI after correction for confounding factors (corrected for age, Killip class and systolic function [WMSI]). — Uncorrected hazard ratio (with 95% CI). – Corrected hazard ratio (with 95% CI). (Courtesy of Hills GS, Møller JE, Pellikka PA, et al: Prognostic significance of echocardiographically defined mitral regurgitation early after acute myocardial infarction. *Am Heart J* 150:1268-1275. Copyright Elsevier 2005.)

their index admission were identified. Patients were followed up a median of 19 months later. The study end point was all-cause mortality.

*Results.*—The prevalence of MR increased with age. It was more common in women, in patients with non-ST-elevation MI, and in those with a history of diabetes, hypertension, prior MI, or previous revascularization. Patients with MR had worse left ventricular (LV) systolic function, more LV dilatation, and more clinical evidence of LV failure. Patients with moderate or severe MR had worse survival than those with no or mild MR (hazard ratio 2.3, 95% CI 1.6-3.2, $P < .0001$). Even mild MR predicted a higher mortality when compared with no MR (hazard ratio 1.7, 95% CI 1.2-2.4, $P = .004$). Mild or moderate MR was not independently predictive of outcome, although, in multivariable analyses, a trend toward worse survival was maintained in patients with severe MR.

*Conclusions.*—Mitral regurgitation, identified by echocardiography, early after acute MI predicts poorer survival after acute MI. However, if mild or moderate, it is not an independent prognostic indicator (Figs 1 and 4).

▶ The prognostic significance of mitral regurgitation (MR) after an acute myocardial infarction (AMI) is still controversial. Among 727 patients in the Survival and Ventricular Enlargement (SAVE) study who had ventriculography, MR was an independent predictor of cardiovascular mortality.[1] In the Controlled Abciximab and Device Investigation to Lower Late Angioplasty Complications (CADILLAC) study,[2] even mild MR was an independent predictor of 30-day mortality. However, Tcheng et al[3] failed to find MR in the early postinfarct period an independent predictor of morality. In this study, Hillis et al, by using color Doppler imaging to define degrees of MR after AMI, found in univariate analysis that MR was a significant predictor of mortality. However, in multivariate analysis after accounting for other significant predictors of mortality such as age, administration of reperfusion therapy, Killip class on admission, and wall motion score index, MR was not found to be an independent predictor of mortality. MR is probably related to the severity of the myocardial damage and the decrease in ventricular function, rather than independently influencing mortality. Although this study brings into question the importance of attempting to repair mild-to-moderate MR at the time of coronary surgery, the median follow-up time after the AMI was only 19 months. Perhaps a longer follow-up might reveal that moderate-to-severe MR does independently increase mortality. The final answer as to what should be done with mild-to-moderate MR at the time of coronary surgery is still controversial.

**M. D. Cheitlin, MD**

*References*

1. Lamas GA, Mitchell GF, Flaker GC, et al: Clinical significance of mitral regurgitation after acute myocardial infarction: Survival and Ventricular Enlargement Investigators. *Circulation* 96:827-833, 1997.
2. Pellizzon GG, Grines CL, Cox DA, et al: Importance of mitral regurgitation in-patients undergoing percutaneous coronary intervention for acute myocardial infarction: The Controlled Abciximab and Device Investigation to Lower Late Angioplasty Complications (CADILLAC) trial. *J Am Coll Cardiol* 43:1368-1374, 2004.
3. Tcheng JE, Jackman JD Jr, Nelson CL, et al: Outcome of patients sustaining acute ischemic mitral regurgitation during myocardial infarction. *Ann Intern Med* 117:18-24, 1992.

## Percutaneous Aortic Valve Implantation Retrograde From the Femoral Artery

Webb JG, Chandavimol M, Thompson CR, et al (St Paul's Hosp, Vancouver, BC, Canada)
*Circulation* 113:842-850, 2006
5–40

*Background.*—Percutaneous aortic valve implantation by an antegrade transvenous approach has been described but is problematic. Retrograde prosthetic aortic valve implantation via the femoral artery has potential advantages. Percutaneous prosthetic aortic valve implantation via the femoral arterial approach is described and the initial experience reported.

*Method and Results.*—The valve prosthesis is constructed from a stainless steel stent with an attached trileaflet equine pericardial valve and a fabric cuff. After routine aortic balloon valvuloplasty, a 22F or 24F sheath is advanced from the femoral artery to the aorta. A steerable, deflectable catheter facilitates manipulation of the prosthesis around the aortic arch and through the stenotic valve. Rapid ventricular pacing is used to reduce cardiac output while the delivery balloon is inflated to deploy the prosthesis within the annulus. Percutaneous aortic prosthetic valve implantation was attempted in 18 patients (aged 81±6 years) in whom surgical risk was deemed excessive because of comorbidities. Iliac arterial injury, seen in the first 2 patients, did not recur after improvement in screening and access site management. Implantation was successful in 14 patients. After successful implantation, the aortic valve area increased from 0.6±0.2 to 1.6±0.4 cm². There were no intraprocedural deaths. At follow-up of 75±55 days, 16 patients (89%) remained alive.

*Conclusions.*—This initial experience suggests that percutaneous transarterial aortic valve implantation is feasible in selected high-risk patients with satisfactory short-term outcomes.

---

**Percutaneous Transvenous Mitral Annuloplasty: Initial Human Experience With Device Implantation in the Coronary Sinus**
Webb JG, Harnek J, Munt BI, et al (Univ of British Columbia, Vancouver, Canada; Univ Hosp of Lund, Sweden)
*Circulation* 113:851-855, 2006                                                    5–41

---

*Background.*—Mitral annuloplasty is the most common surgical procedure performed for ischemic mitral regurgitation (MR). Surgical mitral annuloplasty is limited by morbidity, mortality, and MR recurrence. We evaluated the safety and feasibility of a transvenous catheter-delivered implantable device to provide a percutaneous alternative to surgical mitral annuloplasty.

*Method and Results.*—Five patients with chronic ischemic MR underwent percutaneous transvenous implantation of an annuloplasty device in the coronary sinus. Implantation was successful in 4 patients. Baseline MR in the entire group was grade 3.0±0.7 and was reduced to grade 1.6±1.1 at the last postimplantation visit when the device was intact or the last postprocedural visit in the patient in whom the device was not successfully implanted. Separation of the bridge section of the device occurred in 3 of 4 implanted devices and was detected at 28 to 81 days after implantation. There were no postprocedural device-related complications.

*Conclusions.*—Percutaneous implantation of a device intended to remodel the mitral annulus is feasible. Initial experience suggests a possible favorable effect on MR. Percutaneous transvenous mitral annuloplasty warrants further evaluation as a less invasive alternative to surgical annuloplasty.

▶ Surgery for valvular aortic stenosis in patients more than 75 to 80 years of age, especially with comorbidities, carries a substantial perioperative mortality.[1,2] Balloon valvuloplasty in such patients may result in temporary symptom improvement, but restenosis rapidly occurs regularly.[2,3] Percutaneous aortic valve replacement has recently been developed, although there are technical problems with manipulating a large-profile device either antegrade transvenously by transseptal puncture or retrograde around a tortuous atherosclerotic aorta. This article reports implantation of an aortic valve prosthesis retrograde across the calcified aortic valve in 18 patients (aged 81 ± 6 years), with 14 implantations successful. Techniques for navigating the tortuous aorta are given. There were no deaths. Proper sizing of the prosthesis and problems with prosthesis positioning remain. Percutaneous aortic valve replacement continues to be developed successfully. In the future it may find use in younger patients and replace surgery in at least patients with comorbidities and high operative risk.

A second article[3] describes a percutaneous transvenous mitral annuloplasty technique transcoronary sinus in patients with chronic ischemic mitral regurgitation.

An editorial by Feldman[3] reviews the history of transcutaneous valve replacement and highlights current and future challenges.

**M. D. Cheitlin, MD**

*References*

1. Task Force: Guidelines for the management of patients with valvular heart disease: Executive summary. *Circulation* 98:1949-1984, 1998.
2. Otto CM, Mickel MC, Kennedy JW, et al: Three-year outcome after balloon aortic valvuloplasty: Insights into prognosis of valvular aortic stenosis. *Circulation* 89:642-650, 1994.
3. Feldman T: Percutaneous valve repair and replacement. *Circulation* 113:771-773, 2006.

---

**Valve replacement in patients with critical aortic stenosis and depressed left ventricular function: predictors of operative risk, left ventricular function recovery, and long term outcome**
Vaquette B, Corbineau H, Laurent M, et al (Univ Hosp, Rennes, France)
*Heart* 91:1324-1329, 2005                                                                 5–42

---

*Objectives.*—To identify predictors of operative and postoperative mortality and of functional reversibility after aortic valve replacement (AVR) in patients with aortic stenosis (AS) and severe left ventricular (LV) systolic dysfunction.

*Method and Results.*—Between 1990 and 2000, 155 consecutive patients (mean (SD) age 72 (9) years) in New York Heart Association (NYHA) heart failure functional class III or IV (n = 138) and with LV ejection fraction (LVEF) $\leq 30\%$ underwent AVR for critical AS (mean (SD) valve area index 0.35 (0.09) $cm^2/m^2$). Thirty day mortality was 12%. NYHA class (3.7 (0.6) v 3.2 (0.7), p = 0.004), cardiothoracic ratio (CTR) (0.63 (0.07) v 0.56 (0.06), p < 0.0001), pulmonary artery systolic pressure (63 (25) v 50 (19) mm Hg, p = 0.03), and prevalence of complete left bundle branch block (22% v 8%, p = 0.03) and of renal insufficiency (p = 0.001) were significantly higher in 18 non-survivors than in 137 survivors. In multivariate analysis, the only independent predictor of operative mortality was a CTR $\geq 0.6$ (odds ratio (OR) 12.2, 95% confidence interval (CI) 5.4 to 27.4, p = 0.002). The difference between preoperative and immediate postoperative LVEF (early-$\Delta$EF) was > 10 ejection fraction units (EFU) in 55 survivors. In multivariate analysis, CTR (OR 5.95, 95% CI 3.0 to 11.6, p = 0.006) and mean transaortic gradient (OR 1.05, 95% CI 1.0 to 1.1, p < 0.05) were independent predictors of an early-ΔEF > 10 EFU. During a mean (SD) follow up of 4.6 (3) years, 50 of 137 (36%) 30 day survivors died, 31 of non-cardiac causes. Diabetes (OR 3.8, 95% CI 2.4 to 6.0, p = 0.003), age ≥ 75 years (OR 2.6, 95% CI 2.1 to 4.5, p = 0.004), and early-ΔEF ≤ 10 EFU (OR 0.96, 95% CI 0.94 to 0.97, p = 0.01) were independent predictors of long term mortality. Among 127 survivors, the percentage of patients in NYHA functional class III or IV decreased from 89% preoperatively to 3% at one year. The decrease in functional class was significantly greater in patients with an early-ΔEF > 10 EFU than patients with an early-ΔEF ≤ 10 EFU (p = 0.02). In addition, the mean (SD) LVEF at one year was 53 (11)% in patients with an early-ΔEF > 10 EFU and 42 (11)% in patients with early-ΔEF ≤ 10 EFU (p < 0.001).

*Conclusions.*—Despite a relatively high operative mortality, AVR for AS and severely depressed LVEF was beneficial in the majority of patients. Early postoperative recovery of LV function was associated with significantly greater relief of symptoms and longer survival.

▶ The patient with critical aortic stenosis and severely depressed left ventricular function presents a problem in assessing the probability of benefit from surgery. Aortic stenosis presents a severe afterload burden on the left ventricle (LV) and can result in a depressed LV ejection fraction, which, if the myocardial function remains normal, can be expected to reverse after surgery and removal of the increased LV wall stress. Aortic stenosis also results in myocardial ischemia and ultimately in LV fibrosis, predominantly in the subendocardial region of the LV, that can also cause depressed LV function and a reduced LV ejection fraction that cannot expected to be reversed after valve replacement. The current large series of patients aged 72 ± 9 years with critical aortic stenosis (aortic valve area 0.35 ± 0.09 cm²) and LV ejection fraction ≤30% who underwent aortic valve replacement lends insight into the independent predictors of operative mortality (cardiothoracic ratio ≤0.6 with odds ratio 12.2) representing a dilated left ventricle and left atrium that is seen in the very late stages of the natural history of severe aortic stenosis and late mortality (36% at 4.6 years), diabetes, age ≥75 years, and early change in LVEF preoperatively to postoperatively of ≤10 ejection fraction units. The really difficult patients are those with aortic stenosis, a low LVEF, and a low transvalvular gradient. The surgery was very effective in reducing symptoms from 89% functional class III and IV to 3% at 1 year. The patients in this series had for the most part retained an adequate stroke volume because only 11% had a transvalvular gradient of ≤30 mm Hg.

**M. D. Cheitlin, MD**

## Mitral mechanical replacement in young rheumatic women: Analysis of long-term survival, valve-related complications, and pregnancy outcomes over a 3707–patient-year follow-up

De Santo LS, Romano G, Della Corte A, et al (Second Univ of Naples, Italy; V Monaldi Hosp, Naples, Italy)
*J Thorac Cardiovasc Surg* 130:13-19, 2005                          5–43

*Objective.*—A follow-up study was performed to assess long-term survival, valve-related complications, and pregnancy outcomes in young rheumatic women undergoing isolated mitral mechanical replacement. The influence of prosthetic type on outcomes was also investigated.

*Methods.*—Between 1975 and 2003, 267 isolated mitral mechanical prostheses were implanted. Follow-up reached 3707.8 patient-years.

*Results.*—Actuarial survival at 1, 5, 10, 15, 20, and 25 years was 97% ± 0.01%, 90.4% ± 0.017%, 85.3% ± 0.023%, 82.3% ± 0.025%, 71.7% ± 0.036%, and 70.2% ± 0.038%, respectively. At multivariate analysis, atrial fibrillation at follow-up was identified as an independent risk factor for late mortality, whereas left ventricular ejection fraction at 12 postoperative months proved to be a protective factor. Freedom from thromboembolism at 1, 5, 10, 15, 20, and 25 years was 98.1% ± 0.01%, 94.1% ± 0.015%, 89.1% ± 0.021%, 85.9% ± 0.025%, 81.1% ± 0.031%, and 75.3% ± 0.063%, respectively. Atrial fibrillation and Carbomedics device were significantly associated with an increase in thromboembolic events. Freedom from reoperation at 1, 5, 10, 15, 20, and 25 years was 99.2% ± 0.005%, 95% ± 0.014%, 91.6% ± 0.018%, 88.6% ± 0.022%, and 85.7% ± 0.041%. Type of prosthesis (tilting disc) was identified as a predictor of reoperation. At the end of the study, 208 patients were still alive: 94.7% were in New York Heart Association class I or II. When receiving warfarin therapy, no patient undertaking pregnancy (n = 35) experienced adverse cardiac or valve-related events. Fetal events were significantly less frequent with a daily warfarin dose less than 5 mg.

*Conclusions.*—Mechanical devices provided excellent performance, safety, and durability. The prognostic role of left ventricular function and

TABLE 5.—Multivariate Analysis for Late Death, Reoperation, and Thromboembolic Events

| Risk Factor | β | HR | 95% CI | P Value |
|---|---|---|---|---|
| Late death | | | | |
| EF at 12 months | −.08 | 0.89 | 0.88-0.92 | <.001 |
| Postoperative AF | 1.87 | 6.50 | 1.52-27.87 | <.001 |
| Reoperation | | | | |
| Type of prosthesis: tilting disc | 2.8 | 16.63 | 2.25-122.8 | .004 |
| Thromboembolism | | | | |
| Postoperative AF | 2.4 | 11.27 | 3.67-34.67 | <.001 |
| Prosthetic model: Carbomedics | 1.6 | 4.82 | 1.45-15.99 | .01 |

*AF,* Atrial fibrillation; *EF,* ejection fraction; *HR,* hazard ratio; *CI,* confidence interval.

TABLE 7.—Univariate and Multivariate Analysis of Pregnancy Outcomes

| Variable | No Adverse Fetal Events | Adverse Fetal Events | P Value |
|---|---|---|---|
| Mean INR | 2.6 ± 0.3 | 2.4 ± 0.1 | <.001 |
| Mean warfarin dose | 4.8 ± 1.4 | 7.3 ± 1.6 | <.001 |
| Warfarin dose (mg/d) | | | <.001 |
| >5 | 4 (19%) | 17 (85.2%) | |
| ≤5 | 23 (81%) | 2 (8%) | |
| Order of pregnancy | | | |
| First | 25 (71.4%) | 10 (28.6%) | .003 |
| Subsequent | 2 (18.2%) | 9 (81.8%) | |
| **Exact Logistic Regression Model Covariate*** | **β** | **OR (exact 95% CI)** | **P Value** |
| Warfarin dose >5 vs <5 mg | 3.7 | 41.7 (5.8-298.4) | <.001 |
| Subsequent vs first pregnancy | −.21 | 0.75 (0.25-6.2) | .65 |

Categorical data are presented as: conts (percentages). No significant difference was found for maternal age and prosthetic model. *INR*, International normalized ratio; *OR*, odds ratio; *CI*, confidence interval. $*r^2 = 0.687$.

(Reprinted from De Santo LS, Romano G, Della Corte A, et al: Mitral mechanical replacement in young rheumatic women: Analysis of long-term survival, valve-related complications, and pregnancy outcomes over a 3707–patient-year follow-up. *J Thorac Cardiovasc Surg* 130:13-19. Copyright Elsevier 2005.)

atrial fibrillation overwhelmed any differences that might exist between different prosthetic designs. Pregnancies entail virtually no maternal risk and predictable fetal complications (Tables 5 and 7).

▶ This is a large series of young women with rheumatic heart disease involving the mitral valve and who are undergoing mechanical valve replacement. The average age at surgery was about 30 years of age and the follow-up time ranged up to 27 years. The perioperative mortality rate was low and the long-term survival excellent with freedom from reoperation at 25 years of 85.7%. In the United States most mitral valve surgery is for myxomatous degeneration and the majority of these patients have mitral valve repair rather than replacement. Many large series of patients with mechanical valves are elderly so that part of the long-term problems is related to concomitant coronary artery disease and other comorbidities. This series is unusual in that the majority of the patients are female and young.

In this study there were 267 women aged 15 to 40 years old. There were 37 women with 48 pregnancies, all but one of whom were managed during the pregnancy on warfarin and none of whom had adverse cardiac or valve-related events during the pregnancy. There were 16 spontaneous abortions, 22 stillbirths, and 1 infant with a small ventricular septal defect. The mean annual rate of spontaneous abortion in this series was 12.9%. In the Italian population, the Ministry of Health reports the annual rate as 4.4%, so there is probably an increased rate of spontaneous abortions in these patients with mechanical valves on warfarin. There is no controlled clinical trial of management of anticoagulation during pregnancy that demonstrates the safest regimen for mother and fetus. This same group has reported the relative safety of warfarin during pregnancy as long as the mean warfarin daily dose required to maintain a therapeutic INR is 5 mg or less.[1,2]

The other major problem with mechanical valves is that of thromboembolism. In this series the targeted range of INR for caged ball and tilting prostheses was 3.0 to 4.0 and for bileaflet prostheses was 2.5 to 3.5. Freedom from thromboembolism at 5 years was 94.1%, at 10 years 89.1%, and at 25 years 75.3%. The rhythm at the time of embolism was atrial fibrillation in 88.5%, and only 5.7% were deemed to be inadequately anticoagulated. This series in relatively young patients shows that the currently available mechanical valves properly managed have an excellent long-term safety and effectiveness.

**M. D. Cheitlin, MD**

*References*

1. Vitale N, De Feo M, De Santo LS, et al: Dose-dependent fetal complications of warfarin in pregnant women with mechanical heart valves. *J Am Coll Cardiol* 33:1637-1641, 1999.
2. Cotrufo M, De Feo M, De Santo LS, et al: Risk of warfarin during pregnancy with mechanical valve prostheses. *Obstet Gynecol* 99:35-40, 2002.

## Impact of Prosthesis-Patient Mismatch on Cardiac Events and Midterm Mortality After Aortic Valve Replacement in Patients With Pure Aortic Stenosis

Tasca G, Mhagna Z, Perotti S, et al (Private Nonprofit Hosp Poliambulanza, Brescia, Italy; Laval Univ, Sainte-Foy, Quebec, Canada)
*Circulation* 113:570-576, 2006                                                    5–44

*Background.*—Prosthesis-patient mismatch (PPM) occurs when the effective orifice area (EOA) of the prosthesis being implanted is too small in relation to body size, thus causing abnormally high transvalvular pressure gradients. The objective of this study was to examine the midterm impact of PPM on overall mortality and cardiac events after aortic valve replacement in patients with pure aortic stenosis.

*Method and Results.*—The indexed EOA (EOAi) was estimated for each type and size of prosthesis being implanted in 315 consecutive patients with pure aortic stenosis. PPM was defined as an EOAi $\leq 0.80$ cm$^2$/m$^2$ and was correlated with overall mortality and cardiac events. PPM was present in 47% of patients. The 5-year overall survival and cardiac event-free survival were $82\pm3$% and $75\pm4$%, respectively, in patients with PPM compared with $93\pm3$% and $87\pm4$% in patients with no PPM ($P\leq0.01$). In multivariate analysis, PPM was associated with a 4.2-fold (95% CI, 1.6 to 11.3) increase in the risk of overall mortality and 3.2-fold (95% CI, 1.5 to 6.8) increase in the risk of cardiac events. The other independent risk factors were history of heart failure, NHYA class III-IV, severe left ventricular hypertrophy, and absence of normal sinus rhythm before operation.

*Conclusions.*—PPM is an independent predictor of cardiac events and midterm mortality in patients with pure aortic stenosis undergoing aortic valve replacement. As opposed to other risk factors, PPM may be avoided or its severity may be reduced with the use of a preventive strategy at the time of operation.

▶ The effect on mortality in patients with aortic stenosis (AS) of PPM, defined as EOA that is too small in relation to the patient's body size, has been the subject of great controversy and varied results in different studies.[1-4] There are studies that conclude that PPM increases subsequent mortality[1,2] and others that conclude that prosthesis size and PPM has no effect on subsequent mortality.[3,4]

Logically, if the patient had symptoms and increased mortality because of AS with a small effective orifice, then replacing that valve with a prosthetic valve of similar small orifice should have adverse effects. One possible reason for the discrepancy in the studies is the differing definition of PPM. Some use the geometric internal orifice area (GOA) of the prosthetic valve that is static instead of the EOA, the measurement of which is made dynamically. The GOA overestimates the EOA especially in biological valve prostheses. It has been shown that the GOA cannot be used to predict postoperative gradients,[5]. The only parameter demonstrated as valid to define PPM is the EOA indexed to the body surface area (EOSi).[6,7]

In this article, 315 consecutive patients with severe AS had a prosthetic valve implanted. PPM as defined by an EOAi of $\leq 0.8$ cm$^2$/m$^2$ was present after valve implantation in 47% of patients. The 5-year overall survival and cardiac event-free survival rates were better in those without PPM. PPM was associated with a 4.2-fold increase in overall mortality and a 3.2-fold increase in the risk of cardiac events. Since the EOA of prosthetic valves are known by the manufacturer, it is possible to know before implantation whether PPM will result. Efforts to prevent this would include the use of a valve with a larger EOA, such as a bileaflet valve or a stentless bioprosthesis, or an increase in the size of the aortic ring where the valve will be placed.[8-10]

**M. D. Cheitlin, MD**

*References*

1. Rao V, Jamieson WR, Ivanov J, et al: Prosthesis-patient mismatch affects survival after aortic valve replacement *Circulation* 102: 5S-9S, 2000.
2. Blais C, Dumesnil JG, Baillot R, et al: Impact of valve prosthesis-patient mismatch on short-term mortality after aortic valve replacement. *Circulation* 108:983-988, 2003.
3. Hanayama N, Christakis GT, Mallidi HR, et al: Patient prosthesis mismatch is rare after aortic valve replacement: Valve size may be irrelevant. *Ann Thorac Surg* 73:1822-1829, 2002.
4. Blackstone EH, Cosgrove DM, Jamieson WR, et al: Prosthesis size and long-term survival after aortic valve replacement. *J Thorac Cardiovasc Surg* 126:783-796, 2003.
5. Koch CG, Khandwala F, Estafanous FG, et al: Impact of prosthesis-patient size on functional recovery after aortic valve replacement. *Circulation* 111:3221-3229, 2005.
6. Pibarot P, Dumesnil JG, Jobin J, et al: Usefulness of the indexed effective orifice area at rest in predicting an increase in gradient during maximum exercise in patients with a bioprosthesis in the aortic valve position. *Am J Cardiol* 83:542-546, 1999.

7. Pibarot P, Dumesnil JG, Jobin J, et al: Hemodynamic and physical performance during maximal exercise in patients with an aortic bioprosthetic valve: Comparison of stentless versus stented bioprostheses. *J Am Coll Cardiol* 34:1609-1617, 1999.
8. Castro LJ, Arcidi JM Jr, Fisher AL, et al: Routine enlargement of the small aortic root: A preventive strategy to minimize mismatch. *Ann Thorac Surg* 74:31-36, 2002.
9. Bach DS, Sakwa MP, Goldbach M, et al: Hemodynamics and early clinical performance of the St. Jude Medical Regent mechanical aortic valve. *Ann Thorac Surg* 74:2003-2009, 2002.
10. Gelsomino S, Morocutti G, Frassani R, et al: Usefulness of the Cryolife O'Brien stentless suprannular aortic valve to prevent prosthesis-patient mismatch in the small aortic root. *J Am Coll Cardiol* 39:1845-1851, 2002.

## Outcome of Watchful Waiting in Asymptomatic Severe Mitral Regurgitation

Rosenhek R, Rader F, Klaar U, et al (Med Univ of Vienna)
*Circulation* 113:2238-2244, 2006                                                 5–45

*Background.*—The management of asymptomatic severe mitral regurgitation remains controversial. The aim of this study was to evaluate the outcome of a watchful waiting strategy in which patients are referred to surgery when symptoms occur or when asymptomatic patients develop left ventricular (LV) enlargement, LV dysfunction, pulmonary hypertension, or recurrent atrial fibrillation.

*Method and Results.*—A total of 132 consecutive asymptomatic patients (age 55±15 years, 49 female) with severe degenerative mitral regurgitation (flail leaflet or valve prolapse) were prospectively followed up for 62±26 months. Patients underwent serial clinical and echocardiographic examinations and were referred for surgery when the criteria mentioned above were fulfilled. Overall survival was not statistically different from expected survival either in the total group or in the subgroup of patients with flail leaflet. Eight deaths were observed. Thirty-eight patients developed criteria for surgery (symptoms, 24; LV criteria, 9; pulmonary hypertension or atrial fibrillation, 5). Survival free of any indication for surgery was 92±2% at 2 years, 78±4% at 4 years, 65±5% at 6 years, and 55±6% at 8 years. Patients with flail leaflet tended to develop criteria for surgery slightly but not significantly earlier. There was no operative mortality. Postoperative outcome was good with regard to survival, symptomatic status, and postoperative LV function.

*Conclusions.*—Asymptomatic patients with severe degenerative mitral regurgitation can be safely followed up until either symptoms occur or currently recommended cutoff values for LV size, LV function, or pulmonary hypertension are reached. This management strategy is associated with good perioperative and postoperative outcome but requires careful follow-up.

▶ Rosenhek and colleagues have prospectively managed 132 consecutive asymptomatic patients with severe mitral regurgitation (MR) due to myxomatous valve disease according to the American College of Cardiology/American Heart Association (ACC/AHA) Guidelines for the Management of Patients with

Valvular Heart Disease.[1] The patients were followed up at yearly intervals for the onset of symptoms and by echocardiography for LV function. Intervals were shortened to every 3 to 6 months if no prior evidence of stability was available, or if there were changes with previous measurements, or if measurements were close to the predefined cutoff values. Referral to surgery occurred if there was the onset of even mild symptoms, or, if asymptomatic, the development of 1 or more of the following: (1) LV end-systolic diameter (LVESD) equal to 45 or more; (2) LV end-systolic diameter equal to or more than 26 mm/m[2]; (3) fractional shortening less than 0.32; (4) ejection fraction equal to or less than 0.60; (5) systolic pulmonary artery pressure more than 50 mm Hg, and (6) recurrent atrial fibrillation. The median follow-up time was 69.2 months. During follow-up, one or more criteria for surgery developed in 38 patients with symptoms developing in 2 of 38. Compared with the mortality rate of the general population of similar age, the survival of all patients by 8 years was identical to the expected survival.

This is an important validation of the ACC/AHA guideline's recommendations. However, the same detailed follow-up, including periodic echocardiograms, must be done. Also, of the 38 patients sent to surgery, 29 (83%) had mitral valve repair whereas only 6 (17%) had mitral valve replacement. Therefore, the expertise of the surgeons accomplishing mitral valve repair is an important element in the success of this approach since mitral valve replacement is associated with a higher perioperative and late mortality rate than is mitral valve repair. Other studies[2,3] have recommended early surgery for severe MR even without symptoms of signs of decreased ventricular function. Both these studies found better survival in patients with early surgery than with continued medical management, but the patients were not randomized and were followed up, and therapeutic decisions were made by the patient's private physicians. Also, the surgery was done at the Mayo Clinic. The present study if patients are followed up closely, is more generalizable to all asymptomatic patients with severe myxomatous MR.

An editorial by BP Griffin[4] accompanies this article and is well worth reading.

**M. D. Cheitlin, MD**

*References*

1. Bonow RO, Carabello BA, Kanu C, et al: ACC/AHA 2006 guidelines for the management of patients with valvular heart disease: A report of the American College of Cardiology/American Heart Association Task Force on Practice Guidelines (writing committee to revise the 1998 Guidelines for the Management of Patients With Valvular Heart Disease Circulation. 2006;114:e84-231.
2. Enriquez-Sarano M, Avierinos JF, Messika-Zeitoun D, et al: Quantitative determinants of the outcome of asymptomatic mitral regurgitation. *N Engl J Med* 352:875-883, 2005.
3. Ling LH, Enriquez-Sarano M, Seward JB, et al: Early surgery in patients with mitral regurgitation due to flail leaflets: A long-term outcome study. *Circulation* 96:1819-1825, 1997.
4. Griffin BP: Timing of surgical intervention in chronic mitral regurgitation (editorial). *Circulation* 113:2169-2172, 2006.

## Utility of Plasma N-Terminal Brain Natriuretic Peptide as a Marker of Functional Capacity in Patients With Chronic Severe Mitral Regurgitation

Yusoff R, Clayton N, Keevil B, et al (South Manchester Univ, Wythenshawe, England)

Am J Cardiol 97:1498-1501, 2006                                          5–46

Plasma levels of N-terminal pro-brain natriuretic peptide (NT–pro-BNP) are elevated in severe mitral regurgitation, but their relation to functional capacity and cardiac remodeling is not well defined. We evaluated the role of NT–pro-BNP as a marker of functional capacity, symptoms, and cardiac remodeling in 38 patients with severe degenerative mitral regurgitation and preserved left ventricular ejection fraction. The NT–pro-BNP levels increased progressively with New York Heart Association (NYHA) functional class: NYHA class I (geometric mean [GM] 97.1 pg/ml), NYHA class II (GM 169.8 pg/ml), and NYHA III (GM 457.6 pg/ml; p = 0.015). The end-systolic volume index (r = 0.52, p = 0.001), end-diastolic volume index (r = 0.46, p = 0.003), left atrial volume index (r = 0.4, p = 0.01), regurgitant volume index (r = 0.38, p = 0.02), regurgitant fraction (r = 0.46, p = 0.003), and end-diastolic sphericity index (r = 0.56, p <0.001) all correlated significantly with NT–pro-BNP. The NT–pro-BNP levels correlated significantly with the exercise parameters: maximum oxygen uptake (r = −0.6, p <0.001), exercise time (r = -0.52, p <0.001), and oxygen pulse (r = −0.57, p <0.001). In

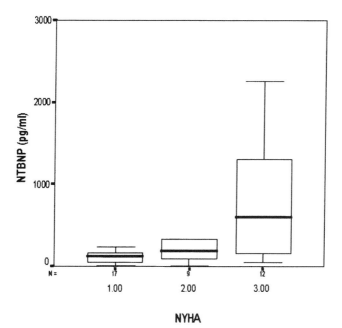

**NYHA**

FIGURE 1.—Plasma NT–pro-BNP levels according to NYHA functional class. Values are shown as mean ± SEM. (Reprinted by permission of the publisher from Yusoff R, Clayton N, Keevil B, et al: Utility of plasma N-Terminal brain natriuretic peptide as a marker of functional capacity in patients with chronic severe mitral regurgitation. *Am J Cardiol* 97:1498-1501. Copyright Elseiver 2006.)

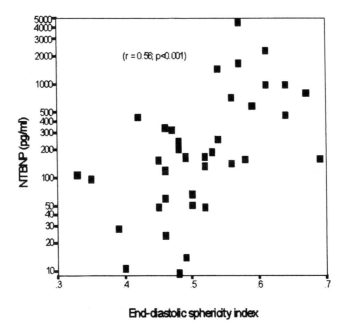

**FIGURE 2.**—Correlation between sphericity index and plasma NT–pro-BNP. (Reprinted by permission of the publisher from Yusoff R, Clayton N, Keevil B, et al: Utility of plasma N-Terminal brain natriuretic peptide as a marker of functional capacity in patients with chronic severe mitral regurgitation. *Am J Cardiol* 97:1498-1501. Copyright Elseiver 2006.)

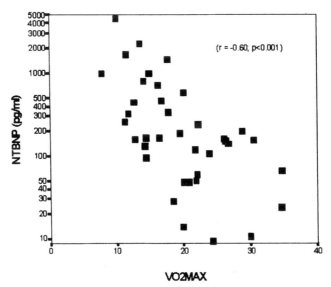

**FIGURE 3.**—Correlation between maximum oxygen uptake (VO$_2$max) and plasma NT–pro-BNP. (Reprinted by permission of the publisher from Yusoff R, Clayton N, Keevil B, et al: Utility of plasma N-Terminal brain natriuretic peptide as a marker of functional capacity in patients with chronic severe mitral regurgitation. *Am J Cardiol* 97:1498-1501. Copyright Elseiver 2006.)

contrast, only weak correlations were obtained between the exercise and echocardiographic variables. NT–pro-BNP was a strong independent predictor of maximum oxygen uptake (p = 0.001). In conclusion, the results of this study have demonstrated that NT–pro-BNP increases progressively with worsening symptoms, is linked to the extent of LV remodeling, and is an independent predictor of functional capacity. NT–pro-BNP may have a role in the optimal treatment of patients with severe mitral regurgitation (Figs 1, 2, and 3).

---

### Association of B-Type Natriuretic Peptide Activation to Left Ventricular End-Systolic Remodeling in Organic and Functional Mitral Regurgitation

Detaint D, Messika-Zeitoun D, Chen, HH, et al (Mayo Clinic, Rochester, Minn)
*Am J Cardiol* 97:1029-1034, 2006                                                          5–47

---

B-type natriuretic peptide (BNP) is activated with mitral regurgitation (MR), but it is unclear whether BNP activation is uniform in organic and functional MR and whether it merely reflects symptoms or is a biomarker of left ventricular (LV) geometric and functional alterations. Comprehensive Doppler echocardiography and hormonal measurements were performed prospectively in 99 patients, 50 with organic MR, 28 with functional MR (with similar LV enlargement 130 ± 21 vs 141 ± 40, p = 0.18, and age 64 ± 13 vs 66 ± 12 years, p = 0.56) and 21 controls subjects of similar age. Compared with the controls, the patients with MR displayed LV remodeling and BNP activation. In those with functional MR compared with those with organic MR, despite a lower regurgitant volume (25 ± 25 vs 96 ± 29 ml), higher BNP levels were noted (385 ± 388 vs 70 ± 97 pg/ml, p <0.0001), even after stratification by functional class (class I 120 ± 122 vs 33 ± 40, class II 318 ± 470 vs

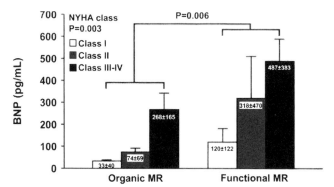

FIGURE 1.—BNP levels in patients stratified according to New York Heart Association (NYHA) functional class I, II, and III or IV separately in groups of patients with organic (*left bar graph*) and functional (*right bar graph*) MR. *Bar height*, mean value in each group, with SEM graphically indicated; ± SD in each bar. Statistical significance by analysis of variance indicated below NYHA functional class. *Top of figure*, stratified comparison of organic and functional MR. (Reprinted by permission of the publisher from Detaint D, Messika-Zeitoun D, Chen, HH, et al: Association of B-type natriuretic peptide activation to left ventricular end-systolic remodeling in organic and functional mitral regurgitation. *Am J Cardiol* 97:1029-1034. Copyright Elseiver 2006.)

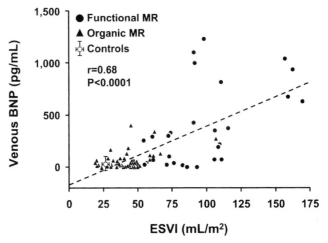

FIGURE 5.—Scatter plot with regression line (*dashed line*) plot of BNP level as a dependent variable (*y axis*) and LV ESVI as an independent variable (*x axis*). *Dots*, patients with functional MR; *triangles*, patients with organic MR; and *open dots with cross markers*, means ± SDs in normal controls; *left upper corner*, correlation and its significance. (Reprinted by permission of the publisher from Detaint D, Messika-Zeitoun D, Chen, HH, et al: Association of B-type natriuretic peptide activation to left ventricular end-systolic remodeling in organic and functional mitral regurgitation. *Am J Cardiol* 97:1029-1034. Copyright Elseiver 2006.)

74 ± 69, class III to IV 487 ± 383 vs 268 ± 165 pg/ml, p = 0.006). The major determinant of BNP activation was the LV end-systolic volume index (p <0.0001), independent of MR etiology, symptoms, other hormonal activation, and hemodynamic characteristics. The BNP level is a biomarker of LV alteration in patients with MR, independent of MR etiology. With BNP >90 pg/ml, the odds ratio of an end-systolic volume index value of ≥60 ml/m² was 16 (95% confidence interval 5.5 to 45). In conclusion, BNP acti-

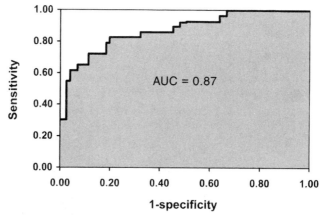

FIGURE 6.—Receiver-operating characteristics curve for diagnosis of LV ESVI ≥60 ml/m², using BNP level. Note, large area under curve (AUC) of 0.87. (Reprinted by permission of the publisher from Detaint D, Messika-Zeitoun D, Chen, HH, et al: Association of B-type natriuretic peptide activation to left ventricular end-systolic remodeling in organic and functional mitral regurgitation. *Am J Cardiol* 97:1029-1034. Copyright Elseiver 2006.)

vation with MR is more pronounced in those with functional than those with organic MR, even after stratification for functional class, and independently reflects the severity of the LV alteration. Pronounced BNP activation is linked to a higher end-systolic volume index, for which it is a biomarker, irrespective of MR etiology and symptoms (Figs 1, 5, and 6).

▶ In the article by Yusoff et al (Abstract 5–47), patients with severe "degenerative" mitral regurgitation (MR) and preserved left ventricular ejection fraction evaluated NT–pro-BNP as a marker for symptoms, functional capacity, and cardiac remodeling compared with that of echocardiographic parameters. They found that NT–pro-BNP increased as functional class, left ventricular end-diastolic volume (LVEDV), left ventricular end-systolic volume (LVESV), and regurgitant volume increased. NT–pro-BNP correlated with exercise parameters, such as maximal oxygen uptake and exercise time better than that of echocardiographic parameters. The patients all had primary mitral valve disease, many with subsequent ventricular remodeling.

In the article by Detaint et al (Abstract 5–48), BNP is evaluated in 99 patients, 50 with organic MR and 28 with functional MR with similar LV enlargement and age. They found that the major determinants of BNP activation were the LVESV index independent of MR etiology, symptoms, other hormonal activation, and hemodynamic characteristics. With a BNP more than 90 pg/mL the odds ratio of an LVESV index of 60 mL/m² or more was 16 (95% confidence interval [CI], 5.5-45). They concluded that BNP activation with MR is more pronounced in those with functional MR than in those with organic MR, even after stratification for functional class and this outcome independently reflects the severity of the LV remodeling.

**M. D. Cheitlin, MD**

---

**Surgical Management of Infective Endocarditis: Early Predictors of Short-Term Morbidity and Mortality**
Jassal DS, Neilan TG, Pradhan AD, et al (Harvard Med School)
*Ann Thorac Surg* 82:525-529, 2006                                          5–48

---

*Background.*—Infective endocarditis is a diagnostic and therapeutic challenge that ultimately requires surgical intervention in 20% of all cases. Early determinants of morbidity and mortality in this high risk population are not well described.

*Methods.*—The aim of this study was to determine preoperative clinical, microbiological, electrocardiographic, and echocardiographic variables that predicted the need for permanent pacemaker implantation and in-hospital death in a surgical cohort of patients with active infective endocarditis.

*Results.*—We identified 91 patients (61 males and 30 females, mean age 58 ± 16 years) who underwent surgical intervention for active culture-positive infective endocarditis as defined by the Duke criteria. Native valve infective endocarditis was present in 78 (85.7%) and prosthetic valve endo-

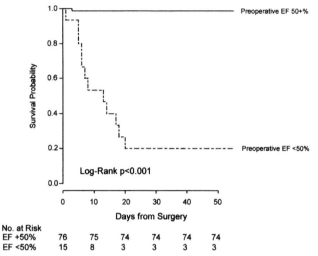

FIGURE 1.—Kaplan-Meier Survival curves according to preoperative ejection fraction (EF). (Courtesy of Jassal DS, Neilan TG, Pradhan AD, et al: Surgical management of infective endocarditis: early predictors of short-term morbidity and mortality. *Ann Thorac Surg* 82:525-529. Copyright Elsevier 2006.)

carditis in 13 (14.3%) of cases. The aortic valve was infected in 61 (67.0%), the mitral in 35 (38.5%), and multiple valves in 8 patients (8.8%). The most common indication for surgical intervention was intractable heart failure. Twenty-two patients (24.2%) required pacemakers, while there were 14 (15.4%) in-hospital deaths. In age-adjusted and gender-adjusted analyses, the presence of left bundle branch block on preoperative electrocardiogram (ECG) and presence of depressed left ventricular systolic function (ejection fraction [EF] < 50%) predicted the need for a permanent pacemaker implantation, while the presence of depressed left ventricular function predicted in-hospital mortality.

*Conclusions.*—Preoperative ECG findings of left bundle branch block and reduced left ventricular function may allow for early risk stratification of this high risk population (Fig 1).

▶ The timing of surgery in patients with acute infective endocarditis is at times difficult. The indications for surgery despite adequate antibiotics occur in 20% of cases[1] and of these patients, 10% require permanent pacemakers. By far the most frequent indication for surgery in patients with infective endocarditis is congestive heart failure,[2] but the development of annular abscesses, persistent bacteremia, recurrent embolization, and the presence of prosthetic material have all been considered indications for surgery.

In the present study, the variables that predict the need for permanent pacemaker implantation and the in-hospital mortality rate were identified in 91 patients with infective endocarditis who underwent surgical intervention. The presence of left bundle branch block in the preoperative ECG and a reduced left ventricular ejection fraction of less than 50% predicted the need for a permanent pacemaker, and a reduced ejection fraction predicted the risk of in-hospital mortality.

Although a periannular abscess in patients with aortic valve infective endo-carditis is believed to have a poor prognosis and require surgical intervention, an article from the International Collaboration on Endocarditis Merged data-base by Anguera et al[3] analyzed 311 patients with aortic endocarditis and found 67 (22%) with a periannular abscess. Patients with abscesses were more likely to undergo surgery (84% vs 36%), and their in-hospital mortality rate was higher (19% vs 11%, $P = .09$). On multivariate analysis of prognostic factors for mortality rate in aortic endocarditis, age (odds ratio [OR] 1.6), and *Staphylococcus aureus* (OR, 2.9) were independently associated with in-creased risk of death. Periannular abscess formation showed a nonsignificant trend toward increased risk of death [OR 1.93 (95% confidence interval [CI] 0.9-3.8). Multivariate analysis of prognostic factors of mortality in aortic endo-carditis with abscess formation identified *S aureus* (OR, 6.9) as independently associated with increased risk of death. In the era of transesophageal echocar-diography (TEE) where periannular abscesses are found more readily and where there is greater use of surgery, periannular abscess formation in aortic valve endocarditis is not an independent risk for mortality.

**M. D. Cheitlin, MD**

*References*

1. Bayer AS, Schled WM: Endocarditis and intravascular infections, in Mandell GL, Bennett JE, Dolin R (eds): *Principles of Infectious Diseases, ed 5.* Edinburgh, *Churchill Livingston, 2000, pp 857-902.*
2. Bonow RO, Carabello BA, Kanu C, et al: ACC/AHA 2006 guidelines for the management of patients with valvular heart disease: A report of the American College of Cardiology/American Heart Association Task Force on Practice Guide-lines (writing committee to revise the 1998 Guidelines for the Management of Patients With Valvular Heart Disease): developed in collaboration with the Society of Cardiovascular Anesthesiologists: endorsed by the Society for Cardiovascular Angiography and Interventions and the Society of Thoracic Surgeons. *Circulation* 114:84S-231S, 2006.
3. Anguera I, Miro JM, Cabell CH, et al: ICE-MD investigators. Clinical character-istics and outcome of aortic endocarditis with periannular abscess in the Interna-tional Collaboration on Endocarditis Merged Database. *Am J Cardiol* 96:976-981, 2005.

---

**Immediate and Long-Term Results of Mitral Balloon Valvotomy for Reste-nosis Following Previous Surgical or Balloon Mitral Commissurotomy**
Fawzy ME, Hassan W, Shoukri M, et al (King Faisal Specialist Hosp, Riyadh, Saudi Arabia)
*Am J Cardiol* 96:971-975, 2005                                                5–49

---

This study compared immediate with long-term results of mitral balloon valvotomy (MBV) in patients who underwent MBV as an initial procedure versus those who underwent repeat MBV. Fifty-six patients who were a mean age of $28 \pm 8.8$ years (group A) and had mitral restenosis after surgical

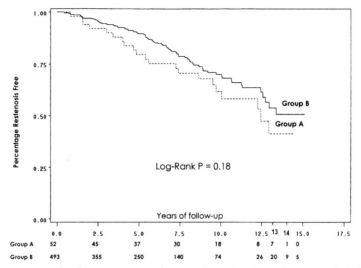

FIGURE 1.—Freedom from restenosis according to Kaplan-Meier estimates for patients who had repeat MBV (group A) and those who had MBV as an initial procedure (group B). Numbers at the bottom represent patients who were alive and uncensored at each year of follow-up. (Courtesy of Fawzy ME, Hassan W, Shoukri M, et al: Immediate and long-term results of mitral balloon valvotomy for restenosis following previous surgical or balloon mitral commissurotomy. *Am J Cardiol* 96:971-975. Copyright Elsevier 2005.)

or balloon commissurotomy underwent MBV and were compared with 524 patients who were a mean age of 31 ± 11 years (group B) and underwent MBV as an initial procedure. Prospective data obtained included demographic, hemodynamic, echocardiographic, and clinical follow-up for 0.5 to 15 years after MBV. No deaths or technical failure were encountered after MBV. Mitral regurgitation >2/4 occurred in 1 patient (2%) in group A and in 9 patients (2%) in group B (p = 0.24). Fifty-two of 56 patients (93%) in group A had good immediate results (mitral valve area ≥1.5 cm², mitral regurgitation <2/4), as did 504 of 524 patients (96%) in group B (p = 0.4). Actuarial values for freedom from restenosis at 10 years were 58 ± 7% for group A versus 69 ± 3% for group B (p = 0.18). Ten-year event-free survival rate was 54 ± 7% for group A versus 80 ± 3% for group B (p <0.005). The predictors of event-free survival were age (p = 0.003), echocardiographic score (p <0.0001), and baseline atrial fibrillation (p = 0.01). In conclusion, MBV is safe and provides good immediate results in patients who have restenosis. Long-term results are inferior compared with de novo mitral stenosis but is still satisfactory. More than 50% of patients remained improved at 10 years, thus enabling the operation or reoperation to be deferred (Fig 1).

▶ In patients with severe mitral stenosis (MS) and a flexible, minimal or no calcification, minimal or no mitral regurgitation, and a nonobstructive subvalvular apparatus, balloon valvotomy (BV) is the treatment of choice.[1] In patients who have had restenosis after previous commissurotomy, the possibility and immediate results of BV have been documented,[1-3] but there is a paucity of long-term results. This study evaluates the safety and immediate and long-term results of a repeat BV in patients who have had a first successful BV or surgical commissurotomy and who subsequently had symptomatic restenosis. The results of 56 patients (group A) with BV for restenosis after a previous successful BV or surgical valvotomy were compared to the results of 524 patients who had BV as the initial procedure (group B). A good result (mitral valve area 1.5 cm² or more, mitral regurgitation less than 2/4)was achieved in 93% of group A and 96% ofgroup B patients ($P$ = 0.18). Freedom from restenosis at 10 years was similar in the 2 groups, but the 10-year event-free survival rate was lower (54±7%) for group A than for group B (80±3%) ($P$< 0.005). The immediate results of BV for restenosis therefore are similar to those of primary BV. The late results were worse for the patients with BV for recurrent stenosis. The risk factors for restenosis after BV were echo score and postprocedural mitral valve area of less than 2.0 cm². The risk factors for event-free survival were young age, echo score 8 or less and baseline atrial fibrillation. Still, the long-term results were satisfactory in group A in that the survival rate without surgery and an NYHA class I or II was present in 54% at 10 years, thus enabling the majority of patients to avoid surgery during the follow-up, attended by a second surgical operation by increased mortality[4] and complications. Since the patients in this series were young, the results cannot be extrapolated to older postcommissurotomy patients who have had restenosis.

**M. D. Cheitlin, MD**

*References*

1. Davidson CJ, Bashore TM, Mickel M, et al: Balloon mitral commissurotomy after previous surgical commissurotomy. The National Heart, Lung, and Blood Institute Balloon Valvuloplasty Registry participants. *Circulation* 86:91-99, 1992.
2. Jang IK, Block PC, Newell JB, et al: Percutaneous mitral balloon valvotomy for recurrent mitral stenosis after surgical commissurotomy. *Am J Cardiol* 75:601-605, 1995.
3. Iung B, Garbarz E, Michaud P, et al: Immediate and mid-term results of repeat percutaneous mitral commissurotomy for restenosis following earlier percutaneous mitral commissurotomy. *Eur Heart J* 21:1683-1689, 2000.
4. John S, Bashi VV, Jairaj PS,et al: Closed mitral valvotomy: Early results and long-term follow-up of 3724 consecutive patients. *Circulation* 68:891-896, 1983.

## Myocarditis and Cardiomyopathy

**Survival in biopsy-proven myocarditis: A long-term retrospective analysis of the histopathologic, clinical, and hemodynamic predictors**
Magnani JW, Danik HJS, Dec GW, et al (Massachusetts Gen Hosp, Boston; Brigham and Women's Hosp, Boston; Vanderbilt Med Ctr, Nashville, Tenn)
*Am Heart J* 151:463-470, 2006                                    5–50

*Objective.*—We hypothesized that histopathology predicts survival without cardiac transplantation in patients with biopsy-proven myocarditis.

*Background.*—The role of endomyocardial biopsy in diagnosing myocarditis remains controversial. Histopathology has been integrated with

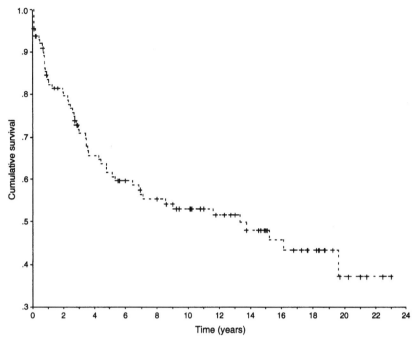

**FIGURE 1.**—Kaplan Meier survival analysis of 112 cases of histopathologically confirmed myocarditis, adjusted for study end point of death or cardiac transplantation, 1978-2002, at Massachusetts General Hospital, Boston, MA. + indicated censored event. (Courtesy of Magnani JW, Kanik HJS, Dec GW, et al: Survival in biopsy-proven myocarditis: A long-term retrospective analysis of the histopathologic, clinical, and hemodynamic predictors. *Am Heart J* 151:463-470. Copyright Elsevier 2006.)

clinical and hemodynamic features to predict prognosis. However, the influence of histopathology on survival >5 years has not been explored.

*Methods.*—We retrospectively identified 112 consecutive patients with histopathologic confirmation of myocarditis. We examined these patients' clinical presentation, hemodynamic assessment, hospital course, and treatment. We selected 14 variables that might influence survival without cardiac transplantation.

*Results.*—A total of 62 (55%) of 112 patients had lymphocytic myocarditis; 88 (79%) and 63 (56%) were alive without cardiac transplantation at 1 and 5 years, respectively. Median follow-up was a mean 95.5 months and median 74.5 months. Among the 55 with complete data of the 14 candidate predictor variables, age, sex, and clinical presentation with congestive heart failure and ventricular (ventricular tachycardia or fibrillation) or atrial arrhythmias (atrial fibrillation or flutter) did not predict the study end point of death or need for transplantation. In univariate analysis, pulmonary capillary wedge pressure $\geq 15$ mm Hg significantly predicted the study end point. In multivariate analysis, pulmonary capillary wedge pressure $\geq 15$ mm Hg and histopathology of lymphocytic, granulomatous, or giant cell myocarditis each significantly predicted mortality or transplant ($P = .047$,

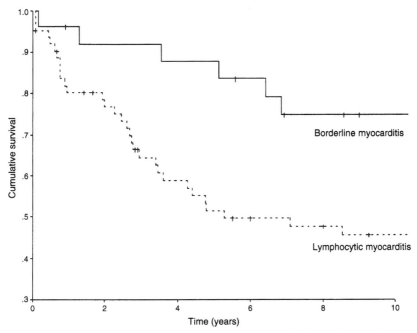

**FIGURE 2.**—Kaplan Meier analysis of survival free of the end point of death or cardiac transplantation stratified by histopathologic subtype (lymphocytic vs borderline myocarditis). $P = .0234$ by Breslow test for equality of survival distributions. + indicates censored event. (Courtesy of Magnani JW, Kanik HJS, Dec GW, et al: Survival in biopsy-proven myocarditis: A long-term retrospective analysis of the histopathologic, clinical, and hemodynamic predictors. *Am Heart J* 151:463-470. Copyright Elsevier 2006.)

$P = .013$, and $P = .054$, respectively) on cumulative survival without cardiac transplantation.

*Conclusions.*—Histopathology predicts long-term survival in patients with myocarditis. Clinical presentation, including presentation with congestive heart failure, ventricular tachycardia/ventricular fibrillation, or atrial fibrillation/atrial flutter, does not predict survival without transplantation. Endomyocardial biopsy can play a role in predicting transplant-free survival in patients with myocarditis (Figs 1 and 2).

▶ The prognosis of patients with acute myocarditis is difficult to predict. The role of endomyocardial biopsy is questionable, possibly because there is confusion about whether the limited look at the myocardium obtained by biopsy can rule out the diagnosis if cellular infiltration is not found, and also because there is evidence that trained pathologists could not agree on the diagnosis given the same slides to examine.[1,2] This article reported a retrospective study of 112 consecutive patients with biopsy-proved myocarditis followed up for a mean of 9.5 months and showed that the survival without cardiac transplantation was predicted not by the clinical presentation but by the histopathologic examination results. In multivariate analysis only pulmonary capillary pressure ≥15 mm Hg and histopathology of lymphocytic, granulomatous, or giant cell myocarditis each predicted death or transplant. It is significant that neither clinical presentation, including heart failure, evidence of severe left ventricular dysfunction, or malignant arrhythmias, was predictive of long-term outcome. In this retrospective study, no search for viral genomes in the myocardial DNA was made. They conclude that myocardial biopsy is helpful in predicting prognosis. What is not clearly proved is that clearing the histopathologic myocarditis with immunologic suppressive drugs will alter the prognosis. The best randomized study we have is that of Mason et al[3] that concluded that using the Dallas criteria, that neither steroids, cyclosporine, or azathioprine altered the 1- and 5-year survival or 28-week rejection fraction compared with placebo. Since that article, there have been other reports that have implicated the presence of viral genomes in the myocardial biopsy or the presence of antiheart antibodies as responsible for the failure of immunosupression[4]. New criteria for the diagnosis of myocarditis are needed, including histopathology, immunohistochemistry, viral polymerase chain reaction, cardiac antibody assessment, and nuclear magnetic resonance imaging that better predict the response to immunotherapy.

An interesting article by Kühl et al[4] showed that in 172 consecutive patients with viral myocarditis on myocardial biopsy all with viral genomes, that after a 6.8 month follow-up one third of the patients cleared the viral genomes spontaneously on repeat biopsy. These patients improved their left ventricular ejection fraction, whereas those with persistent viral genomic sequences had continued deterioration of the ejection fraction. The benefit of elimination of the viral genomes was seen with ejection fractions both above and below 45%.

**M. D. Cheitlin, MD**

*References*

1. Shanes JG, Ghali J, Billingham ME, et al: Interobserver variability in the pathologic interpretation of endomyocardial biopsy results. *Circulation* 75:401-405, 1987.
2. Baughman KL: Diagnosis of myocarditis. Death of Dallas criteria. *Circulation* 113:593-595, 2006.
3. Mason JW, O'Connell JB, Herskowitz A, et al: A clinical trial of immunosuppressive therapy for myocarditis: The Myocarditis Treatment Trial Investigators. *N Engl J Med* 333:269-275, 1995.
4. Frustaci A, Chimenti C, Calabrese F, et al: Immunosuppressive therapy for active lymphocytic myocarditis: Virological and immunologic profile of responders versus nonresponders. *Circulation* 107:857-863, 2003.

---

**Are Implantable Cardioverter Defibrillator Shocks a Surrogate for Sudden Cardiac Death in Patients With Nonischemic Cardiomyopathy?**
Ellenbogen KA, for the Defibrillators in Non-Ischemic Cardiomyopathy Treatment Evaluation (DEFINITE) Investigators (Med College of Virginia, Richmond; et al)
*Circulation* 113:776-782, 2006                                             5–51

---

*Background.*—Ventricular tachyarrhythmias long enough to cause implantable cardioverter defibrillator (ICD) shocks are generally thought to progress to cardiac arrest. In previous ICD trials, shocks have been considered an appropriate surrogate for sudden cardiac death (SCD) because the number of shocks has been thought to be equivalent to the mortality excess in patients without ICDs. The practice of equating ICD shocks with mortality is controversial and has not been validated critically.

*Method and Results.*—The Defibrillators in Non-Ischemic Cardiomyopathy Treatment Evaluation (DEFINITE) trial was a prospective, randomized, multicenter trial of ICD therapy in 458 patients with nonischemic cardiomyopathy. Patients were randomized to receive standard medical therapy (STD) or STD plus an ICD. Shock electrograms were reviewed, and the cause of death was evaluated by a separate blinded events committee. There were 15 SCD or cardiac arrests in the STD group and only 3 in the ICD arm. In contrast, of the 229 patients randomized to an ICD, 33 received 70 appropriate ICD shocks and 47 patients received 86 inappropriate shocks. Patients in the ICD arm were more likely to have an arrhythmic event (ICD shock plus SCD) than patients in the STD arm (hazard ratio 2.12, 95% CI 1.153 to 3.893, $P$=0.013). The number of arrhythmic events when one includes syncope as a potential arrhythmic event was similar in both groups (hazard ratio 1.20, 95% CI 0.774 to 1.865, $P$=0.414). Approximately the same number of total events was noted in each arm when we compared syncope plus SCD/cardiac arrest in the STD arm with SCD plus ICD shocks plus syncope in the ICD arm.

*Conclusions.*—Appropriate ICD shocks occur more frequently than SCD in patients with nonischemic cardiomyopathy. This suggests that episodes of nonsustained ventricular tachycardia frequently terminate spontaneously in such patients.

▶ The Defibrillators in Non-Ischemic Cardiomyopathy Treatment Evaluation (DEFINITE) trial showed that implantable cardioverter defibrillators (ICD) decreased the incidence of sudden death in patients with nonischemic cardiomyopathy.[1] In many trials of the effectiveness of ICDs, the presence on interrogation of the ICD of appropriate shocks has been taken as a surrogate for sudden death; that is, if the ICD had not been present and defibrillated a run of sustained ventricular tachycardia or fibrillation, then that patient would have died suddenly. This study showed that patients with nonischemic cardiomyopathy and implantation of an ICD for primary prevention had approximately twice as many shocks as the number of fatal events in the control standard treatment group (STG). An increased number of episodes of syncope in the STG balanced the excessive number of ICD shocks in the ICD group so that the total number of events (sudden death + syncope) in the STG almost exactly equaled the number of cardiac events (sudden death + syncope + appropriate shocks) in the ICD group.

The implication is that many episodes of ventricular tachycardia or fibrillation in patients with nonischemic cardiomyopathy resolve spontaneously and would not have resulted in sudden death. The PAIN-FREE II trial[2] showed that one third of fast monomorphic ventricular tachycardia episodes terminated spontaneously before antitachycardia pacing therapy could begin. This study shows that many episodes of polymorphic ventricular tachycardia and fibrillation will also terminate spontaneously. The findings of this study cannot be assumed to be true for patients with ischemic cardiomyopathy where superimposition of additional myocardial ischemia during the ventricular tachycardia may initiate or maintain the ventricular tachycardia to the point of sudden death.

It is apparent that appropriate firing of an ICD is not an appropriate surrogate end point for assessing the impact of ICD therapy on the mortality rate, and therefore counting appropriate shocks in a study is not equivalent to counting lives saved by the ICD therapy.

**M. D. Cheitlin, MD**

*References*

1. Kadish A, Dyer A, Daubert JP, et al: Defibrillators in Non-Ischemic Cardiomyopathy Treatment Evaluation (DEFINITE) Investigators: Prophylactic defibrillator implantation in patients with nonischemic dilated cardiomyopathy. *N Engl J Med* 350:2151-2158, 2004.
2. Wathen MS, DeGroot PJ, Sweeney MO, et al: PainFREE Rx II Investigators. Prospective randomized multicenter trial of empirical antitachycardia pacing versus shocks for spontaneous rapid ventricular tachycardia in patients with implantable cardioverter-defibrillators: Pacing Fast Ventricular Tachycardia Reduces Shock Therapies (PainFREE Rx II) trial results. *Circulation* 110:2591-2596, 2004.

---

**Delayed Gadolinium-Enhanced Cardiac Magnetic Resonance in Patients With Chronic Myocarditis Presenting With Heart Failure or Recurrent Arrhythmias**

De Cobelli F, Pieroni M, Esposito A, et al (Università Vita-Salute San Raffaele, Milan, Italy; La Sapienza Univ Rome)
*J Am Coll Cardiol* 47:1649-1654, 2006
5–52

---

*Objectives.*—We evaluated the effectiveness of contrast-enhanced cardiac magnetic resonance (CE-CMR) in detecting chronic myocarditis (CM).

*Background.*—Chronic myocarditis represents a common evolution of acute myocarditis. Although CE-CMR has been revealed to be effective in identifying areas of myocardial damage in acute myocarditis, its role in the diagnosis of chronic myocardial inflammation has not yet been investigated.

*Methods.*—Twenty-three patients with CM underwent CE-CMR and endomyocardial biopsy (EMB). Chronic myocarditis was defined by the presence of: 1) chronic (>6 months) heart failure symptoms and/or repetitive ventricular arrhythmias; 2) no history of recent flu-like symptoms or infections; and 3) histologic evidence of active myocarditis (AM) or borderline myocarditis (BM) according to Dallas criteria. Contrast-enhanced cardiac magnetic resonance included black-blood T2-weighted (BBT2w) images without and with fat saturation and delayed three-dimensional T1 turbo field-echo inversion-recovery sequences obtained 15 min after gadolinium injection.

*Results.*—Histology showed AM in 14 patients and BM in 9 patients. FatSat BBT2w revealed the presence of edema in five (36%) patients with

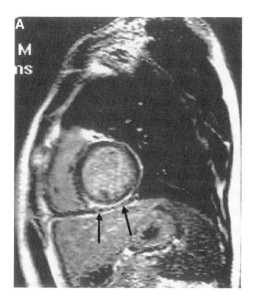

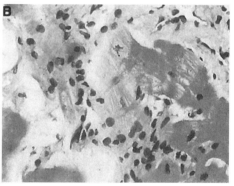

FIGURE 1.—Patient with active myocarditis. Contrast-enhanced cardiac magnetic resonance short-axis imaging (**A** shows a subepicardial late-enhancement stria in the posteroinferior left ventricular wall (**arrows**). (**B**) Left ventricular myocardial biopsy shows clusters of lymphocytic inflammatory infiltrates associated with necrosis of adjacent myocytes (hematoxylin and eosin, original magnification ×400). (Courtesy of De Cobelli F, Pieroni M, Esposito A, et al: Delayed gadolinium-enhanced cardiac magnetic resonance in patients with chronic myocarditis presenting with heart failure or recurrent arrhythmias. *J Am Coll Cardiol* 47:1649-1654. Copyright Elsevier 2006.)

AM but not in BM patients. Areas of late enhancement (LE) were observed in 12 (84%) subjects with AM and in 4 (44%) cases with BM. A mid-wall LE pattern was the most frequent finding in both groups while a subepicardial distribution of LE was observed only in patients with AM.

*Conclusions.*—Contrast-enhanced cardiac magnetic resonance identified areas of myocardial inflammation in up to 70% of patients with biopsy-proven CM. We suggest that CE-CMR may be a useful non-invasive diagnostic tool in patients with CM, and it may indicate and even guide the execution of left ventricular EMB with relevant prognostic and therapeutic implications (Fig 1).

▶ The diagnosis of acute myocarditis can be relatively easy in patients with fever, elevated troponins and elevated inflammatory markers. The diagnosis of CM manifested by congestive heart failure (CHF) and/or recurrent ventricular arrhythmias can be more difficult. There is evidence that on myocardial biopsy, with demonstration of cellular infiltration and the presence of segments of viral genome, that immunosuppressive therapy,[1] high-dose immunoglobulin,[2] or β-interferon[3] may promote recovery of cardiac function. Therefore, the identification of patients with CHF and/or recurrent ventricular arrhythmias who might have active or CM has important therapeutic implications.

Contrast-enhanced cardiac magnetic resonance (CE-CMR) imaging has been shown to be useful in the noninvasive recognition of myocardial inflammation in patients with acute myocarditis.[4,5] This study investigated whether CE-CMR could noninvasively detect myocardial inflammation in patients with CM. They showed that delayed gadolinium CE-CMR identified regions of inflammation in the myocardial wall in 70% of patients with biopsy-proven CM. Since other reasons for myocardial inflammation, such as necrosis, after an acute myocardial infarction can also cause delayed CE-CMR, coronary artery disease must be ruled out.[6] This noninvasive technique could select patients who might benefit from endomyocardial biopsy to identify those patients who could respond to immunosuppressive therapy.

**M. D. Cheitlin, MD**

*References*

1. Frustaci A, Chimenti C, Calabrese F, et al: Immunosuppressive therapy for active lymphocytic myocarditis: virological and immunologic profile of responders versus nonresponders. *Circulation* 107:857-863, 2003.
2. McNamara DM, Rosenblum WD, Janosko KM, et al: Intravenous immune globulin in the therapy of myocarditis and acute cardiomyopathy. *Circulation* 95:2476-2478, 1997.
3. Kuhl U, Pauschinger M, Schwimmbeck PL, et al: Interferon-beta treatment eliminates cardiotropic viruses and improves left ventricular function in patients with myocardial persistence of viral genomes and left ventricular dysfunction. *Circulation* 107:2793-2798, 2003.
4. Mahrholdt H, Goedecke C, Wagner A,, et al: Cardiovascular magnetic resonance assessment of human myocarditis: A comparison to histology and molecular pathology. *Circulation* 109:1250-1258, 2004.
5. Abdel-Aty H, Boye P, Zagrosek A, et al: Diagnostic performance of cardiovascular magnetic resonance in patients with suspected acute myocarditis: Comparison of different approaches. *J Am Coll Cardiol* 45:1815-1822, 2005.
6. Ibrahim T, Nekolla SG, Hornke M, et al: Quantitative measurement of infarct size by contrast-enhanced magnetic resonance imaging early after acute myocardial infarction: Comparison with single-photon emission tomography using Tc99m-sestamibi. *J Am Coll Cardiol* 45:544-552, 2005.

**Improved outcomes in peripartum cardiomyopathy with contemporary**
Amos AM, Jaber WA, Russell SD, et al (Duke Univ, Durham, NC; Johns Hopkins Hosp, Baltimore, Md)
*Am Heart J* 152:509-513, 2006                                                  5–53

*Background.*—Prior studies have shown both high morbidity and mortality for patients with peripartum cardiomyopathy (PPCM). These studies were small and predated current advances in heart failure treatment. We sought to determine the outcomes of women with PPCM in the contemporary era and to determine predictors of poor outcome.

*Methods.*—Patients with PPCM from 1990 to 2003 were identified retrospectively through screening of heart failure clinics and echocardiography records. Their records were reviewed, and current clinical status was determined.

*Results.*—Fifty-five patients were identified with an average follow-up of 43 months. Their mean initial ejection fraction (EF) was 20%. Compared with their initial EF, 62% of patients improved, 25% were unchanged, and 4% declined. No patients died, and 10% eventually required transplant. At 2 months after diagnosis, 75% of those who eventually recovered had an EF >45%. Factors associated with lack of recovery at initial assessment were a left ventricular (LV) end-diastolic dimension >5.6 cm, the presence of LV thrombus, and African-American race. Recovery of LV function was not predicted by the initial EF. Among patients who recovered, the withdrawal of heart failure medications was not associated with decompensation over a follow-up of 29 months.

*Conclusions.*—The morbidity related to PPCM is less than previously reported. Initial LV end-diastolic dimension and EF at 2 months predict long-term outcomes. The discontinuation of heart failure medications after recovery did not lead to decompensation (Fig 1).

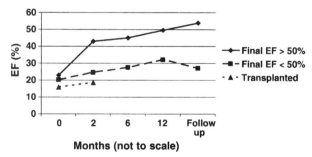

FIGURE 1.—Trend in EF according to the final outcome. (Courtesy of Amos AM, Jaber WA, Russell SD, et al: Improved outcomes in peripartum cardiomyopathy with contemporary. *Am Heart J* 152:509-513. Copyright Elsevier 2006.)

### Frequency of Peripartum Cardiomyopathy

Mielniczuk LM, Williams K, Davis DR, et al (Brigham and Women's Hosp, Boston; Univ of Ottawa, Ont, Canada)

*Am J Cardiol* 97:1765-1768, 2006                                    5–54

Reports from case series have estimated the incidence of peripartum cardiomyopathy (PC) at 1 case/1,485 live births to 1 case/15,000 live births and probable mortality rates of 7% to 60%. The objective of this study was to produce the first population-based study of the incidence, mortality, and risk factors for PC. The National Hospital Discharge Survey was used. Discharge information was available for 3.6 million patient discharges from 1990 to 2002. There were an estimated 16,296 cases of PC from 1990 to 2002. During this period, there were 51,966,560 live births in the United States. Thus, the incidence of PC was 1 case/3,189 live births. There was a trend toward an increase in PC incidence during the study period, with an estimate for the years 2000 to 2002 of 1 case/2,289 live births. The in-hospital mortality rate was 1.36% (95% confidence interval 0% to 10.2%). The total mortality rate was 2.05% (95% confidence interval 0.29% to 10.8%). Patients with PC were older (mean age 29.7 vs 26.9 years), were more likely to be black (32.2% vs 15.7%), and had a higher incidence of pregnancy associated hypertensive disorders (22.5% vs 5.87%) compared with national data. In conclusion, the incidence of PC is relatively uncommon, occurring at an average frequency of 1 case/3,189 live births from 1990 to 2002. The estimated mortality of 1.36% to 2.05% (95% confidence interval 0.29% to 10.8%) is less than previously reported from most case series.

▶ PC is defined as a cardiomyopathy that develops in the last month of pregnancy or within 5 months of delivery without preexisting heart failure.[1] The incidence of PC from case report series varies from about 1 case/1500 to 1 case/15,000 live births.[2] The mortality rate has also varied in the literature from 7% to 60 %, mostly from small series of cases.[3,4] In the largest series of 100 cases reported by Elkayam and colleagues[5] from a survey among US hospitals, the mortality rate was 9%. Most patients reported were from an era before contemporary therapy for heart failure. In the article by Amos et al (Abstract 5–54), 55 patients with PC were identified with an average follow-up of 43 months. The mean initial left ventricular EF was 20%, and, on follow-up, compared with their initial EF, 62% improved, 25% were unchanged, and 4% declined. There were no deaths, and 10% required transplantation. The initial EF was not predictive of lack of recovery. On recovery of EF, withdrawal of heart failure medications did not result in decompensation in a follow-up of 29 months.

The article by Mielniczuk and colleagues (Abstract 5–55) reported the first population-based study of the incidence, mortality, and risk factors for PC using the National Hospital Discharge Survey. The incidence of PC was 1 case per 3189 live births and the in-hospital mortality rate was 2.05% (95% Confidence interval [CI], 0%-10.2%). The total mortality rate was 2.05% (95% CI, 0.29%-10.8%). Patients with PC were more likely to be black (32.2% vs

15.7%) and had a higher incidence of pregnancy-associated hypertension (2.5% vs 5.87%). In both these studies, the incidence and mortality of patients with PC is lower than has been previously reported.

**M. D. Cheitlin, MD**

*References*

1. Pearson GD, Veille JC, Rahimtoola S, et al: Peripartum cardiomyopathy: National Heart, Lung, and Blood Institute and Office of Rare Diseases (National Institutes of Health) workshop recommendations and review. *JAMA* 283:1183-1188, 2000.
2. Lampert MB, Lang RM: Peripartum cardiomyopathy. *Am Heart J* 130:860-870, 1995.
3. Elkayam U, Akhter MW, Singh H, et al: Pregnancy-associated cardiomyopathy: Clinical characteristics and a comparison between early and late presentation. *Circulation* 111:2050-2055, 2005.
4. Felker GM, Jaeger CJ, Klodas E, et al: Myocarditis and long-term survival in peripartum cardiomyopathy. *Am Heart J* 140:785-791, 2000.
5. Cunningham FG, Pritchard JA, Hankins GD, et al: Peripartum heart failure: Idiopathic cardiomyopathy or compounding cardiovascular events? *Obstet Gynecol* 67:157-168, 1986.

## Mineralocorticoid Receptor Antagonism Ameliorates Left Ventricular Diastolic Dysfunction and Myocardial Fibrosis in Mildly Symptomatic Patients With Idiopathic Dilated Cardiomyopathy: A Pilot Study

Izawa H, Murohara T, Nagata K, et al (Nagoya Univ, Japan; Mie Univ, Tsu, Japan)
*Circulation* 112:2940-2945, 2005                5–55

*Background.*—Mineralocorticoid receptor antagonism reduces mortality associated with heart failure by mechanisms that remain unclear. The effects of the mineralocorticoid receptor antagonist spironolactone on left ventricular (LV) function and chamber stiffness associated with myocardial fibrosis were investigated in mildly symptomatic patients with idiopathic dilated cardiomyopathy (DCM).

*Method and Results.*—Twenty-five DCM patients with a New York Heart Association functional class of I or II were examined before and after treatment with spironolactone for 12 months. LV pressures and volumes were measured simultaneously, and LV endomyocardial biopsy specimens were obtained. Serum concentrations of the carboxyl-terminal propeptide (PIP) and carboxyl-terminal telopeptide (CITP) of collagen type I were measured. The patients were divided into 2 groups on the basis of the serum PIP/CITP ratio ($\leq$35, group A, n=12; >35, group B, n=13), an index of myocardial collagen accumulation. LV diastolic chamber stiffness, the collagen volume fraction, and abundance of collagen type I and III mRNAs in biopsy tissue were greater and the LV early diastolic strain rate (tissue Doppler echocardiography) was smaller in group B than in group A at baseline. These differences and the difference in PIP/CITP were greatly reduced after treatment of patients in group B with spironolactone, with treatment having no effect on these parameters in group A. The collagen volume fraction was significantly correlated with PIP/CITP, LV early diastolic strain rate, and LV diastolic chamber stiffness for all patients before and after treatment with spironolactone.

*Conclusions.*—Spironolactone ameliorated LV diastolic dysfunction and reduced chamber stiffness in association with regression of myocardial fibrosis in mildly symptomatic patients with DCM. These effects appeared limited, however, to patients with increased myocardial collagen accumulation.

▶ Almost half of the elderly patients with congestive heart failure have diastolic dysfunction as the major problem with relative preservation of LV systolic function. Even patients with decreased LV systolic function have a substantial number with concomitant diastolic dysfunction. Diastolic dysfunction is manifested by decreased LV compliance and increased LV stiffness. The approach to treatment of diastolic dysfunction is as yet uncertain. This article explores the mechanism by which diastolic dysfunction occurs in mildly symptomatic patients with idiopathic DCM with LV ejection fraction less than 45% and the effects of blocking mineralocorticoid receptors with spironolactone. They found that the patients could be divided into 2 groups using an index of myocardial collagen accumulation: the PIP/CITP ratio less than or equal to 35 and more than 35. Those with a high index after 1 year of treatment with spironolactone had a decrease in LV stiffness, collagen volume fraction, and early diastolic strain rate, whereas those with the lower ratio had no changes in these parameters. Spironolactone ameliorated LV diastolic dysfunction and reduced LV chamber stiffness with regression in myocardial fibrosis, but only in patients with increased myocardial collagen accumulation. If these findings are true for congestive heart failure from other etiologies, such as hypertension, the implication of this study is that mineralocorticoid receptor antagonism with spironolactone or eplerenone should be started early after the onset of symptomatic congestive heart failure and continued long-term to possibly delay or prevent the development of diastolic dysfunction.

**M. D. Cheitlin, MD**

---

### Effects of Statin Therapy on Arrhythmic Events and Survival in Patients With Nonischemic Dilated Cardiomyopathy

Goldberger JJ, for the DEFINITE Investigators (Northwestern Mem Hosp, Chicago; et al)
*J Am Coll Cardiol* 48:1228-1233, 2006                     5–56

---

*Objectives.*—We sought to evaluate whether statins were associated with a survival benefit and significant attenuation in life-threatening arrhythmias in patients with nonischemic dilated cardiomyopathy.

*Background.*—Statins are associated with a reduction in appropriate implantable cardioverter-defibrillator (ICD) therapy in patients with coronary artery disease and improved clinical status in nonischemic dilated cardiomyopathy.

*Methods.*—The effect of statin use on time to death or resuscitated cardiac arrest and time to arrhythmic sudden death was evaluated in 458 patients enrolled in the DEFINITE (DEFIbrillators in Non-Ischemic cardiomyopathy Treatment Evaluation) study. The effect of statin use on time to first appropriate shock was analyzed only in the 229 patients who were randomized to ICD therapy.

*Results.*—The unadjusted hazard ratio (HR) for death among patients on versus those not on statin therapy was 0.22 (95% confidence interval [CI] 0.09 to 0.55; p = 0.001). When controlled for statin effects, ICD therapy was associated with improved survival (HR 0.61; 95% CI 0.38 to 0.99; p = 0.04). There was one arrhythmic sudden death in the 110 patients receiving statin therapy (0.9%) versus 18 of 348 patients not receiving statins (5.2%; p = 0.04). The unadjusted HR for arrhythmic sudden death among patients on versus those not on statin therapy was 0.16 (95% CI 0.022 to 1.21; p = 0.08). The HR for appropriate shocks among patients on versus those not on statin therapy was 0.78 (95% CI 0.34 to 1.82) after adjustment for baseline differences in the two groups.

*Conclusions.*—Statin use in the DEFINITE study was associated with a 78% reduction in mortality. This reduction was caused, in part, by a reduction in arrhythmic sudden death. These findings should be confirmed in a prospective, randomized clinical trial.

▶ Statins have a been found to have beneficial effects on protection against atrial fibrillation[1] and on clinical improvement in patients with heart failure,[2,3] independent of lipid-lowering effects. These so-called pleiotropic effects have been attributed to the statins anti-inflammatory, antioxidant and autonomic effects as well as possible other effects.[4] In patients with coronary artery disease and implantable cardioverter-defibrillators (ICD) for secondary prevention of ventricular arrhythmias, treatment with lipid-lowering drugs resulted in a substantial reduction in appropriate shocks, 22% in those on lipid-lowering drugs, and 57% in those not so treated.[5] Other studies in patients with coronary artery disease showed similar reduction in the need for ICD therapy in those on statins,[6] and in the Antiarrhythmics Versus Implantable Defibrillators (AVID) trial,[7] there was a 40% reduction in relative hazard ratio for recurrence of ventricular tachycardia/fibrillation.

In the present study, a substudy of the DEFINITE study (Defibrillators in Non-Ischemic Cardiomyopathy Treatment Evaluation), a 78% reduction in mortality rate was observed in patients with nonischemic cardiomyopathy for those on statins versus those not so treated. As part of this reduction, a reduction was also seen in the unadjusted hazard ratio for arrhythmic sudden death among those on statins versus those not on statins (0.16) and a nonsignificant reduction in appropriate shocks for those on statins—hazard ratio of 0.78 after adjusting for baseline differences in the 2 groups.

The mechanism by which this antiarrhythmic effect is achieved is not understood but is probably related to the pleiotropic effects of statins mentioned previously. If this finding in nonischemic cardiomyopathy patients is confirmed in randomized trials, with the benefits of statins already shown in these patients, statin therapy in the absence of contraindications, should be added to βblockers and angiotension-converting enzyme (ACE) inhibitors in all such patients.

In an article by Foody et al,[8] evaluating more than 61,000 Medicare beneficiaries, 65 years or older with heart failure, statins were associated with an improvement in 3-year mortality rate with a hazard ratio of 0.82 (95% confidence interval [CI], 0.79-0.85) regardless of cholesterol level or coronary artery disease status. In an article by Scirica et al,[9] in 4162 patients hospitalized with acute coronary syndrome (ACS), in a mean follow-up of 24 months, treatment with 80-mg atorvastatin reduced subsequent hospitalizations for heart failure with a hazard ratio of 0.55 (95% CI, 0.35-0.85) with most benefit in patients with the highest BNP. In an article by Go and colleagues,[10] more than 24,000 patients with heart failure not using statins were studied. More than 12,000 patients were discharged on statins. On follow-up, statin use was independently associated with lower risks of death and rehospitalization in patients with and without coronary artery disease. An article by Anker and colleagues from 2 observational studies with 5200 patients found that statins decreased mortality rate, independent of cholesterol levels, disease etiology and clinical status.[11]

**M. D. Cheitlin, MD**

*References*

1. Young-Xu Y, Jabbour S, Goldberg R, et al: Usefulness of statin drugs in protecting against atrial fibrillation in patients with coronary artery disease. *Am J Cardiol* 92:1379-1383, 2003.
2. Node K, Fujita M, Kitakaze M, et al: Short-term statin therapy improves cardiac function and symptoms in patients with idiopathic dilated cardiomyopathy. *Circulation* 108:839-843, 2003.
3. Sola S, Mir MQ, Lerakis S, et al: Atorvastatin improves left ventricular systolic function and serum markers of inflammation in nonischemic heart failure. *J Am Coll Cardiol* 47:332-337, 2006.
4. Pham M, Oka RK, Giacomini JC: Statin therapy in heart failure. *Curr Opin Lipidol* 16:630-634, 2005.
5. De Sutter J, Tavernier R, De Buyzere M, et al: Lipid lowering drugs and recurrences of life-threatening ventricular arrhythmias in high-risk patients. *J Am Coll Cardiol* 36:766-772, 2000.
6. Chiu JH, Abdelhadi RH, Chung MK, et al: Effect of statin therapy on risk of ventricular arrhythmia among patients with coronary artery disease and an implantable cardioverter-defibrillator. *Am J Cardiol* 95:490-491, 2005.
7. Mitchell LB, Powell JL, Gillis AM, et al: AVID Investigators. Are lipid-lowering drugs also antiarrhythmic drugs? An analysis of the Antiarrhythmics versus Implantable Defibrillators (AVID) trial. *J Am Coll Cardiol* 42:81-87, 2003.
8. Foody JM, Shah R, Galusha D, et al: Statins and mortality among elderly patients hospitalized with heart failure. *Circulation* 113:1086-1092, 2006.
9. Scirica BM, Morrow DA, Cannon CP, et al: PROVE IT-TIMI 22 Investigators. Intensive statin therapy and the risk of hospitalization for heart failure after an acute coronary syndrome in the PROVE IT-TIMI 22 study. *J Am Coll Cardiol* 47:2326-2331, 2006.
10. Go AS, Lee WY, Yang J, et al: Statin therapy and risks for death and hospitalization in chronic heart failure. *JAMA* 296:2105-2111, 2006.
11. Anker SD, Clark AL, Winkler R, et al: Statin use and survival in patients with chronic heart failure—results from two observational studies with 5200 patients. *Int J Cardiol* 112:234-242, 2006.

## Miscellaneous

### Patent Foramen Ovale: Innocent or Guilty? Evidence From a Prospective Population-Based Study

Meissner I, Khandheria BK, Heit JA, et al (Mayo Clinic, Rochester, Minn)
*J Am Coll Cardiol* 47:440-445, 2006                                                  5–57

*Objectives.*—We sought to determine the association between patent foramen ovale (PFO), atrial septal aneurysm (ASA), and stroke prospectively in a unselected population sample.

*Background.*—The disputed relationship between PFO and stroke reflects methodologic weaknesses in studies using invalid controls, unblinded transesophageal echocardiography examinations, and data that are unadjusted for age or comorbidity.

*Methods.*—The use of transesophageal echocardiography to identify PFO was performed by a single echocardiographer using standardized definitions in 585 randomly sampled, Olmsted County (Minnesota) subjects age 45 years or older participating in the Stroke Prevention: Assessment of Risk in a Community (SPARC) study.

*Results.*—A PFO was identified in 140 (24.3%) subjects and ASA in 11 (1.9%) subjects. Of the 140 subjects with PFO, 6 (4.3%) had an ASA; of the 437 subjects without PFO, 5 had an ASA (1.1%, two-sided Fisher exact test, p = 0.028). During a median follow-up of 5.1 years, cerebrovascular events (cerebrovascular disease-related death, ischemic stroke, transient ischemic attack) occurred in 41 subjects. After adjustment for age and comorbidity, PFO was not a significant independent predictor of stroke (hazard ratio 1.46, 95% confidence interval 0.74 to 2.88, p = 0.28). The risk of a cerebrovascular event among subjects with ASA was nearly four times higher than

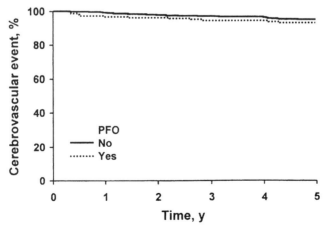

FIGURE 1.—Kaplan-Meier estimate of survival free of cerebrovascular events in 577 subjects according to presence of patent foramen ovale (PFO). (Reprinted with permission from the American College of Cardiology from Meissner I, Khandheria BK, Heit JA, et al: Patent foramen ovale: Innocent or guilty? Evidence from a prospective population-based study. *J Am Coll Cardiol* 47:440-445. Copyright Elsevier 2006.)

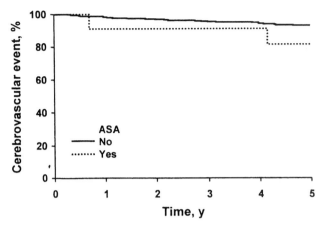

FIGURE 2.—Kaplan-Meier estimate of survival free of cerebrovascular events in 583 subjects according to presence of atrial septal aneurysm (ASA). (Reprinted with permission from the American College of Cardiology from Meissner I, Khandheria BK, Heit JA, et al: Patent foramen ovale: Innocent or guilty? Evidence from a prospective population-based study. *J Am Coll Cardiol* 47:440-445. Copyright Elsevier 2006.)

that in those without ASA (hazard ratio 3.72, 95% confidence interval 0.88 to 15.71, p = 0.074).

*Conclusions.*—These prospective population-based data suggest that, after correction for age and comorbidity, PFO is not an independent risk factor for future cerebrovascular events in the general population. A larger study is required to test the putative stroke risk associated with ASA (Figs 1 and 2).

▶ The argument as to the role of a patent foramen ovale (PFO) in paradoxic embolism has become more important now that catheter closure of the PFO is possible. There is no doubt that paradoxic embolism through a PFO occurs because instances of a thrombus straddling the PFO at autopsy are well established. Because PFOs are present in 15% to 25% of the population, the question is can we identify risk factors making it more likely that a recurrent embolism will occur and what the incidence of recurrence is. The current article is a population-based study of 585 randomly sampled individuals, 45 years of age and older, who had a transesophageal echocardiogram as a part of the Stroke Prevention: Assessment of Risk in a Community (SPARC) study. A PFO was seen in 140 (24.3%) of subjects, 6 (4.3%) of whom had an atrial septal aneurysm (ASA). After a median follow-up of 5.1 years, there were 41 subjects with a cerebrovascular event (cerebrovascular disease death, ischemic stroke, transient ischemic attack [TIA]). After adjustment for age and comorbidities, a PFO was not a significant independent predictor of a subsequent cerebrovascular event. The presence of an ASA almost quadrupled the risk in patients with a PFO. This study illustrates, at least in the short-term follow-up, that there is no difference in the incidence of cerebrovascular events in patients with a PFO than without. The apparent increased risk of the presence of a PFO and an ASA is consistent with other studies.[1,2]

In most retrospective observational studies, patients with a cryptogenic stroke have an increased prevalence of PFO compared with an echocardiographic control group. A meta-analysis of case-controlled studies from the literature[3] reported an association of PFO with all strokes with an odds ratio of 3, which increased to 5 if only cryptogenic strokes were considered. Why the different results? The current study was population based, the incidence of cerebrovascular events small, and the follow-up relatively short. Also, the subjects did not start out with a previous cerebrovascular event.

Other studies report that patients with a stroke or TIA and a PFO, at least on aspirin therapy, are at no greater risk of recurrence than those without a PFO.[1,2] Mas et al[1] reported 581 patients 55 years old and younger with an ischemic stroke of unclear origin within the preceding 3 months. All patients received 300 mg of aspirin prophylactically. After 4 years follow-up the risk of recurrent stroke in patients with a solitary PFO was 2.3% (95% CI 0.3%-4.3%), among patients with a PFO and ASA 15.2% (95% CI 1.8%-28.6%), and patients neither of these abnormalities 4.2% (95% CI 1.8%-6.6%). The presence of both a PFO and an ASA was a significant risk factor for recurrent stroke even with the patient on aspirin, but not for the patient with an isolated PFO.

It appears that in the patient with a cryptogenic cerebrovascular event and a PFO that aspirin rather than closure is the appropriate therapy. If the PFO is large or associated with an ASA, consideration for closure should be given.

An interesting editorial by Meier[4] accompanies the article.

**M. D. Cheitlin, MD**

*References*

1. Mas JL, Arquizan C, Lamy C, et al: Patent Foramen Ovale and Atrial Septal Aneurysm Study Group: Recurrent cerebrovascular events associated with patent foramen ovale, atrial septal aneurysm, or both. *N Engl J Med* 345:1740-1746, 2001.
2. Homma S, Sacco RL, Di Tullio MR, et al: PFO in Cryptogenic Stroke Study (PICSS) Investigators: Effect of medical treatment in stroke patients with patent foramen ovale: patent foramen ovale in Cryptogenic Stroke Study. *Circulation* 105:2625-2631, 2002.
3. Overell JR, Bone I, Lees KR: Interatrial septal abnormalities and stroke: A meta-analysis of case-control studies. *Neurology* 55:1172-1179, 2000.
4. Meier B: Patent foramen ovale, guilty but only as a gang member and for a lesser crime. *J Am Coll Cardiol* 47:446-448, 2006.

---

**Effect of the oral endothelin antagonist bosentan on the clinical, exercise, and haemodynamic status of patients with pulmonary arterial hypertension related to congenital heart disease**

Apostolopoulou SC, Manginas A, Cokkinos DV, et al (Onassis Cardiac Surg Centre, Athens, Greece)
*Heart* 91:1447-1452, 2005                                                                5–58

---

*Objective.*—To evaluate the clinical, exercise, and haemodynamic effects of chronic oral administration of the non-selective endothelin receptor antagonist bosentan on patients with pulmonary arterial hypertension (PAH) related to congenital heart disease (CHD).

*Design.*—Prospective non-randomised open clinical study.

*Setting.*—Cardiology tertiary referral centre.

*Patients.*—21 patients with a mean (SEM) age of 22 (3) years with chronic PAH related to CHD (15 with Eisenmenger's syndrome). Patients were in World Health Organization (WHO) class II to IV with oxygen saturation 87 (2)%.

*Intervention.*—Patients underwent clinical, exercise, and haemodynamic evaluations at baseline and after 16 weeks of treatment.

*Results.*—Bosentan improved ($p < 0.01$) WHO class, peak oxygen consumption from 16.8 (1.4) to 18.3 (1.4) ml/kg/min, exercise duration from 9.0 (0.8) to 10.7 (0.6) minutes during the treadmill test, walking distance from 416 (23) to 459 (22) m, and Borg dyspnoea index from 2.8 (0.2) to 2.0 (0.1) during the six minute walk test. Bosentan treatment improved ($p < 0.05$) mean pulmonary artery pressure from 87 (4) to 81 (4) mm Hg, pulmonary blood flow index from 3.2 (0.4) to 3.7 (0.5) l/min/m², pulmonary to systemic blood flow ratio from 1.2 (0.2) to 1.4 (0.2), and pulmonary vascular resistance index from 2232 (283) to 1768 (248) dyn·.s·.cm$^{-5}$. Two patients died, presumably of arrhythmic causes, who were in WHO class IV at baseline and who had improved during treatment.

*Conclusions.*—Bosentan induces short and mid term clinical, exercise, and haemodynamic improvements in patients with PAH related to CHD. Larger studies with long term endothelin receptor antagonism are needed to assess the safety and possible treatment role of bosentan in this population.

▶ Pulmonary hypertension in patients with congenital heart disease is generally thought to be irreversible. Endothelin is a promoter of cellular proliferation and a vasoconstrictor through enothelin A and B receptors on smooth muscle cells and a vasodilator through endothelin B receptors on the endothelium. The current study reports on the effects of bosentan, a nonselective endothelin antagonist in a small series of patients with congenital heart disease and severe pulmonary hypertension, with or without surgical repair and a pulmonary vascular resistance of >500 dyn · sec · cm$^{-5}$. Fifteen of the 21 patients had Eisenmenger's syndrome. After 4 months of treatment there were significant clinical, exercise, and hemodynamic improvements. The study was too small to see any differences in adverse events. This is a group of patients with minimal choices of therapy and with a markedly poor prognosis. This study justifies a larger, longer trial of bosentan in these relatively young patients.

**M. D. Cheitlin, MD**

## Relationship of Pulmonary Arterial Capacitance and Mortality in Idiopathic Pulmonary Arterial Hypertension

Mahapatra S, Nishimura RA, Sorajja P, et al (Mayo Clinic, Rochester, Minn)
*J Am Coll Cardiol* 47:799-803, 2006                                                      5–59

*Objectives.*—The purpose of this study was to determine if pulmonary vascular capacitance predicts survival in patients with idiopathic pulmonary arterial hypertension (IPAH).

*Background.*—The prognosis of patients with IPAH is difficult to predict, despite knowledge of clinical and hemodynamic parameters previously identified as predictors.

*Methods.*—We proposed a capacitance index of stroke volume divided by pulmonary pulse pressure (SV/PP) and prospectively gathered data on IPAH patients who underwent a right heart catheterization. SV/PP was analyzed as a predictor of mortality after adjusting for other modifiers of risk.

*Results.*—During 4-year follow-up of 104 patients, 21 patients died. When compared with conventional markers, SV/PP was the strongest univariate predictor of mortality (hazard ratio 17.0 per ml·mm Hg$^{-1}$ decrease, 95% confidence interval 13.0 to 22.0; p < 0.0001). In successive bivariate analysis, SV/PP was the only predictor of mortality. In quartile analysis, the lowest SV/PP quartile had a 4-year mortality of 61%; the highest SV/PP had no deaths.

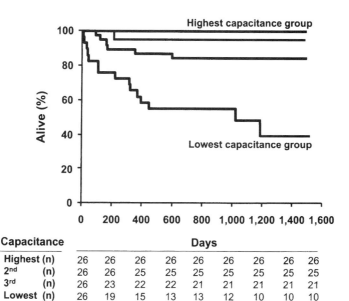

| Capacitance | | | | | Days | | | | |
|---|---|---|---|---|---|---|---|---|---|
| Highest (n) | 26 | 26 | 26 | 26 | 26 | 26 | 26 | 26 | 26 |
| 2nd    (n) | 26 | 26 | 25 | 25 | 25 | 25 | 25 | 25 | 25 |
| 3rd    (n) | 26 | 23 | 22 | 22 | 21 | 21 | 21 | 21 | 21 |
| Lowest (n) | 26 | 19 | 15 | 13 | 13 | 12 | 10 | 10 | 10 |

FIGURE 2.—Kaplan-Meier survival curves by pulmonary vascular capacitance quartiles. (Reprinted with permission from the American College of Cardiology from Mahapatra S, Nishimura RA, Sorajja P, et al: Relationship of pulmonary artrial capacitance and mortality in idiopathic pulmonary arterial hypertension. *J Am Coll Cardiol* 47:799-803. Copyright Elsevier 2006.)

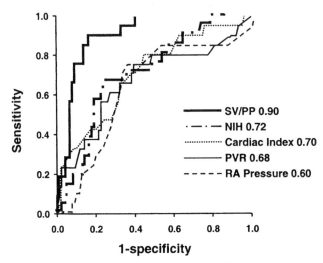

FIGURE 4.—Receiver-operator curves for potential predictors. Abbreviations as in Figure 1. (Reprinted with permission from the American College of Cardiology from Mahapatra S, Nishimura RA, Sorajja P, et al: Relationship of pulmonary arterial capacitance and mortality in idiopathic pulmonary arterial hypertension. *J Am Coll Cardiol* 47:799-803. Copyright Elsevier 2006.)

*Conclusions.*—The capacitance index (SV/PP) is a strong independent predictor of mortality in patients with IPAH (Figs 2 and 4).

▶ Predicting mortality in patients with idiopathic pulmonary arterial hypertension (IPAH) is difficult. Although the parameters of cardiac index, pulmonary artery pressure, and right atrial mean pressure used in the National Institutes of Health (NIH) IPAH Registry[1] predict survival, it is cumbersome and has not been validated in prospective studies in the era of vasodilators, especially prostenoids. Survival in IPAH is dependent on right ventricular function. Capacitance of the pulmonary arterial system, as reflected by the ratio of stroke volume over pulmonary artery pulse pressure (SV/PP), is inversely proportional to right ventricular work-load.[2] This study in patients with IPAH on modern medical therapy followed up for 4 years showed that the capacitance index SV/PP is the best independent predictor of mortality in patients with IPAH. The finding of a reliable prognostic indicator is valuable in helping to select the proper timing for a lung transplant. SV/PP could also be used as a surrogate end point in future studies of possible therapies for IPAH.

**M. D. Cheitlin, MD**

*References*

1. D'Alonzo GE, Barst RJ, Ayres SM,, et al: Survival in patients with primary pulmonary hypertension: Results from a national prospective registry. *Ann Intern Med* 115:343-349, 1991.
2. Linehan JH, Dawson CA, Rickaby DA, et al: Pulmonary vascular compliance and viscoelasticity. *J Appl Physiol* 61:1802-1814, 1986.

## Colchicine in Addition to Conventional Therapy for Acute Pericarditis: Results of the COlchicine for acute PEricarditis (COPE) Trial

Imazio M, Bobbio M, Cecchi E, et al (Maria Vittorio Hosp, Turin, Italy; Univ of Turin, Italy)
*Circulation* 112:2012-2016, 2005                                                    5–60

*Background.*—Colchicine is effective and safe for the treatment and prevention of recurrent pericarditis and might ultimately serve as the initial mode of treatment, especially in idiopathic cases. The aim of this work was to verify the safety and efficacy of colchicine as an adjunct to conventional therapy for the treatment of the first episode of acute pericarditis.

*Method and Results.*—A prospective, randomized, open-label design was used. A total of 120 patients (mean age $56.9\pm18.8$ years, 54 males) with a first episode of acute pericarditis (idiopathic, viral, postpericardiotomy syndromes, and connective tissue diseases) were randomly assigned to conventional treatment with aspirin (group I) or conventional treatment plus colchicine 1.0 to 2.0 mg for the first day and then 0.5 to 1.0 mg/d for 3 months (group II). Corticosteroid therapy was restricted to patients with aspirin contraindications or intolerance. The primary end point was recurrence rate. During the 2873 patient-month follow-up, colchicine significantly reduced the recurrence rate (recurrence rates at 18 months were, respectively, 10.7% versus 32.3%; $P=0.004$; number needed to treat=5) and symptom persistence at 72 hours (respectively, 11.7% versus 36.7%; $P=0.003$). After multivariate analysis, corticosteroid use (OR 4.30, 95% CI 1.21 to 15.25; $P=0.024$) was an independent risk factor for recurrences. Colchicine was discontinued in 5 cases (8.3%) because of diarrhea. No serious adverse effects were observed.

*Conclusions.*—Colchicine plus conventional therapy led to a clinically important and statistically significant benefit over conventional treatment, decreasing the recurrence rate in patients with a first episode of acute pericarditis. Corticosteroid therapy given in the index attack can favor the occurrence of recurrences.

▶ The most important and difficult to treat complication of acute pericarditis is the development of recurrent pericarditis, occurring in 15% to 50% of cases.[1,2] Although the primary occurrence of acute pericarditis is usually viral,[3] the mechanism of recurrence is generally believed to be an autoimmune process.[4] Colchicine has been used to treat recurrent episodes of pericarditis.[1] The mechanism of colchicine's action is not fully understood. Its pharmacologic action on cells involved in inflammation seems to be related to its capacity to interrupt microtubules by binding with tubulin and inhibiting movement of intercellular granules and secretion of various substances,[5,6] thus inhibiting various leukocyte functions. This current prospective, randomized open-labeled study provides evidence that in the first episode of acute pericarditis that colchicines added to aspirin or corticosteroids if aspirin is contraindicated or not tolerated can shorten the duration of the acute episode and significantly reduce the recurrence rate by a factor of 3-fold compared with treatment with conventional anti-inflammatory agents. The study also found that recurrence rate was higher in those patients treated with corticosteroids, possibly because the steroids may exacerbate and prolong the viral-induced pericardial injury.[3]

**M. D. Cheitlin, MD**

*References*

1. Adler Y, Finkelstein Y, Guindo J, et al: Colchicine treatment for recurrent pericarditis: A decade of experience. *Circulation* 97:2183-2185, 1998.
2. Troughton R, Asher CR, Klein AL: Pericarditis. *Lancet* 363:717-727, 2004.
3. Lange RA, Hillis LD: Acute pericarditis. *N Engl J Med* 351:2195-2202, 2004.
4. Soler-Soler J, Sagrista-Sauleda J, Permanyer-Miralda G: Relapsing pericarditis. *Heart* 90:1364-1368, 2004.
5. Molad Y: Update on colchicine and its mechanism of action. *Curr Rheumatol Rep* 4:252-256, 2002.
6. Lange U, Schumann C, Schmidt KL: Current aspects of colchicine therapy—Classical indications and new therapeutic uses. *Eur J Med Res* 6:150-160, 2001.

**Long-Term Outcomes in Difficult-to-Treat Patients With Recurrent Pericarditis**

Brucato A, Brambilla G, Moreo A, et al (Ospedale Niguarda, Milano, Italy; Univ of Padua, Italy; Sheba Med Ctr, Tel-Hashomer, Israel; et al)
*Am J Cardiol* 98:267-271, 2006                                    5–61

Patients with many recurrences of acute pericarditis are commonly alarmed by the fear of constriction. We studied their long-term outcome and the possible presence of systemic diseases. Sixty-one Italian patients (36 men) were followed for an average of 8.3 years according to a predefined protocol, including testing for autoimmune diseases and familial Mediterranean fever. Symptomatic pericarditis lasted from 1 to 43 years (mean 5.4 years). Fifty-two patients had been referred to us after failure of previous therapies, including steroids. We observed 378 attacks with a mean of 1.6 per patient per year and 156 hospital admissions. Thirteen patients had a post-cardiac injury syndrome. In 43 (70.5%), the pericarditis remained idiopathic, whereas we made a new diagnosis of rheumatoid arthritis in 1 and of Sjogren's syndrome in 4 patients, but in these patients pericarditis represented the dominant clinical manifestation. Cardiac tamponade occurred during the initial attacks in 4 patients (6.5%) but never recurred. Pleural effusions were present during the first attack in 22 patients (36.0%) and liver involvement in 5 (8%). No patients developed constrictive pericarditis. Echocardiographic examination produced no evidence of chronic myocardial disease. Response to therapy was good. Thirty-one patients (50.8%) are in sustained remission, without any therapy; their total observation period has averaged 10.3 years. In idiopathic patients, antinuclear antibodies were present in 56.2% and anti-Ro/SSA in 8.3%. Mutations linked to familial Mediterranean fever were absent. In conclusion, in this large series of difficult patients with recurrent acute pericarditis and a very long follow-up, the long-term prognosis is good.

▶ Recurrent acute pericarditis can be a difficult therapeutic problem. This is an observational study of 61 patients with recurrent acute pericarditis, 85.2% of whom were on steroids when referred to this pericarditis clinic. They were treated with indomethacine 75-150 mg, aspirin 1500-2400 mg, slow withdrawal of steroids, and colchicines 0.5-1.0 mg per day. The patients were followed up for the longest period reported in the literature, an average of 8.3 years. Although 4 were seen with cardiac tamponade, it never recurred, and there were no instances of constrictive pericarditis. Over one half the patients were in sustained remission without therapy. The long-term prognosis appears to be very good. Those patients who went into remission had a longer total mean observation period than those who were not in remission, suggesting that the disease activity ultimately spontaneously "burns out."

**M. D. Cheitlin, MD**

---

**Low-Pressure Cardiac Tamponade: Clinical and Hemodynamic Profile**
Sagristà-Sauleda J, Angel J, Sambola A, et al (Hosp Gen Universitari Vall d'Hebron, Barcelona)
*Circulation* 114:945-952, 2006                                                    5–62

---

*Background.*—Low-pressure cardiac tamponade is a form of cardiac tamponade in which a comparatively low pericardial pressure results in cardiac compression because of low filling pressure. This syndrome is poorly characterized because only isolated cases have been reported. We conducted a study of its clinical and hemodynamic profiles.

*Methods and Results.*—From 1986 through 2004, we evaluated all patients at our institution with combined pericardiocentesis and cardiac catheterization. We identified those patients who fulfilled catheterization-based criteria of low-pressure cardiac tamponade and compared their clinical and catheterization data with those of patients with classic tamponade. A total of 1429 patients with pericarditis were evaluated, 279 of whom underwent combined pericardiocentesis and catheterization. Criteria of low-pressure cardiac tamponade were met in 29, whereas 114 had criteria of classic cardiac tamponade. Patients with low-pressure tamponade less frequently had clinical signs of tamponade, but the rate of constitutional symptoms, use of diuretics, and echocardiographic findings of tamponade were similar in both groups. Patients with low-pressure tamponade showed a significant increase in cardiac output after pericardiocentesis, but they usually had less severe cardiac tamponade compared with patients with classic tamponade. Prognosis was related mainly to the underlying disease.

*Conclusions.*—Low-pressure cardiac tamponade was identified in 20% of patients with catheterization-based criteria of tamponade. Clinical recognition may be difficult because of the absence of typical physical findings of tamponade in most patients. Although some patients are critically ill, most show a stable clinical condition. However, these patients obtain a clear benefit from pericardiocentesis.

▶ Occasional case reports of patients with cardiac tamponade have been reported where extravascular volume depletion was found to be responsible for the absence of the classical signs of tamponade. This article reports the experience from the Mayo Clinic gathered during 18 years from 1429 patients with pericarditis, 279 of whom had combined pericardiocentesis and cardiac catheterization. Of 143 patients with cardiac tamponade, 114 had the classic clinical features of cardiac tamponade (Gp I) and 29 (20%) had low-pressure cardiac tamponade (L-P CT) (Gp II). There is no agreed-upon definition of L-P CT. The authors decided that the criteria for the diagnosis for L-P CT were the equalization of intrapericardial pressure and right atrial (RA) pressure, with the RA transmural pressure less than 2 mm Hg. Therefore, L-P CT was diagnosed when the intrapericardial pressure was less than 7 mm Hg before pericardiocentesis and the RA pressure became less than 4 mm Hg after intrapericardial pressure had been lowered to near 0 mm Hg after pericardiocentesis.

## Clinical Findings

| | Gp I | Gp II | | Gp I | Gp II |
|---|---|---|---|---|---|
| Asymptomatic | 21% | 15% | Amount pericardial effusion | 30% | 34% |
| Rest Dyspnea | 17% | 33% | No collapses | 27% | 21% |
| Exertional dyspnea | 48% | 41% | RA collapse | 74% | 76% |
| Chest pain, fever, | 40% | 52% (N.S.) | Exaggerated respiratory Δ | 54% | 59% |
| Friction rub | | | mitral-tricuspid flow | | |
| Clinical tamponade | 24% | 71% (p=0.0001) | | (All N.S.) | |
| Jugular venous | 22% | 55% (p=0.003) | | | |
| Pulsus paradoxus | 7% | 50% (p=0.0001) | | | |

This experience suggests that L-P CT is not rare. Its recognition requires a high index of suspicion in patients who are hemodynamically compromised with suspected pericardial disease, in spite of the absence of the classical clinical findings of cardiac tamponade.

**M. D. Cheitlin, MD**

# 6 Cardiac Arrhythmias, Conduction Disturbances, and Electrophysiology

## Introduction

CARDIAC ARRHYTHMIAS, CONDUCTION DISTURBANCES, AND ELECTROPHYSIOLOGY

Atrial fibrillation continues to dominate the arrhythmia field in 2006. Significant has been the advancement of the empiric approach to catheter ablation, with success rates now in the range where it has become a second line treatment option for atrial fibrillation in selected patients. The technique is still used primarily in younger patients (mean age in the middle 50s), and mostly to treat paroxysmal atrial fibrillation in the absence of structural heart disease. However, advances continue to be made in its use in patients with chronic atrial fibrillation of the persistent and permanent types, as well as in the presence of structural heart disease. No doubt yet greater advances will be made when the missing pieces related to understanding the mechanism of atrial fibrillation will be more fully known. We also continue to learn more about treatment of patients with atrial fibrillation who have risk factors for stroke and systemic embolism. The early stopping of the ACTIVE W trial (clopidogrel and aspirin versus warfarin in patients with atrial fibrillation at risk for stroke) provide important new data emphasizing the efficacy of warfarin, and the relative inefficacy of antiplatelet agents. More data continue to accumulate indicating that atrial fibrillation is probably most often caused by a driver mechanism, ie, an area or areas in the atria that have very rapid rates that drive the rest of the atria in a manner that they cannot follow 1:1, resulting in fibrillatory conduction. Device therapy also continues to mature in important ways. Biventricular pacing in appropriate patients with congestive heart failure continues to evolve because of important clinical trials demonstrating efficacy, particularly, the CARE-HF trial. Similarly, we continue to refine our understanding of the use of implantable cardioverter

417

defibrillator devices (ICDs), alone or in combination with biventricular pacemakers. Antiarrhythmic drug therapy has maintained a low profile. But the continued demonstration that ACE inhibitors (ACEIs), angiotension II receptor blockers (ARBs), and statins favorably affect the prevalence of atrial fibrillation, suggest that these drugs probably need to be incorporated into standard management in ways that will decrease the prevalence of atrial fibrillation in patients at risk for its development, particularly the elderly. All in all, it was another good year for clinical cardiac electrophysiology.

Albert L. Waldo, MD

## Atrial Fibrillation and Anticoagulation

### Risk of Thromboembolic Events After Percutananeous Left Atrial Radio-frequency Ablation of Atrial Fibrillation

Oral H, Chugh A, Özaydin M, et al (Univ of Michigan, Ann Arbor)
*Circulation* 114:759-765, 2006                                                     6–1

*Background.*—In patients with atrial fibrillation (AF), the risk of thromboembolic events (TEs) is variable and is influenced by the presence and number of comorbid conditions. The effect of percutaneous left atrial radiofrequency ablation (LARFA) of AF on the risk of TEs is unclear.

*Method and Results.*—LARFA was performed in 755 consecutive patients with paroxysmal (n = 490) or chronic (n = 265) AF. Four hundred eleven patients (56%) had ≥1 risk factor for stroke. All patients were anti-coagulated with warfarin for ≥3 months after LARFA. A TE occurred in 7 patients (0.9%) within 2 weeks of LARFA. A late TE occurred 6 to 10 months after ablation in 2 patients (0.2%), 1 of whom still had AF, despite therapeutic anticoagulation in both. Among 522 patients who remained in sinus rhythm after LARFA, warfarin was discontinued in 79% of 256 patients without risk factors and in 68% of 266 patients with ≥1 risk factor. Patients older than 65 years or with a history of stroke were more likely to remain anticoagulated despite a successful outcome from LARFA. None of the patients in whom anticoagulation was discontinued had a TE during 25 ± 8 months of follow-up.

*Conclusions.*—The risk of a TE after LARFA is 1.1%, with most events occurring within 2 weeks after the procedure. Discontinuation of anticoagulant therapy appears to be safe after successful LARFA, both in patients without risk factors for stroke and in patients with risk factors other than age >65 years and history of stroke. Sufficient safety data are as yet unavailable to support discontinuation of anticoagulation in patients older than 65 years or with a history of stroke.

▶ The Oral et al article is the best paper on this subject. It relates to what we should do in the way of warfarin therapy in patients who have had ostensibly successful catheter ablation of their atrial fibrillation. The issues are that we have not yet had good, long-term data on recurrence of atrial fibrillation, nor on the incidence of asymptomatic atrial fibrillation in these patients. The Oral et al article has limitations in terms of the group of patients we are most interested in, namely, those with one or more high risk factors for stroke or 2 or more moderate risk factors for stroke (ie, the atrial fibrillation patient group identified as in need of warfarin therapy by the 2006 ACC/AHA/ESC Atrial Fibrillation Treatment Guidelines). Of the 755 patients studied by Oral et al, 411 had 1 or more stroke risk factors. However, although we know that 2 risk factors were present in 115 of these 755 patients (15%), we don't know postablation how many were in sinus rhythm, how many had recurrent atrial fibrillation, nor how many were on oral anticoagulation. Moreover, there were 23 patients (3%) of the 755 patients who had 3 stroke risk factors. But again, we don't know who among them were in sinus rhythm and on no oral anticoagulation, in sinus rhythm and on oral anticoagulation, had recurrent atrial fibrillation with no oral anticoagulation, or had recurrent atrial fibrillation with oral anticoagulation. So, critical data are missing with regard to invoking the 2006 ACC/AHA/ESC Atrial Fibrillation Treatment Guideline recommendations regarding warfarin therapy. We do know that there is at least a 5% recurrence rate of atrial fibrillation from year 1 to year 2 postablation, as demonstrated in the Oral et al article and by Pappone et al[1]. But of those patients who had recurrence, we do not know in which stroke risk category they fit. Moreover, the possibility of asymptomatic recurrence of atrial fibrillation is a real, but not well-characterized, issue in these patients. These imponderables all have to be factored into decisions about the use of warfarin therapy in patients with stroke risk factors post ablation.

Although there is a paucity of long-term data, especially from large, randomized clinical trials or from large series of data rigorously obtained regarding oral anticoagulation after apparent successful radiofrequency ablation of atrial fibrillation, there are probably some areas of general agreement, perhaps even consensus. Thus, if a patient had no risk factors for stroke before the ablation, it seems reasonable at some time, probably 3 to 6 months after ostensibly successful cure of atrial fibrillation with radiofrequency ablation, to stop warfarin. However, if there is no apparent recurrence of atrial fibrillation, but antiarrhythmic drug therapy is needed for the atrial fibrillation suppression, warfarin should be continued in the presence of 1 or more high stroke risk factors or 2 or more moderate stroke risk factors. If less validated or weaker stroke risk factors are present or 1 moderate stroke risk factor is present, the risk of thromboembolic events must be weighed against the risks of warfarin therapy per se. If there is recurrent atrial fibrillation in the presence of 1 or more high risk factors or 2 or more moderate risk factors, again, warfarin therapy should be continued. If there is no apparent recurrence of atrial fibrillation in the presence of 1 or more high risk factors or 2 or more moderate risk factors, the question then pertains as to how good is the evidence that there is no silent or asymptomatic atrial fibrillation. This editor believes that warfarin should be maintained for at least 1 year, and then its continued use should be reevaluated. The latter is an area much in need of data. And finally, if sinus rhythm is present, or even if atrial fibrillation is present, but there are only less validated or weaker stroke risk factors present or only 1 moderate stroke risk factor is present, per the 2006 ACC/AHA/ESC Guidelines, one must weigh the risks of thromboembolic events versus the risks of warfarin.

**A. L. Waldo, MD**

*Reference*

1. Pappone C, Rosanio S, Augello G, et al: Mortality, morbidity, and quality of life after circumferential pulmonary vein ablation for atrial fibrillation: outcomes from a controlled nonrandomized long-term study. *J Am Coll Cardiol* 42:185-197, 2003.

---

**Association of Atrial Fibrillation and Focal Neurologic Deficits With Impaired Cognitive Function in Hospitalized Patients ≥65 Years of Age**
Jozwiak A, Guzik P, Mathew A, et al (Univ of Med Sciences, Poznan, Poland)
*Am J Cardiol* 98:1238-1241, 2006                                          6–2

---

Atrial fibrillation (AF) is a risk factor for cerebrovascular diseases and can manifest as impaired cognitive function (ICF). ICF may be accompanied by various focal neurologic deficits (FNDs). This study evaluated cognitive function and the risk for ICF in patients aged ≥65 years hospitalized for any reason and grouped according to the presence of AF and/or FNDs. Data on 2,314 conscious patients aged ≥65 years (1,506 women) were analyzed. Physical examination, electrocardiography at rest, and the Mini-Mental State Examination were performed at admission. The median Mini-Mental State Examination score was 25 in patients without AF or FNDs (63.4%), 23 in those with AF alone (23.6%), 21 in those with FNDs alone (8.9%), and 18 in those with AF and FNDs (4.1%). On multivariate logistic regression (adjusted for age and gender), the risk for ICF was increased in patients with AF alone (p <0.0001), in those with FNDs alone (p <0.0001), and in those with AF and FNDs (p <0.0001). In conclusion, hospitalized patients aged ≥65 years with AF and/or FNDs at admission are at increased risk for ICF. The influences of AF and FNDs on the risk for ICF are independent of each other.

---

**Atrial Fibrillation Is Associated With Lower Cognitive Performance in the Framingham Offspring Men**
Elias MF, Sullivan LM, Elias PK, et al (Boston Univ; Univ of Maine, Mt Desert; NIH, Bethesda, Md)
*J Stroke Cerebrovasc Dis* 15:214-222, 2006                                6–3

---

The purpose of this study was to investigate the association of atrial fibrillation (AFIB) with multiple measures of cognitive performance in a large community-based sample extensively characterized for vascular risk factors. Our primary analysis included 1011 Framingham Offspring Study (Framingham, Mass) men, mean age = 61.0 (37-89) years, free of clinical stroke and dementia. Using multivariable linear regression models, we related the presence (n = 59) versus absence (n = 952) of AFIB in men to a global measure of performance and multiple measures of specific cognitive abilities assessed an average of 8 months after the AFIB surveillance period. Adjusting for age, education, multiple cardiovascular risk factors, and cardiovascular disease, men with AFIB exhibited significantly lower mean levels of cognitive performance compared with men in normal sinus rhythm. Men with AFIB exhibited lower performance on global cognitive ability and cognitive abilities including Similarities (abstract reasoning), Visual Reproductions-Immediate Recall, Visual Reproductions-Delayed Recall, Visual Organization, Logical Memory-Delayed Recall, and Trail Making A (scanning and tracking) and Trail Making B (scanning, tracking, and executive functioning). Further studies leading to a better understanding of the mechanisms underlying the relation between AFIB and cognitive performance are important.

▶ These 2 articles (Abstracts 6–2 and 6–3) are of considerable interest, particularly to this editor, because they again document the association of atrial fibrillation with important impaired cognitive function in patients with atrial fibrillation. The reason for this is not clear. Although patients in the older age range not uncommonly present with impaired cognitive function regardless of the presence or absence of atrial fibrillation, it is clear that the presence of atrial fibrillation adds significantly to this. One notion is that this may be due to multiple, small embolic strokes in areas of the brain that, in the presence of an ischemic event, do not manifest either motor or sensory deficit. Such so-called silent or asymptomatic stroke is well recognized in patients with atrial fibrillation.

The Jozwiak et al article (Abstract 6–2) does not address this issue at all, and the Elias et al article (Abstract 6–3) only mentions it rather obliquely. Of note, in the latter article, although the mean age was 68.1 years, only 39% of the patients were being treated with anticoagulation. And, we don't know how many of those patients had an INR in the therapeutic range, clearly an important marker for efficacy in stroke prevention in these patients. And then one must also consider that emboli from the left atrium may be pencil point sized. Thus, the notion that multiple small strokes can be associated with cognitive dysfunction is important. And because the elderly are less likely to get anticoagulated in the presence of atrial fibrillation, this potential role of atrial fibrillation in the development and exacerbation of cognitive dysfunction should be considered.

**A. L. Waldo, MD**

### Relationship of Atrial Fibrillation and Stroke After Coronary Artery Bypass Graft Surgery: When is Anticoagulation Indicated?

Kollar A, Lick SD, Vasquez KN, et al (Univ of Texas, Galveston)
Ann Thorac Surg 82:515-523, 2006                                    6–4

*Background.*—Atrial fibrillation (AF) is considered as a risk factor for stroke after coronary artery bypass grafting operations.

*Methods.*—A retrospective search in our hospital's medical record database was done to identify patients with postoperative strokes who underwent coronary artery bypass grafting operations from January 1, 1993, until December 31, 2004. All cases were individually reviewed, and the temporal relationship between neurologic event and postoperative episodes of AF was determined. During the study period it was our consistent policy to use only Coumadin anticoagulation limited to patients who had persistent AF or were to be discharged in AF.

*Results.*—Of the 2,964 coronary artery bypass grafting operations, 576 patients (19.4%) had AF and 32 patients (1.1%) suffered stroke. Seventeen stroke patients maintained normal sinus rhythm during their hospital stay. Of the remaining 15 patients, 9 presented with neurologic deficit before the first episode of AF, with 5 having intraoperative and 4 having postoperative stroke. Of the 6 patients with AF before neurologic event, three strokes occurred within 1 week after spontaneous conversion to normal sinus rhythm. One patient with preoperative and also with intraoperative AF who underwent emergency coronary artery bypass grafting woke up with stroke. In the remaining two cases, the AF or atrial flutter episodes lasted less than 6 hours each before the neurologic event. More aggressive anticoagulation as suggested in the published guidelines could not have prevented strokes in any of these 6 patients.

*Conclusions.*—This retrospective analysis does not support the use of aggressive anticoagulation, particularly full intravenous heparinization as a bridging therapy to decrease the already low incidence of postoperative strokes after routine coronary artery bypass grafting surgery.

▶ This article is of a very large series from one institution with a conservative, but reasonable, approach to anticoagulation in patients who have atrial fibrillation after coronary artery bypass graft surgery. The key is that if patients have atrial fibrillation for 48 hours or more, therapy is initiated with warfarin and is maintained through discharge. Second, there is no aggressive cardioversion policy. One should recall that cardioversion, per se, in the presence of atrial fibrillation without anticoagulation is associated with a small, but important incidence, of stroke. It is curious that the authors do not report anything regarding valve therapy or the like. That may be because with the presence of a prosthetic valve, anticoagulation is used early on. But in patients with atrial fibrillation after mitral valve repair, one would like to have known what their anticoagulation policy was and what their stroke incidence was. So, this study does not answer all the questions but provides very sound data for a very simple, but, seemingly, most appropriate method to treat patients with atrial fibrillation in the immediate period after coronary artery bypass graft surgery.

**A. L. Waldo, MD**

---

**Clopidogrel plus aspirin versus oral anticoagulation for atrial fibrillation in the Atrial fibrillation Clopidogrel Trial with Irbesartan for prevention of Vascular Events (ACTIVE W): a randomised controlled trial**
Connolly SJ, for The ACTIVE Writing Group for the ACTIVE Investigators (Hamilton Health Sciences Corp, Ont, Canada; et al)
*Lancet* 367:1903-1912, 2006                                                    6–5

---

*Background.*—Oral anticoagulation therapy reduces risk of vascular events in patients with atrial fibrillation. However, long-term monitoring is necessary and many patients cannot achieve optimum anticoagulation. We assessed whether clopidogrel plus aspirin was non-inferior to oral anticoagulation therapy for prevention of vascular events.

*Methods.*—Patients were enrolled if they had atrial fibrillation plus one or more risk factor for stroke, and were randomly allocated to receive oral anticoagulation therapy (target international normalised ratio of 2.0–3.0; n=3371) or clopidogrel (75 mg per day) plus aspirin (75–100 mg per day recommended; n=3335). Outcome events were adjudicated by a blinded committee. Primary outcome was first occurrence of stroke, non-CNS systemic embolus, myocardial infarction, or vascular death. Analyses were by intention-to-treat. This study is registered with ClinicalTrials.gov, number NCT00243178.

*Results.*—The study was stopped early because of clear evidence of superiority of oral anticoagulation therapy. There were 165 primary events in patients on oral anticoagulation therapy (annual risk 3.93%) and 234 in those on clopidogrel plus aspirin (annual risk 5.60%; relative risk 1.44 (1.18–1.76; p=0.0003). Patients on oral anticoagulation therapy who were already receiving this treatment at study entry had a trend towards a greater reduction in vascular events (relative risk 1.50, 95% CI 1.19–1.89) and a significantly (p=0.03 for interaction) lower risk of major bleeding with oral anticoagulation therapy (1.30; 0.94–1.79) than patients not on this treatment at study entry (1.27, 0.85–1.89 and 0.59, 0.32–1.08, respectively).

*Conclusion.*—Oral anticoagulation therapy is superior to clopidogrel plus aspirin for prevention of vascular events in patients with atrial fibrillation at high risk of stroke, especially in those already taking oral anticoagulation therapy.

▶ This important trial should put to rest the notion that antiplatelet agents, per se, provide effective prevention of thromboembolic events in patients with atrial fibrillation at risk for stroke. Recall that clots in the left atrium are fiber rich, whereas clots associated with coronary artery ischemia and infarction are platelet rich. Thus, the difference in efficacy of these 2 medications in preventing clot formation in atrial fibrillation versus coronary artery disease may be as simple as that. Also, these trial data are consistent with data from several prior trials that have demonstrated that aspirin has remarkably little efficacy in preventing stroke in patients with atrial fibrillation. Of note, the other thing that this study highlighted was the risk of bleeding associated with the initiation of warfarin therapy. Many other studies have also shown that, but this study really did highlight that. To this editor, an obvious implication is that the onset of oral anticoagulation therapy with warfarin in patients should be very closely and frequently monitored, and an appropriate treatment initiation algorithm should be developed.

**A. L. Waldo, MD**

---

### Clinical classification schemes for predicting hemorrhage: Results from the National Registry of Atrial Fibrillation (NRAF)

Gage BF, Yan Y, Milligan PE, et al (Washington Univ, St Louis; Yale-New Haven Health, Conn)
*Am Heart J* 151:713-719, 2006                                      6–6

---

*Background.*—Although warfarin and other anticoagulants can prevent ischemic events, they can cause hemorrhage. Quantifying the rate of hemorrhage is crucial for determining the risks and net benefits of prescribing antithrombotic therapy. Our objective was to find a bleeding classification scheme that could quantify the risk of hemorrhage in elderly patients with atrial fibrillation.

*Methods.*—We combined bleeding risk factors from existing classification schemes into a new scheme, HEMORR$_2$HAGES, and validated all bleeding classification schemes. We scored HEMORR$_2$HAGES by adding 2 points for a prior bleed and 1 point for each of the other risk factors: hepatic or renal disease, ethanol abuse, malignancy, older (age > 75 years), reduced platelet count or function, hypertension (uncontrolled), anemia, genetic factors, excessive fall risk, and stroke. We used data from quality improvement orga-

---

TABLE 2.—Risk of Major Bleeding in NRAF Participants Prescribed Warfarin, Stratified by HEMORR$_2$HAGES Score

| HEMORR$_2$HAGES Score* | n | No. of Bleeds | Bleeds Per 100 Point-years Warfarin (95% CI) |
|---|---|---|---|
| 0 | 209 | 4 | 1.9 (0.6-4.4) |
| 1 | 508 | 11 | 2.5 (1.3-4.3) |
| 2 | 454 | 20 | 5.3 (3.4-8.1) |
| 3 | 240 | 13 | 8.4 (4.9-13.6) |
| 4 | 106 | 9 | 10.4 (5.1-18.9) |
| ≥5 | 87 | 8 | 12.3 (5.8-23.1) |
| Any score | 1604 | 67 | 4.9 (3.9-6.3) |

*HEMORR$_2$HAGES is scored by adding 1 point for each bleeding risk factor: hepatic or renal disease, ethanol abuse, malignancy, older (age > 75 years), reduced platelet count or function, rebleeding risk (2 points), hypertension (uncontrolled), anemia, genetic factors (not available in this study), excessive fall risk, and stroke.

(Courtesy of Gage BF, Yan Y, Milligan PE, et al: Clinical classification of schemes for predicting hemorrhage: Results from the National Registry of Atrial Fibrillation (NRAF). *Am Heart J* 151:713-719. Copyright Elsevier 2006.)

nizations representing 7 states to assemble a registry of 3791 Medicare beneficiaries with atrial fibrillation.

*Results.*—There were 162 hospital admissions with an *International Classification of Diseases, Ninth Revision, Clinical Modification* code for hemorrhage. With each additional point, the rate of bleeding per 100 patient-years of warfarin increased: 1.9 for 0, 2.5 for 1, 5.3 for 2, 8.4 for 3, 10.4 for 4, and 12.3 for $\geq 5$ points. In patients prescribed warfarin, HEMORR$_2$HAGES had greater predictive accuracy ($c$ statistic 0.67) than other bleed prediction schemes ($P < .001$).

*Conclusions.*—Adaptations of existing classification schemes, especially a new bleeding risk scheme, HEMORR$_2$HAGES, can quantify the risk of hemorrhage and aid in the management of antithrombotic therapy (Table 2).

▶ The value of this article is the use of the HEMORR$_2$HAGES scheme for bleeding risk factors in patients with atrial fibrillation undergoing therapy with warfarin, aspirin, or neither. The HEMORR$_2$HAGES score works quite well in identifying patients at most risk for bleeding. As the authors point out, this permits the clinician with the patient to consider the potential benefits versus the potential risks of warfarin therapy by comparing the stroke risk schemes (eg, CHADS$_2$) with the bleeding risk (HEMORR$_2$HAGES). Also of note, and similar to the ACTIVE W trial and other previous clinical atrial fibrillation trials that used warfarin for stroke prevention, the bleeding risk with warfarin therapy is particularly noted with the onset of therapy. Again, there is a need to take great care in the initiation and establishment of a maintenance dose of warfarin so that bleeding is minimized.

**A. L. Waldo, MD**

---

**Age and the Risk of Warfarin-Associated Hemorrhage: The Anticoagulation and Risk Factors In Atrial Fibrillation Study**

Fang MC, Go AS, Hylek EM, et al (Univ of California at San Francisco; Kaiser Permanente of Northern California, Oakland; Boston Univ; et al)
*J Am Geriatr Soc* 54:1231-1236, 2006                                      6–7

---

*Objectives.*—To assess whether older age is independently associated with hemorrhage risk in patients with atrial fibrillation, whether or not they are taking warfarin therapy.

*Design.*—Cohort study.

*Setting.*—Integrated healthcare delivery system. Thirteen thousand five hundred fifty-nine adults with nonvalvular atrial fibrillation.

*Measurements.*—Patient data were collected from automated clinical and administrative databases using previously validated search algorithms. Medical charts were reviewed from patients hospitalized were for major hemorrhage (intracranial, fatal, requiring $\geq 2$ units of transfused blood, or involving a critical anatomic site). Age was categorized into four categories (<60, 60–69, 70–79, and $\geq 80$), and multivariable Poisson regression was

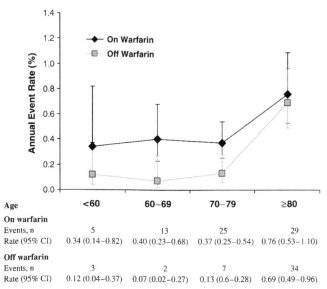

| Age | <60 | 60–69 | 70–79 | ≥80 |
|---|---|---|---|---|
| **On warfarin** | | | | |
| Events, n | 5 | 13 | 25 | 29 |
| Rate (95% CI) | 0.34 (0.14–0.82) | 0.40 (0.23–0.68) | 0.37 (0.25–0.54) | 0.76 (0.53–1.10) |
| **Off warfarin** | | | | |
| Events, n | 3 | 2 | 7 | 34 |
| Rate (95% CI) | 0.12 (0.04–0.37) | 0.07 (0.02–0.27) | 0.13 (0.6–0.28) | 0.69 (0.49–0.96) |

FIGURE 1.—Unadjusted age-specific rates of intracranial hemorrhage in 13,559 patients with nonvalvular atrial fibrillation taking and not taking warfarin. CI = confidence interval. (Courtesy of Fang MC, Go AS, Hylek EM, et al: Age and the risk of warfarin-associated hemorrhage: The Anticoagulation and Risk Factors in Atrial Fibrillation Study. *J Am Geriatr Soc* 54:1231-1236, 2006. Reprinted by permission of Blackwell Publishing.)

used to assess whether major hemorrhage rates increased with age, stratified by warfarin use and adjusted for other clinical risk factors for hemorrhage.

*Results.*—A total of 170 major hemorrhages were identified during 15,300 person-years of warfarin therapy and 162 major hemorrhages during 15,530 person-years off warfarin therapy. Hemorrhage rates rose with older age, with an average increase in hemorrhage rate of 1.2 (95% confidence interval (CI) 1.0–1.4) per older age category in patients taking warfarin and 1.5 (95% CI=1.3–1.8) in those not taking warfarin. Intracranial hemorrhage rates were significantly higher in those aged 80 and older (adjusted rate ratio=1.8, 95% CI=1.1–3.1 for those taking warfarin, adjusted rate ratio=4.7, 95% CI=2.4–9.2 for those not taking warfarin) than in those younger than 80.

*Conclusion.*—Older age increases the risk of major hemorrhage, particularly intracranial hemorrhage, in patients with atrial fibrillation, whether or not they are taking warfarin. Hemorrhage rates were generally comparable with those reported in previous randomized trials, indicating that carefully monitored warfarin therapy can be used with reasonable safety in older patients (Fig 1).

▶ This editor would like to emphasize the authors' conclusion that their study indicated " . . . that carefully monitored warfarin therapy can be used with reasonable safety in older patients." In fact, the most feared of the hemorrhages, intracranial hemorrhage, was remarkably constant (annual event rate of 0.04% or less) across the decades until the age of 80 years. At age 80 years or higher, there was virtually no difference in the annual event rate between people taking warfarin or not taking warfarin who had an intracranial hemorrhage, and even at that, the rate was only 0.8% per year.

**A. L. Waldo, MD**

---

**The use of enoxaparin compared with unfractionated heparin for short-term antithrombotic therapy in atrial fibrillation patients undergoing transoesophageal echocardiography-guided cardioversion: Assessment of Cardioversion Using Transoesophageal Echocardiography (ACUTE) II randomized multicentre study**
Klein AL, for The ACUTE II Steering and Publications Committee For the ACUTE II Investigators (Univ of Pittsburgh, Pa; et al)
*Eur Heart J* 27:2858-2865, 2006                                                          6–8

---

*Aims.*—To compare the feasibility and safety of transoesophageal echocardiograpy-guided cardioversion (CV) with enoxaparin and unfractionated heparin (UFH) in patients with atrial fibrillation (AF).

*Method and Results.*—The Assessment of Cardioversion Using Transoesophageal Echocardiography (ACUTE) II pilot trial compared the safety and efficacy of enoxaparin with UFH in 155 patients with AF who were scheduled for transoesophageal echocardiography (TEE)-guided CV. Safety outcomes over a 5-week period were ischaemic stroke, major or minor bleeding, and death. Efficacy outcomes were length of stay (LOS) and return to normal sinus rhythm (NSR). Of the 76 patients assigned to the enoxaparin group, 72 (94.7%) had a transoesophageal echocardiogram and 63 (82.9%) had early CV, of which 59 (93.7%) were successful. Of the 79 UFH patients, 66 (83.5%) had a transoesophageal echocardiogram and 58 (73.4%) had early CV, of which 54 (98.2%) were successful. There were no significant differences in embolic events, bleeding, or deaths between groups. The enoxaparin group had shorter median LOS compared with the UFH group [3(2–4) vs. 4(3–5)] days; $P < 0.0001$). There was also more NSR at 5 weeks in the enoxaparin group (76 vs. 57%; $P = 0.013$).

*Conclusion.*—In the ACUTE II trial, there were no differences in safety outcomes between the two strategies. However, the enoxaparin group had a shorter LOS. Thus, the TEE-guided enoxaparin strategy may be considered a safe and effective alternative strategy for AF. The shorter LOS may translate to lower costs using the enoxaparin TEE-guided approach.

▶ This trial confirms and expands the data from the anticoagulation in cardioversion using enoxaparin (ACE) trial.[1] The bottom line is that when one decides on an aggressive protocol for cardioversion of atrial fibrillation, low-molecular-weight heparin administration is clearly the equal of and has some several advantages over the use of unfractionated heparin.

**A. L. Waldo, MD**

*Reference*

1. Hemmings DG, Veeraready S, Baker PN, et al: Increased myogenic responses in uterine but not mesenteric arteries from pregnant offspring of diet-restricted rat dams. *Circulation* 109:997-1003, 2004.

## Reversal of Elevated International Normalized Ratios and Bleeding with Low-Dose Recombinant Activated Factor VII in Patients Receiving Warfarin

Dager WE, King JH, Regalia RC, et al (Univ of California, Sacramento; VA Northern California Health Care System, Mather)
*Pharmacotherapy* 26:1091-1098, 2006                                6–9

*Study Objective.*—To assess the effectiveness of using low-dose recombinant activated factor VII (rFVIIa) to reverse the effects of warfarin in critically ill patients with major bleeding events.

*Design.*—Prospective observational study.

*Setting.*—Intensive care unit of a 500-bed university-affiliated hospital.

*Patients.*—Sixteen nonhemophiliac patients who had been receiving warfarin and had an acute major bleeding event.

*Intervention.*—Patients received rFVIIa 1.2 mg for reversal of anticoagulation.

*Measurements and Main Results.*—Patients were identified from clinical pharmacology consult service electronic tracking records, and their data were cross-checked with the pharmacy information system. Information collected for each patient included extent of bleeding and magnitude of elevation in international normalized ratio (INR). A mean ± SD dose of rFVIIa 16.3 ± 4.1 µg/kg (range 11–25 µg/kg) reduced the mean INR from 2.8 ± 1.6 (range 1.44–6.34) to 1.07 ± 0.27 (range 0.86–1.92, p<0.001). A rapid onset of response for achieving a desirable hemostatic effect was observed in 14 of the 16 patients.

*Conclusion.*—Low-dose rFVIIa appears to be an effective, rapid reversal modality for major bleeding events in the presence of warfarin and an elevated INR. The agent's response is quicker than that expected with fresh frozen plasma combined with vitamin K. In emergency situations, rFVIIa 1.2 mg can be used to reverse the anticoagulant effect of warfarin and other vitamin K antagonists without inducing a hypercoagulable state; the product, however, is expensive.

▶ This small study demonstrated that low-dose rFVIIa was rapidly effective in reversing abnormal INR values in the presence of serious hemorrhage. This editor agrees with the authors' conclusion that "administration of rFVIIa 1.2 mg in combination with FFP [fresh-frozen plasma] and vitamin K may be particularly useful in patients with life-threatening bleeding, in whom FFP treatment may not be immediately available or in whom the volume expansion may be detrimental." However, as the authors also caution, "rFVIIa should be reserved for patients in whom FFP with or without intravenous vitamin K is either insufficient or unlikely to provide the clotting factors needed to attain hemostasis."

**A. L. Waldo, MD**

## Catheter Ablation of Atrial Fibrillation and Flutter

### Circumferential Pulmonary-Vein Ablation for Chronic Atrial Fibrillation
Oral H, Pappone C, Chugh A, et al (Univ of Michigan, Ann Arbor; San Raffaele Univ, Milan, Italy)
*N Engl J Med* 354:934-941, 2006                                                    6–10

*Background.*—We conducted a randomized, controlled trial of circumferential pulmonary-vein ablation for the treatment of chronic atrial fibrillation.

*Methods.*—A total of 146 patients with a mean (±SD) age of 57±9 years who had chronic atrial fibrillation were randomly assigned to receive amiodarone and undergo two cardioversions during the first three months alone (the control group) or in combination with circumferential pulmonary-vein ablation. Cardiac rhythm was assessed with daily telephonic transmissions for one year. The left atrial diameter and the severity of symptoms were assessed at 12 months.

*Results.*—Among the 77 patients assigned to undergo circumferential pulmonary-vein ablation, ablation was repeated because of recurrent atrial fibrillation in 26 percent of patients and atypical atrial flutter in 6 percent. An intention-to-treat analysis showed that 74 percent of patients in the ablation group and 58 percent of those in the control group were free of recurrent atrial fibrillation or flutter without antiarrhythmic-drug therapy at one year (P=0.05). Among the 69 patients in the control group, 53 (77 percent) crossed over to undergo circumferential pulmonary-vein ablation for recurrent atrial fibrillation by one year and only 3 (4 percent) were in sinus rhythm without antiarrhythmic-drug therapy or ablation. There were significant decreases in the left atrial diameter (12±11 percent, P<0.001) and the symptom severity score (59±21 percent, P<0.001) among patients who remained in sinus rhythm after circumferential pulmonary-vein ablation. Except for atypical atrial flutter, there were no complications attributable to circumferential pulmonary-vein ablation.

*Conclusions.*—Sinus rhythm can be maintained long term in the majority of patients with chronic atrial fibrillation by means of circumferential pulmonary-vein ablation independently of the effects of antiarrhythmic-drug therapy, cardioversion, or both. The maintenance of sinus rhythm is associated with a significant decrease in both the severity of symptoms and the left atrial diameter.

▶ This is an impressive study that clearly demonstrates that in patients with chronic atrial fibrillation defined as atrial fibrillation that had been present for more than 6 months without intervening spontaneous episodes of sinus rhythm that recur within 1 week of cardioversion, ablation was most effective, particularly compared with therapy with amiodarone. Of note, and really part and parcel of most studies of ablation therapy, exclusion criteria included patients over the age of 70 years. That clearly excludes the majority of patients with atrial fibrillation, in whom standard rate versus rhythm treatment approaches apply. In addition, most of these patients had no structural heart disease (only 6 in each group). Nevertheless, the data remain quite impressive.

**A. L. Waldo, MD**

## A Tailored Approach to Catheter Ablation of Paroxysmal Atrial Fibrillation

Oral H, Chugh A, Good E, et al (Univ of Michigan, Ann Arbor)
*Circulation* 113:1824-1831, 2006                                                      6–11

*Background.*—Because the genesis of atrial fibrillation (AF) is multifactorial and variable, an ablation strategy that involves pulmonary vein isolation and/or a particular set of ablation lines may not be equally effective or efficient in all patients with AF. A tailored strategy that targets initiators and drivers of AF is a possible alternative to a standardized lesion set.

*Method and Results.*—Catheter ablation was performed in 153 consecutive patients (mean age, 56±11 years) with symptomatic paroxysmal AF with the use of an 8-mm tip radiofrequency ablation catheter. The esophagus was visualized with barium. The pulmonary veins and left atrium were mapped during spontaneous or induced AF. Arrhythmogenic pulmonary veins were isolated or encircled. If AF was still present or inducible, complex electrograms in the left atrium, coronary sinus, and superior vena cava were targeted for ablation. The end point of ablation was absence of frequent atrial ectopy and spontaneous AF during isoproterenol infusion and noninducibility of AF. Routine energy applications near the esophagus were avoided. During follow-up, left atrial flutter developed in 19% of patients and was still present in 10% at <12 weeks of follow-up. A repeat ablation procedure was performed in 18% of patients. During a mean follow-up of 11±4 months, 77% of patients were free from AF and/or atrial flutter without antiarrhythmic drug therapy. Pericardial tamponade or transient neurological events occurred in 2% of procedures.

*Conclusions.*—A tailored ablation strategy that only targets triggers and drivers of AF is feasible and eliminates paroxysmal AF in approximately 80% of patients.

▶ Once again, the results are impressive. Once again, the editor wishes to note that the mean age of the subjects was 56 years. And ultimately, it is also important to note that almost 20% of the patients developed an atypical atrial flutter after the ablation, of which about half disappeared spontaneously. Also, 18% of the patients required a repeat ablation procedure, either for recurrent atrial fibrillation or for atypical atrial flutter. And finally, although the data seem to continue to improve, critical pieces of the puzzle for understanding more completely the mechanism of atrial fibrillation are still missing. Ultimately, we need to remain aware that the current approach to ablation of atrial fibrillation is empirical, and its mechanism(s), particularly the relationship between trigger and atrial substrate, are still in need of more enlightenment. As we more fully understand these factors (mechanism, trigger, substrate, etc), we should anticipate improved treatment of atrial fibrillation, including improved application of ablation.

**A. L. Waldo, MD**

---

**Long-Term Safety and Efficacy of Circumferential Ablation with Pulmonary Vein Isolation**
Cheema A, Dong J, Dalal D, et al (Johns Hopkins Univ, Baltimore, Md)
*J Cardiovasc Electrophysiol* 17:1080-1085, 2006                    6–12

---

*Background.*—Each of the two main approaches to catheter ablation of atrial fibrillation (AF, segmental and circumferential) is associated with moderate long-term efficacy.

*Objective.*—To report the long-term outcomes of a modified technique that combines circumferential ablation with pulmonary vein (PV) isolation, determined by a circular mapping catheter and to determine the relationship between complete PV isolation and long-term efficacy.

*Methods.*—The patient population was composed of 64 consecutive patients (47 men [73%]; age 59 ± 11 years) with AF who underwent catheter ablation. AF was paroxysmal in 29 (45%) and nonparoxysmal in 35 (55%). Each patient was followed for a minimum of 12 months.

*Results.*—After a mean follow-up of 13 ± 1 months, the long-term single-procedure success rate was 45% (n = 29) with an additional 4% (n = 3) of patients demonstrating improvement. With repeat procedures in 19 patients, the overall long-term success rate was 62% (n = 40) with 9% (n = 6) demonstrating improvement. All the patients who underwent repeat ablations had recovered PV conduction. Incomplete PV isolation was the only independent predictor of failure. A major complication occurred in four (6%) patients, including three patients with vascular complications and one with cardiac tamponade.

*Conclusion.*—Our results suggest that the long-term single-procedure efficacy of circumferential ablation with PV isolation in a cohort of patients with predominantly nonparoxysmal AF approaches 50%. Repeat procedures involving re-isolation of the PVs result in a significant improvement in outcomes. Complete electrical isolation of the PVs has a significant impact on the long-term efficacy of the procedure.

▶ This article from the group at Johns Hopkins is of note because the results are not as good as those reported from the University of Michigan and several other centers in a patient cohort with both paroxysmal and nonparoxysmal atrial fibrillation. The long-term single procedure efficacy of the authors' approach when applied to a cohort of patients with predominantly nonparoxysmal atrial fibrillation was only 45%. The authors emphasize the importance of isolation of the pulmonary veins and the need for a second procedure. This confirms what appears to be an accepted axiom by those doing these procedures. Nevertheless, the efficacy rates here are noticeably lower than other reports, and the reality of these sorts of data from a fine laboratory should be understood.

**A. L. Waldo, MD**

---

**Left Atrial Ablation Versus Biatrial Ablation for Persistent and Permanent Atrial Fibrillation: A Prospective and Randomized Study**
Calò L, Lamberti F, Loricchio ML, et al (Policlinico Casilino, Rome; Sant'Eugenio Hosp, Rome; Sandro Pettini Hosp, Rome; et al)
*J Am Coll Cardiol* 47:2504-2512, 2006                                     6–13

---

*Objectives.*—The aim of this study was to compare—in patients with persistent and permanent atrial fibrillation (AF)—the efficacy and safety of left atrial ablation with that of a biatrial approach.

*Background.*—Left atrium-based catheter ablation of AF, although very effective in the paroxysmal form of the arrhythmia, has an insufficient efficacy in patients with persistent and permanent AF.

*Methods.*—Eighty highly symptomatic patients (age, $58.6 \pm 8.9$ years) with persistent (n = 43) and permanent AF (n = 37), refractory to antiarrhythmic drugs, were randomized to two different ablation approaches guided by electroanatomical mapping. A procedure including circumferential pulmonary vein, mitral isthmus, and cavotricuspid isthmus ablation was performed in 41 cases (left atrial ablation group). In the remaining 39 patients (biatrial ablation group), the aforementioned approach was integrated by the following lesions in the right atrium: intercaval posterior line, intercaval septal line, and electrical disconnection of the superior vena cava.

*Results.*—During follow-up (mean duration $14 \pm 5$ months), AF recurred in 39% of patients in the left atrial ablation group and in 15% of patients in the biatrial ablation group (p = 0.022). Multivariable Cox regression analysis showed that ablation technique was an independent predictor of AF recurrence during follow-up.

*Conclusions.*—In patients with persistent and permanent AF, circumferential pulmonary vein ablation, combined with linear lesions in the right atrium, is feasible, safe, and has a significantly higher success rate than left atrial and cavotricuspid ablation alone.

▶ These data from a well-known Italian group again present another aspect of the breadth of the data being reported on ablation of AF. These data indicate that a biatrial approach to ablation was more efficacious. But, to this editor, it just emphasizes the empiric nature of the approach. Why some of these ablation lesions used by the authors makes the therapy more effective is unclear, at least mechanistically. One can speculate as to why that is, but in fact it just underlines the issue that the relation between trigger and substrate needs still better understanding. In the meantime, we are faced with the reality that an empiric approach is really what this is about, with improvements clearly being made but not always understood why.

**A. L. Waldo, MD**

---

**Results From the Loire-Ardèche-Drôme-Isère-Puy-de-Dôme (LADIP) Trial on Atrial Flutter, a Multicentric Prospective Randomized Study Comparing Amiodarone and Radiofrequency Ablation After the First Episode of Symptomatic Atrial Flutter**
Da Costa A, for the Loire-Ardèche-Drôme-Isère-Puy-de-Dôme (LADIP) Trial of Atrial Flutter Investigators (Centre Hospitalier Universitaire de Saint-Etienne, France; et al)
*Circulation* 114:1676-1681, 2006                                           6–14

---

*Background.*—There is no published randomized study comparing amiodarone therapy and radiofrequency catheter ablation (RFA) after only 1 episode of symptomatic atrial flutter (AFL). The aim of the Loire- Ardèche-Drôme-Isère-Puy-de-Dôme (LADIP) Trial of Atrial Flutter was 2-fold: (1) to prospectively compare first-line RFA (group I) versus cardioversion and amiodarone therapy (group II) after only 1 AFL episode; and (2) to determine the impact of both treatments on the long-term risk of subsequent atrial fibrillation (AF).

*Method and Results.*—From October 2002 to February 2006, 104 patients (aged 78±5 years; 20 women) with AFL were included, with 52 patients in group I and 52 patients in group II. The cumulative risk of AFL or AF was interpreted with the use of Kaplan-Meier curves and compared by the log-rank test. Clinical presentation, echocardiographic data, and follow-up were as follows: age (78.5±5 versus 78±5 years), history of AF (27% versus 21.6%); structural heart disease (58% versus 65%), left ventricular ejection fraction (56±14% versus 54.5±14%), left atrial size (43±7 versus 43±6 mm), mean follow-up (13±6 versus 13±6 months; *P*=NS), recurrence of AFL (3.8% versus 29.5%; *P*<0.0001), and occurrence of significant AF beyond 10 minutes (25% versus 18%; *P*=0.3). Five complications (10%) were noted in group II (sick sinus syndrome in 2, hyperthyroidism in 1, and hypothyroidism in 2) and none in group I (0%) (*P*=0.03).

*Conclusions.*—RFA should be considered a first-line therapy even after the first episode of symptomatic AFL. There is a better long-term success rate, the same risk of subsequent AF, and fewer secondary effects.

▶ This randomized study confirms what has been a general impression, namely that in most instances radiofrequency ablation to treat classic AFL is indicated after a single presenting event and is far better than drug therapy. Of note, and of particular interest to this editor, the rate of atrial fibrillation occurrence after successful ablation of AFL is not a surprise. Because a transient period of atrial fibrillation precedes AFL in almost all instances, the functional components necessary for the AFL reentrant circuit form during the transient period of atrial fibrillation.[1] In other words, the AFL reentrant circuit is not an anatomic circuit waiting to be engaged by a premature atrial beat. Rather, critical functional components of this reentrant circuit, principally the line of block between the venae cavae, have to form before there is a stable AFL reentrant circuit present and that is not subject to short circuiting. So, with the successful ablation of AFL, it should be no surprise that in patients in whom atrial fibrillation ordinarily advanced to AFL, post AFL ablation, the atrial fibrillation will now simply remain in some, even many, patients.

**A. L. Waldo, MD**

*Reference*

1. Waldo AL: Inter-relationships between atrial flutter and atrial fibrillation. *Pacing Clin Electrophysiol* 26:1583-1596, 2003.

## Surgical Ablation of Atrial Fibrillation

**Surgery for Paroxysmal Atrial Fibrillation in the Setting of Mitral Valve Disease: A Role for Pulmonary Vein Isolation?**
Gillinov AM, Bakaeen F, McCarthy PM, et al (Cleveland Clinic Found, Ohio)
*Ann Thorac Surg* 81:19-28, 2006                                         6–15

*Background.*—It is unknown whether pulmonary vein isolation or a complete Cox-Maze procedure is needed to ablate paroxysmal atrial fibrillation in patients with mitral valve disease. Our objective was to assess the impact of different surgical treatments for this arrhythmia in patients undergoing mitral valve surgery.

*Methods.*—From July 1993 to January 2004, 152 patients underwent combined surgical treatment of paroxysmal atrial fibrillation and mitral valve disease. Ablation procedures included pulmonary vein isolation alone (n = 31, 20%), pulmonary vein isolation with left atrial connecting lesions (n = 80, 53%), and Cox-Maze (n = 41, 27%). The latter had longer durations of atrial fibrillation than the former ($p < 0.0001$). Rhythm documented on 1,225 postoperative electrocardiograms was used to estimate prevalence of, and risk factors for, atrial fibrillation across time. Ablation failure was defined as occurrence of atrial fibrillation any time beyond 6 months after operation.

*Results.*—Prevalence of postoperative atrial fibrillation peaked at 22% at 2 weeks and declined to 9% at 1 year. Risk factors included older age ($p = 0.09$), larger left atrium ($p = 0.05$), and rheumatic ($p = 0.003$) and degenerative etiologies (p = 0.03). Freedom from ablation failure was 84% at one year. Ablation procedure did not affect prevalence of atrial fibrillation or incidence of ablation failure.

*Conclusions.*—Pulmonary vein isolation alone may be adequate treatment for patients with paroxysmal atrial fibrillation undergoing mitral valve surgery, particularly when it is of short duration. A randomized trial is necessary to examine this strategy, especially in patients with longer duration of paroxysmal atrial fibrillation.

▶ This is a large series from a group with a large experience in surgical ablation to treat atrial fibrillation. This study compared 3 modifications of the MAZE operation and got similar results in all 3. And while the overall response rates seem good, for this editor, this report highlights some of the problems with all the ablation approaches, including the surgical approach. First, the nature of the long-term follow-up is less than desirable in terms of how absence of atrial fibrillation is documented. In this study, it was largely through single ECGs recorded at long intervals, but not always available in all patients. In addition, of 103 patients who had an ECG obtained 6 months or more after ablation, atrial fibrillation or atrial flutter occurred in 24 patients (almost 25%). Clearly, there is a great need to understand atrial fibrillation better so that more precise ablation procedures, both medical and surgical, can be performed with increased expectation for success.

**A. L. Waldo, MD**

---

## Freedom from atrial arrhythmias after classic maze III surgery: A 10-year experience

Ballaux PKEW, Geuzebroek GSC, van Hemel NM, et al (Heart Lung Ctr Utrecht, The Netherlands; St Antonius Hosp, Nieuwegein, The Netherlands)
*J Thorac Cardiovasc Surg* 132:1433-1440, 2006 6–16

---

*Objectives.*—We studied the persistence of favorable outcome, the occurrence of new atrial arrhythmias, and sinus node dysfunction in patients who underwent the maze III procedure.

*Methods.*—Preoperative, in-hospital, and follow-up data of 203 patients who underwent the maze III procedure between June 1993 and June 2003 were collected. A total of 139 patients underwent the maze procedure for lone atrial fibrillation, and 64 patients underwent the maze procedure and concomitant cardiac surgery.

*Results.*—There was no 30-day postoperative mortality. During a mean follow-up of $4.0 \pm 2.6$ years, 12 patients (6%) died (2 cardiac related). At the end of follow-up, freedom from supraventricular arrhythmias was 80% for the lone atrial fibrillation group and 64% for the concomitant atrial fibrillation group. Freedom from stroke during follow-up was 100% in the lone atrial fibrillation group and 97% in the concomitant group. Multivariate analysis revealed that rhythm at 1-year follow-up ($P < .001$; odds ratio 9.56, 95% confidence limits 3.92-23.31) and preoperative left atrium dimension ($P = .028$; odds ratio 1.06 for every millimeter, 95% confidence limits 1.01-1.12) were predictors of success at the end of follow-up.

*Conclusions.*—This study shows that the favorable results of the maze III procedure in terms of freedom from supraventricular arrhythmias persist in most patients for at least 4 years.

▶ This is a large single series with a 4-year mean follow-up that included patients with symptomatic paroxysmal atrial fibrillation or chronic atrial fibrillation. Moreover, the procedure was the classic MAZE III operation without any of its modifications that are currently in use. Of note, the majority (68%) of patients underwent the MAZE procedure simply for lone atrial fibrillation. The rest of the patients had the MAZE procedure along with surgery for another indication. Much as with cardiac catheterization, patients who did best were those with lone atrial fibrillation (80.1% success rate vs 64.5% success rate for the concomitant surgery group). For this editor, these results again point to the limits of an empiric approach to this therapy.

**A. L. Waldo, MD**

---

**Left Ventricular Dysfunction in Atrial Fibrillation: Restoration of Sinus Rhythm by the Cox-Maze Procedure Significantly Improves Systolic Function and Functional Status**
Stulak JM, Dearani JA, Daly RC, et al (Mayo Clinic, Rochester, Minn)
*Ann Thorac Surg* 82:494-501, 2006                                               6–17

---

*Background.*—Atrial flutter or fibrillation with rapid, uncontrolled ventricular response may lead to left ventricular dysfunction, and conversion to sinus rhythm with control of heart rate can improve left ventricular ejection fraction. Little is known about the effects of the Cox-maze procedure on this form of tachycardia-induced cardiomyopathy.

*Methods.*—Four hundred forty-three patients underwent the Cox-maze procedure from 1993 to 2002. Ninety-nine had atrial flutter or fibrillation without associated valvular or congenital heart disease, and 37 (37%) had decreased left ventricular function (ejection fraction < 0.35 in 11 [severe], ejection fraction 0.36 to 0.45 in 8 [moderate], and ejection fraction 0.46 to 0.55 in 18 [mild]). Ages of these 37 patients (34 male) ranged from 35 to 74 years (median, 55 years).

*Results.*—Atrial flutter or fibrillation was present for 3 months to 19 years (median, 48 months) preoperatively, and 24 patients (65%) exhibited symptoms of heart failure. Preoperative ejection fraction ranged from 0.25 to 0.55 (median, 0.45). At last follow-up (median, 63 months), the Cox-maze procedure eliminated atrial flutter or fibrillation in all but 1 patient, and the greatest improvement was observed in patients with severe preoperative impairment (0.31 to 0.53; $p = 0.01$, preoperative versus follow-up), and patients with preoperative chronic atrial flutter or fibrillation (0.43 to 0.55; $p < 0.05$ preoperative versus follow-up). This improvement was observed immediately postoperatively and was sustained at last follow-up. Further, improvement in left ventricular function correlated with enhancement of functional status.

*Conclusions.*—In some patients, atrial flutter or fibrillation may be the cause rather than the consequence of left ventricular dysfunction. Importantly, systolic function and functional status can be significantly improved with the restoration of sinus rhythm by the Cox-maze procedure.

▶ These data seem very much to mimic the data from catheter ablation of atrial fibrillation in that there is improvement of ventricular function in patients after a successful MAZE procedure. Of note, the patients who were helped the most were those with nonvalvular atrial fibrillation who had severe left ventricular dysfunction and those with chronic rather than paroxysmal atrial fibrillation.

**A. L. Waldo, MD**

## Mechanisms of Atrial Tachyarrhythmias Following Surgical Atrial Fibrillation Ablation

Magnano AR, Argenziano M, Dizon JM, et al (Columbia Univ, New York)
*J Cardiovasc Electrophysiol* 17:366-373, 2006                              6–18

*Introduction.*—Typical and atypical atrial flutters (AFLs) and atrial tachycardias (ATs) have been reported in patients with prior surgical atrial fibrillation ablation. The underlying mechanisms for this group of atrial tachyarrhythmias have not been well characterized and the efficacy of catheter ablation in their treatment is unknown.

*Method and Results.*—Twenty patients (6 females) with a surface ECG diagnosis of AFL or AT following surgical atrial fibrillation ablation underwent 26 electrophysiology studies. Patients manifesting sustained, organized, and beat-by-beat reproducible atrial electrical activity underwent complete right and left atrial catheter mapping and catheter ablation. One patient had no inducible tachyarrhythmia, while 5 patients had nonmappable arrhythmias. Nineteen of the 31 potentially mappable atrial tachyarrhythmias were completely characterized in 14 patients. The underlying mechanisms were macro-reentrant left AFL (n = 9), focal left AT (n = 3), typical right AFL (n = 6), and atypical right AFL (n = 1). Of the 19 completely characterized atrial arrhythmias, catheter ablation was performed for 18, and the procedure was successful for 13 of these. After a mean follow-up of 15 ± 10 months, 15 of 20 patients (75%) were in sinus rhythm including 10 of 13 patients (77%) with AT/flutter ablation. Ten patients, including 6 following ablation, were maintaining sinus rhythm without antiarrhythmic medications.

*Conclusions.*—Patients with an ECG diagnosis of AFL or AT following surgical atrial fibrillation ablation may have multiple tachycardia mechanisms with the right or left atrium as the site of origin. Many of these rhythms may resolve with further maturation of surgical atrial fibrillation ablation (SAFA) lesions or be treatable with antiarrhythmic medication. However, persistent tachyarrhythmias can often be treated successfully with catheter mapping and ablation.

▶ This article serves as a reminder that much as with atrial fibrillation ablation using catheter techniques, ATs, particularly atypical AFL in the left atrium, may be a consequence of the surgical ablation procedure. The lesions made during the procedure have the potential to provide a line of block around which a reentrant circuit can travel. They also may serve as a boundary protecting the reentrant circuit from short circuiting.

A. L. Waldo, MD

**Atrial Arrhythmias After Surgical Maze: Findings During Catheter Ablation**
Wazni OM, Saliba W, Fahmy T, et al (Cleveland Clinic Found, Ohio)
*J Am Coll Cardiol* 48:405-409, 2006                                              6–19

*Objectives.*—We describe the clinical and electrophysiologic characteristics and management of post "cut and sew" Maze arrhythmias in symptomatic patients.

*Background.*—The Cox Maze procedure was developed as a surgical treatment of atrial fibrillation. Until recently, invasive electrophysiologic studies in patients with symptomatic post-operative arrhythmias in this patient population have not been described.

*Methods.*—The management and clinical course of consecutive patients with post-Maze arrhythmias refractory to antiarrhythmic drugs (AADs) between January 2000 and December 2003 are presented.

*Results.*—Twenty-three patients (15 men) presented $14 \pm 14$ months after Maze surgery for treatment of atrial fibrillation (AF). Eight patients underwent "cut and sew" Maze for lone AF with no other surgical indication. Fifteen patients underwent the "cut and sew" Maze procedure in addition to another surgical procedure: mitral valve surgery (11 patients) and coronary artery bypass graft surgery (4 patients). Eight patients (35%) had recurrent AF secondary to recovered conduction around the lines encircling the pulmonary veins. Five patients were documented to have focal atrial tachycardia, which was mapped to the coronary sinus in 3 patients, to the posterolateral right atrium in 1 patient, and to the left atrial (LA) septum in 1 patient. Four patients had right atrium incisional atrial flutter (AFL), and 6 had LA incisional AFL, which was mapped around the mitral valve annulus in 4 patients and around the right pulmonary veins in 2 patients. Twenty-two of the 23 patients were treated successfully with radiofrequency ablation. At 1-year follow-up, 19 patients were arrhythmia-free and taking no AADs.

*Conclusions.*—After surgical "cut and sew" Maze, approximately one-third of patients experiencing atrial arrhythmias have AF secondary to pulmonary vein-left atrium conduction recovery. Moreover, incisional AFL seems to be a common finding in this group of patients. Catheter-based mapping and ablation of these arrhythmias seems to be feasible and effective.

▶ This study deals with "cut and sew" MAZE procedures. Interestingly enough, the authors found that in approximately one third of the patients who experienced atrial arrhythmias after the procedure, the rhythm was recurrent AFL. Furthermore, in these instances, there appeared often to be a reconnection between the pulmonary veins and the LA. One has to wonder how then could be a reconnection across a scar that forms from a "cut and sew" lesion? One suspects that the cryo-lesions placed to bridge the "gaps" between the surgical incisions may not have been through-and-through lesions or may only temporarily have damaged tissue so that the reconnection was really a reawakening of the connection already present. In addition, the incidence of incisional AFL was 48%, again recognizing that the procedure can produce arrhythmias of clinical consequence not previously present.

**A. L. Waldo, MD**

---

**Atrial Incision Affects the Incidence of Atrial Tachycardia After Mitral Valve Surgery**
Lukac P, Hjortdal VE, Pedersen AK, et al (Skejby Univ, Aarhus, Denmark)
*Ann Thorac Surg* 81:509-513, 2006           6–20

---

*Background.*—Atrial fibrillation is common after mitral valve surgery. We do not know the incidence of atrial tachycardia and how it depends on the surgical approach used.

*Methods.*—The subjects of the study were 213 consecutive patients who had surgery for mitral valve disease from January 1, 2001, through January 26, 2004. The surgeons used either the superior transseptal approach (69 patients, group A) or left atrial approach (144 patients, group B). An investigator, blinded for the approach used, analyzed all 12-lead electrocardiograms taken during the admission after the operation. The data were analyzed using the Cox regression analysis as time from the operation until documentation of atrial tachycardia or atrial fibrillation on a 12-lead electrocardiogram. Hazard ratio (95% confidence interval) is reported.

*Results.*—The superior transseptal approach (2.0 [1.1 to 3.5], $p = 0.023$), age 60 years or more (2.3 [1.2 to 4.6], $p = 0.015$), and male sex (2.6 [1.3 to 5.2], $p = 0.007$) were independent predictors of atrial tachycardia. Age 60 years or more was the only independent predictor of atrial fibrillation (2.0 [1.2 to 3.3], $p = 0.007$). Although atrial tachycardia was less frequent than atrial fibrillation in group B ($p < 0.001$), atrial tachycardia was as common as atrial fibrillation in group A ($p = 0.149$).

*Conclusions.*—The superior transseptal approach has a higher risk of atrial tachycardia than the left atrial approach. Atrial tachycardia has different predictors than atrial fibrillation and constitutes a significant problem, especially after the superior transseptal approach. These results emphasize the need to distinguish between atrial tachycardia and atrial fibrillation— two entities with different pathophysiology, therapy, and also epidemiology.

▶ The atrial tachycardia in this report is really atrial flutter. An understanding of why atrial flutter may develop after these lesions is shown in a study by Tomita et al,[1] in which it was shown that a long enough surgical incision in a critical area between the venae cavae can develop a functional extension to one or both the superior or inferior venae cavae. This permits the development of the atrial flutter macro-reentrant circuit of typical atrial flutter. Alternatively, one can simply get reentry around the lesion itself. The hope would be that these patients with these rhythms could be prevented by a different surgical approach that wouldn't create lesions conducive to the formation of atrial flutter.

**A. L. Waldo, MD**

*Reference*

1. Tomita Y, Matsuo K, Sahadevan J, et al: Role of functional block extension in lesion-related atrial flutter. *Circulation* 103:1025-1030, 2001.

## Epidemiology and Mechanisms of Atrial Fibrillation

### Secular Trends in Incidence of Atrial Fibrillation in Olmsted County, Minnesota, 1980 to 2000, and Implications on the Projections for Future Prevalence

Miyasaka Y, Barnes ME, Gersh BJ, et al (Mayo Clinic, Rochester, Minn)
*Circulation* 114:119-125, 2006                                    6–21

*Background.*—Limited data exist on trends in incidence of atrial fibrillation (AF). We assessed the community-based trends in AF incidence for 1980 to 2000 and provided prevalence projections to 2050.

*Method and Results.*—The adult residents of Olmsted County, Minnesota, who had ECG-confirmed first AF in the period 1980 to 2000 (n=4618) were identified. Trends in age-adjusted incidence were determined and used to construct model-based prevalence estimates. The age- and sex-adjusted incidence of AF per 1000 person-years was 3.04 (95% CI, 2.78 to 3.31) in 1980 and 3.68 (95% CI, 3.42 to 3.95) in 2000. According to Poisson regression with adjustment for age and sex, incidence of AF increased significantly ($P=0.014$), with a relative increase of 12.6% (95% CI, 2.1 to 23.1) over 21 years. The increase in age-adjusted AF incidence did not differ between men and women ($P=0.84$). According to the US population projections by the US Census Bureau, the number of persons with AF is projected to be 12.1 million by 2050, assuming no further increase in age-adjusted incidence of AF, but 15.9 million if the increase in incidence continues.

*Conclusions.*—The age-adjusted incidence of AF increased significantly in Olmsted County during 1980 to 2000. Whether or not this rate of increase continues, the projected number of persons with AF for the United States will exceed 10 million by 2050, underscoring the urgent need for primary prevention strategies against AF development.

▶ This study is similar to an article by Go et al[1] on the incidence of AF in adults, which projects the incidence out to the year 2050. The difference is that the current study projects a significant increase in the age-adjusted incidence of AF over the period studied, essentially tripling the prevalence of AF. Much of this is because people are living longer. And because approximately 10% of patients in their 80s develop AF, perhaps this is no surprise. However, the Framingham data,[2] which were gathered beginning after World

War II, indicate that about 1 of every 4 Americans will develop AF at some time. The enormity of these epidemiological statistics and their clinical implications are obvious. We need to understand this arrhythmia much more. Most important would be finding ways to minimize this incidence, although treating it more successfully would, of course, also be useful.

**A. L. Waldo, MD**

*References*

1. Go AS, Hyleck EM, Phillips KA, et al: Prevalence of diagnosed atrial fibrillation in adults: National implications for rhythm management and stroke prevention: The AnTicoagulation and Risk Factors in Atrial Fibrillation (ATRIA) Study. *JAMA* 285:2370-2375, 2001.
2. (Lloyd-Jones DM, Wang TJ, Leip EP, et al: Lifetime risk for development of atrial fibrillation: The Framingham Heart Study. *Circulation* 110:1042-1046, 2004.)

---

**Atrioventricular Nodal Reentrant Tachycardia in Patients Referred for Atrial Fibrillation Ablation: Response to Ablation That Incorporates Slow-Pathway Modification**
Sauer WH, Alonso C, Zado E, et al (Univ of Pennsylvania, Philadelphia)
*Circulation* 114:191-195, 2006                                                    6–22

---

*Background.*—Although the most common sites of atrial ectopy that trigger atrial fibrillation (AF) are in or around the pulmonary veins (PVs), atrioventricular nodal reentrant tachycardia (AVNRT) can also cause or coexist with AF. We sought to characterize patients with AF and AVNRT and assess clinical outcomes after ablation.

*Method and Results.*—To determine the prevalence of concomitant AVNRT and AF, 629 consecutive patients referred for catheter ablation between November 1998 and March 2005 were studied. Electrophysiological studies with programmed stimulation during isoproterenol infusion identified atrial ectopy that initiated AF and the presence of inducible AVNRT. AF ablation consisted of proximal isolation of PVs and elimination of any non-PV trigger of AF, including AVNRT. There were 27 patients (4.3%) who had inducible AVNRT at the time of AF ablation. Of these, 13 underwent AVNRT ablation without PV isolation. Compared with the rest of the cohort, patients with AVNRT and AF were younger at the time of symptom onset (age 36.8±13.8 versus 48.2±11.7 years; *P*<0.01). Freedom from AF with or without previously ineffective antiarrhythmic medication was similar in both groups (96.3% versus 90.7%; mean follow-up 21.4±9.4 months); however, patients with AVNRT targeted for ablation were more likely to be AF free while not taking any antiarrhythmic medication after a single procedure during the follow-up period (87.5% versus 54.7%; *P*<0.01) and had fewer complications (0% versus 2.5%; *P*=0.30). Twelve of the 13 patients who underwent slow-pathway ablation without left atrial ablation remained AF free without the need for antiarrhythmic medication after a single procedure.

*Conclusions.*—AVNRT is an uncommon AF trigger seen more frequently in younger patients. Ablation of AVNRT in patients with AF was associated with improved outcomes compared with those with other triggers of AF.

▶ The concept of tachycardia-induced tachycardia is very important and often underappreciated. This study demonstrated once again that AF may be preceded by another tachycardia, in this case AVNRT. Why AVNRT would predispose to AF is of interest and relates to the rapid atrial rate, per se, during the tachycardia. Although not really discussed in this study, this editor suggests this critically involves the concept of facilitation. During AVNRT, the rapid rates cause a physiological shortening of the atrial refractory period. Shortening the atrial refractory period makes the atria vulnerable to premature beats from the PVs, which then precipitate the AF. The notion is that after the AVNRT stops, usually spontaneously, PV potentials that previously were "parasystolic" because of their very short cycle length (often 120 ms or even less), can now escape the PVs and activate the atria, causing AF. Although not stated in this report, the association of AVNRT with AF is also another example of a tachycardia-induced tachycardia due to the same process. The AVNRT predisposes the AF, which in turn evolves to atrial flutter. The latter, which has been well described, results from the fact that the critical components of the atrial flutter reentrant circuit sometimes form during AF.[1] The most critical part of that is the development of a line of block between the venae cavae. When that occurs, AF can become atrial flutter. Thus the association of AVNRT with atrial flutter. Curing the AVNRT also cures the atrial flutter in that instance because it also cures the AF. It should be noted, however, that because the PV potentials still remain, some of these patients do later on develop AF.

**A. L. Waldo, MD**

*Reference*

1. Waldo AL: Inter-relationships between atrial flutter and atrial fibrillation. *Pacing Clin Electrophysiol* 26:1583-1596, 2003.

---

**Localized Sources Maintaining Atrial Fibrillation Organized by Prior Ablation**
Haïssaguerre M, Hocini M, Sanders P, et al (Univ Victor Segalen, Bordeaux, France)
*Circulation* 113:616-625, 2006                                       6–23

---

*Background.*—Endocardial mapping of localized sources driving atrial fibrillation (AF) in humans has not been reported.

*Method and Results.*—Fifty patients with AF organized by prior pulmonary vein and linear ablation were studied. AF was considered organized if mapping during AF showed irregular but discrete atrial complexes exhibiting consistent activation sequences for >75% of the time using a 20-pole catheter with 5 radiating spines covering 3.5-cm diameter or sequential conventional mapping. A site or region centrifugally activating the remaining atrial tissue defined a source. During AF with a cycle length of 211±32 ms, activation mapping identified 1 to 3 sources at the origin of atrial wavefronts in 38 patients (76%) predominantly in the left atrium, including the coronary sinus region. Electrograms at the earliest area varied from discrete centrifugal activation to an activity spanning 75% to 100% of the cycle length in 42% of cases, the latter indicating complex local conduction or a reentrant circuit. A gradient of cycle length (>20 ms) to the surrounding atrium was observed in 28%. Local radiofrequency ablation prolonged AF cycle length by 28±22 ms and either terminated AF or changed activation sequence to another organized rhythm. In 4 patients, the driving source was isolated, surrounded by the atrium in sinus rhythm, and still firing at high frequency (228±31 ms) either permanently or in bursts.

*Conclusions.*—AF associated with consistent atrial activation sequences after prior ablation emanates mostly from localized sources that can be mapped and ablated. Some sources harbor electrograms suggesting the presence of localized reentry.

---

### Frequency Mapping of the Pulmonary Veins in Paroxysmal Versus Permanent Atrial Fibrillation

Sanders P, Nalliah CJ, Dubois R, et al (Université Victor Segalen Bordeaux II, France)

*J Cardiovasc Electrophysiol* 17:965-972, 2006                6–24

---

*Introduction.*—The pulmonary veins (PVs) are a dominant source of triggers initiating atrial fibrillation (AF). While recent evidence implicates these structures in the maintenance of paroxysmal AF, their role in permanent AF is not known. The current study aims to compare the contribution of PV activity to the maintenance of paroxysmal and permanent AF.

*Method and Results.*—Thirty-four patients with paroxysmal AF (n = 20) or permanent AF (n = 14) undergoing ablation were studied. Prior to ablation, 32 seconds of electrograms were acquired from each PV and the coronary sinus (CS). The frequency of activity of each PV and CS was defined as the highest amplitude frequency on spectral analysis. The effects of ablation on the AF cycle length (AFCL) and frequency and on AF termination were determined. Significant differences were observed between paroxysmal and permanent AF. Paroxysmal AF demonstrates higher frequency PV activity (11.0 ± 3.1 vs 8.8 ± 3.0 Hz; P = 0.0003) but lower CS frequency (5.8 ± 1.2 vs 6.9 ± 1.4 Hz; P = 0.01) and longer AFCL (182 ± 17 vs 158 ± 21 msec; P = 0.002), resulting in greater PV to atrial frequency gradient (7.2 ± 2.2 vs 4.2 ± 2.9 Hz; P = 0.006). PV isolation in paroxysmal AF resulted in a greater decrease in atrial frequency (1.0 ± 0.7 vs −0.05 ± 0.4 Hz; P < 0.0001), greater prolongation of the AFCL (49 ± 35 vs 5 ± 6 msec; P < 0.0001), and more frequent AF termination (11/20 vs 0/14; P = 0.0007) compared to permanent AF.

*Conclusion.*—Paroxysmal AF is associated with higher frequency PV activity and lesser CS frequency compared to permanent AF. Isolation of the

PVs had a greater impact on the fibrillatory process in paroxysmal AF compared to permanent AF, suggesting that while the PVs have a role in maintaining paroxysmal AF, these structures independently contribute less to the maintenance of permanent AF.

## Fibrillating Areas Isolated within the Left Atrium after Radiofrequency Linear Catheter Ablation

Rostock T, Rotter M, Sanders P, et al (Université Victor Segalen Bordeaux II, France)

*J Cardiovasc Electrophysiol* 17:807-812, 2006                      6–25

*Introduction.*—Nonpulmonary vein sources have been implicated as potential drivers of atrial fibrillation (AF). This observational study describes regions of fibrillating atrial tissue isolated inadvertently from the left atrium (LA) following linear catheter ablation for AF.

*Method and Results.*—We report four patients with persistent/permanent AF who underwent pulmonary vein isolation with additional linear lesions and who presented with recurrent AF (mean AF cycle length [AFCL] 175–270 ms). Further catheter ablation resulted in the inadvertent electrical isolation of significant areas of the LA in which AF persisted at the same AFCL as was measured prior to disconnection, despite the restoration of sinus rhythm (SR) in all other left and right atrial areas, strongly suggesting that these islands were driving the remaining atria into fibrillation. The disconnected areas were located in the lateral LA, including the left atrial appendage (LAA) in three patients (limited to the LAA in one) and in the posterior LA in one patient. These isolated fibrillating regions represented 15–24% of the global LA surface, as estimated by electroanatomic mapping.

*Conclusion.*—Fibrillation can be maintained within electrically isolated regions of the LA following catheter ablation of AF, demonstrating the importance of atrial drivers in the maintenance of AF. Further mapping of these drivers is needed to characterize their mechanism and thereby allow for a more specific ablation strategy.

## Organization of Frequency Spectra of Atrial Fibrillation: Relevance to Radiofrequency Catheter Ablation

Takahashi Y, Sanders P, Jaïs P, et al (Univ Victor Segalen Bordeaux 2, France)

*J Cardiovasc Electrophysiol* 17:382-388, 2006                      6–26

*Introduction.*—We hypothesized that the frequency spectra of fibrillatory electrograms may reflect the complexity of activities perpetuating atrial fibrillation (AF). To test this hypothesis, we evaluated the frequency spectra in patients with paroxysmal AF in relation to catheter ablation.

*Method and Results.*—This study comprised two protocols: 25 patients undergoing pulmonary vein (PV) isolation in protocol I, and 20 patients undergoing mitral isthmus linear ablation after PV isolation in protocol II. The mean of dominant frequency (DF) and organization index (the ratio of the area under the DF and its harmonics to the total power) were determined from 32-second recordings in the coronary sinus. In protocol I, a PV was considered "driver" of AF if isolation of the PV resulted in termination or slowing of AF (decrease in DF by $\geq 0.25$ Hz). Twenty-one patients had AF termination during four PV isolation. Among these 21 patients, 13 patients with single driving PV showed significantly higher baseline organization index than eight patients with multiple driving PVs ($0.45 \pm 0.08$ vs $0.35 \pm 0.07$, $P = 0.009$). Patients with multiple driving PVs showed a significant increase in the organization index to $0.45 \pm 0.11$ ($P < 0.05$) after isolation of the initial driving PVs. In protocol II, the baseline organization index was significantly higher in seven patients who had termination of AF during mitral isthmus ablation than 13 patients who did not ($0.50 \pm 0.10$ vs $0.38 \pm 0.07$, $P < 0.008$). The baseline DF was not associated with outcomes of ablation in both protocols.

*Conclusions.*—A higher organization index of atrial electrograms is associated with termination of AF during limited ablation. This parameter may be useful to anticipate the extent of ablation.

▶ These 4 reports (Abstracts 6–23 through 6–26) are all variations on the same theme. The authors have used either fast Fourier transform analysis or beat-to-beat cycle length analysis and identified areas of an apparent driver or drivers that seem to generate the AF. This really gets into the nature of what causes or maintains AF. The notion is that there are sources (probably reentrant, the authors suggest, but the mechanism is uncertain) that are so fast that they cause fibrillatory conduction and maintain the AF. They may be a single source, or they may be multiple sources. This is important, as this seems likely the dominant mechanism of AF, whether it be paroxysmal, persistent, or permanent. For this editor, the notion of multiple reentrant wavelets without a driver ("source") is probably not the most important or even the most frequent mechanism of AF. These studies also serve to focus on the need to understand better the mechanism of AF and hopefully target these drivers more carefully. It is important to understand how the trigger(s) induces the driver(s) because that, once again, might provide insights into a vulnerable part of the substrate for ablation and thereby cure of AF. And sometimes it seems that the triggers and drivers are one and the same.

**A. L. Waldo, MD**

## Use of Fast Fourier Transform Analysis of Atrial Electrograms for Rapid Characterization of Atrial Activation—Implications for Delineating Possible Mechanisms of Atrial Tachyarrhythmias

Ryu K, Sahadevan J, Khrestian CM, et al (Case Western Reserve Univ, Cleveland, Ohio)

*J Cardiovasc Electrophysiol* 17:198-206, 2006                6–27

*Introduction.*—Different analysis techniques have been developed to help understand and characterize the mechanisms responsible for atrial arrhythmias. We tested the hypothesis that Fast Fourier Transform (FFT) analysis of recorded atrial electrograms (AEGs) will rapidly and accurately identify regular and irregular patterns of atrial activation, and, thereby, may provide evidence suggestive of underlying mechanisms of atrial tachyarrhythmias.

*Method and Results.*—During induced atrial tachyarrhythmias in both the canine sterile pericarditis model and canine rapid ventricular pacing-induced congestive heart failure model; 380–404 AEGs were recorded simultaneously from epicardial electrodes on both atria. From AEGs, atrial activation sequences were determined during atrial flutter (AFL), focal atrial tachycardia (AT), and atrial fibrillation (AF). Four-second recording segments of each AEG were subjected to FFT analysis. Frequencies found during FFT analyses in all studies precisely corresponded to the cycle lengths of the AEGs. In AFL and AT, one dominant frequency peak was found throughout both atria. In AF due to multiple unstable reentry circuits, multiple and broad frequency peaks were found in both atria. In AF due to a stable rapid rhythm (driver) in the left atrium with fibrillatory conduction to the rest of the atria, one dominant frequency peak in areas with 1:1 conduction from the driver, and multiple and/or broad frequency peaks in areas with fibrillatory conduction produced by the driver were found. Computation time for all FFT analyses took <5 minutes.

*Conclusion.*—FFT analysis accurately and rapidly identifies global atrial activation patterns during AFL, AT, and AF, thereby assisting in determining arrhythmia mechanisms.

▶ This study in animal models of AF from the editor's laboratory again serves to document and support the notion that it is drivers of very short cycle length that are responsible for most AF. The authors used FFT, a simple technique that can be applied clinically, to identify the areas of shortest cycle length, and by mapping the atria with FFT were able to distinguish the areas of fibrillatory conduction from the area(s) of the driver.

**A. L. Waldo, MD**

## Shortening of Fibrillatory Cycle Length in the Pulmonary Vein During Vagal Excitation

Takahashi Y, Jaïs P, Hocini M, et al (Université Victor Segalen Bordeaux 2, France)

*J Am Coll Cardiol* 47:774-780, 2006                     6–28

*Objectives.*—The goal of the present prospective study is to evaluate the impact of vagal excitation on ongoing atrial fibrillation (AF) during pulmonary vein (PV) isolation.

*Background.*—The role of vagal tone in maintenance of AF is controversial in humans.

*Methods.*—Twenty-five patients (18 with paroxysmal AF, 7 with chronic AF) were selected by occurrence of vagal excitation during AF (atrioventricular [AV] block: R-R interval >3 s) produced by PV isolation. Fibrillatory cycle length (CL) in the targeted PV and coronary sinus (CS) were determined before, during, and after vagal excitation. The CL was available at PV ostium during vagal excitation in 11 patients.

*Results.*—Forty-eight episodes of vagal excitation were observed. During vagal excitation, CL abruptly decreased both in CS and PV (CS, 164 ± 20 ms to 155 ± 23 ms, p < 0.0001; PV, 160 ± 22 ms to 143 ± 28 ms, p < 0.0001), and both returned to the baseline value with resumption of AV conduction. The decrease in PVCL occurred earlier (2.5 ± 1.5 s vs. 4.0 ± 2.6 s, p < 0.01) and was of greater magnitude than that in CSCL (16 ± 16 ms vs. 8 ± 9 ms, p < 0.01). A sequential gradient of CL was observed from PV to PV ostium and CS during vagal excitation (138 ± 29 ms, 149 ± 24 ms, and 159 ± 26 ms, respectively). The decrease in CL was significantly greater in paroxysmal than in chronic AF (CS, 11 ± 9 ms vs. 5 ± 7 ms, p < 0.05; PV, 23 ± 25 ms vs. 8 ± 14 ms, p < 0.05).

*Conclusions.*—Vagal excitation is associated with shortening of fibrillatory CL. This occurs earlier in PV with a sequential gradient to PV ostium and CS, suggesting that vagal excitation enhances a driving role of PV.

▶ Once again, this report from Haïssaguerre's group provides more evidence for the concept that facilitation is an important part of understanding inception and maintenance of AF. By causing shortening of atrial effective refractory period, vagal stimulation permits PV potentials of very short cycle length to exit to the atria and cause fibrillatory conduction. Isolating the PVs prevents this.

**A. L. Waldo, MD**

## Drug Therapy

### Effect of *Atorvastatin* on the Recurrence Rates of Atrial Fibrillation After Electrical Cardioversion

Ozaydin M, Varol E, Aslan SM, et al (Suleyman Demirel Univ, Turkey; State Hosp, Isparta, Turkey)

*Am J Cardiol* 97:1490-1493, 2006                                                                6–29

To study the effect of atorvastatin on recurrence of atrial fibrillation (AF) after electrical cardioversion (EC), 48 patients with AF lasting 48 hours who were scheduled for EC were randomized to the atorvastatin (group I) and control (group II) groups. Six patients in group I (25%) and 2 patients in group II (8.3%) had spontaneous conversion before EC (p >0.05). The end point was the recurrence of AF during 3 months of follow-up. Eighteen patients in group I (12.5%) and 11 patients in group II (45.8%) had recurrence (p = 0.01, log-rank test). With the Cox proportional model, the predictors of recurrence included a body mass index of 25 to 30 kg/m$^2$ (relative risk [RR] 0.07, 95% confidence interval [CI] 0.008 to 0.59), body mass index ≥30 kg/m$^2$ (RR 0.24, 95% CI 0.08 to 0.72), AF duration of ≥3 months (RR 0.28, 95% CI 0.09 to 0.83), diabetes mellitus (RR 0.34, 95% CI 0.12 to 0.98), and left atrial diameter of ≥ 45 mm (RR 0.23, 95% CI 0.07 to 0.74). Atorvastatin was associated with a significantly reduced risk of developing AF (unadjusted RR 0.23, 95% CI 0.064 to 0.82, p = 0.024). This association remained significant after adjustment for these predictors (adjusted RR 0.19, 95% CI 0.052 to 0.72, p = 0.01). High-sensitivity C-reactive protein levels at baseline were not different between the 2 groups (p = 0.92). Although the high-sensitivity C-reactive protein levels decreased significantly 48 hours after EC compared with the baseline levels in group I (2.82 ± 1.46 vs 2.56 ± 1.3 mg/dl, p = 0.02), no significant change occurred in group II (2.87 ± 0.8 vs 2.84 ± 0.8 mg/dl, p = 0.09). In conclusion, atorvastatin decreased the recurrence rate of AF after EC.

▶ There continue to be reports of the efficacy of the statins in preventing the new onset or recurrence of AF. This prospective trial shows the same thing occurs after DC cardioversion.

**A. L. Waldo, MD**

### Meta-analysis: Inhibition of renin-angiotensin system prevents new-onset atrial fibrillation

Anand K, Mooss AN, Hee TT, et al (Creighton Univ, Omaha, Neb)

*Am Heart J* 152:217-222, 2006                                                                6–30

*Background.*—Epidemiologic studies suggest that inhibition of renin-angiotensin system with angiotensin-converting enzyme inhibitors and angiotensin receptor blockers may prevent development of atrial fibrillation (AF).

*Objective.*—The objective of the study was to assess if there is significant indication for using angiotensin-converting enzyme inhibitors and angiotensin receptor blockers in the prevention of new-onset AF and to identify the target patient population.

*Methods.*—PubMed and Cochrane clinical trials database were searched from 1980 through March 2005 together with the review of citations. Nine randomized controlled human trials reporting the prevention of new-onset AF by inhibition of renin-angiotensin system were identified. Information about study design, follow-up, intervention, population, outcomes, and methodology quality was extracted.

*Results.*—The mean follow-up of the studies ranged from 6 months to 6.1 year. The pooled estimate using random effects model was 0.82 (95% CI 0.70-0.97) for prevention of new-onset AF and 0.61 (95% CI 0.46-0.83) for primary prevention of AF. The angiotensin-converting enzyme inhibitors (0.75, 95% CI 0.57-0.99) had greater protective effect than angiotensin receptor blockers (0.81, 95% CI 0.62-1.06). Patients with heart failure benefited the most (0.57, 95% CI 0.37-0.89). The test for heterogeneity between studies was significant. There was no consistent visual or statistical evidence of publication bias.

*Conclusion.*—The use of angiotensin-converting enzyme inhibitors and angiotensin receptor blockers had an overall effect of 18% risk reduction in new-onset AF across the trials and 43% risk reduction in patients with heart failure.

▶ Although this meta-analysis has some problems that the authors outline well, the summary pooled estimate using the random effects model from the 9 randomized trials included in the meta-analysis shows an 18% risk reduction in new-onset AF. In the 5 primary prevention trials, there was a 31% risk reduction in the incidence of AF. Thus, the analysis showed that the angiotensin-converting enzyme inhibitors work better in prevention of new-onset AF. This finding is different from results from a previous meta-analysis in which the angiotensin-converting enzyme inhibitors and angiotensin-receptor blockers were equally efficacious. The bottom line is that these drugs do seem to have an impact and are probably worthy of consideration for use as treatment. The question is, should these drugs now be used prophylactically in patients, such as the elderly or those with risk factors for AF to try to prevent its occurrence?

**A. L. Waldo, MD**

---

**Prevention of atrial fibrillation in patients with symptomatic chronic heart failure by candesartan in the Candesartan in Heart failure: Assessment of Reduction in Mortality and morbidity (CHARM) program**
Ducharme A, for the CHARM Investigators (Montreal Heart Inst; et al)
*Am Heart J* 152:86-92, 2006
6–31

---

*Background.*—Atrial fibrillation (AF) is frequent in patients with chronic heart failure (CHF). Experimental and small patient studies have demonstrated that blocking the renin-angiotensin-aldosterone system may prevent AF. In the CHARM program, the effects of the angiotensin receptor blocker candesartan on cardiovascular mortality and morbidity were evaluated in a broad spectrum of patients with symptomatic CHF. CHARM provided the opportunity to prospectively determine the effect of candesartan on the incidence of new AF in this CHF population.

*Methods.*—7601 patients with symptomatic CHF and reduced or preserved left ventricular systolic function were randomized to candesartan (target dose 32 mg once daily, mean dose 24 mg) or placebo in the 3 component trials of CHARM. The major outcomes were cardiovascular death or CHF hospitalization and all-cause mortality. The incidence of new AF was a prespecified secondary outcome. Median follow-up was 37.7 months. A conditional logistic regression model for stratified data was used.

*Results.*—6379 patients (83.9%) did not have AF on their baseline electrocardiogram. Of these, 392 (6.15%) developed AF during follow-up, 177 (5.55%) in the candesartan group and 215 (6.74%) in the placebo group (odds ratio 0.812, 95% CI 0.662-0.998, $P = .048$). After adjustment for baseline covariates, the odds ratio was 0.802 (95% CI 0.650-0.990, $P = .039$). There was no heterogeneity of the effects of candesartan in preventing AF between the 3 component trials ($P = .57$).

*Conclusions.*—Treatment with the angiotensin receptor blocker candesartan reduced the incidence of AF in a large, broadly-based, population of patients with symptomatic CHF.

▶ This is the first study to demonstrate a reduction in the incidence of AF with an angiotensin II receptor blocker in such a wide spectrum of patients with symptomatic CHF, including those with preserved as well as reduced left ventricular systolic function, many of whom were also treated with an angiotensin-converting enzyme inhibitor. Importantly, this was not a retrospective part of the CHARM analysis, but a prespecified analysis, adding to the importance of the observation. But to this editor, the importance of these prospectively obtained data is that the angiotensin-receptor blocker candesartan had this effect on top of all the other drugs, including angiotensin-converting enzyme inhibitors and statins that these patients were taking.

**A. L. Waldo, MD**

---

**Comparison of β-Blockers, Amiodarone Plus β-Blockers, or Sotalol for Prevention of Shocks From Implantable Cardioverter Defibrillators: The OPTIC Study: A Randomized Trial**

Connolly SJ, for the Optimal Pharmacological Therapy in Cardioverter Defibrillator Patients (OPTIC) Investigators (McMaster Univ, Hamilton, Ont, Canada; et al)
*JAMA* 295:165-171, 2006                                                                6–32

---

*Context.*—Implantable cardioverter defibrillator (ICD) therapy is effective but is associated with high-voltage shocks that are painful.

*Objective.*—To determine whether amiodarone plus β-blocker or sotalol are better than β-blocker alone for prevention of ICD shocks.

*Design, Setting, and Patients.*—A randomized controlled trial with blinded adjudication of events of 412 patients from 39 outpatient ICD clinical centers located in Canada, Germany, United States, England, Sweden, and Austria, conducted from January 13, 2001, to September 28, 2004. Patients were eligible if they had received an ICD within 21 days for inducible or spontaneously occurring ventricular tachycardia or fibrillation.

*Intervention.*—Patients were randomized to treatment for 1 year with amiodarone plus β-blocker, sotalol alone, or β-blocker alone.

*Main Outcome Measure.*—Primary outcome was ICD shock for any reason.

*Results.*—Shocks occurred in 41 patients (38.5%) assigned to β-blocker alone, 26 (24.3%) assigned to sotalol, and 12 (10.3%) assigned to amiodarone plus β-blocker. A reduction in the risk of shock was observed with use of either amiodarone plus β-blocker or sotalol vs β-blocker alone (hazard ratio [HR], 0.44; 95% confidence interval [CI], 0.28-0.68; $P<.001$). Amiodarone plus β-blocker significantly reduced the risk of shock compared with β-blocker alone (HR, 0.27; 95% CI, 0.14-0.52; $P<.001$) and sotalol (HR, 0.43; 95% CI, 0.22-0.85; $P=.02$). There was a trend for sotalol to reduce shocks compared with β-blocker alone (HR, 0.61; 95% CI, 0.37-1.01; $P=.055$). The rates of study drug discontinuation at 1 year were 18.2% for amiodarone, 23.5% for sotalol, and 5.3% for β-blocker alone. Adverse pulmonary and thyroid events and symptomatic bradycardia were more common among patients randomized to amiodarone.

*Conclusions.*—Despite use of advanced ICD technology and treatment with a β-blocker, shocks occur commonly in the first year after ICD implant. Amiodarone plus β-blocker is effective for preventing these shocks and is more effective than sotalol but has an increased risk of drug-related adverse effects.

▶ This useful study demonstrated that amiodarone plus β-blockers significantly reduced shocks in patients with ICDs. However, sotalol, while not as good as amiodarone, almost reached statistical significance ($P = .055$). This editor would prefer to start with sotalol and a β-blocker because of the lower incidence of adverse effects than that associated with amiodarone. One can always later administer amiodarone if needed.

**A. L. Waldo, MD**

### Verapamil Versus Digoxin and Acute Versus Routine Serial Cardioversion for the Improvement of Rhythm Control for Persistent Atrial Fibrillation

Hemels MEW, Van Noord T, Crijns HJGM, et al (Univ of Groningen, The Netherlands; Univ Hosp, Maastricht, The Netherlands; Trial Coordination Ctr, Groningen, The Netherlands; et al)

*J Am Coll Cardiol* 48:1001-1009, 2006 6–33

*Objectives.*—The VERDICT (Verapamil Versus Digoxin and Acute Versus Routine Serial Cardioversion Trial) is a prospective, randomized study to investigate whether: 1) acutely repeated serial electrical cardioversions (ECVs) after a relapse of atrial fibrillation (AF); and 2) prevention of intracellular calcium overload by verapamil, decrease intractability of AF.

*Background.*—Rhythm control is desirable in patients suffering from symptomatic AF.

*Methods.*—A total of 144 patients with persistent AF were included. Seventy-four (51%) patients were randomized to the *acute* (within 24 h) and 70 (49%) patients to the *routine* serial ECVs, and 74 (51%) patients to verapamil and 70 (49%) patients to digoxin for rate control before ECV and continued during follow-up ($2 \times 2$ factorial design). Class III antiarrhythmic drugs were used after a relapse of AF. Follow-up was 18 months.

*Results.*—At baseline, there were no significant differences between the groups, except for beta-blocker use in the verapamil versus digoxin group (38% vs. 60%, respectively, $p = 0.01$). At follow-up, no difference in the occurrence of permanent AF between the acute and the routine cardioversion groups was observed (32% [95% confidence intervals (CI)] 22 to 44) vs. 31% [95% CI 21 to 44], respectively, $p = NS$), and also no difference between the verapamil- and the digoxin-randomized patients (28% [95% CI 19 to 40] vs. 36% [95% CI 25 to 48] respectively, $p = NS$). Multivariate Cox regression analysis revealed that lone digoxin use was the only significant predictor of failure of rhythm control treatment (hazard ratio 2.2 [95% CI 1.1 to 4.4], $p = 0.02$).

*Conclusions.*—An acute serial cardioversion strategy does not improve long-term rhythm control in comparison with a routine serial cardioversion strategy. Furthermore, verapamil has no beneficial effect in a serial cardioversion strategy.

▶ This study had all to do with so-called remodeling of the atria by AF. There are 3 useful conclusions to this prospective study. First, the study shows that an acute serial cardioversion strategy does not improve the outcome of rhythm control therapy. Thus, the rush to acute cardioversion is not critical. Also, in a serial cardioversion strategy, verapamil does not have any beneficial effects. Finally, and importantly, digoxin monotherapy should not be instituted in patients in whom a rhythm control strategy is indicated or is the therapy of choice.

**A. L. Waldo, MD**

## Serial Cardioversion by Class IC Drugs During 4 Months of Persistent Atrial Fibrillation in the Goat

Eijsbouts S, Ausma J, Blaauw Y, et al (Maastricht Univ, The Netherlands)
*J Cardiovasc Electrophysiol* 17:648-654, 2006                    6–34

*Introduction.*—The success rate of pharmacological cardioversion of atrial fibrillation (AF) in patients depends on the duration of AF. It is unknown to what extent AF-induced structural atrial remodeling contributes to this loss of efficacy.

*Method and Results.*—In 10 goats, persistent AF was induced by repetitive burst pacing. During a time period of 16 weeks, the efficacy of flecainide and cibenzoline to cardiovert AF was investigated by serial cardioversion. The drugs were administered intravenously at a rate of 0.1 mg/kg/min. AF cycle length (AFCL) was continuously monitored. Drug infusion was continued until AF was successfully cardioverted or the QRS duration was prolonged about twofold. The average atrial cycle length during persistent AF was 104 ± 10 msec and did not change during the 16-week period. The success rate of cardioversion by flecainide and cibenzoline decreased with the duration of AF from 60% to 17% and from 80% to 63%. In goats that failed to cardiovert, sinus rhythm was not restored despite a twofold prolongation of the AF cycle length (respectively from 96 ± 5 msec to 168 ± 30 msec (flecainide) and 203 ± 26 msec (cibenzoline)). The sensitivity of AF for Class IC drugs was not altered with time, and the dose-dependent effect on AFCL remained the same (flecainide: 8 ± 5 vs 7 ± 2 msec/mg/kg (P = 0.70) and cibenzoline: 13 ± 3 vs 13 ± 5 msec/mg/kg (P = 0.95)). In animals in which cardioversion remained possible, the critical AFCL at which cardioversion occurred increased from 96 ± 5 msec to 211 msec (flecainide) and 189 ± 24 msec (cibenzoline).

*Conclusions.*—The progressive loss of efficacy of Class IC drugs to cardiovert AF of longer duration is not due to a decrease in the sensitivity of remodeled atrial myocardium for Class IC drugs. Failure of cardioversion was due to an increase in the critical AF cycle length required for pharmacological cardioversion.

▶ This is a basic science study dealing with a well-known clinical question, namely the difficulty in achieving cardioversion with drug therapy, in this case with a class IC agent late after onset of AF. This study does implicate remodeling as the problem, particularly structural anatomic changes, including dilation of the atria. Thus, although the article from the VERDICT study (Abstract 6–33) indicates that acute cardioversion is not required for the long-term implementation and efficacy of a rhythm control strategy; the ease of cardioversion, particularly with drug therapy, clearly is affected.

**A. L. Waldo, MD**

## Device Therapy

### Safety of Sports Participation in Patients with Implantable Cardioverter Defibrillators: A Survey of Heart Rhythm Society Members

Lampert R, Cannom D, Olshansky B (Yale Univ, New Haven, Conn; Los Angeles Cardiology Associates; Univ of Iowa, Iowa City)
*J Cardiovasc Electrophysiol* 17:11-15, 2006                    6–35

*Introduction.*—The safety of sports participation for patients with implantable cardioverter defibrillators (ICDs) is unknown, and recommendations among physicians may vary widely. The purposes of this study were to determine current practice among patients with ICDs and their physicians regarding sports participation, and to determine how many physicians have cared for patients who have sustained adverse events during sports participation.

*Method and Results.*—A survey was mailed to all 1,687 U.S. physician members of the Heart Rhythm Society. Among 614 respondent physicians, recommendations varied widely. Only 10% recommended avoidance of all sports more vigorous than golf. Seventy-six percent recommended avoidance of contact, and 45% recommend avoidance of competitive sports. Most (71%) based restrictions on patients' underlying heart disease. Regardless of recommendations, most physicians (71%) reported caring for patients who participated in sports, including many citing vigorous, competitive sports, most commonly cited were basketball, running, and skiing. ICD shocks during sports were common, cited by 40% of physicians. However, few adverse consequences were reported. One percent of physicians reported known injury to patient (all but 3 minor); 5%, injury to the ICD system, and <1%, failure of shocks to terminate arrhythmia. The most common adverse event reported was lead damage attributed to repetitive-motion activities, most commonly weightlifting and golf.

*Conclusions.*—Physician recommendations for sports participation for patients with ICDs varies widely. Many patients with ICDs do participate in vigorous and even competitive sports. While shocks were common, significant adverse events were rare.

▶ This area is controversial, to say the least. What is reassuring is that although shocks in this patient population were not uncommon, significant adverse effects were rare. One should also note that such patients who want to participate in sports often do what they want to do in any event.

**A. L. Waldo, MD**

## Cardiovascular Outcomes With Atrial-Based Pacing Compared With Ventricular Pacing: Meta-Analysis of Randomized Trials, Using Individual Patient Data

Healey JS, Toff WD, Lamas GA, et al (McMaster Univ, Hamilton, Ont, Canada; Univ of Leicester, England; Mount Sinai Med Ctr, Miami Beach, Fla; et al)
*Circulation* 114:11-17, 2006             6–36

*Background.*—Several randomized trials have compared atrial-based (dual-chamber or atrial) pacing with ventricular pacing in patients with bradycardia. No trial has shown a mortality reduction, and only 1 small trial suggested a reduction in stroke. The goal of this review was to determine whether atrial-based pacing prevents major cardiovascular events.

*Method and Results.*—A systematic review was performed of publications since 1980. For inclusion, trials had to compare an atrial-based with a ventricular-based pacing mode; use a randomized, controlled, parallel design; and have data on mortality, stroke, heart failure, or atrial fibrillation. Individual patient data were obtained from 5 of the 8 identified studies, representing 95% of patients in the 8 trials, and a total of 35 000 patient-years of follow-up. There was no significant heterogeneity among the results of the individual trials. There was no significant reduction in mortality (hazard ratio [HR], 0.95; 95% confidence interval [CI], 0.87 to 1.03; $P=0.19$) or heart failure (HR, 0.89; 95% CI, 0.77 to 1.03; $P=0.15$) with atrial-based pacing. There was a significant reduction in atrial fibrillation (HR, 0.80; 95% CI, 0.72 to 0.89; $P=0.00003$) and a reduction in stroke that was of borderline significance (HR, 0.81; 95% CI, 0.67 to 0.99; $P=0.035$). There was no convincing evidence that any patient subgroup received special benefit from atrial-based pacing.

*Conclusions.*—Compared with ventricular pacing, the use of atrial-based pacing does not improve survival or reduce heart failure or cardiovascular death. However, atrial-based pacing reduces the incidence of atrial fibrillation and may modestly reduce stroke.

▶ This is a useful meta-analysis. However, as is noted in the discussion by the authors, single-chamber atrial pacing seems to offer many advantages over dual-chamber pacing or ventricular pacing, particularly in the face of ventricular dysfunction, as evidenced by such trials as the DAVID trial[1] and the MOST trial.[2] These days, it is usually desirable in all patients that whenever possible and clinically reasonable, atrial pacing alone is preferable, with some form of VVI backup pacing as needed, but only at a sufficiently low rate that ventricular pacing is infrequent.

**A. L. Waldo, MD**

*References*

1. Wilcock BL, Cook JR, Epstein AE, et al: Dual-chamber pacing or ventricular backup pacing in patients with an implantable defibrillator: The Dual Chamber and VVI Implantable Defibrillator (DAVID) Trial. *JAMA* 288:3115-3123, 2002.

2. Sweeney MO, Hellkamp AS, Ellenbogen KA, et al: Adverse effect of ventricular pacing on heart failure and atrial fibrillation among patients with normal baseline QRS duration in a clinical trial of pacemaker therapy for sinus node dysfunction. *Circulation* 107:2932-2937, 2003.

---

**Pacemaker and ICD Generator Malfunctions: Analysis of Food and Drug Administration Annual Reports**
Maisel WH, Moynahan M, Zuckerman BD, et al (Harvard Med School; US Food and Drug Administration, Rockville, Md)
*JAMA* 295:1901-1906, 2006                                    6–37

---

*Context.*—Pacemakers and implantable cardioverter-defibrillators (ICDs) are complex medical devices proven to reduce mortality in specific high-risk patient populations. It is not known if increasing device complexity is associated with decreased reliability.

*Objectives.*—To analyze postapproval annual reports submitted to the US Food and Drug Administration (FDA) by manufacturers of pacemakers and ICDs to determine the reported number and rate of pacemaker and ICD malfunctions and to assess trends in device performance.

*Design and Setting.*—Pacemaker and ICD annual reports submitted to the FDA for the years 1990-2002 were reviewed. A pacemaker or ICD generator was defined as having malfunctioned if it was explanted due to an observed malfunction, returned to the manufacturer, and confirmed by the manufacturer to be functioning inappropriately. Leads and biventricular devices were not included in the study. Deaths were attributed to device malfunction only if they were witnessed, the malfunction immediately led to the death, and the malfunction was confirmed by the manufacturer.

*Main Outcome Measures.*—Number of implanted pacemaker and ICD generators; number of reported malfunctions; and annual malfunction replacement rates. Generator malfunction replacement rates were defined as the annual number of replacements due to confirmed malfunction divided by the annual number of implants.

*Results.*—During the study period, 2.25 million pacemakers and 415,780 ICDs were implanted in the United States. Overall, 17,323 devices (8834 pacemakers and 8489 ICDs) were explanted due to confirmed malfunction. Battery/capacitor abnormalities (4085 malfunctions [23.6%]) and electrical issues (4708 malfunctions [27.1%]) accounted for half of the total device failures. The annual pacemaker malfunction replacement rate per 1000 implants decreased significantly during the study, from a peak of 9.0 in 1993 to a low of 1.4 in 2002 ($P=.006$ for trend). In contrast, the ICD malfunction replacement rate per 1000 implants, after decreasing from 38.6 in 1993 to 7.9 in 1996, increased markedly during the latter half of the study, peaking in 2001 at 36.4 ($P=.04$ for trend). More than half of the reported ICD malfunctions occurred in the last 3 years of the study. Overall, the annual ICD malfunction replacement rate was significantly higher than the pacemaker malfunction replacement rate (mean [SD], 20.7 [11.6] vs 4.6 [2.2] replacements per 1000 implants; $P<.001$; rate ratio, 5.9 [95% confidence interval,

2.7-9.1]). Sixty-one deaths (30 pacemaker patients, 31 ICD patients) were attributable to device malfunction.

*Conclusions.*—This study demonstrates that thousands of patients have been affected by pacemaker and ICD malfunctions, the pacemaker malfunction replacement rate has decreased, the ICD malfunction replacement rate increased during the latter half of the study, and the ICD malfunction replacement rate is significantly higher than that for pacemakers. Although pacemakers and ICDs are important life-sustaining devices that have saved many lives, careful monitoring of device performance is still required.

▶ This is an important report simply for what it puts together in quantitative form. As the authors note, pacemakers and ICDs are complex medical devices, clinically proven to reduce mortality rates effectively in specific high-risk patient populations. But they are, after all, manmade, and despite all the intense efforts to make them the best possible, there is an inevitability about their problems. This report puts all this in perspective. The importance of these devices to medical care is clearly established. Nevertheless, the importance of vigilance, principally in the form of monitoring, but also in an informed patient, remains very important.

**A. L. Waldo, MD**

---

## Complications Associated With Implantable Cardioverter-Defibrillator Replacement in Response to Device Advisories

Gould PA, for the Canadian Heart Rhythm Society Working Group on Device Advisories (Univ of Western Ontario, London, Canada)
*JAMA* 295:1907-1911, 2006        6–38

*Context.*—Recent implantable cardioverter-defibrillator (ICD) advisories and recalls have caused management dilemmas for physicians, particularly because there are no specific guidelines or data on outcomes from current management strategies. The risk of ICD generator replacement has not been assessed in this population.

*Objective.*—To determine the complication rate associated with ICD generator replacement for the current ICD advisories.

*Design and Setting.*—Seventeen ICD implanting centers in Canada were surveyed to assess complication rates as a result of generator replacements because of ICD advisories from October 2004 to October 2005.

*Main Outcome Measure.*—Complications associated with elective ICD generator replacement for current device advisories.

*Results.*—At the 17 surveyed centers, 2915 patients had recall devices, including 533 (18.3%) who had advisory ICDs replaced a mean (SD) of 26.5 (11.5) months after their initial implant. Of these patients, 66% had a secondary prevention ICD, and 45% had received a previous appropriate shock. During a mean (SD) of 2.7 (2.8) months' follow-up after ICD generator replacement, complications occurred in 43 patients (8.1%). Major complications attributable to advisory device replacement requiring reoperation occurred in 31 patients (5.8%), with death in 2 patients after extraction for pocket infection. Minor complications occurred in 12 patients (2.3%). There were 3 (0.1%) advisory-related device malfunctions reported, without clinical consequences.

*Conclusions.*—ICD generator replacement in patients with advisory devices is associated with a substantial rate of complications, including death. These complications need to be considered in the development of guidelines determining the appropriate treatment of patients with advisory devices.

▶ This is an important compliment to the report by Maisel et al (Abstract 6–37), and it is from the Canadian Heart Rhythm Society Working Group on Device Advisories. As the authors point out, these data raise important concerns for advisory committees. Most important is the recognition that there is a potential for the risks associated with device failure to be less than the complication risks associated with device replacement. As Tennyson said, "Knowledge comes, but wisdom lingers . . . "

**A. L. Waldo, MD**

---

**Withdrawing Implantable Defibrillator Shock Therapy in Terminally Ill Patients**
Lewis WR, Luebke DL, Johnson NJ, et al (Case Western Reserve Univ, Cleveland, Ohio; MetroHealth Med Ctr, Cleveland, Ohio)
*Am J Med* 119:892-896, 2006                                    6–39

---

*Purpose.*—The purpose of this study is to review a multidisciplinary strategy used to identify patients with terminal illnesses and initiate withdrawal of implantable cardioverter defibrillator (ICD) shock therapy as part of a comprehensive comfort care approach. With indications for ICDs increasing, more patients are receiving devices. Once protected from an arrhythmic death, these patients may develop other terminal diseases such as cancer or congestive heart failure. It is appropriate to withdraw defibrillator shock therapy when such patients desire only comfort care.

*Methods.*—The charts of ICD patients who had died were reviewed. Two groups emerged: Group 1 (20) included patients whose defibrillator was turned off through the comprehensive comfort care approach. Group 2 (43) included patients whose clinical course was so rapid that the defibrillator was not turned off. Pacing therapy was not withdrawn in either group.

*Results.*—Defibrillator discharges, cause of death, and time from ICD discharge to death were compared. Group 2 patients died more acutely than Group 1. Group 1 experienced fewer shocks prior to death when compared to Group 2. Comparing pacemaker dependent and non-dependent patients, there was no difference in the time between therapy discontinuation and death.

*Conclusion.*—This is the largest study to date to review the characteristics of patients with ICDs and terminal illness. Only one-third of terminally ill patients with ICDs were able to have shock therapy withdrawn as part of a comfort care strategy. These patients experienced fewer shocks in the final days of their illness.

▶ This is a very good and thoughtful report that would be good to be read by anyone taking care of patients who have an ICD. Decisions about withdrawing ICD therapy can sometimes be difficult, but most of the time should not be. This report provides a database and a thoughtful discussion on which to consider this problem.

**A. L. Waldo, MD**

---

**Causes and Consequences of Heart Failure After Prophylactic Implantation of a Defibrillator in the Multicenter Automatic Defibrillator Implantation Trial II**
Goldenberg I, for the Multicenter Automatic Defibrillator Implantation Trial (MADIT) II Investigators (Univ of Rochester, NY; et al)
*Circulation* 113:2810-2817, 2006                                                    6–40

---

*Background.*—Implantable cardioverter-defibrillator (ICD) therapy may be associated with an increased risk for heart failure (HF). The present study evaluated the frequency, causes, and consequences of HF after ICD implantation.

*Method and Results.*—We performed a retrospective analysis of the clinical factors and outcomes associated with postenrollment HF events in 1218 patients enrolled in the Multicenter Automatic Defibrillator Implantation Trial II. The adjusted hazard ratios (HRs) of ICD:conventional therapy for first and recurrent HF events were 1.39 ($P$=0.02) and 1.58 ($P$<0.001), respectively. The risk was increased among patients who received single-chamber or dual-chamber ICDs. Development of HF was associated with an increased mortality risk (HR, 3.80; $P$<0.001). Among patients who received a single-chamber ICD, there was a similar survival benefit before and after the development of HF (HR, 0.59 and 0.61, respectively; $P$=0.92 for difference), whereas among patients with dual-chamber devices, there was a significant reduction in survival benefit after HF (HR, 0.26 and 0.83, respectively; $P$=0.01 for difference). Within the defibrillator arm of the trial, patients who received life-prolonging therapy from the ICD had an increased risk for first and recurrent HF events (HR, 1.90; $P$=0.01 and 1.74; $P$<0.001, respectively).

*Conclusions.*—Patients with chronic ischemic heart disease who are treated with either single-chamber or dual-chamber ICDs have improved survival but an increased risk of HF. The present data suggest that ICD therapy transforms sudden death risk to a subsequent HF risk. These findings should direct more attention to the prevention of HF in patients who receive an ICD.

▶ This study is of interest, especially in light of the DAVID trial.[1] The majority of patients in the MADIT II trial got dual-chamber ICDs in which there was a significant amount of right ventricular pacing. As with the DAVID trial, no doubt this contributed to heart failure. Interestingly enough, with single-chamber ICDs, ventricular pacing was minimal, and still there was a problem with long-term heart failure. So, the "DAVID type" data do not explain all aspects of the prominence of heart failure as the cause of death in the MADIT II trial. The likely explanation for these data is that the ICD prevents sudden cardiac death, allowing death from heart failure per se to become manifest.

**A. L. Waldo, MD**

*Reference*

1. Wilkoff BL, Cook JR, Epstein AE, et al: Dual-chamber pacing or ventricular backup pacing in patients with an implantable defibrillator: the Dual Chamber and VVI Implantable Defibrillator (DAVID) Trial. *JAMA* 288:3115-3123, 2002.

---

**Time Dependence of Defibrillator Benefit After Coronary Revascularization in the Multicenter Automatic Defibrillator Implantation Trial (MADIT)-II**

Goldenberg I, for the MADIT-II Investigators (Univ of Rochester, NY; et al)
*J Am Coll Cardiol* 47:1811-1817, 2006                                    6–41

*Objectives.*—The study was designed to assess the effect of elapsed time from coronary revascularization (CR) on the benefit of the implantable cardioverter-defibrillator (ICD) and the risk of sudden cardiac death (SCD) in patients with ischemic left ventricular dysfunction.

*Background.*—The ICD improves survival in appropriately selected high-risk cardiac patients by 30% to 54%. However, in the Coronary Artery By-pass Graft (CABG)-Patch trial no evidence of improved survival was shown among a similar population of patients in whom an ICD was implanted pro-phylactically at the time of elective CABG.

*Methods.*—The outcome by time from CR was analyzed in 951 patients in whom a revascularization procedure was performed before enrollment in the Multicenter Automatic Defibrillator Implantation Trial (MADIT)-II.

*Results.*—The adjusted hazard ratio (HR) of ICD versus conventional therapy was 0.64 (p = 0.01) among patients enrolled more than six months after CR, whereas no survival benefit with ICD therapy was shown among patients enrolled six months or earlier after CR (HR = 1.19; p = 0.76). In the conventional therapy group, the risk of cardiac death increased significantly with increasing time from CR (p for trend = 0.009), corresponding mainly to a six-fold increase in the risk of SCD among patients enrolled more than six months after CR.

*Conclusions.*—In patients with ischemic left ventricular dysfunction, the efficacy of ICD therapy after CR is time dependent, with a significant life-saving benefit in patients receiving device implantation more than six months after CR. The lack of ICD benefit when implanted early after CR may be related to a relatively low risk of SCD during this time period.

▶ This report presents another interesting result from the MADIT-II trial. It may also explain what has been a poorly understood result of the CABG-Patch trial in which no evidence of improved survival was shown among patients with coronary artery disease, a depressed left ventricular ejection fraction, and an abnormal signal-averaged ECG in whom an ICD was implanted prophylactically at the time of surgery. In the end, these data do not change the fact that the ICD in the MADIT-II population is indicated. These data also confirm the importance of coronary artery revascularization in the face of ischemic heart disease as important for prognosis.

**A. L. Waldo, MD**

---

**Predictive Value of Ventricular Arrhythmia Inducibility for Subsequent Ventricular Tachycardia or Ventricular Fibrillation in Multicenter Automatic Defibrillator Implantation Trial (MADIT) II Patients**
Daubert JP, for the MADIT II Study Investigators (Univ of Rochester, NY; et al)
*J Am Coll Cardiol* 47:98-107, 2006                                                      6–42

---

In the Multicenter Automatic Defibrillator Implantation Trial (MADIT) II, implantable cardioverter-defibrillator (ICD)-randomized patients underwent electrophysiologic testing. Both inducible and noninducible patients received an ICD. We correlated inducibility with the occurrence of subsequent ventricular tachycardia (VT) or ventricular fibrillation (VF). Intracardiac ICD electrograms for subsequent events were analyzed to categorize the spontaneous arrhythmia as VT or VF. The two-year Kaplan-Meier event rate for VT in inducible patients was 29.0% versus 19.3% in noninducible patients. However, ICD therapy for spontaneous VF was less common at two years in inducible patients (3.2%) than in noninducible patients (8.6%). In the MADIT II study, inducibility predicted an increased likelihood of VT but decreased VF.

*Objectives.*—We correlated electrophysiologic inducibility with spontaneous ventricular tachycardia (VT) or ventricular fibrillation (VF) in the Multicenter Automatic Defibrillator Implantation Trial (MADIT) II.

*Background.*—In the MADIT II study, 593 (82%) of 720 implantable cardioverter-defibrillator (ICD) randomized patients underwent electrophysiologic testing. Patients received an ICD whether they were inducible or not.

*Methods.*—A "standard" inducibility definition included sustained monomorphic or polymorphic VT induced with three or fewer extrastimuli or VF induced with two or fewer extrastimuli. We compared a narrow inducibility definition (only monomorphic VT) and a broad definition (standard definition plus VF with three extrastimuli). We used ICD-stored electrograms to categorize spontaneous VT or VF.

*Results.*—Inducible patients (standard definition) had a greater likelihood of experiencing ICD therapy for VT than noninducible patients (p = 0.023). Unexpectedly, ICD therapy for spontaneous VF was less common (p = 0.021) in inducible patients than in noninducible patients. The two-year Kaplan-Meier event rate for VT or VF was 29.4% for inducible patients and 25.5% for noninducible patients. Standard inducibility did not predict the combined end point of VT or VF (p = 0.280, by log-rank analysis). The narrow inducibility definition outperformed the standard definition, whereas the broad definition appeared inferior to the standard definition.

*Conclusions.*—In the MADIT II study patients, inducibility was associated with an increased likelihood of VT. Noninducible MADIT II study subjects using this electrophysiologic protocol had a considerable VT event rate and a higher VF event rate than inducible patients. Induction of polymorphic VT or VF, even with double extrastimuli, appears less relevant than induction of monomorphic VT.

▶ Importantly, this study demonstrates that electrophysiologic testing probably adds little to the indication for an ICD in the MADIT II patient population. Also, these MADIT II data are consistent with data from the MUSTT study.[1]

**A. L. Waldo, MD**

*Reference*

1. Buxton AE, Lee KL, Hafley GE, et al: Relation of ejection fraction and inducible ventricular tachycardia to mode of death in patients with coronary artery disease: an analysis of patients enrolled in the multicenter unsustained tachycardia trial. *Circulation* 106:2466-2472, 2002.

## Microvolt T-Wave Alternans and the Risk of Death or Sustained Ventricular Arrhythmias in Patients With Left Ventricular Dysfunction

Bloomfield DM, Bigger JT, Steinman RC, et al (Columbia Univ, New York; Univ of South Florida, Tampa; Case Western Reserve Univ, Cleveland, Ohio; et al)
*J Am Coll Cardiol* 47:456-463, 2006                                    6–43

*Objectives.*—This study hypothesized that microvolt T-wave alternans (MTWA) improves selection of patients for implantable cardioverter-defibrillator (ICD) prophylaxis, especially by identifying patients who are not likely to benefit.

*Background.*—Many patients with left ventricular dysfunction are now eligible for prophylactic ICDs, but most eligible patients do not benefit; MTWA testing has been proposed to improve patient selection.

*Methods.*—Our study was conducted at 11 clinical centers in the U.S. Patients were eligible if they had a left ventricular ejection fraction (LVEF) ≤0.40 and lacked a history of sustained ventricular arrhythmias; patients were excluded for atrial fibrillation, unstable coronary artery disease, or New York Heart Association functional class IV heart failure. Participants underwent an MTWA test and then were followed for about two years. The primary outcome was all-cause mortality or non-fatal sustained ventricular arrhythmias.

*Results.*—Ischemic heart disease was present in 49%, mean LVEF was 0.25, and 66% had an abnormal MTWA test. During 20 ± 6 months of follow-up, 51 end points (40 deaths and 11 non-fatal sustained ventricular arrhythmias) occurred. Comparing patients with normal and abnormal MTWA tests, the hazard ratio for the primary end point was 6.5 at two years (95% confidence interval 2.4 to 18.1, p < 0.001). Survival of patients with normal MTWA tests was 97.5% at two years. The strong association between MTWA and the primary end point was similar in all subgroups tested.

*Conclusions.*—Among patients with heart disease and LVEF ≤0.40, MTWA can identify not only a high-risk group, but also a low-risk group unlikely to benefit from ICD prophylaxis.

▶ The data from this study are most impressive, but there are some difficulties. One is that this test is not always easy to do. And, there seems to be a learning curve in understanding how to do and interpret the test. But the data still are impressive. The reader should be advised that this test can really help in providing patients with alternatives to simply implanting an ICD because a patient's LVEF is low and he or she has structural heart disease. We do know that a large number of such patients who get an ICD prophylactically never use the device. While that is fortunate for them, one would still like to have a method to identify patients in whom maybe one could save the cost and whatever else is involved with the risk of implanting an ICD. The MTWA test does offer an objective test that, if negative, makes the risk of sudden cardiac arrhythmic death very low indeed.

**A. L. Waldo, MD**

---

**The PROTECT AF (WATCHMAN Left Atrial Appendage System for Embolic PROTECTion in Patients with Atrial Fibrillation) Trial**
Fountain RB, Holmes DR, Chandrasekaran K, et al (Mayo Clinic, Rochester, Minn; Minneapolis Heart Inst; Cooper Univ, Camden, NJ)
*Am Heart J* 151:956-961, 2006                                             6–44

---

*Background.*—Atrial fibrillation (AF) is the most common sustained cardiac arrhythmia and is the primary cardiac abnormality associated with embolic stroke. The left atrial appendage (LAA) is the major location of thrombi in patients with AF. Warfarin therapy is effective at reducing the risk of stroke, but chronic anticoagulation presents many problems of safety and acceptability for many patients. The WATCHMAN Left Atrial Appendage System is a novel device designed to prevent the embolization of thrombi that may form in the LAA. It is hypothesized that it may prevent ischemic stroke and systemic thromboembolization in patients with AF. The purpose of this study is to demonstrate the safety and efficacy of the WATCHMAN implant.

*Methods.*—The study is a multicenter, prospective, randomized study comparing patients with the WATCHMAN implant with control patients receiving long-term therapy alone. The implant procedure is performed under local or general anesthesia. Patients are monitored in the hospital for at least 24 hours and continue on warfarin for at least 45 days. If warfarin is discontinued at this time, clopidogrel, 75 mg daily, is then prescribed until completion of the 6-month follow-up visit, and aspirin is prescribed for the duration of the trial. Control and implant patients are evaluated by a neurologist at the 6- and 12-month follow-up visits and at annual clinical follow-up visits for the 5-year length of the trial. An independent core laboratory will be used to interpret all echocardiographic data and chest radiographs gathered on all WATCHMAN study patients. All statistical analyses will be by intention-to-treat, with each patient analyzed as being part of their group regardless of actual treatment received.

*Conclusions.*—The Protect AF trial is the only randomized trial of a percutaneous LAA isolation device. The purpose of the trial is the evaluation of the relative merits of this type of device compared with the standard therapy with warfarin.

▶ This is an interesting and potentially very important trial, in this editor's judgment, because it is comparing warfarin versus the placement of an occlusive device using catheter techniques in the LAA to, it is hoped, prevent any left atrial clots from forming and becoming systemic emboli. The trial is well underway and has the potential of offering an effective alternative to warfarin therapy. It is recognized that warfarin therapy is very effective, but it is also recognized that it is quite difficult to use, as all patients know who take the drug. So, the limitations of warfarin are such that physicians have been looking for an alternative to warfarin therapy in patients with AF at risk for stroke. The WATCHMAN trial will be watched carefully to see whether we will have that alternative.

**A. L. Waldo, MD**

---

### Evaluation of a novel device for left atrial appendage exclusion: The second-generation atrial exclusion device

Kamohara K, Fukamachi K, Ootaki Y, et al (Cleveland Clinic Found, Ohio)
*J Thorac Cardiovasc Surg* 132:340-346, 2006                                   6–45

---

*Background.*—The left atrial appendage is a frequent source of thromboemboli in patients with atrial fibrillation. Exclusion of the left atrial appendage may reduce the risk of stroke in patients with atrial fibrillation. The atrial exclusion device, previously developed to perform left atrial appendage exclusion on a beating heart, was modified to accommodate different anatomic patterns of the human left atrial appendage and to ensure uniform pressure and occlusion. The purpose of this study was to evaluate this second-generation atrial exclusion device during a midterm period in a canine model.

*Methods.*—Ten mongrel dogs (mean weight 28.9 ± 4.6 kg) were used in this study. The atrial exclusion device, constructed from two parallel and rigid titanium tubes and two nitinol springs with a knit-braided polyester fabric, was implanted at the base of the left atrial appendage through a left thoracotomy on a beating heart using a specially designed delivery tool.

Dogs were evaluated at 30 days (n = 4) and 90 days (n = 6) by epicardial echocardiography, left atrial and coronary angiography, gross pathology, and histologic inspection.

*Results.*—Device implantation was performed without complications in all dogs. Complete left atrial appendage exclusion without device migration or hemodynamic instability was confirmed, and there was no damage to the left circumflex artery or pulmonary artery. Macroscopic and microscopic assessments revealed favorable biocompatibility during midterm follow-up.

*Conclusion.*—The atrial exclusion device enabled rapid, reliable, and safe exclusion of the left atrial appendage. Clinical application may provide a new therapeutic option for reducing the risk of stroke in patients with atrial fibrillation.

▶ The efficacy and the apparent safety of this device in the animal model seem clear. There is hope that this would provide yet another alternative to warfarin therapy in that an occlusive device can be applied surgically, and by minimally invasive surgery, to fully occlude the left atrial appendage and thereby prevent systemic emboli in patients with atrial fibrillation at risk for stroke. We await further developments of this exciting new approach to therapy.

**A. L. Waldo, MD**

---

**Biventricular Versus Conventional Right Ventricular Stimulation for Patients With Standard Pacing Indication and Left Ventricular Dysfunction: The Homburg Biventricular Pacing Evaluation (HOBIPACE)**
Kindermann M, Hennen B, Jung J, et al (Universitätsklinikum des Saarlandes, Homburg/Saar, Germany; Innere Klinik I, Worms, Germany)
*J Am Coll Cardiol* 47:1927-1937, 2006                                    6–46

---

*Objectives.*—The Homburg Biventricular Pacing Evaluation (HOBIPACE) is the first randomized controlled study that compares the biventricular (BV) pacing approach with conventional right ventricular (RV) pacing in patients with left ventricular (LV) dysfunction and a standard indication for antibradycardia pacing in the ventricle.

*Background.*—In patients with LV dysfunction and atrioventricular block, conventional RV pacing may yield a detrimental effect on LV function.

*Methods.*—Thirty patients with standard indication for permanent ventricular pacing and LV dysfunction defined by an LV end-diastolic diameter ≥60 mm and an ejection fraction ≤40% were included. Using a prospective, randomized crossover design, three months of RV pacing were compared with three months of BV pacing with regard to LV function, N-terminal pro-B-type natriuretic peptide (NT-proBNP) serum concentration, exercise capacity, and quality of life.

*Results.*—When compared with RV pacing, BV stimulation reduced LV end-diastolic ($-9.0\%$, p = 0.022) and end-systolic volumes ($-16.9\%$, p <

0.001), NT-proBNP level (−31.0%, p < 0.002), and the Minnesota Living with Heart Failure score (−18.9%, p = 0.01). Left ventricular ejection fraction (+22.1%), peak oxygen consumption (+12.0%), oxygen uptake at the ventilatory threshold (+12.5%), and peak circulatory power (+21.0%) were higher (p < 0.0002) with BV pacing. The benefit of BV over RV pacing was similar for patients with (n = 9) and without (n = 21) atrial fibrillation. Right ventricular function was not affected by BV pacing.

*Conclusions.*—In patients with LV dysfunction who need permanent ventricular pacing support, BV stimulation is superior to conventional RV pacing with regard to LV function, quality of life, and maximal as well as submaximal exercise capacity.

▶ The results of this study are really intuitive, so it is very nice to see the results. This investigator-driven, prospective, randomized, single-blinded crossover comparison trial between RV and BV pacing provides most interesting results. It is a study in a small number of patients (n = 33), but the data are quite striking. The data make a compelling case that in patients with LV dysfunction who require ventricular pacing support for bradycardia in the presence of impaired atrioventricular conduction, atrial BV or BV pacing should be considered because in this study it was associated with better LV function, better quality of life, and better exercise capacity.

**A. L. Waldo, MD**

---

**Four-Year Efficacy of Cardiac Resynchronization Therapy on Exercise Tolerance and Disease Progression: The Importance of Performing Atrioventricular Junction Ablation in Patients With Atrial Fibrillation**
Gasparini M, Auricchio A, Regoli F, et al (IRCCS Instituto, Milan, Italy; IRCCS Policlinico San Matteo, Pavia, Italy; Univ Hosp, Magdeburg, Germany; et al)
*J Am Coll Cardiol* 48:734-743, 2006                                    6–47

---

*Objectives.*—The goal of this study was to investigate the effects of cardiac resynchronization therapy (CRT) in heart failure patients with permanent atrial fibrillation (AF) and the role of atrioventricular junction (AVJ) ablation.

*Background.*—Cardiac resynchronization therapy has been proven effective in heart failure patients with sinus rhythm (SR). However, little is known about the effects of CRT in heart failure patients with permanent AF.

*Methods.*—Efficacy of CRT on ventricular function, exercise performance, and reversal of maladaptive remodeling process was prospectively compared in 48 patients with permanent AF in whom ventricular rate was controlled by drugs, thus resulting in apparently adequate delivery of biventricular pacing (>85% of pacing time), and in 114 permanent AF patients, who had undergone AVJ ablation (100% of resynchronization therapy delivery). The clinical and echocardiographic long-term outcomes of both groups were compared with those of 511 SR patients treated with CRT.

*Results.*—Both SR and AF groups showed significant and sustained improvements of all assessed parameters (model p < 0.001 for all parameters). However, within the AF group, only patients who underwent ablation showed a significant increase of ejection fraction (p < 0.001), reverse remodeling effect (p < 0.001), and improved exercise tolerance (p < 0.001); no improvements were observed in AF patients who did not undergo ablation.

*Conclusions.*—Heart failure patients with ventricular conduction disturbance and permanent AF treated with CRT showed large and sustained long-term (up to 4 year) improvements of left ventricular function and functional capacity, similar to patients in SR, only if AVJ ablation was performed.

▶ This is the first long-term, prospectively designed study demonstrating the importance of AVJ ablation in patients with AF treated with CRT. An important part of the conclusions from the data is that among patients with permanent AF, only those undergoing ablation of the AVJ demonstrated a significant symptomatic benefit and improved left ventricular function with CRT therapy.

**A. L. Waldo, MD**

---

**Effect of Cardiac Resynchronization on the Incidence of Atrial Fibrillation in Patients With Severe Heart Failure**
Hoppe UC, Casares JM, Eiskjær H, et al (Univ of Cologne, Germany; Hosp Reina Sofia, Cordoba, Spain; Aarhus Univ, Denmark; et al)
*Circulation* 114:18-25, 2006                                                6–48

---

*Background.*—Atrial fibrillation/flutter (AF) and heart failure often coexist; however, the effect of cardiac resynchronization therapy (CRT) on the incidence of AF and on the outcome of patients with new-onset AF remains undefined.

*Method and Results.*—In the CArdiac REsynchronisation in Heart Failure (CARE-HF) trial, 813 patients with moderate or severe heart failure were randomly assigned to pharmacological therapy alone or with the addition of CRT. The incidence of AF was assessed by adverse event reporting and by ECGs during follow-up, and the impact of new-onset AF on the outcome and efficacy of CRT was evaluated. By the end of the study (mean duration of follow-up 29.4 months), AF had been documented in 66 patients in the CRT group compared with 58 who received medical therapy only (16.1% versus 14.4%; hazard ratio 1.05; 95% confidence interval, 0.73 to 1.50; *P*=0.79). There was no difference in the time until first onset of AF between groups. Mortality was higher in patients who developed AF, but AF was not a predictor in the multivariable model (hazard ratio 1.17; 95% confidence interval, 0.82 to 1.67; *P*=0.37). In patients with new-onset AF, CRT significantly reduced the risk for all-cause mortality and all other predefined end points and improved ejection fraction and symptoms (no interaction between AF and CRT; all *P*>0.2).

*Conclusions.*—Although CRT did not reduce the incidence of AF, CRT improved the outcome regardless of whether AF developed.

▶ Of note, in this further analysis of the CARE-HF trial, CRT did not influence the incidence of AF. However, new onset of AF did not diminish the beneficial effects of cardiac resynchronization on the combined primary end point of the main trial or, more fundamentally, on all-cause mortality. Interestingly enough, there were no differences in the nature of mitral regurgitation, left ventricular ejection fraction, or end-systolic volume index between the 2 groups. However, left atrial systolic and diastolic area was significantly larger in patients with AF than in those who didn't have AF, looking at both the medical therapy alone group and the medical therapy plus CRT group. Clearly there is more to understanding the relationships of heart failure and AF. But left atrial size is one of the important ones.

**A. L. Waldo, MD**

## Miscellaneous

**Activation and depolarization of the normal human heart under complete physiological conditions**
Ramanathan C, Jia P, Ghanem R, et al (Case Western Reserve Univ, Cleveland, Ohio; Washington Univ, St Louis)
*Proc Natl Acad Sci U S A* 103:6309-6314, 2006                6–49

Knowledge of normal human cardiac excitation stems from isolated heart or intraoperative mapping studies under nonphysiological conditions. Here, we use a noninvasive imaging modality (electrocardiographic imaging) to study normal activation and repolarization in intact unanesthetized healthy adults under complete physiological conditions. Epicardial potentials, electrograms, and isochrones were noninvasively reconstructed. The normal electrophysiological sequence during activation and repolarization was imaged in seven healthy subjects (four males and three females). Electrocardiographic imaging depicted salient features of normal ventricular activation, including timing and location of the earliest right ventricular (RV) epicardial breakthrough in the anterior paraseptal region, subsequent RV and left ventricular (LV) breakthroughs, apex-to-base activation of posterior LV, and late activation of LV base or RV outflow tract. The repolarization sequence was unaffected by the activation sequence, supporting the hypothesis that in normal hearts, local action potential duration (APD) determines local repolarization time. Mean activation recovery interval (ARI), reflecting local APD, was in the typical human APD range (235 ms). Mean LV apex-to-base ARI dispersion was 42 ms. Average LV ARI exceeded RV ARI by 32 ms. Atrial images showed activation spreading from the sinus node to the rest of the atria, ending at the left atrial appendage. This study provides previously undescribed characterization of human cardiac activation and repolarization under normal physiological conditions. A common sequence of activation was identified, with interindividual differences in specific patterns. The repolarization sequence was determined by local repolarization properties rather than by the activation sequence, and significant dispersion of repolarization was observed between RV and LV and from apex to base.

▶ The importance of this report lies in the fact that ECG imaging is now here, and this editor would think here to stay, as a new tool in looking at and understanding normal and abnormal sequences of activation in all chambers of the heart to better understand and even treat disorders of cardiac rhythm and conduction. The importance of ECG imaging lies in its ease of application, the fact that it is noninvasive, the fact that it is reliable, and the fact that it really only requires 1 beat to look at activation sequence. Of course, it can be used for consecutive beats as well. But especially in this era of use of ablation to treat supraventricular arrhythmias and, more increasingly, ventricular arrhythmias, ECG imaging can be used to know when ventricular arrhythmias come from the epicardium of the ventricles, to know where drivers may be in atrial fibrillation, etc. There are a host of potential applications for this technique, and we look forward to an exciting future with this new technology.

**A. L. Waldo, MD**

# Subject Index

## A

Ablation, for atrial fibrillation
  with atrioventricular nodal reentrant
    tachycardia, clinical outcomes, 441
  catheter
    vs. amiodarone, after first episode of
      symptomatic atrial flutter, 433
    circumferential pulmonary-vein, 429
    circumferential with pulmonary vein
      isolation, 431
    fibrillating areas isolated within the
      left atrium after, 444
    left atrial vs. biatrial, 432
    relevance of organization of
      frequency spectra, 444
    tailored strategy targeting initiators
      and drivers, 430
    thromboembolic event risk after, 418
  in heart failure patients, cardiac
    resynchronization therapy after,
    466
  surgical
    atrial arrhythmias after "cut and
      sew" MAZE procedures, 438
    classic MAZE III procedure, freedom
      from atrial arrhythmias after, 435
    Cox-Maze procedure and
      improvements in systolic function
      and functional status, 436
    mechanisms of atrial
      tachyarrhythmias following, 437
    during mitral valve surgery, role of
      pulmonary vein isolation, 434
Acadesine
  for adenosine regulation in
    post-reperfusion myocardial
    infarction, long-term survival with,
    258
Acupuncture
  for hypertension, 88
Acute myocardial infarction (*see*
    Myocardial infarction)
Age
  (*see also* Older adults)
  cardiovascular disease risk and, in men
    and women with and without
    diabetes, 278
Amiodarone
  with β-blockers vs. sotalol alone for
    prevention of shocks from ICDs,
    451
  vs. radiofrequency ablation after first
    episode of symptomatic atrial
    flutter, 433

Amlodipine
  fasting glucose levels and incident
    diabetes mellitus in older
    nondiabetic adults and, 77
  vs. lisinopril in high-risk hypertensive
    patients, clinical events incidence
    with, 75
  vs. ramipril or metoprolol in
    hypertensive kidney disease,
    diabetes mellitus incidence and, 83
Anemia
  biomarkers of increased heart failure
    risk and, as predictors of mortality,
    310
  chronic kidney disease and, as predictor
    of outcomes in chronic heart
    failure, 324
  in heart failure, clinical correlates and
    consequences, 325
Aneurysm
  aortic root, long-term results of aortic
    valve-sparing surgery for, 183
  atrial septal, cerebrovascular event risk
    and, 407
Angina
  refractory, enhanced external
    counterpulsation for, 359
  stable, B-type natriuretic peptide for
    prediction of long-term outcome,
    238
Angiography
  after CABG, indications for, 158
Angioplasty
  cutting balloon, for pulmonary vein
    in-stent stenosis, 142
  door-to-balloon time and mortality in
    ST-segment elevation myocardial
    infarction, 230
  effects on early and late infarct size and
    left ventricular wall characteristics,
    232
  rescue, after failed thrombolytic therapy
    for myocardial infarction, 213
  with vs. without stenting,
    cardiovascular risk of noncardiac
    surgery following, 256
Angiotensin-converting enzyme (ACE)
    inhibitor(s)
  atrial fibrillation prevention and, 448
  vs. calcium channel blockers
    in high-risk hypertensive patients,
      clinical events incidence with, 75
    or β-blockers in hypertensive kidney
      disease, diabetes mellitus incidence
      and, 82

471

# Author Index